P9-BZU-399

EMERGING INFECTIONS 7

EMERGING INFECTIONS 7

Edited by
W. Michael Scheld
Division of Infectious Diseases
and International Health
University of Virginia Health System
Charlottesville, Virginia

David C. Hooper
Division of Infectious Diseases
Massachusetts General Hospital
Boston, Massachusetts

James M. Hughes
Division of Infectious Diseases
Department of Medicine
Emory University School of Medicine
Atlanta, Georgia

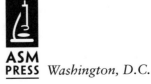

ASM PRESS *Washington, D.C.*

Address editorial correspondence to ASM Press, 1752 N Street NW, Washington,
DC 20036-2904, USA

Send orders to ASM Press, P.O. Box 605, Herndon, VA 20172, USA
Phone: (800) 546-2416 or (703) 661-1593
Fax: (703) 661-1501
E-mail: books@asmusa.org
Online: estore.asm.org

Copyright © 2007 ASM Press
       American Society for Microbiology
       1752 N Street NW
       Washington, DC 20036-2904

ISBN-10 1-55581-377-1
ISBN-13 978-1-55581-377-2

All Rights Reserved
Printed in the United States of America

Cover photo: Electron micrograph of filamentous influenza A (H5N1) virions
forming at the surface of an infected MDCK cell. (Source: C. S. Goldsmith and
R. Bright. Courtesy of Sherif R. Zaki, National Center for Infectious Diseases,
Centers for Disease Control and Prevention.)

In memory of J.-W. Lee, director-general of the World Health Organization from 2003 to 2006, for his outstanding leadership in increasing global preparedness to detect and respond to emerging infectious diseases

CONTENTS

CONTRIBUTORS

Charalampos Antachopoulos • Pediatric Oncology Branch, National Cancer Institute, National Institutes of Health, Bethesda, Maryland 20892

Naomi E. Aronson • Department of Medicine, Infectious Diseases Division, Uniformed Services University of the Health Sciences, Bethesda, Maryland 20814

Michael J. Arrowood • Division of Parasitic Diseases, National Center for Infectious Diseases, Centers for Disease Control and Prevention, U.S. Department of Health and Human Services, Atlanta, Georgia 30341

Susan Boyle-Vavra • Department of Pediatric Infectious Diseases, University of Chicago, 5841 S. Maryland, MC 6054, Chicago, Illinois 60637

Simona Bratu • Division of Infectious Diseases, SUNY Downstate Medical Center, Brooklyn, New York 11203

V. C. C. Cheng • Department of Microbiology, University Pathology Building, Queen Mary Hospital, The University of Hong Kong, Pokfulam Road, Hong Kong Special Administrative Region, People's Republic of China

Susan E. Crawford • Department of Pediatric Infectious Diseases, University of Chicago, 5841 S. Maryland, MC 6054, Chicago, Illinois 60637

Inger Damon • Poxvirus Program, Centers for Disease Control and Prevention, Atlanta, Georgia 30329-4018

Robert S. Daum • Department of Pediatric Infectious Diseases, University of Chicago, 5841 S. Maryland, MC 6054, Chicago, Illinois 60637

Kepler A. Davis • Infectious Disease Service, D. D. Eisenhower Army Medical Center, 300 Hospital Rd., Fort Gordon, Georgia 30905

Ronald Fayer • Environmental Microbial Safety Laboratory, Animal and Natural Resources Institute, Agricultural Research Service, U.S. Department of Agriculture, Beltsville, Maryland 20705

Jay A. Fishman • Transplant Infectious Disease and Compromised Host Program, Infectious Diseases Division, Massachusetts General Hospital, Harvard Medical School, Boston, Massachusetts 02114

Ron A. M. Fouchier • Department of Virology, Erasmus Medical Center, Dr. Molewaterplein 50, 3015 GE Rotterdam, The Netherlands

Vincent A. Fulginiti • University of Colorado Health Sciences Center, Denver, Colorado, and University of Arizona, Tucson, Arizona

Corina E. Gonzalez • Department of Pediatrics, Division of Pediatric Hematology-Oncology, Georgetown University Hospital, Washington, DC 20007

Y. Guan   •   Department of Microbiology, University Pathology Building, Queen Mary Hospital, The University of Hong Kong, Pokfulam Road, Hong Kong Special Administrative Region, People's Republic of China

Walid Heneine   •   Laboratory Branch, Division of HIV/AIDS Prevention, National Center for HIV, Hepatitis, STD, and TB Prevention, Centers for Disease Control and Prevention, MS G-45, Atlanta, Georgia 30333

Michael G. Ison   •   Transplant Infectious Diseases Service, Northwestern University Feinberg School of Medicine, 676 North St. Clair Street, Suite 200, Chicago, Illinois 60611

Keith P. Klugman   •   Hubert Department of Global Health, Rollins School of Public Health, and Division of Infectious Diseases, School of Medicine, Emory University, 1518 Clifton Rd., Rm. 720, Atlanta, Georgia 30322

Shabir A. Madhi   •   Respiratory and Meningeal Pathogens Research Unit, Chris Hani-Baragwanath Hospital, Old Nurses Home, 1st Floor, West Wing, Bertsham, Gauteng 2013, South Africa

Akhilesh Chandra Mishra   •   National Institute of Virology, 20-A Dr. Ambedkar Road, Pune-411 001, India

Kimberly A. Moran   •   Infectious Disease Service, Walter Reed Army Medical Center, 6900 Georgia Avenue NW, Washington, DC 20307

Najih A. Naser   •   TransTech Pharma, 4170 Mendenhall Oaks Parkway, High Point, North Carolina 27265

Saleh A. Naser   •   Department of Molecular Biology and Microbiology, Burnett College for Biomedical Sciences, University of Central Florida, Orlando, Florida 32816

J. M. Nicholls   •   Department of Pathology, University Pathology Building, Queen Mary Hospital, The University of Hong Kong, Pokfulam Road, Hong Kong Special Administrative Region, People's Republic of China

Ynes R. Ortega   •   Center for Food Safety and Quality Enhancement, University of Georgia, 1109 Experiment Street, Griffin, Georgia 30223

Justin R. Ortiz   •   Epidemiology and Surveillance Branch, Influenza Division, National Center for Immunization and Respiratory Diseases, Centers for Disease Control and Prevention, Atlanta, Georgia 30333

Albert D. M. E. Osterhaus   •   Department of Virology, Erasmus Medical Center, Dr. Molewaterplein 50, 3015 GE Rotterdam, The Netherlands

J. S. M. Peiris   •   Department of Microbiology, University Pathology Building, Queen Mary Hospital, The University of Hong Kong, Pokfulam Road, Hong Kong Special Administrative Region, People's Republic of China

Lyle R. Petersen   •   Division of Vector-Borne Infectious Diseases, National Center for Infectious Diseases, Centers for Disease Control and Prevention, Fort Collins, Colorado 80521

L. L. M. Poon   •   Department of Microbiology, University Pathology Building, Queen Mary Hospital, The University of Hong Kong, Pokfulam Road, Hong Kong Special Administrative Region, People's Republic of China

John Quale   •   Division of Infectious Diseases, SUNY Downstate Medical Center, Brooklyn, New York 11203

Joseph Rahimian   •   Department of Infectious Diseases, St. Vincent's Hospital, New York, New York 10011

Shmuel Shoham   •   Division of Infectious Diseases, Washington Hospital Center, Washington, DC 20010

William M. Switzer   •   Laboratory Branch, Division of HIV/AIDS Prevention, National Center for HIV, Hepatitis, STD, and TB Prevention, Centers for Disease Control and Prevention, MS G-45, Atlanta, Georgia 30333

Timothy M. Uyeki   •   Epidemiology and Surveillance Branch, Influenza Division, National Center for Immunization and Respiratory Diseases, Centers for Disease Control and Prevention, Atlanta, Georgia 30333

Bernadette G. van den Hoogen   •   Department of Virology, Erasmus Medical Center, Dr. Molewaterplein 50, 3015 GE Rotterdam, The Netherlands

Thomas J. Walsh   •   Pediatric Oncology Branch, National Cancer Institute, National Institutes of Health, Bethesda, Maryland 20892

Jin-Town Wang   •   Department of Microbiology, National Taiwan University Hospital, Taipei 10016, Taiwan

Nathan D. Wolfe   •   Departments of Epidemiology, International Health, and Molecular Microbiology and Immunology, Bloomberg School of Public Health, Johns Hopkins University, Baltimore, Maryland 21205

Lihua X. Xiao   •   Division of Parasitic Diseases, National Center for Infectious Diseases, Centers for Disease Control and Prevention, U.S. Department of Health and Human Services, Atlanta, Georgia 30341

K. Y. Yuen   •   Department of Microbiology, University Pathology Building, Queen Mary Hospital, The University of Hong Kong, Pokfulam Road, Hong Kong Special Administrative Region, People's Republic of China

FOREWORD

The history of human civilizations has been defined in part by interactions between humans and infectious agents. Major epidemics—including the plague of Athens; the Black Death, which killed a third of Europe's population; the epidemics of smallpox and measles that decimated the Inca and Aztec civilizations and allowed the Spanish to conquer the Americas; the cholera epidemics of 19th-century Europe; and the influenza pandemic of 1918—are but a few of the most prominent history-changing landmarks. Today, other infectious diseases are defining the level of health in many developing countries, with the foremost example being the current scourge of human immunodeficiency virus (HIV) and AIDS in Africa. These diseases adversely affect the well-being, survival, and longevity of affected populations and diminish prospects for economic development.

At the turn of the 20th century, the situation in the United States was much like that of the developing world today. Life expectancy at birth hovered at about 40 years, many of the deaths occurred in infants and children, and few medical or health interventions dramatically improved outcomes. However, in the 20th century, we learned to control many of the diseases of infectious etiology with an arsenal of antibiotics and vaccines; improvements in water, sanitation, and food hygiene; and improved understanding of public health and disease control concepts. Longevity increased, child survival improved, and infections seemed to be well controlled. As a result, the surgeon general of the United States proclaimed in the late 1960s that we had controlled problems due to infectious diseases and could thus focus our efforts on chronic diseases that affect aging populations. Unfortunately, history proved him wrong.

This claim of victory against infectious diseases was the premature call of a surgeon general who did not appreciate the adaptable nature of the enemy, the continuing susceptibility of the population under attack, or the struggle required by the medical community to develop novel weapons to sustain the upper hand in this continuing battle. In the past 40 years, dozens of new infectious agents that place our population at risk have been discovered, and many of the tools to fight these and other pathogens have lost their edge. In the past decade alone, we have seen the emergence of novel pathogens like severe acute respiratory syndrome (SARS) coronavirus, "flesh-eating" bacteria (which cause necrotizing fasciitis), and West Nile virus, and we have experienced the threat of avian influenza and the weaponization of agents, such as the smallpox and anthrax agents, that we thought had been controlled. Remaining unchecked in the developing world are HIV infection, tuberculosis (including drug-resistant strains), and malaria, each of which kills more than a million people every year, and acute respiratory infections and diarrhea, which remain the first and second most common causes, respectively, of childhood deaths worldwide. Clearly, the battle with infectious agents is not over; our enemies are versatile in their ability to find new patterns and mechanisms of spread, and most of these agents are but a few hours or days away from areas conducive to widespread transmission, such as airports, seaports, and food markets. Human behavior has also changed over the centuries. We now crowd the planet with more than 6 billion people who live, work, and play in spaces that are becoming more densely crowded. We travel more than we used to, eat foods from around the world, share food and water sources that are subject to contamination, and interact with unusual pets that can be vectors for disease. Most important, our public health arsenal is not prepared to combat the increasing challenges presented by infectious agents.

This book represents the seventh in a line of volumes that document the changing panorama of emerging diseases that lie before us during the early 21st century. Earlier writers, such as Hans Zinsser, who concluded in his acclaimed book *Rats, Lice and History* (published in 1935) that human history had been marked and shaped by plagues; Paul de Kruif, whose historical narrative *Microbe Hunters* (published in 1926 and 1953) acquaints readers with the early heroes of microbiology; and Richard Krause, whose book *The Restless Tide* (published in 1981) predicted that humans would not see an end to infectious diseases, stood alone in describing the challenges presented by an endless wave of infectious pathogens. When the world awoke to the epidemic of HIV/AIDS, a new appreciation for the threat of emerging infections arose, and the writings of these early authors gained new credence. In 1992, the Institute of Medicine's Committee on Emerging Microbial Threats to Health authored a report titled *Emerging Infections: Microbial Threats to Health in the United States*. The book's editors, Joshua Lederberg, Robert E. Shope, and Stanley C. Oaks, Jr., documented in clear and convincing terms the extent of the continuing challenge between microbes and humans and the changes in human behavior and society that were making us more susceptible to microbial threats. The editors also raised the specter that, with complacency, we could lose the two most powerful weapons in our arsenal: antibiotics, which were losing effectiveness as organisms were becoming resistant to them, and a public health surveillance infrastructure for identifying new challenges to health as they arise. It was clear that we needed new investments and initiatives to understand the problem and put systems in place to ensure an effective response.

What is needed to address the challenges posed by continuously emerging infections? Alert clinicians, effective global surveillance networks, open communications among researchers and public health professionals, state-of-the-art laboratories, investigators who can bring the best science to bear on problems that could be of global proportions, and financial and political support. In short, we need a public health ethic that is global in nature and collaborative in approach, that provides for the rapid recognition of and response to health concerns worldwide, and that is appreciated by public health officials and politicians alike. The current global concern about avian influenza has spotlighted the problems associated with the lack of an effective global surveillance system and highlighted the need for such surveillance. Microbiology and molecular biology have provided us with powerful tools for quickly detecting and characterizing new pathogens, seeking creative solutions for treatment and control, and allowing a global army of scientists to communicate at warp speed and address local problems that could rapidly spread to global proportions. The assembly of a global team of investigators to work together to identify the agent of SARS or to monitor strains of influenza virus in birds and humans represents the beginning of this new modus operandi. This volume provides the latest update on the emerging infections facing us today and the approaches needed to keep us fully engaged in public health efforts for surveillance, research, and control. It is a feast for readers, keeping them abreast of the latest developments in this ongoing struggle.

Roger I. Glass
Director
Fogarty International Center
Associate Director for International Research
National Institutes of Health
Bethesda, Maryland

PREFACE

Despite progress in the prevention and control of infectious diseases during the past several decades, the early years of the 21st century provide continued evidence of the persistence and tenacity of infectious disease threats. The interplay of rapid globalization, demographic shifts, ecologic changes, and unprecedented movement of people and goods, while offering increased benefits in many arenas, also yields unexpected risks to health—often with attendant social and economic repercussions. The emergence and rapid global spread of severe acute respiratory syndrome (SARS), the widespread geographic diffusion of West Nile virus since its introduction into the Western Hemisphere, and the stepped-up preparations for a seemingly imminent outbreak of pandemic influenza provide dramatic evidence of the continued ability of microbes to emerge, spread, adapt, and challenge the global community.

Since 1995, the program committee of the Interscience Conference on Antimicrobial Agents and Chemotherapy (ICAAC) and the leaders of the Infectious Diseases Society of America (IDSA) have organized joint sessions on new and emerging pathogens during ICAAC and the IDSA annual meetings. These sessions are designed to address the spectrum of new and emerging bacteria, viruses, fungi, and parasites of recognized or potential scientific and public health importance, with discussions on strategies for their prevention and control. The chapters in *Emerging Infections 7* are derived from recent sessions and focus on a range of infections that pose challenges for the clinical, laboratory, and public health communities. Some of these are newly recognized diseases, whereas others are previously known pathogens presenting new challenges. Some are described as domestic threats, whereas others affect populations elsewhere. However, as has been clearly demonstrated, infectious agents know no borders: every threat is potentially a global threat.

Our experiences in responding to the outbreaks of the recent past, many of which are of zoonotic origin, provide important lessons for the future. Most important, a global threat requires a global response. In today's world, detection and control of infectious diseases call for a wide-ranging and multifaceted international approach that includes strong leadership and political will; a robust network for global disease detection, monitoring, containment, and control; and cooperation, collaboration, and seamless communication among nations and leaders. Because weakened public health systems and health services in many areas of the world pose threats for all, investments in national public health institutes and systems, health services, and response capacity, as well as workforce development, can yield substantial returns for the health and security of the global community. Finally, in addition to the necessity of managing the immediate and specific risks and vulnerabilities posed by infectious diseases, there is a critical need to tackle the underlying factors that contribute to disease emergence and spread; key among these are poverty, social inequities, malnutrition, and lack of clean water and adequate sanitation.

Future infectious disease challenges are difficult to predict but certainly include continued problems with antimicrobial-resistant infections, diarrheal diseases, and influenza and other respiratory diseases, as well as continued and new threats for immunocompromised populations. Additional links between chronic diseases and infectious agents will likely be discovered, providing new opportunities for disease prevention and treatment. In addition to preparing for naturally occurring infectious disease outbreaks, we will continue to strengthen our ability to detect and respond to potential acts of bioterrorism. This volume, the seventh in the *Emerging Infections* series, should serve as a valuable source of current information for those responsible for these and other microbial threats to global health, economies, and security.

W. Michael Scheld
David C. Hooper
James M. Hughes

ACKNOWLEDGMENTS

We thank everyone who has helped us in preparing this volume. Most important, we thank all of the authors for their outstanding contributions. As editors, we are particularly grateful to the members of the Interscience Conference on Antimicrobial Agents and Chemotherapy (ICAAC) Program Committee who assisted us in coordinating topic and speaker selection for and/or moderating the joint symposia on emerging infections during the 2003 and 2004 ICAAC meetings. Numerous other colleagues provided helpful discussion, advice, and criticisms. We are also grateful to our assistants, Ruth Aldridge, Jenni Crow, Portia Allen, and Allison Greenspan. We thank Ken April of ASM Press for his superb work in coordinating production of the book. And finally, we thank our families for their understanding and support during this undertaking.

Emerging Infections 7
Edited by W. M. Scheld, D. C. Hooper, and J. M. Hughes
© 2007 ASM Press, Washington, D.C.

Chapter 1

Avian Influenza A (H5N1) Virus

Justin R. Ortiz and Timothy M. Uyeki

Since 1997, highly pathogenic avian influenza A (H5N1) viruses have caused unprecedented widespread poultry outbreaks with high mortality in a number of Asian, European, Middle Eastern, and African countries; have infected other animal species; and have caused sporadic, severe, and fatal human infections. In 2005, H5N1 viruses were documented among wild migratory birds in the western People's Republic of China, and the spread of H5N1 into other regions, including Eastern Europe, may be due in part to wild birds (83). H5N1 viruses have also caused severe and fatal illness among leopards (35), tigers (35), and domestic cats (61), but pigs have been asymptomatically infected (17). Asymptomatic infections in ducks and other wild birds have also been reported (36). From 1997 to 4 July 2006, human cases of H5N1 were reported in 10 countries (Azerbaijan; Cambodia; China, including the Hong Kong Special Administrative Region [SAR]; Djibouti; Egypt; Indonesia; Iraq; Thailand; Turkey; and Vietnam), and these cases coincided with outbreaks among poultry. Since the reemergence of H5N1 among poultry in Asia in late 2003, human H5N1 cases have occurred in three apparent waves, the third of which is currently (2006) ongoing. As of 4 July 2006, 229 H5N1 cases with 131 deaths had been reported to the World Health Organization (WHO) since January 2004 (74).

Human illness caused by infection with H5N1 virus is primarily characterized as a severe febrile respiratory disease with high mortality. Most human cases appear to have resulted from sporadic avian-to-human transmission of H5N1 viruses to previously healthy individuals who had direct contact with sick or dead poultry. No specific treatment has yet proven effective, and management is largely supportive. Although clusters of cases have been observed, with an apparent increase during 2005 (49), and probable cases of limited human-to-human transmission of H5N1 have been reported (64), there is no evidence of sustained human-to-human spread of H5N1 to date, and human illness due to H5N1 virus infection remains rare.

The key to reducing the public health impact of H5N1 is to control the spread of H5N1 among poultry. Comprehensive strategies to control H5N1 in poultry and other bird

Justin R. Ortiz and Timothy M. Uyeki • Epidemiology and Surveillance Branch, Influenza Division, National Center for Immunization and Respiratory Diseases, Centers for Disease Control and Prevention, Atlanta, GA 30333.

populations are needed and include active surveillance, culling of infected flocks, disinfecting the environment, vaccinating poultry using standardized inactivated vaccines, compensating farmers, improving hygienic practices in live-poultry markets, and improving biosecurity (9). In the absence of an available efficacious human H5N1 vaccine, infection with H5N1 virus is primarily prevented by avoiding or minimizing exposure to infected poultry, poultry products, and contaminated environments. Persons involved in culling H5N1-infected poultry should wear appropriate personal protective equipment, and antiviral chemoprophylaxis, if available, should be considered for these persons (80). It is recommended that health care workers caring for H5N1 patients receive human influenza vaccine to prevent the potential for coinfection with human influenza A viruses and H5N1, which could lead to genetic reassortment (72). Persons suspected of being infected with H5N1 should be placed in isolation with appropriate infection control precautions; they should be treated by health care personnel who have received antiviral chemoprophylaxis, if available, and who are wearing personal protective equipment (7, 72). Surveillance for suspected human H5N1 cases in areas affected by H5N1 among poultry is critically important.

GENERAL INFLUENZA VIROLOGY

Influenza viruses are single-stranded, negative-sense RNA viruses with eight gene segments that encode 10 proteins and belong to the family *Orthomyxoviridae*. Influenza viruses are divided into types A, B, and C. Influenza A viruses are further categorized into subtypes, and the A subtypes and type B and C viruses are all further subclassified into strains. Influenza A viruses generally infect people and birds but have infected other animal species; influenza B and C viruses primarily infect humans (20). Human influenza A and B viruses primarily infect epithelial cells of the upper respiratory tract, and they can also infect and replicate in lower respiratory tract cells.

Human influenza A and B viruses cause seasonal epidemics among people in temperate climates worldwide each year (30). In the United States, annual epidemics of human influenza are associated with an average of more than 200,000 hospitalizations and 36,000 deaths (59, 60). In tropical and subtropical climates, human influenza viruses may circulate year round. Influenza C virus infections are associated with a mild "cold-like" illness (29). Only novel human influenza A viruses can cause influenza pandemics. All influenza viruses are dynamic and are continuously evolving. Human influenza A viruses preferentially bind to nonciliated epithelial cells bearing receptors for sialic acids with α-2,6 linkages (44). Influenza A viruses are classified into subtypes on the basis of the antigenicity of the surface glycoproteins hemagglutinin and neuraminidase. The natural reservoir for all known influenza A viruses is wild aquatic waterfowl (20). To date, 16 hemagglutinin subtypes and 9 neuraminidase subtypes have been identified (26). The hemagglutinin protein is responsible for the attachment of virus to the host cell surface. It is the major antigen against which the host's protective antibody response is directed (29). Antibody to hemagglutinin confers protection against infection but is strain specific. The neuraminidase protein is less abundant on the viral surface, and its function is related, in part, to the release of virus from infected host cells. Antibody to neuraminidase can modify the spread and severity of influenza virus infection (29). The current circulating human influenza A subtypes are H1N1, H1N2, and H3N2 (30).

Influenza viruses have the propensity for genetic change. Minor genetic changes, called "antigenic drift," are spontaneous uncorrected point mutations in the hemagglutinin and neuraminidase genes of human influenza A and B viruses that result in minor antigenic changes to the corresponding hemagglutinin and neuraminidase surface proteins. Antigenic drift is an ongoing unpredictable process that results in the appearance of new antigenic variant strains. Eventually, one of the newer influenza strains becomes predominant as antibody levels to previous epidemic strains rise in the general population and exert selective evolutionary pressure (20). An epidemic antigenic variant typically predominates for a few years before a significantly different variant emerges to replace it. This is the basis for global strain surveillance, the biannual strain selection process for the composition of the trivalent influenza vaccine used in the northern and southern hemispheres (30). Major changes in the viral genome are called "antigenic shift," which refers to the emergence of an influenza A virus in humans bearing either a novel hemagglutinin or a combination of novel hemagglutinin and neuraminidase proteins. Only influenza A viruses undergo antigenic shift, which has the potential to lead to pandemics, but only if the new influenza A virus subtype is sufficiently transmissible among humans to maintain epidemic activity and is capable of causing disease. Antigenic shift is believed to occur in one of two ways—through genetic reassortment of human and animal influenza A viruses and through direct animal-to-human transmission (46).

Influenza in Animals

A variety of animal species have been infected by influenza viruses. While influenza B viruses have infected seals (50), many animal species have been infected with influenza A viruses, including pigs (68), dogs (21), horses (66), and marine mammals (47). Swine influenza A viruses are primarily an agricultural concern, but infections of humans have been documented (48). Pigs can be infected by avian, swine, and human influenza A viruses (46). They therefore could potentially serve as mixing vessels for genetic reassortment if a pig respiratory tract cell were coinfected with avian and human influenza A viruses and reassortment of gene segments occurred, resulting in the emergence of a novel, hybrid influenza virus.

Most avian influenza A viruses bind to host cell receptors bearing sialic acids with α-2,3 linkages that are found in the respiratory and gastrointestinal tracts of birds (44). Avian influenza A viruses are detectable in respiratory secretions and are excreted in feces of infected birds. Wild birds can be asymptomatically infected with avian influenza A viruses. Avian influenza A viruses have been detected in environmental water samples in arctic climates (32), and some viruses can remain viable for long periods in the environment under low-temperature and low-humidity conditions (33).

Pathogenicity of Avian Influenza A Viruses

Avian influenza A viruses are divided into two classes—low-pathogenic avian influenza (LPAI) A viruses and highly pathogenic avian influenza (HPAI) A viruses. These classifications are determined by specific molecular, as well as pathogenicity, criteria (84).

LPAI viruses usually do not cause illness in wild birds (70). They may cause mild illness in domestic poultry (ruffled feathers, decreased egg production, and weight loss) and are associated with wild birds and poultry outbreaks worldwide. Poultry outbreaks of

LPAI are generally an agricultural problem. However, LPAI viruses have the ability to evolve into highly pathogenic viruses that are threats to both poultry and public health. Human infections with LPAI A viruses have resulted in mild or uncomplicated illness. LPAI viruses documented to infect humans include H9N2 (Hong Kong and China) (5, 51, 65, 86), H7N7 (United Kingdom) (40), and H7N2 (United States) (10).

HPAI viruses have been associated with H5 and H7 subtypes that possess characteristic multibasic amino acid sequences adjacent to the hemagglutinin cleavage site, are associated with high mortality under specific pathogenicity testing, and can grow in the absence of trypsin (84). HPAI viruses do not usually cause illness in wild birds but do cause high-mortality outbreaks among domestic poultry. HPAI virus spreads very rapidly through poultry flocks, causes disease affecting multiple internal organs, and can cause mortality approaching 100%, often within 48 hours (70). HPAI viruses that have caused human illness during poultry outbreaks include H5N1, H7N7, and H7N3. An outbreak of HPAI H7N7 in The Netherlands in 2003 resulted in 89 human cases, most of which were mild illnesses, such as conjunctivitis, among poultry workers, but included one death of a veterinarian (37). In British Columbia, Canada, two people experienced very mild illness with HPAI H7N3 in 2004 (62). Both human H7N3 cases followed close contact with infected poultry and contaminated materials.

Influenza Pandemics

An influenza pandemic can occur only if there is efficient and sustained transmission among humans of a novel influenza A virus subtype to which most of the population lacks immunity and of a virus that causes disease. There were three influenza pandemics during the 20th century and an estimated 10 in the past 300 years (Table 1) (62). The most devastating was the 1918 Spanish flu pandemic, in which the emergence of influenza A (H1N1) caused an estimated 50 million to 100 million deaths worldwide (34). Molecular sequencing analysis has revealed that the 1918–1919 H1N1 pandemic virus was entirely of avian origin (58). In contrast, the emergence of the 1957–1958 H2N2 pandemic virus strain and the 1968–1969 H3N2 pandemic virus strain resulted from reassortment between LPAI

Table 1. Influenza pandemics of the 20th century[a]

Epidemic and dates	Strain	Estimated no. of U.S. deaths	Comments
Spanish flu, 1918–1919	H1N1	500,000	Nearly half of those who died were young, healthy adults. Influenza A (H1N1) viruses still circulate today after being introduced again into the human population in 1977.
Asian flu, 1957–1958	H2N2	70,000	First identified in China in late February 1957, the Asian flu spread to the United States by June 1957.
Hong Kong flu, 1968–1969	H3N2	34,000	This virus was first detected in Hong Kong in early 1968 and spread to the United States later that year. Influenza A (H3N2) viruses still circulate today.

[a]Source: Centers for Disease Control and Prevention (http://www.cdc.gov/flu/pandemic/keyfacts.htm#history).

viruses and human influenza A virus genes. The global human public health impact of the emergence of a pandemic virus is not limited to the year that the pandemic occurs. For example, through antigenic drift, H3N2 viruses have continued to circulate among humans since the 1968–1969 pandemic.

Experts at the WHO and elsewhere believe that the world is now closer to another influenza pandemic than at any time since 1968, when the last of the 20th century's three pandemics occurred. The WHO developed pandemic alert phases to warn the world of the pandemic threat and to aid in global planning for an influenza pandemic (Table 2) (77). As of 4 July 2006, the world was in WHO pandemic alert period phase 3. Between 1997 and July 2006, rare, ongoing, inefficient transmission of H5N1 virus from infected poultry to humans occurred in Africa, Asia, Europe, and the Middle East. There has been one convincing reported instance of limited human-to-human spread of H5N1 virus (64), although there is epidemiologic evidence suggesting limited, inefficient, nonsustained human-to-human transmission (6).

Emergence of H5N1

On 10 May 1997, a 3-year-old boy in Hong Kong developed fever and abdominal pain and was treated as an outpatient with antibiotics and aspirin. The symptoms progressed, and on 13 May he was hospitalized for pneumonia. Despite treatment with broad-spectrum

Table 2. WHO pandemic phases[a]

Period and phase	Description
Interpandemic period[b]	
Phase 1	No new influenza virus subtypes have been detected in humans. An influenza virus subtype that has caused human infection may be present in animals. If present in animals, the risk of human infection or disease is considered to be low.
Phase 2	No new influenza virus subtypes have been detected in humans. However, a circulating animal influenza virus subtype poses a substantial risk of human disease.
Pandemic alert period[c]	
Phase 3	Human infection(s) with a new subtype, but no human-to-human spread or at most rare instances of spread to a close contact
Phase 4	Small cluster(s) with limited human-to-human transmission, but spread is highly localized, suggesting that the virus is not well adapted to humans
Phase 5	Larger cluster(s), but human-to-human spread is still localized, suggesting that the virus is becoming increasingly better adapted to humans but may not yet be fully transmissible (substantial pandemic risk)
Pandemic period	
Phase 6	Pandemic phase: increased and sustained transmission among general population

[a]Source: reference 77.

[b]The distinction between phases 1 and 2 is based on the risk of human infection or disease resulting from circulating strains in animals. The distinction is based on various factors and their relative importance according to current scientific knowledge. Factors may include pathogenicity in animals and humans; occurrence in domesticated animals and livestock or only in wildlife; whether the virus is enzootic or epizootic, geographically localized or widespread; and other scientific parameters.

[c]The distinction among phases 3, 4, and 5 is based on an assessment of the risk of a pandemic. Various factors and their relative importance according to current scientific knowledge may be considered. Factors may include rate of transmission, geographical location and spread, severity of illness, presence of genes from human strains (if derived from an animal strain), and other scientific parameters.

antibiotics, his condition deteriorated; he was transferred to the Queen Elizabeth Hospital in Hong Kong, where he was intubated, developed multiorgan failure, and died on 21 May. Post-mortem pathology was consistent with Reye's syndrome and influenza A pneumonia (38). A viral isolate from this case was confirmed as avian influenza A (H5N1) virus in August 1997.

From March to May 1997, widespread outbreaks of H5N1 infection with high mortality among poultry were reported in chicken farms in northwestern Hong Kong (13). Genetic sequencing of the H5N1 viruses isolated from the index case and from affected chickens revealed that they were virtually identical viruses (57). The infection of the 3-year-old boy remained the only confirmed human H5N1 case until an additional 17 confirmed cases with five deaths were identified after a second outbreak among poultry in wholesale and retail markets (4) in November and December 1997 (54). Overall mortality was 18% in children and 57% in adults. After preliminary investigations suggested that humans were most likely infected directly by poultry and that chickens in Hong Kong live-bird markets were nearly 20% seropositive for anti-H5N1 antibodies (54), the reaction by the Hong Kong SAR was swift. Poultry imports from southern China were suspended, and from 29 to 31 December, authorities orchestrated the culling of 1.5 million chickens and several hundred thousand other domestic fowl in the territory (13). This depopulation of poultry successfully ended the 1997 H5N1 outbreak in Hong Kong.

Hong Kong implemented enhanced surveillance for avian influenza A viruses among animals and humans, prohibited mixing of different bird species in live-poultry markets, and improved biosecurity at poultry farms and markets, including monthly market "rest days" (69). Enhanced surveillance detected human infections with avian influenza A (H9N2) viruses in 1999 and 2003 (5, 51, 65). Sporadic outbreaks of H5N1 infection continued to be detected among poultry in Hong Kong, resulting in poultry culling and market closures (69). However, no human H5N1 cases were identified until February 2003, when Hong Kong confirmed two cases of HPAI H5N1 with one death among five members of a Hong Kong family that visited Fujian Province, China, in late January 2003 (51). This coincided with reports of 305 cases of atypical pneumonia and five deaths, including health care workers, in Guangdong Province, China, in February 2003, and prompted global public health concern about the possible beginning of an influenza pandemic. Instead of an influenza pandemic, the atypical pneumonia was a new disease called severe acute respiratory syndrome (SARS) and was found to be caused by infection with a novel SARS-associated coronavirus. The SARS outbreak resulted in 8,096 probable cases and 774 deaths and spread to 29 countries in 6 months (75). The SARS episode highlighted how quickly a novel infectious disease can emerge and spread worldwide.

It is now known that H5N1 virus emerged in southern China in 1996 and that outbreaks of HPAI H5N1 among poultry have occurred in southern China for several years (55). During 2003, unreported outbreaks of H5N1 infection among poultry occurred in China, Indonesia, Vietnam, and Thailand. These outbreaks signaled the start of an unprecedented epizootic (82). However, poultry outbreaks of H5N1 infection were not officially reported until South Korea confirmed H5N1 infection outbreaks in commercial poultry farms to the World Animal Health Organization in December 2003. In January 2004, Vietnam officially reported poultry outbreaks of H5N1 infection. Other Asian countries reported widespread outbreaks of H5N1 infection among poultry in 2004. By 2005, H5N1 was documented in poultry or migratory birds in additional Asian countries and had been detected in Africa, Europe, and the Middle East as of July 2006 (14, 74). Although migratory waterfowl have been implicated in the global spread of H5N1 (83), recent evidence suggests that the movement of poultry plays a major role in its spread and perpetuation (15). To date, only three countries—Hong Kong SAR, China; South Korea; and Japan—have controlled HPAI H5N1 poultry infection outbreaks. Data from surveillance for H5N1 viruses among poultry in southern China have indicated that H5N1 activity increases among poultry during months with cooler temperatures and lower humidity (14). This finding has been supported by the observed increases in poultry outbreaks in Thailand and Vietnam during the late and early months of 2003 to 2005 and suggests seasonality of H5N1 activity among poultry. Human H5N1 cases have been associated with poultry outbreaks. Nevertheless, H5N1 outbreaks among poultry have occurred during months with high temperatures and high humidity, and human cases have occurred outside cool periods.

Other animal species have been infected with HPAI H5N1 viruses. Tigers and leopards have been infected through consumption of infected poultry, resulting in fatal illness, and tiger-to-tiger transmission has been reported (19). Domestic cats have been experimentally infected with H5N1 viruses with resultant severe illness (39), and pigs have been infected with H5N1 viruses without apparent signs of illness (22, 23).

H5N1 viruses that infected humans from 1997 to 2005 were of the Z genotype, and until 2005, were entirely due to clade 1, 1′, and 3 viruses (Vietnam, Thailand, and Cambodia) (79). In 2005, human H5N1 cases were identified in Indonesia and China and were attributed to clade 2 viruses, antigenically distinct from clade 1, 1′, and 3 viruses (49, 79). It is clear that H5N1 viruses have evolved since their emergence in 1996 and continue to evolve. HPAI H5N1 viruses that infected humans in 1997 were antigenically distinct from the viruses that infected humans in 2003 and those that infected humans in 2004 and 2005.

EPIDEMIOLOGY OF HUMAN DISEASE

As of 4 July 2006, 229 H5N1 cases with 131 deaths had been officially reported to the WHO since January 2004 (Table 3) (74). Since January 2004, 10 countries have reported human H5N1 cases, including Azerbaijan, Cambodia, China, Djibouti, Egypt, Indonesia, Iraq, Thailand, Turkey, and Vietnam (Fig. 1). Cases have occurred in three apparent waves generally corresponding to the early and late parts of the year (Fig. 2). Many of the H5N1 cases have occurred in Vietnam, which reported cases in all three waves. In June 2006, the WHO published a summary of the epidemiology of 205 confirmed human H5N1 cases from 1 December 2003 to 30 April 2006 (81a). The WHO maintains an updated list of H5N1 cases on its website. In early 2006, the Republic of Turkey reported human H5N1 cases and deaths in multiple provinces. These cases were coincident with outbreaks in poultry occurring in several parts of the country. As of 6 February 2006, there have been 12 confirmed cases, with four deaths. Control measures were rapidly implemented, and public health officials are working to better understand the epidemiology of the disease. Preliminary information suggested that the epidemiology of human H5N1 cases in Turkey was similar to that of cases in Southeast Asia.

Surveillance Case Definitions

Surveillance for human H5N1 cases has focused primarily upon hospitalized patients with severe respiratory disease (Fig. 3). A possible case of H5N1 infection was defined by

Table 3. WHO human influenza A (H5N1) confirmed cases and deaths[a]

| Location | 1997, Hong Kong | 2003, Hong Kong and Fujian Province, China | Present epidemic | | | | Total |
			Wave 1 (12/26/03–3/10/04)[b]	Wave 2 (7/19/04–10/8/04)	Wave 3 (12/16/04–present)	Present epidemic total	
Azerbaijan	0 (0)	0 (0)	0 (0)	0 (0)	8 (5)	8 (5)	8 (5)
Cambodia	0 (0)	0 (0)	0 (0)	0 (0)	6 (6)	6 (6)	6 (6)
China (Hong Kong)	18 (6)	2 (1)	0 (0)	0 (0)	19 (12)	19 (12)	39 (19)
Djibouti	0 (0)	0 (0)	0 (0)	0 (0)	1 (0)	1 (0)	1 (0)
Egypt	0 (0)	0 (0)	0 (0)	0 (0)	14 (6)	14 (6)	14 (6)
Indonesia	0 (0)	0 (0)	0 (0)	0 (0)	52 (40)	52 (40)	52 (40)
Iraq	0 (0)	0 (0)	0 (0)	0 (0)	2 (2)	2 (2)	2 (2)
Thailand	0 (0)	0 (0)	12 (8)	5 (4)	5 (2)	22 (14)	22 (14)
Turkey	0 (0)	0 (0)	0 (0)	0 (0)	12 (4)	12 (4)	12 (4)
Vietnam	0 (0)	0 (0)	23 (16)	4 (4)	66 (22)	93 (42)	93 (42)
Total	18 (6)	2 (1)	35 (24)	9 (8)	185 (99)	229 (131)	249 (138)

[a]Source: reference 78.
[b]Dates are given as month/day/year.

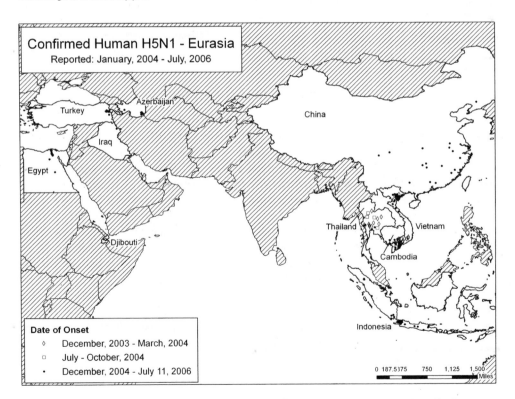

Figure 1. Confirmed human H5N1 cases in Eurasia reported from January 2004 to February 2006. (Source: World Health Organization [http://www.who.int/csr/disease/avian_influenza/updates/en/index.html]. Map by Margaret McCarron.)

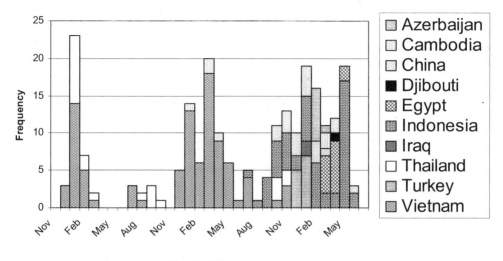

Figure 2. WHO confirmed H5N1 cases as of 4 July 2006. Eleven of 12 Turkish cases are represented. (Source: World Health Organization [http://www.who.int/csr/disease/avian_influenza/country/cases_table_2006_02_06/en/index.html].)

the WHO in Vietnam in 2004 as any individual with influenza-like illness and one or more of the following: laboratory evidence for influenza A by a test that does not subtype the virus, contact during the prior 7 days with a confirmed H5N1 patient, contact during the prior 7 days with birds that had died, or laboratory work during the prior 7 days in which specimens from suspected H5N1 cases were processed (78).

Evidence of Poultry-to-Human Transmission

Epidemiological studies conducted in Hong Kong during the 1997 H5N1 outbreak implicated avian-to-human transmission of H5N1 virus. A case-control study found that the main risk factor associated with H5N1 was visiting a live-poultry market in the week prior to illness (45). Eating poultry, home preparation of fresh poultry, exposure to other birds, recent travel, and recent contact with persons with respiratory illness were not associated with H5N1 infection (45). A study of 1,525 Hong Kong poultry market workers reported an estimated 10% seroprevalence of H5N1 antibodies (4). Risk factors for antibody to H5N1 included working in retail poultry operations, reporting mortality of >10% among poultry with which they worked, butchering poultry, and feeding poultry (4). Among 293 Hong Kong government workers who helped cull infected poultry at commercial farms, the seroprevalence of H5N1 antibodies was 3%, including one asymptomatic seroconversion (4).

Because H5N1 viruses have evolved since 1997 and 2003, there is an urgent need for epidemiological studies to ascertain the risk of avian-to-human transmission of H5N1 since 2003. One limited study of 25 persons in Vietnam who had contact with sick poultry found that none had antibodies to H5N1 in 2004 (2). Field investigations and anecdotal reports in 2004 and 2005 have suggested that in addition to direct contact with sick or dead poultry, other behaviors are potential risk factors for avian-to-human transmission of

Possible H5N1 case

I. Any individual presenting with fever ≥38°C
AND One or more of the following symptoms:
   • cough;
   • sore throat;
   • shortness of breath
AND One or more of the following:
   • laboratory evidence for influenza A by a test that does not subtype the virus;
   • having been in contact during the 7 days prior to the onset of symptoms with a confirmed case of H5N1 while this case was infectious;
   • having been in contact during the 7 days prior to the onset of symptoms with birds, including chickens, that have died of an illness;
   • having worked in a laboratory during the 7 days prior to the onset of symptoms where there is processing of samples from persons or animals that are suspected of having highly pathogenic avian influenza (HPAI) infection
OR
II. Death from an unexplained acute respiratory illness
AND one or more of the following:
   • residing in area where HPAI is suspected or confirmed;
   • having been in contact during the 7 days prior to the onset of symptoms with a confirmed case of H5N1 while this case was infectious

Probable H5N1 case

Any individual presenting with fever ≥38°C
AND one or more of the following symptoms:
   • cough;
   • sore throat;
   • shortness of breath
AND limited laboratory evidence for H5N1 (H5 specific antibodies detected in a single serum specimen)

Confirmed H5N1 case

An individual for whom laboratory testing demonstrates one or more of the following:
   • positive viral culture for H5N1;
   • positive PCR for H5N1;
   • immunofluorescence antibody (IFA) test positive using H5N1 monoclonal antibodies;
   • 4-fold rise in H5N1 specific antibody titer in paired serum samples

* Individuals infected with H5N1 virus are considered to be infectious starting from one day before the onset of symptoms up to 7 days after onset of symptoms. * Laboratory investigations for H5N1 may also be undertaken on deceased individuals and in the context of targeted epidemiological studies. Laboratory confirmed cases identified under these circumstances should also be reported.

Figure 3. WHO H5N1 case definitions used in Vietnam, 2004 (source: reference 78).

H5N1: plucking and preparing of diseased birds, handling cockfighting roosters, playing with poultry, contact with asymptomatically infected ducks, and consumption of duck blood or undercooked poultry (2).

Limited Human-to-Human Transmission

Several studies have assessed the risk of human-to-human transmission of H5N1 viruses among close contacts of case patients and among health care workers. Some studies were limited by the difficulty of distinguishing potential confounding poultry exposures or by the collection of a single serum specimen from which it could not be discerned whether infection occurred in the past through poultry exposure or recently through human contact. Although H5N1 viruses have evolved since 1997, studies suggest that limited human-to-human transmission of H5N1 viruses is very rare to date. One limited study in Vietnam found that none of 51 household contacts had evidence of infection (2). The best evidence for limited human-to-human transmission of H5N1 in Hong Kong was found in cohort studies of health care workers who cared for H5N1 patients. Two nurses who did not have any poultry contact had evidence of seroconversion to H5N1 antibodies (4). One had a mild respiratory illness, and one was asymptomatic. Limited studies conducted in 2004 in Hanoi and Ho Chi Minh City, Vietnam, and Bangkok, Thailand, among health care workers who cared for H5N1 patients suggested that nosocomial transmission did not occur despite initially poor infection control measures (19, 43, 53).

The best evidence to suggest that limited human-to-human transmission of H5N1 has occurred was in a cluster of cases in Thailand in September 2004. An 11-year-old girl was hospitalized with a severe febrile respiratory illness. She lived with her aunt in a village where poultry had recently died. Her mother lived far away and did not have any poultry contact. The mother and the child's aunt provided bedside care to the sick child for 24 h in the hospital before she died. Specimens from the girl were not available for H5N1 testing. However, the mother and aunt became ill 3 and 8 days after the girl's death; both women were confirmed to have H5N1 infection, and the mother subsequently died (64).

Clustering of Cases

The occurrence of clustering of suspected H5N1 cases among contacts always demands rapid epidemiological and virological investigation to assess if human-to-human transmission is likely to have occurred and if the virus suggests greater transmissibility and an increased pandemic threat. In such investigations, the potential roles of confounding animal and environmental exposures must be assessed, because case clustering does not necessarily indicate human-to-human transmission. Clustering could indicate ongoing animal or environmental exposures or variable incubation periods. Clustering with H5N1 has been documented among family members and relatives beginning with the 1997 Hong Kong outbreak. Two confirmed H5N1 case patients in the 1997 outbreak were cousins who had household contact (8). In another family, a father and son were confirmed to have H5N1 infection in 2003 after visiting southern China (51). From January 2004 to July 2005, 15 H5N1 family clusters were noted, although insufficient epidemiological data were available to assess whether human-to-human transmission had occurred (49). Clustering of cases among family members and relatives could also suggest an increased genetic susceptibility to H5N1 virus infection, and this hypothesis should be investigated.

Evidence of Asymptomatic and Mild Infection

Seroprevalence studies among exposed poultry workers in Hong Kong in 1997 found that asymptomatic and mild H5N1 virus infections occurred through avian-to-human transmission much more frequently than through limited person-to-person transmission (4, 6). Few serosurveys have been conducted among persons not known to be exposed to poultry or to H5N1 cases. In the 1997 Hong Kong outbreak, none of 219 healthy people tested had antibodies to H5 (11), and a study of 209 health care workers not exposed to an H5N1 case patient found only 2 persons with evidence of prior infection (6). Since case finding for H5N1 has recently focused upon persons with severe respiratory illness, it is clear that seroepidemiological studies are needed to ascertain the frequency of asymptomatic and mild H5N1 virus infections in Asia.

CLINICAL H5N1 INFECTION

Clinical case reports of H5N1 infection reflect surveillance for severe respiratory illness in hospitals. There are few descriptions of the clinical features of mild or atypical disease.

Incubation Period

The incubation period of H5N1 virus infection is difficult to ascertain unless the true exposure that resulted in infection is known. For ongoing poultry or environmental exposures, this may be difficult to determine. In the 1997 Hong Kong outbreak, most cases occurred within 2 to 4 days of known exposure (87). More recently, the incubation period has been estimated to range from 2 to 8 days (87). Some possible factors affecting the incubation period include the mode of transmission, the infectious dose, and repeated exposures.

Presenting Symptoms

Most ill H5N1 patients present with febrile respiratory disease. In a Thai case series, all 12 patients had fever (>38°C), respiratory symptoms, and abnormal chest radiographs on admission (19). Patients often have severe respiratory abnormalities. In a case series of 10 pediatric and young adult patients in Vietnam, all had profound tachypnea with a median respiratory rate of 55 (range, 28 to 70) breaths per minute (31). Patients rarely have rhinorrhea or conjunctivitis, common findings with human influenza virus infection (2). H5N1 patients are more likely than patients with human influenza to experience gastrointestinal symptoms. Among 10 Vietnamese patients, seven had watery diarrhea, and 50% of the 1997 Hong Kong case patients had abdominal pain, vomiting, or diarrhea (87). There is a case report of an H5N1 patient who had diarrhea preceding respiratory symptoms by 5 days (1).

Laboratory Findings

Leukopenia, lymphopenia, and moderate thrombocytopenia are common findings on presentation and are associated with an increased risk of death (19). In one case series, the median admitting leukocyte count was 2,100/µl, the median lymphocyte count was 700/µl, and the median platelet count was 75,500/µl (31). Slight elevations in hepatic transaminases and creatinine are common (87). Hyperglycemia has been reported but may be due to the use of high-dose corticosteroids (2). Cultures of blood and tracheal aspirates usually do not reveal any bacterial coinfections. Limited clinical data suggest that patients have primarily viral pneumonias on presentation without secondary bacterial pneumonia (2), although ventilator-associated pneumonias have been reported (87).

Radiographic Findings

Most chest radiographs at admission show abnormal but nonspecific findings. Chest X-ray abnormalities have been reported a median of 7 days after the onset of symptoms (19). Major abnormalities reported in one case series included extensive bilateral infiltrates, lobar collapse, focal consolidation, and air bronchograms (2, 31). Pleural effusions appear to be rare (2).

Disease Course

Lower respiratory tract manifestations develop early, and rapid progression of respiratory disease is common (2). Most cases that have progressed to adult respiratory distress syndrome (ARDS) and multiorgan dysfunction have been fatal. A WHO report noted that the median duration from illness onset to hospitalization was 4 days (range, 0 to 18 days) and the median duration from illness onset until death was 9 days (range, 2 to 31 days) (81a).

Complications

Many complications have been reported to have occurred during H5N1 virus infection. Reye's syndrome associated with aspirin ingestion may have contributed to the death of one pediatric H5N1 patient in 1997 (38). Common cardiac complications include cardiac dilatation and supraventricular tachycardia (2). Pneumothorax, pneumomediastinum, pulmonary hemorrhage, and ventilator-associated pneumonia have been reported as complications of mechanical ventilation (2, 18, 28). Many patients with pneumonia progress to ARDS. Pancytopenia and septic shock without bacteremia have also been reported (2).

Atypical Clinical Illness

In February 2004, a healthy 4-year-old boy presented to medical care with seizures 10 days after the death of his 9-year-old sister from encephalitis of unknown origin. Both children had fever, watery diarrhea, and somnolence without respiratory symptoms. The boy's initial chest radiograph was unremarkable. Initial diagnostic workup, including lumbar puncture, was unrevealing, and the child was diagnosed clinically with encephalitis. He subsequently developed bilateral pneumonia and died of respiratory failure. As part of a study of encephalitis of unknown origin, H5N1 virus was isolated from cerebrospinal fluid, fecal, throat, and serum specimens (24). This case suggests the likelihood of H5N1 viremia, penetration into the cerebrospinal fluid, and involvement of the gastrointestinal tract. H5N1 virus was isolated from the plasma of a case in Thailand, also suggesting viremia (19a). Another atypical case of H5N1 infection in which gastrointestinal symptoms preceded respiratory symptoms occurred in a previously healthy 39-year-old Thai woman in March 2004. The woman was admitted with fever, diarrhea, nausea, and vomiting without respiratory symptoms. On her fifth hospital day, she developed respiratory symptoms that progressed to ARDS with a fatal outcome (1).

Autopsy Data

Postmortem data on fatal H5N1 cases are very limited. Autopsy data have demonstrated that H5N1 viruses replicate in the lungs, and type II pneumocytes appear to be the major site of viral replication (63). One postmortem examination of a child who died 16 days after illness onset found evidence of H5N1 viral replication in small- and large-intestinal tissue (63). In addition, negative-stranded RNA was detected in the spleen, suggesting low or absent replication in this site (63). Such findings may explain the prevalence of gastrointestinal symptoms with H5N1 virus infection.

Pathogenesis

The immune response to H5N1 may contribute to disease pathogenesis. When compared with human influenza A (H1N1) virus, H5N1 viruses were shown to be more potent inducers of proinflammatory cytokines and chemokines from primary human macrophages and in vitro human respiratory epithelial cells (12, 16). These findings suggest that cytokine dysregulation may play a role in the pathogenesis of H5N1 infection. These data are the basis for empiric use of immunomodulators, such as corticosteroids, to dampen the immune response to H5N1 in severely ill patients, and they may also explain the diminished efficacy of antiviral treatment in the same patients.

H5N1 virus was shown to attach predominantly to type II pneumocytes, alveolar macrophages, and nonciliated cuboidal epithelial cells in terminal bronchioles of the lower respiratory tract (66a). This suggests that the inability of current H5N1 viruses to attach to human upper respiratory tract tissues may limit human-to-human transmissibility.

Mortality

In the 1997 outbreak, the H5N1 case fatality rate was 33%. With the reemergence of H5N1 in late 2003, the case fatality rate has increased. As of December 2005, the cumulative case fatality rate since January 2004 was 41%. It is very likely that many H5N1 cases have not been identified, especially fatal cases, due to surveillance and laboratory testing limitations. Therefore, the official WHO H5N1 case counts are likely to be an underestimate of all H5N1 cases, including fatal cases. Since H5N1 surveillance has focused on severe respiratory illness and since few mild or asymptomatic infections have been identified, the case fatality rate is likely to be biased upward.

Management

Most patients require supplemental oxygen and ventilatory support. While some have avoided invasive ventilation with continuous positive airway pressure (31), those with respiratory failure have required invasive mechanical ventilation (31). Almost all patients have received empiric broad-spectrum antibiotics. In addition, many of the critically ill patients have been treated with systemic corticosteroids. However, the effectiveness of corticosteroid therapy is unknown. Hyperglycemia has occurred in some patients, likely as a complication of glucose dysregulation due to steroids, and insulin has been used to maintain glycemic control.

Antiviral Therapy

The adamantanes (amantadine and rimantadine) and the neuraminidase inhibitors (oseltamivir and zanamivir) are two classes of antiviral medications with activity against influenza A viruses. While all H5N1 virus isolates from the 1997 Hong Kong outbreak were adamantane sensitive, most H5N1 viruses isolated from human cases in 2004 and 2005 are resistant to amantadine and rimantadine (2). Therefore, treatment of H5N1 patients with neuraminidase inhibitors is recommended (2). There is laboratory evidence that neuraminidase inhibitors have activity against H5N1 (27, 42), and their early administration is associated with better clinical outcomes with human influenza (19). In mouse models of H5N1 infection, there is a dose-dependent response to oseltamivir, with the longest survival seen with high-dose therapy (85). However, no prospective studies have been performed to assess their efficacy in human cases of H5N1, especially as late treatment of severely ill patients. Almost all H5N1 virus isolates obtained have been sensitive to neuraminidase inhibitors. One H5N1 viral isolate was reported that had mixed properties of reduced susceptibility to oseltamivir (41). It was collected from a child who was a contact of a known case patient, had been receiving oseltamivir chemoprohylaxis, and had only mild disease. In contrast, two highly resistant H5N1 viral isolates were collected from two Vietnamese patients during or shortly after they received therapeutic doses of oseltamivir (25). Both patients subsequently died. These findings could have implications for treatment of secondary limited person-to-person transmission cases. In May 2006, the WHO published guidelines on pharmacological management of human H5N1 cases (81b). More research is needed to understand the development of neuraminidase-resistant H5N1 viruses, their transmissibility, and the optimal antiviral therapy for H5N1 infection.

DIAGNOSIS

The "gold standard" for laboratory diagnosis of H5N1 is isolation of virus from respiratory specimens, using either embryonated hen's eggs or tissue cell culture under enhanced biosafety level (BSL) 3 conditions. Detection of H5N1 RNA by conventional or real-time PCR testing of respiratory specimens using H5-specific primers under BSL2 laboratory conditions is the most common method of H5N1 diagnosis. However, since H5N1 viruses are continuously evolving and humans have been infected by at least two distinct clades, it is very important to update the primers used for real-time PCR. The optimal respiratory specimen for detection of H5N1 is not currently known, but it appears that lower respiratory tract and throat specimens had a much higher yield than nasopharynx or nasal specimens during 2004 and 2005. To maximize detection of H5N1 virus in suspected cases, collection of multiple respiratory specimens from different sites (upper and lower respiratory tract) on different days is recommended. The duration of viral shedding appears to be longer than with human influenza virus, and H5N1 RNA has been detected in infected patients up to 15 days from illness onset. Confirmation of H5N1 should be done at a WHO H5N1 reference laboratory (73).

Serological diagnosis of H5N1 virus infection can be ascertained by the detection of H5N1 neutralizing antibodies in paired or convalescent sera by microneutralization assay. The microneutralization assay requires the use of live H5N1 virus and must be done under enhanced BSL3 laboratory conditions. Additionally, confirmatory testing using a Western blot assay should be done (52). Traditional hemagglutination inhibition serological testing is insensitive and nonspecific for detection of H5N1, and although a modified horse red blood cell hemagglutination inhibition assay has been devised (56), it has not been sufficiently validated and is therefore only a screening test.

Use of rapid influenza diagnostic tests is not recommended for the purpose of detecting H5N1 for many reasons (81). Such tests are currently very insensitive for detecting H5N1 and also are not specific. A positive test result could be a false positive, indicate human influenza A virus infection, or indicate H5N1 infection. Since human influenza viruses circulate worldwide, including among people in countries with H5N1 poultry outbreaks, and since human influenza is much more common than H5N1, a positive test result is much more likely to indicate infection with human influenza viruses than with H5N1.

PREVENTION

Reducing Poultry Exposure

The key to preventing human infections with H5N1 virus is to avoid unprotected direct contact with diseased and dead poultry, materials contaminated by poultry feces, and uncooked or inadequately cooked poultry or poultry products. Community education to raise public awareness about H5N1 and to promote risk reduction behavior is essential where poultry outbreaks have occurred, especially in rural areas. Personal protective equipment should be provided to persons involved in poultry culling, disposal, and environmental disinfection activities to minimize human exposure to H5N1 virus.

Recommendations for Hospital Infection Control

There is a risk of transmission of H5N1 in hospital settings. Human influenza is spread primarily via large respiratory droplets; therefore, standard and droplet precautions are recommended for the care of human influenza patients (3). Additionally, vaccination against human influenza virus is recommended for all health care workers (30). The modes of transmission of H5N1 are not entirely elucidated. Transmission of the virus in a health care setting may occur by inhalation of aerosolized respiratory droplets, contact with virus-containing secretions, or laboratory exposure to H5N1 isolates (3). The uncertainty about the modes of transmission of H5N1 among humans has led the WHO to recommend additional precautions for health care workers. In addition to standard precautions, which apply to all patients hospitalized for pandemic influenza, WHO recommends droplet precautions and respirators during respiratory-aerosol-producing procedures (71). Further infection control recommendations include contact and airborne precautions, including negative-pressure isolation rooms when they are available (2, 72). Infection control guidelines are based on the best available evidence and are subject to change as more data become available.

Vaccine Development

There were no commercially available H5N1 vaccines as of 4 July 2006, but many are under development, and one has been tested in phase I and II clinical trials (76). Currently, manufacturing capacity is inadequate to produce enough vaccine to meet pandemic demands. Additionally, no vaccine will be available for widespread use against H5N1 in the near future (76). There are several challenges to producing a pandemic influenza vaccine. Aside from the problems with production capacity and distribution, three additional challenges to creating an H5N1 vaccine are antigenic drift, immunogenicity, and vaccine pathogenicity to embryonated chicken eggs. Antigenic drift may significantly alter a pandemic virus. Since a vaccine is tailored for a particular strain or strains of virus, large-scale vaccine production cannot precede pandemic virus emergence (76). Additionally, some experimental H5N1 vaccines were poorly immunogenic, and an efficacious H5N1 vaccine might require multiple doses, high antigen content, or adjuvants to mount a significant immunologic response. These issues increase the cost and complexity of large-scale vaccination. In 2006, an unadjuvanted clade 1 H5N1 virus vaccine was shown to be safe in adults, but it required high doses to promote immunogenicity (61a). Finally, traditional influenza vaccine production in embryonated chicken eggs has not been possible due to vaccine virulence. However, researchers have recently shown that they could produce an avirulent H5N1 vaccine on a human influenza A virus backbone in 4 months, showing the promise for this technique to produce a pandemic vaccine (67). Because of reverse genetics and other techniques, more recent vaccines have had more encouraging results (2).

CONCLUSION

Human infection with H5N1 virus has been a rare event through July 2006, but given the widespread and expanding H5N1 epizootic among avian populations, exposure to this potentially lethal virus will continue and new human H5N1 cases are expected. Although there is some evidence of rare, limited, unsustained human-to-human transmission, H5N1 infection remains primarily an animal disease at this time, with sporadic avian-to-human H5N1 virus transmission. Spontaneous mutations of virus genes or reassortment of H5N1 genes with human influenza A virus genes could lead to increased and sustained transmission among humans. Such developments could initiate the first influenza pandemic since 1968. Whether H5N1 viruses will evolve to cause a pandemic is unknown, but the current situation is extremely worrisome, and government pandemic planning and international cooperation are prudent. Improvement of surveillance for H5N1 infection among animals and people is urgently needed.

There are many unanswered questions about the epidemiology, virology, and clinical aspects of human infection with H5N1 virus. Further studies are needed to determine the prevalence and risk of H5N1 infection among people in countries that have experienced outbreaks of H5N1 infection in poultry and to explore behavioral risk factors and potential susceptibility. Better clinical data are needed about H5N1-infected patients, including mild and severe cases, and about the efficacies of antivirals and other drugs used for treatment of H5N1 infection. Development of simple, accurate, and inexpensive H5N1 diagnostics and new treatments for H5N1 infection are urgently needed. Currently, there is no available human H5N1 vaccine; development of vaccines that protect against both clade 1 and 2 H5N1 virus infections are needed, and rapid tissue cell culture-based vaccine production technology should be encouraged. Prevention efforts must focus urgently upon controlling H5N1 infection among poultry flocks and minimizing human exposure to infected poultry, poultry products, and contaminated environments.

REFERENCES

1. **Apisarnthanarak, A., R. Kitphati, K. Thongphubeth, P. Patoomanunt, P. Anthanont, W. Auwanit, P. Thawatsupha, M. Chittaganpitch, S. Saeng-Aroon, S. Waicharoen, P. Apisarnthanarak, G. A. Storch, L. M. Mundy, and V. J. Fraser.** 2004. Atypical avian influenza (H5N1). *Emerg. Infect. Dis.* **10:** 1321–1324.

2. **Beigel, J. H., J. Farrar, A. M. Han, F. G. Hayden, R. Hyer, M. D. de Jong, S. Lochindarat, T. K. Nguyen, T. H. Nguyen, T. H. Tran, A. Nicoll, S. Touch, and K. Y. Yuen.** 2005. Avian influenza A (H5N1) infection in humans. *N. Engl. J. Med.* **353:**1374–1385.

3. **Bridges, C. B., M. J. Kuehnert, and C. B. Hall.** 2003. Transmission of influenza: implications for control in health care settings. *Clin. Infect. Dis.* **37:**1094–1101.

4. **Bridges, C. B., W. Lim, J. Hu-Primmer, L. Sims, K. Fukuda, K. H. Mak, T. Rowe, W. W. Thompson, L. Conn, X. Lu, N. J. Cox, and J. M. Katz.** 2002. Risk of influenza A (H5N1) infection among poultry workers, Hong Kong, 1997–1998. *J. Infect. Dis.* **185:**1005–1010.

5. **Butt, K. M., G. J. Smith, H. Chen, L. J. Zhang, Y. H. Leung, K. M. Xu, W. Lim, R. G. Webster, K. Y. Yuen, J. S. Peiris, and Y. Guan.** 2005. Human infection with an avian H9N2 influenza A virus in Hong Kong in 2003. *J. Clin. Microbiol.* **43:**5760–5767.

6. **Buxton Bridges, C., J. M. Katz, W. H. Seto, P. K. Chan, D. Tsang, W. Ho, K. H. Mak, W. Lim, J. S. Tam, M. Clarke, S. G. Williams, A. W. Mounts, J. S. Bresee, L. A. Conn, T. Rowe, J. Hu-Primmer, R. A. Abernathy, X. Lu, N. J. Cox, and K. Fukuda.** 2000. Risk of influenza A (H5N1) infection among health care workers exposed to patients with influenza A (H5N1), Hong Kong. *J. Infect. Dis.* **181:**344–348.

7. **Centers for Disease Control and Prevention.** 2004. Interim recommendations for infection control in health-care facilities caring for patients with known or suspected avian influenza. [Online.] http://www.cdc.gov/flu/avian/professional/infect-control.htm.

8. **Centers for Disease Control and Prevention.** 1997. Isolation of avian influenza A(H5N1) viruses from humans—Hong Kong, May–December 1997. *Morb. Mortal. Wkly. Rep.* **46:**1204–1207.

9. **Centers for Disease Control and Prevention.** 2004. Overview of biosecurity and avian influenza. [Online.] http://www.cdc.gov/flu/pp/biosecurity_on_farm_11_2004.pdf.

10. **Centers for Disease Control and Prevention.** 2004. Update: influenza activity—United States and worldwide, 2003–04 season, and composition of the 2004–05 influenza vaccine. *Morb. Mortal. Wkly. Rep.* **53:**547–552.

11. **Centers for Disease Control and Prevention.** 1998. Update: isolation of avian influenza A(H5N1) viruses from humans—Hong Kong, 1997–1998. *Morb. Mortal. Wkly. Rep.* **46:**1245–1247.

12. **Chan, M. C., C. Y. Cheung, W. H. Chui, G. S. Tsao, J. M. Nicholls, Y. O. Chan, R. W. Chan, H. T. Long, L. L. Poon, Y. Guan, and J. S. Peiris.** 2005. Proinflammatory cytokine responses induced by influenza A (H5N1) viruses in primary human alveolar and bronchial epithelial cells. *Respir. Res.* **6:**135.

13. **Chan, P. K.** 2002. Outbreak of avian influenza A(H5N1) virus infection in Hong Kong in 1997. *Clin. Infect. Dis.* **34**(Suppl. 2)**:**S58–S64.

14. **Chen, H., G. J. Smith, S. Y. Zhang, K. Qin, J. Wang, K. S. Li, R. G. Webster, J. S. Peiris, and Y. Guan.** 2005. Avian flu: H5N1 virus outbreak in migratory waterfowl. *Nature* **436:**191–192.

15. **Chen, H., G. J. D. Smith, K. S. Li, J. Wang, X. F. Fan, J. M. Rayner, D. Vijaykrishna, J. X. Zhang, C. T. Guo, C. L. Cheung, K. M. Xu, L. Duan, K. Huang, K. Qin, Y. H. C. Leung, W. L. Wu, H. R. Lu, Y. Chen, N. S. Xia, S. P. Naipospos, K. Y. Yuen, S. S. Hassan, S. Bahri, T. D. Nguyen, R. G. Webster, J. S. M. Peiris, and Y. Guan.** 2006. Establishment of multiple sub-lineages of H5N1 influenza virus in Asia—implications for pandemic control. *Proc. Natl. Acad. Sci. USA* **103:**2845–2850.

16. **Cheung, C. Y., L. L. Poon, A. S. Lau, W. Luk, Y. L. Lau, K. F. Shortridge, S. Gordon, Y. Guan, and J. S. Peiris.** 2002. Induction of proinflammatory cytokines in human macrophages by influenza A (H5N1) viruses: a mechanism for the unusual severity of human disease? *Lancet* **360:**1831–1837.

17. **Choi, Y. K., T. D. Nguyen, H. Ozaki, R. J. Webby, P. Puthavathana, C. Buranathal, A. Chaisingh, P. Auewarakul, N. T. Hanh, S. K. Ma, P. Y. Hui, Y. Guan, J. S. Peiris, and R. G. Webster.** 2005. Studies of H5N1 influenza virus infection of pigs by using viruses isolated in Vietnam and Thailand in 2004. *J. Virol.* **79:**10821–10825.

18. **Chokephaibulkit, K., M. Uiprasertkul, P. Puthavathana, P. Chearskul, P. Auewarakul, S. F. Dowell, and N. Vanprapar.** 2005. A child with avian influenza A (H5N1) infection. *Pediatr. Infect. Dis. J.* **24:**162–166.

19. **Chotpitayasunondh, T., K. Ungchusak, W. Hanshaoworakul, S. Chunsuthiwat, P. Sawanpanyalert, R. Kijphati, S. Lochindarat, P. Srisan, P. Suwan, Y. Osotthanakorn, T. Anantasetagoon, S. Kanjanawasri, S. Tanupattarachai, J. Weerakul, R. Chaiwirattana, M. Maneerattanaporn, R. Poolsavathitikool, K. Chokephaibulkit, A. Apisarnthanarak, and S. F. Dowell.** 2005. Human disease from influenza A (H5N1), Thailand, 2004. *Emerg. Infect. Dis.* **11:**201–209.

19a. **Chutinimitkul, S., P. Bhattarakosol, S. Srisuratanon, A. Eiamudomkan, K. Kongsomboon, S. Damrongwatanapokin, A. Chaisingh, K. Suwannakarn, T. Chieochansin, A. Theamboonlers, and Y. Poovorawan.** 2006. H5N1 influenza A virus and infected human plasma. *Emerg. Infect. Dis.* **12:**1041–1043.

20. **Cox, N. J., and K. Subbarao.** 1999. Influenza. *Lancet* **354:**1277–1282.
21. **Crawford, P. C., E. J. Dubovi, W. L. Castleman, I. Stephenson, E. P. Gibbs, L. Chen, C. Smith, R. C. Hill, P. Ferro, J. Pompey, R. A. Bright, M. J. Medina, C. M. Johnson, C. W. Olsen, N. J. Cox, A. I. Klimov, J. M. Katz, and R. O. Donis.** 2005. Transmission of equine influenza virus to dogs. *Science* **310:**482–485.
22. **Cyranoski, D.** 2004. Bird flu data languish in Chinese journals. *Nature* **430:**955.
23. **Cyranoski, D.** 2005. Bird flu spreads among Java's pigs. *Nature* **435:**390–391.
24. **de Jong, M. D., V. C. Bach, T. Q. Phan, M. H. Vo, T. T. Tran, B. H. Nguyen, M. Beld, T. P. Le, H. K. Truong, V. V. Nguyen, T. H. Tran, Q. H. Do, and J. Farrar.** 2005. Fatal avian influenza A (H5N1) in a child presenting with diarrhea followed by coma. *N. Engl. J. Med.* **352:**686–691.
25. **de Jong, M. D., T. T. Thanh, T. H. Khanh, V. M. Hien, G. J. D. Smith, N. V. Chau, B. V. Cam, P. T. Qui, D. Q. Ha, Y. Guan, J. S. M. Peiris, T. T. Hien, and J. Farrar.** 2005. Oseltamivir resistance during treatment of influenza A (H5N1) infection. *N. Engl. J. Med.* **353:**2667–2672.
26. **Fouchier, R. A., V. Munster, A. Wallensten, T. M. Bestebroer, S. Herfst, D. Smith, G. F. Rimmelzwaan, B. Olsen, and A. D. Osterhaus.** 2005. Characterization of a novel influenza A virus hemagglutinin subtype (H16) obtained from black-headed gulls. *J. Virol.* **79:**2814–2822.
27. **Govorkova, E. A., I. A. Leneva, O. G. Goloubeva, K. Bush, and R. G. Webster.** 2001. Comparison of efficacies of RWJ-270201, zanamivir, and oseltamivir against H5N1, H9N2, and other avian influenza viruses. *Antimicrob. Agents Chemother.* **45:**2723–2732.
28. **Grose, C., and K. Chokephaibulkit.** 2004. Avian influenza virus infection of children in Vietnam and Thailand. *Pediatr. Infect. Dis. J.* **23:**793–794.
29. **Harper, S., A. Klimov, T. Uyeki, and K. Fukuda.** 2002. Influenza. *Clin. Lab. Med.* **22:**863–882, vi.
30. **Harper, S. A., K. Fukuda, T. M. Uyeki, N. J. Cox, and C. B. Bridges.** 2005. Prevention and control of influenza. Recommendations of the Advisory Committee on Immunization Practices (ACIP). *Morb. Mortal. Wkly. Rep. Recomm. Rep.* **54:**1–40.
31. **Hien, T. T., M. de Jong, and J. Farrar.** 2004. Avian influenza—a challenge to global health care structures. *N. Engl. J. Med.* **351:**2363–2365.
32. **Hinshaw, V. S., R. G. Webster, and B. Turner.** 1979. Water-borne transmission of influenza A viruses? *Intervirology* **11:**66–68.
33. **Ito, T., K. Okazaki, Y. Kawaoka, A. Takada, R. G. Webster, and H. Kida.** 1995. Perpetuation of influenza A viruses in Alaskan waterfowl reservoirs. *Arch. Virol.* **140:**1163–1172.
34. **Johnson, N. P., and J. Mueller.** 2002. Updating the accounts: global mortality of the 1918–1920 "Spanish" influenza pandemic. *Bull. Hist. Med.* **76:**105–115.
35. **Keawcharoen, J., K. Oraveerakul, T. Kuiken, R. A. Fouchier, A. Amonsin, S. Payungporn, S. Noppornpanth, S. Wattanodorn, A. Theamboonlers, R. Tantilertcharoen, R. Pattanarangsan, N. Arya, P. Ratanakorn, D. M. Osterhaus, and Y. Poovorawan.** 2004. Avian influenza H5N1 in tigers and leopards. *Emerg. Infect. Dis.* **10:**2189–2191.
36. **Kishida, N., Y. Sakoda, N. Isoda, K. Matsuda, M. Eto, Y. Sunaga, T. Umemura, and H. Kida.** 2005. Pathogenicity of H5 influenza viruses for ducks. *Arch. Virol.* **150:**1383–1392.
37. **Koopmans, M., B. Wilbrink, M. Conyn, G. Natrop, H. van der Nat, H. Vennema, A. Meijer, J. van Steenbergen, R. Fouchier, A. Osterhaus, and A. Bosman.** 2004. Transmission of H7N7 avian influenza A virus to human beings during a large outbreak in commercial poultry farms in the Netherlands. *Lancet* **363:**587–593.
38. **Ku, A. S., and L. T. Chan.** 1999. The first case of H5N1 avian influenza infection in a human with complications of adult respiratory distress syndrome and Reye's syndrome. *J. Paediatr. Child Health* **35:**207–209.
39. **Kuiken, T., G. Rimmelzwaan, D. van Riel, G. van Amerongen, M. Baars, R. Fouchier, and A. Osterhaus.** 2004. Avian H5N1 influenza in cats. *Science* **306:**241.
40. **Kurtz, J., R. J. Manvell, and J. Banks.** 1996. Avian influenza virus isolated from a woman with conjunctivitis. *Lancet* **348:**901–902.
41. **Le, Q. M., M. Kiso, K. Someya, Y. T. Sakai, T. H. Nguyen, K. H. Nguyen, N. D. Pham, H. H. Nguyen, S. Yamada, Y. Muramoto, T. Horimoto, A. Takada, H. Goto, T. Suzuki, Y. Suzuki, and Y. Kawaoka.** 2005. Avian flu: isolation of drug-resistant H5N1 virus. *Nature* **437:**1108.
42. **Leneva, I. A., N. Roberts, E. A. Govorkova, O. G. Goloubeva, and R. G. Webster.** 2000. The neuraminidase inhibitor GS4104 (oseltamivir phosphate) is efficacious against A/Hong Kong/156/97 (H5N1) and A/Hong Kong/1074/99 (H9N2) influenza viruses. *Antivir. Res.* **48:**101–115.

43. **Liem, N. T., and W. Lim.** 2005. Lack of H5N1 avian influenza transmission to hospital employees, Hanoi, 2004. *Emerg. Infect. Dis.* **11:**210–215.
44. **Matrosovich, M. N, T. Y. Matrosovich, T. Gray, N. A. Roberts, and H. D. Klenk.** 2004. Human and avian influenza viruses target different cell types in cultures of human airway epithelium. *Proc. Natl. Acad. Sci. USA* **101:**4620–4624.
45. **Mounts, A. W., H. Kwong, H. S. Izurieta, Y. Ho, T. Au, M. Lee, C. Buxton Bridges, S. W. Williams, K. H. Mak, J. M. Katz, W. W. Thompson, N. J. Cox, and K. Fukuda.** 1999. Case-control study of risk factors for avian influenza A (H5N1) disease, Hong Kong, 1997. *J. Infect. Dis.* **180:**505–508.
46. **Nicholson, K. G., J. M. Wood, and M. Zambon.** 2003. Influenza. *Lancet* **362:**1733–1745.
47. **Ohishi, K., A. Ninomiya, H. Kida, C. H. Park, T. Maruyama, T. Arai, E. Katsumata, T. Tobayama, A. N. Boltunov, L. S. Khuraskin, and N. Miyazaki.** 2002. Serological evidence of transmission of human influenza A and B viruses to Caspian seals (Phoca caspica). *Microbiol. Immunol.* **46:**639–644.
48. **Olsen, C. W., L. Brammer, B. C. Easterday, N. Arden, E Belay, I. Baker, and N. J. Cox.** 2002. Serologic evidence of H1 swine influenza virus infection in swine farm residents and employees. *Emerg. Infect. Dis.* **8:**814–819.
49. **Olsen, S. J., K. Ungchusak, L. Sovann, T. M. Uyeki, S. F. Dowell, N. J. Cox, W. Aldis, and S. Chunsut-tiwat.** 2005. Family clustering of avian influenza A (H5N1). *Emerg. Infect. Dis.* **11:**1799–1801.
50. **Osterhaus, A. D., G. F. Rimmelzwaan, B. E. Martina, T. M. Bestebroer, and R. A. Fouchier.** 2000. Influenza B virus in seals. *Science* **288:**1051–1053.
51. **Peiris, J. S., W. C. Yu, C. W. Leung, C. Y. Cheung, W. F. Ng, J. M. Nicholls, T. K. Ng, K. H. Chan, S. T. Lai, W. L. Lim, K. Y. Yuen, and Y. Guan.** 2004. Re-emergence of fatal human influenza A subtype H5N1 disease. *Lancet* **363:**617–619.
52. **Rowe, T., R. A. Abernathy, J. Hu-Primmer, W. W. Thompson, X. Lu, W. Lim, K. Fukuda, N. J. Cox, and J. M. Katz.** 1999. Detection of antibody to avian influenza A (H5N1) virus in human serum by using a combination of serologic assays. *J. Clin. Microbiol.* **37:**937–943.
53. **Schultsz, C., V. C. Dong, N. V. V. Chau, N. T. H. Le, W. Lim, T. T. Thanh, C. Dolecek, M. D. de Jong, T. T. Hien, and J. Farrar.** 2005. Avian influenza H5N1 and healthcare workers. *Emerg. Infect. Dis.* **11:**1158–1159.
54. **Shortridge, K. F.** 1999. Poultry and the influenza H5N1 outbreak in Hong Kong, 1997: abridged chronology and virus isolation. *Vaccine* **17**(Suppl. 1):S26–S29.
55. **Sims, L. D., J. Domenech, C. Benigno, S. Kahn, A. Kamata, J. Lubroth, V. Martin, and P. Roeder.** 2005. Origin and evolution of highly pathogenic H5N1 avian influenza in Asia. *Vet. Rec.* **157:**159–164.
56. **Stephenson, I., J. M. Wood, K. G. Nicholson, A. Charlett, and M. C. Zambon.** 2004. Detection of anti-H5 responses in human sera by HI using horse erythrocytes following MF59-adjuvanted influenza A/Duck/Singapore/97 vaccine. *Virus Res.* **103:**91–95.
57. **Suarez, D. L., M. L. Perdue, N. Cox, T. Rowe, C. Bender, J. Huang, and D. E. Swayne.** 1998. Comparisons of highly virulent H5N1 influenza A viruses isolated from humans and chickens from Hong Kong. *J. Virol.* **72:**6678–6688.
58. **Taubenberger, J. K., A. H. Reid, R. M. Lourens, R. Wang, G. Jin, and T. G. Fanning.** 2005. Characterization of the 1918 influenza virus polymerase genes. *Nature* **437:**889–893.
59. **Thompson, W. W., D. K. Shay, E. Weintraub, L. Brammer, C. B. Bridges, N. J. Cox, and K. Fukuda.** 2004. Influenza-associated hospitalizations in the United States. *JAMA* **292:**1333–1340.
60. **Thompson, W. W., D. K. Shay, E. Weintraub, L. Brammer, N. Cox, L. J. Anderson, and K. Fukuda.** 2003. Mortality associated with influenza and respiratory syncytial virus in the United States. *JAMA* **289:**179–186.
61. **Tiensin, T., P. Chaitaweesub, T. Songserm, A. Chaisingh, W. Hoonsuwan, C. Buranathai, T. Paraka-mawongsa, S. Premashthira, A. Amonsin, M. Gilbert, M. Nielen, and A. Stegeman.** 2005. Highly pathogenic avian influenza H5N1, Thailand, 2004. *Emerg. Infect. Dis.* **11:**1664–1672.
61a. **Treanor, J. J., J. D. Campbell, K. M. Zangwill, T. Rowe, and M. Wolff.** 2006. Safety and immunogenicity of an inactivated subvirion influenza A (H5N1) vaccine. *N. Engl. J. Med.* **354:**1343–1351.
62. **Tweed, S. A., D. M. Skowronski, S. T. David, A. Larder, M. Petric, W. Lees, Y. Li, J. Katz, M. Krajden, R. Tellier, C. Halpert, M. Hirst, C. Astell, D. Lawrence, and A. Mak.** 2004. Human illness from avian influenza H7N3, British Columbia. *Emerg. Infect. Dis.* **10:**2196–2199.
63. **Uiprasertkul, M., P. Puthavathana, K. Sangsiriwut, P. Pooruk, K. Srisook, M. Peiris, J. M. Nicholls, K. Chokephaibulkit, N. Vanprapar, and P. Auewarakul.** 2005. Influenza A H5N1 replication sites in humans. *Emerg. Infect. Dis.* **11:**1036–1041.

64. **Ungchusak, K., P. Auewarakul, S. F. Dowell, R. Kitphati, W. Auwanit, P. Puthavathana, M. Uiprasertkul, K. Boonnak, C. Pittayawonganon, N. J. Cox, S. R. Zaki, P. Thawatsupha, M. Chittaganpitch, R. Khontong, J. M. Simmerman, and S. Chunsutthiwat.** 2005. Probable person-to-person transmission of avian influenza A (H5N1). *N. Engl. J. Med.* **352:**333–340.

65. **Uyeki, T. M., Y. H. Chong, J. M. Katz, W. Lim, Y. Y. Ho, S. S. Wang, T. H. Tsang, W. W. Au, S. C. Chan, T. Rowe, J. Hu-Primmer, J. C. Bell, W. W. Thompson, C. B. Bridges, N. J. Cox, K. H. Mak, and K. Fukuda.** 2002. Lack of evidence for human-to-human transmission of avian influenza A (H9N2) viruses in Hong Kong, China 1999. *Emerg. Infect. Dis.* **8:**154–159.

66. **van Maanen, C., and A. Cullinane.** 2002. Equine influenza virus infections: an update. *Vet. Q.* **24:**79–94.

66a. **van Riel, D., V. J. Munster, E. de Wit, G. F. Rimmelzwaan, R. A. Fouchier, A. D. Osterhaus, and T. Kuiken.** 2006. H5N1 virus attachment to lower respiratory tract. *Science* **312:**399.

67. **Webby, R. J., D. R. Perez, J. S. Coleman, Y. Guan, J. H. Knight, E. A. Govorkova, L. R. McClain-Moss, J. S. Peiris, J. E. Rehg, E. I. Tuomanen, and R. G. Webster.** 2004. Responsiveness to a pandemic alert: use of reverse genetics for rapid development of influenza vaccines. *Lancet* **363:**1099–1103.

68. **Webby, R. J., K. Rossow, G. Erickson, Y. Sims, and R. Webster.** 2004. Multiple lineages of antigenically and genetically diverse influenza A virus co-circulate in the United States swine population. *Virus Res.* **103:**67–73.

69. **Webster, R. G.** 2004. Wet markets—a continuing source of severe acute respiratory syndrome and influenza? *Lancet* **363:**234–236.

70. **World Health Organization.** 2005. Avian influenza frequently asked questions. [Online.] http://www.who.int/csr/disease/avian_influenza/avian_faqs/en/.

71. **World Health Organization.** 2005. Clarification. Use of masks by health-care workers in pandemic settings. [Online.] http://www.who.int/csr/resources/publications/influenza/Mask%20Clarification10_11.pdf.

72. **World Health Organization.** 2004. Influenza A (H5N1): WHO interim infection control guidelines for health care facilities. [Online.] http://www.who.int/csr/disease/avian_influenza/guidelines/Guidelines_for_health_care_facilities.pdf.

73. **World Health Organization.** 2005. Recommended laboratory tests to identify avian influenza A virus in specimens from humans. [Online.] http://www.who.int/csr/disease/avian_influenza/guidelines/labtests/en/index.html.

74. **World Health Organization.** 2005. Situation updates—avian influenza. [Online.] http://www.who.int/csr/disease/avian_influenza/updates/en/index.html.

75. **World Health Organization.** 2003. Summary of probable SARS cases with onset of illness from 1 November 2002 to 31 July 2003. [Online.] http://www.who.int/csr/sars/country/table2004_04_21/en/index.html.

76. **World Health Organization.** 2005. Vaccine research and development: current status. [Online.] http://www.who.int/csr/disease/avian_influenza/vaccineresearch2005_11_3/en/index.html.

77. **World Health Organization.** 2005. WHO global influenza preparedness plan. [Online.] http://www.who.int/csr/resources/publications/influenza/GIP_2005_5Eweb.pdf.

78. **World Health Organization.** 2004. WHO guidelines for global surveillance of influenza A/H5. [Online.] http://www.who.int/csr/disease/avian_influenza/guidelines/globalsurveillance.pdf.

79. **World Health Organization.** 2005. WHO intercountry-consultation. Influenza A/H5N1 in humans in Asia. Manila, Philippines 6–7 May 2005. [Online.] http://www.who.int/csr/resources/publications/influenza/WHO_CDS_CSR_GIP_2005_7_04.pdf.

80. **World Health Organization.** 2004. WHO interim recommendations for the protection of persons involved in the mass slaughter of animals potentially infected with highly pathogenic influenza viruses. [Online.] http://www.who.int/csr/disease/avian_influenza/guidelines/Avian%20Influenza.pdf.

81. **World Health Organization.** 2005. WHO recommendations on the use of rapid testing for influenza diagnosis. [Online.] http://www.who.int/csr/disease/avian_influenza/guidelines/RapidTestInfluenza_web.pdf.

81a. **World Health Organization.** 2006. Epidemiology of WHO-confirmed human cases of avian influenza A (H5N1) infection. *Wkly. Epidemiol. Rec.* **81:**249–257.

81b. **World Health Organization.** May 2006. WHO Rapid Advice Guidelines on pharmacological management of humans infected with avian influenza A (H5N1) virus. [Online.] http://www.who.int/medicines/publications/WHO_PSM_PAR_2006.6.pdf.

82. **World Health Organization Global Influenza Program Surveillance Network.** 2005. Evolution of H5N1 avian influenza viruses in Asia. *Emerg. Infect. Dis.* **11:**1515–1521.

83. **World Organisation for Animal Health.** 2005. *Highly Pathogenic Avian Influenza in Romania.* Follow-up report no. 3. [Online.] http://www.oie.int/eng/info/hebdo/AIS_48.HTM#Sec1.

84. **World Organisation for Animal Health.** 2005. *Manual of Diagnostic Tests and Vaccines for Terrestrial Animals.* [Online.] http://www.oie.int/eng/normes/mmanual/A_00037.htm.
85. **Yen, H. L., A. S. Monto, R. G. Webster, and E. A. Govorkova.** 2005. Virulence may determine the necessary duration and dosage of oseltamivir treatment for highly pathogenic A/Vietnam/1203/04 influenza virus in mice. *J. Infect. Dis.* **192:**665–672.
86. **Yuanji, G.** 2002. Influenza activity in China: 1998–1999. *Vaccine* **20**(Suppl. 2)**:**S28–S35.
87. **Yuen, K. Y., and S. S. Wong.** 2005. Human infection by avian influenza A H5N1. *Hong Kong Med. J.* **11:**189–199.

Emerging Infections 7
Edited by W. M. Scheld, D. C. Hooper, and J. M. Hughes
© 2007 ASM Press, Washington, D.C.

Chapter 2

Severe Acute Respiratory Syndrome (SARS)

J. S. M. Peiris, Y. Guan, L. L. M. Poon, V. C. C. Cheng, J. M. Nicholls, and K. Y. Yuen

Severe acute respiratory syndrome (SARS) first emerged in Guangdong Province of the People's Republic of China in late 2002. The disease was characterized by a severe atypical pneumonia syndrome with clusters of disease in the family or hospital setting. There was no response to conventional antibiotic therapy (189). Initial case clusters were reported in November and December 2002 in Foshan and Heyuan, respectively, both cities in Guangdong Province. The index case of the latter outbreak was a chef working in Shenzhen involved in the wild-game-animal restaurant trade. It came to global attention in February 2003 following a large outbreak of pneumonia in Guangzhou, the provincial capital of Guangdong. A total of 305 cases had been documented between November 2002 and 9 February 2003, 105 of them in health care workers (174, 189, 190). A physician who acquired infection while treating patients in Guangzhou travelled to Hong Kong and stayed in a hotel (hotel M) for 1 day before being hospitalized in Hong Kong. During that day, he inadvertently infected a number of other hotel guests, predominantly those residing on the same floor of the hotel. They, in turn, carried infection with them to their destinations, initiating outbreaks of disease in Toronto, Singapore, and Vietnam and within Hong Kong (8). Within weeks, the disease spread to affect 29 countries and five continents. Globally, 8,096 patients were affected, with 774 fatalities, a case fatality rate of 9.6%. Unusually, hospitals served as a major focus of disease transmission, and health care workers were major victims; globally, 21% of all cases were in health care workers (http://www.who.int/csr/sars/country/table2004_04_21/en). In Hong Kong, the overall attack rate among health care workers was 1.2%, and this was correlated with the number of SARS patients admitted to hospitals (75).

While good clinical case descriptions had been compiled by the physicians in Guangdong (189), they were not widely available internationally at the time of the Hong Kong

J. S. M. Peiris, Y. Guan, L. L. M. Poon, V. C. C. Cheng, and K. Y. Yuen • Department of Microbiology, University Pathology Building, Queen Mary Hospital, The University of Hong Kong, Pokfulam Road, Hong Kong Special Administrative Region, People's Republic of China. *J. M. Nicholls* • Department of Pathology, University Pathology Building, Queen Mary Hospital, The University of Hong Kong, Pokfulam Rd., Hong Kong Special Administrative Region, People's Republic of China.

outbreak. Carlo Urbani, who helped investigate the disease cluster in Hanoi in late February 2003, provided the first clinical case description of SARS to the World Health Organization (WHO) and the international community. Sadly, he succumbed to the disease himself, one of many health care workers who died of SARS. By 10 March, there were reports of a cluster of cases in a hospital in Hong Kong. On 12 March, the WHO issued a global health alert. Suspected cases then began to be reported from Canada and Singapore, leading to decisive action by the WHO, which issued a travel advisory in relation to affected regions with the aim of interrupting further global spread (54, 168). The disease was formally given a name, severe acute respiratory syndrome, and a preliminary case definition was provided (Table 1).

Table 1. Chronology of events[a]

Date	Key event(s)
November 2002	Unusual atypical pneumonia documented in Foshan, Guangdong Province, China
January 2003	Pneumonia outbreaks in Guangzhou (capital city of Guangdong Province)
11 February 2003	WHO receives reports of an outbreak of respiratory disease in Guangdong, with 305 cases and 5 deaths.
21 February 2003	A 65-year-old doctor from Guangdong arrives and checks in at hotel M in Hong Kong (Hong Kong index case). He had been ill since 15 February. His health deteriorates further, and he is admitted to the hospital on 22 February. He infects other guests and visitors at the hotel, some of whom travel on to Vietnam, Singapore, and Toronto, where they initiate local clusters of transmission.
26 February 2003	A hotel M contact is admitted to a private hospital in Hanoi and is the source of an outbreak there. Seven health care workers are ill by 5 March.
4 March 2003	A hotel M contact is admitted to Prince of Wales Hospital, Hong Kong. By 7 March, health care workers at this hospital report a respiratory illness.
5 March 2003	A hotel M contact dies in Toronto. Five family members are affected.
12 March 2003	WHO issues global alert.
14 March 2003	Singapore and Toronto report clusters of atypical pneumonia. In retrospect, both groups have epidemiological links to hotel M. One of the doctors who had treated patients in Singapore develops symptoms while traveling and is isolated in transit on arrival in Germany.
15 March 2003	WHO has received reports of over 150 cases of the new disease, now named SARS. A travel advisory is issued.
17 March 2003	WHO multicenter laboratory network is established for the study of SARS causation and diagnosis.
21–27 March 2003	A novel coronavirus is identified in patients with SARS.
12 April 2003	Mapping of the full genome of SARS CoV is completed.
16 April 2003	WHO announces that SARS CoV is the causative agent of SARS.
June 2003	A virus related to SARS CoV is isolated from animals.
5 July 2003	Absence of further transmission in Taiwan signals the end of the human SARS outbreak.
September 2003	Laboratory-acquired SARS, Singapore
December 2003	Laboratory-acquired SARS, Taiwan
December 2003–January 2004	Reemergence of SARS infecting humans from animal markets
February 2004	Laboratory-acquired SARS leads to community transmission in Beijing and Anhui Province.

[a]Modified from reference 121.

The WHO initiated a virtual network of laboratories to identify the cause of this new disease (168). Subsequently, this international collaboration was extended to other networks focusing on clinical features and epidemiology, respectively. By the end of the outbreak in July 2003, over 152 experts from institutions in 17 countries had demonstrated the possibility of close collaboration and sharing of information to serve global public health (54, 168). Between 21 and 24 March, the etiological agent of SARS was identified. Its characteristics were rapidly defined, and early diagnostic tests were put into use in affected countries by early April. In parallel, an aggressive effort to detect and isolate suspected cases based on a clinical case definition and epidemiological linkages led to the interruption of community transmission. By 5 July, it was possible for the WHO to declare that all known chains of human-to-human transmission had been interrupted (http://www.who.int/features/2003/07/en/)—a historic triumph for international and global public health.

Since early 2003, SARS has reemerged on a number of occasions. Three were laboratory-associated infections, one of which led to further transmission within the community (93, 102, 118; http://www.who.int/csr/don/2004_05_18a/en/index.html). In addition to infections originating in the laboratory, SARS coronavirus (CoV) infection was detected in four patients with no possible laboratory exposure during December 2003 and January 2004. These four epidemiologically unrelated patients likely acquired the infection through exposure to infected animals in live-game-animal markets in Guangdong. They had mild disease and did not transmit infection to others (92).

THE VIRUS: ITS RECEPTOR, ORIGINS, AND EVOLUTION

A number of possible agents were detected in the course of investigating patients with suspected SARS, including human metapneumovirus and chlamydia (168). However, these were only detected in a few patient cohorts. A novel coronavirus was isolated in culture in Vero-E6 cells and FRhK-4 cells (Fig. 1), and its presence was consistently demonstrated by molecular detection and serology in patients with SARS in many parts of the world (34, 70, 72, 119). Experimental infection of cynomolgus macaques provided evidence of virus replication and significant lung pathology (37). The sharing of information and viruses within the WHO laboratory network allowed a consensus to be reached that this novel coronavirus was the etiological agent of SARS (SARS CoV) (Fig. 1). *Causitive*

Coronaviruses are enveloped viruses with a single-stranded positive-sense genome of 2,732 kb, the largest genome found among RNA viruses. They are subdivided into three groups, with the two previously recognized human coronaviruses, 229E and OC43, belonging to groups 1 and 2, respectively (57) (Fig. 2A). The 229E and OC43 viruses were known to be causes of upper respiratory disease and the common cold and have rarely been identified as a cause of severe human disease.

The genetic sequence of the SARS coronavirus was fully determined within weeks of the virus being isolated (99, 131). This confirmed that SARS CoV was a novel coronavirus, distinct from all other human and animal coronaviruses but distantly related to the group 2 coronaviruses (137). It is now designated a group 2b coronavirus. The genome organization of SARS CoV is summarized in Fig. 2 (140).

Patients with SARS invariably seroconverted to this novel virus in immunofluorescent assays, enzyme-linked immunosorbent assays, and neutralization tests (9, 70, 119). However, the general population had no antibody to SARS CoV, suggesting that it was a novel

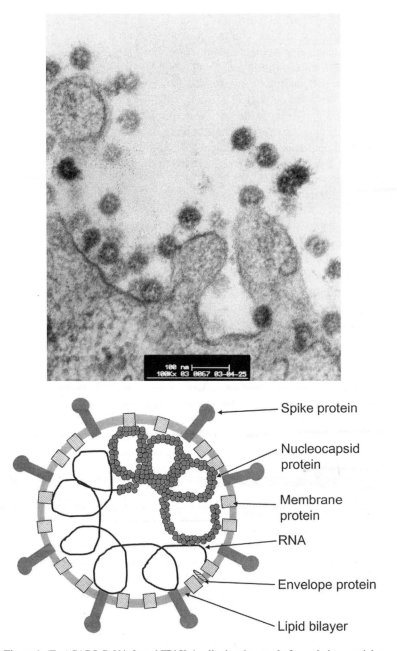

Figure 1. (Top) SARS CoV-infected FRhK-4 cells showing newly formed virus particles. (Bottom) Schematic view of a SARS CoV particle. The four structural proteins, spike, envelope, membrane, and nucleocapsid, and the viral genomic RNA are indicated. Within the virion, the viral RNA is encapsulated with nucleoprotein (shown in part). The drawing is not to scale.

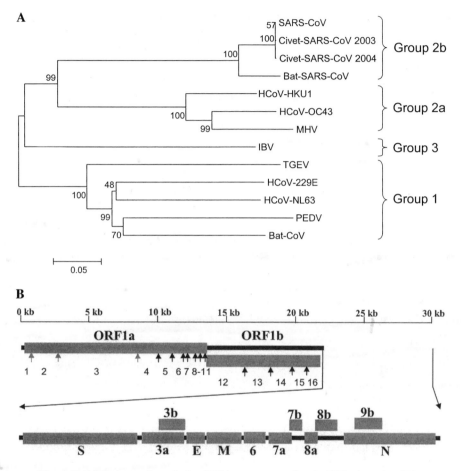

Figure 2. (A) Phylogenetic analysis of RNA sequences coding for RNA-dependent RNA polymerase (partial sequence). Phylogenetic trees were constructed by the neighbor-joining method, and bootstrap values were determined by 1,000 replicates. Human SARS CoV (SARS-CoV) (GenBank accession number NC004718), SARS CoVs isolated from palm civets in 2003 (AY304487) and 2004 (AY686863) and SARS CoV-related virus from bats (Bat-SARS-CoV; DQ022305) were aligned with reference sequences as indicated. The reference sequences used in the study were transmissible gastroenteritis virus (TGEV) (NC002306), human coronavirus (HCoV) HCoV-229E (AF304460), HCoV-NL63 (AY567487), HCoV-OC43 (NC005147), HCoV-HKU1 (NC006577), porcine epidemic diarrhea virus (PEDV) (AF353511), infectious bronchitis virus (IBV) (NC005147), mouse hepatitis virus (MHV) (NC001846), and group 1 Bat-CoV (AY864196). (B) Genome organization of SARS CoV. ORFs 1 to 9 are indicated. Polyproteins encoded by ORFs 1a and 1b are cleaved by papain-like cysteine proteinase (nsp 3) and 3C-like cysteine proteinase (nsp 5) to generate 16 nonstructural polyproteins (nsp 1 to 16). The cleavage sites for papain-like cysteine proteinase and 3C-like cysteine proteinase are indicated by gray and black arrows, respectively. ORFs 2, 4, 5, and 9a encode the viral structural proteins, S, E, M, and N, respectively. Subgenomic mRNAs 3, 7, 8, and 9 are believed to express two viral proteins.

virus that recently emerged in the human population, very likely from an animal reservoir. Some of the patients with SARS-like disease in the early stages of the outbreak had occupational exposure to live game animals held within markets serving the restaurant trade in Guangdong (174). Testing of animals in live-game-animal markets in Guangdong led to the detection of a SARS-like coronavirus in a number of small mammal species, including Himalayan palm civets (*Paguma larvata*) and raccoon dogs (*Nyctereutes procyonides*) (45). Furthermore, those directly involved in the live-animal trade within these markets had high seroprevalence to SARS-like viruses, although they gave no history of SARS-like disease (45). These findings suggested that the animal markets might be the interface at which interpecies transmission to humans occurred. Civets are susceptible to experimental infection with the human SARS coronavirus (171). However, SARS CoV antibody has not been consistently detected in civet farms that supply the live-animal markets (155). There are few data on wild-caught civets, but from the limited available data, it does not appear that these animals are endemically infected in the wild (122). It appears likely that the role of the civets and other small mammals (e.g., raccoon dogs) is as amplifier hosts within the animal markets rather than as the natural reservoir of the virus. In such markets, animals are continually removed for consumption while new animals are added, providing a continuous supply of susceptible animals. A parallel is provided by live-poultry markets, which are known to amplify and perpetuate avian influenza viruses within them (74). More recently, a novel SARS-like coronavirus was detected in *Rhinolophus* bats (77, 89) in mainland China and Hong Kong, suggesting that these species are more likely to be the natural reservoir from which SARS coronavirus emerged. Such bats are also sold for consumption in the same live-animal markets, together with civets and other small mammals, and this possibly explains the introduction of these viruses into the live-animal market setting.

Studies on the molecular evolution of SARS CoV have revealed that viruses in the early phase of the human SARS outbreak were more closely related to viruses detected in palm civets and other small mammals in the live-animal markets. The virus was under strong positive selection in the early phase of outbreak, suggesting a process of adaptation to the new human host (20, 46, 179). Interestingly, the virus was also evolving rapidly in palm civets, an observation that is compatible with the idea that civets may not be the natural reservoir of the virus (138). The virus detected in the four patients with SARS CoV infections in December 2003 and January 2004 (see above) was phylogenetically more closely related to SARS coronavirus-like viruses identified in civets than to the viruses associated with the global outbreak in early 2003, suggesting that these infections were new introductions from the animal reservoir. Many human viruses in the later stages of the outbreak in 2003 had deletions in the open reading frame (ORF) 8 region of the genome, while most animal viruses do not have this deletion (20, 45). The functional significance of the deletion, if any, is presently unclear.

The virus spike protein mediates virus attachment and entry into susceptible cells (136). The receptor for SARS CoV has been identified as angiotensin-converting enzyme 2 (ACE2) (91, 158). SARS CoV replication in the lungs of ACE2 knockout mice is markedly suppressed, proving the importance of this receptor in vivo, at least in mice (71). ACE2 expression is detectable on pneumocytes, enterocytes, vascular endothelial cells, and smooth muscle cells (49, 150). The finding of ACE2 on respiratory and intestinal epithelium is compatible with the known tropism of the virus. However, not all cells that express ACE2 are susceptible to virus infection (e.g., endothelial cells). A number of other molecules, such as L-SIGN and DC-SIGN, have been demonstrated to bind SARS CoV (62, 178). DC-SIGN serves as a binding receptor and may be relevant in transferring infectious virus bound to the surfaces of dendritic cells from one site to another. L-SIGN mediates binding and entry of SARS CoV. However, rather than leading to productive viral replication, virus uptake by L-SIGN leads to proteasome-dependent viral degradation (10a).

The spike protein of SARS CoV (Tor 2, a virus from the later phase of the outbreak in 2003) interacts efficiently with ACE2 of human and civet origins (90). This is in agreement with the finding that human SARS CoV can infect civets. In contrast, SARS CoV spike protein of civet origin binds well to ACE2 of civets but poorly to human ACE2. This suggests that, without prior adaptation, the civet SARS CoV is not well adapted to replicate in human cells. This explains why the SARS CoV-like virus found in civets cannot be maintained in culture in primate cell lines that effectively support the replication of the human SARS CoV (unpublished data). It may also explain the mild disease and low transmissibility observed when SARS CoV reemerged from its animal reservoir to infect humans in December 2003 and January 2004 (see above).

An infectious clone of SARS CoV is now available and is likely to rapidly enhance understanding of the virulence determinants of the virus (181).

TRANSMISSION

Transmission is thought to occur through the deposition of virus-laden respiratory droplets from an infected patient onto the respiratory or conjunctival mucosal epithelium of a susceptible individual. Entry via the gastrointestinal tract may also play a role, although there is no direct evidence for this. Virus has been cultured from respiratory secretions, feces, and urine and detected by reverse transcription (RT)-PCR in tears (9, 70, 96, 119). All of these may provide sources of infectious virus for transmission. Given that the virus remains viable for many days on inanimate surfaces (35, 126), it is possible that contaminated surfaces and fomites may play roles in virus transmission. The role of true airborne spread remains more controversial, but it has clearly occurred in some instances. Aerosol-generating procedures, such as the use of nebulizers, high-flow oxygen, suction, and intubation, have been associated with transmission within hospital settings (22, 82, 102, 157). An unusual community outbreak at the Amoy Gardens housing estate in Hong Kong appears to have been associated with aerosolization of infected feces in the sewage system, leading to the infection of over 300 persons (182). One instance of transmission within an airliner was attributed to airborne spread (116). However, contaminated surfaces in communal areas, for example, contamination of the airplane toilet, may also have contributed to transmission in this instance.

The incubation period of the disease is estimated as 2 to 14 days (85, 95, 128). Although a few cases were responsible for large numbers of secondary cases (so called superspreading incidents) (82, 135, 182), the majority of patients did not transmit at all. A number of superspreading incidents provided the impetus for the explosive transmission observed with SARS. While host-related factors may have played some part, it is relevant that each of these incidents had a unique combination of circumstances that played a major role in determining the extent of the transmission (102). The most unusual and dramatic of these was the transmission at Amoy Gardens in Hong Kong, as mentioned above. In contrast with these superspreading incidents, only a minority (e.g., 15% in Hong Kong) of households had evidence of secondary transmission (102). The overall basic reproduction number (R_0) of SARS, i.e., the average number of secondary cases from each patient, is estimated to be approximately 2 to 4 (95, 128). This is not dissimilar to that of pandemic influenza (104) but markedly less than the transmissibility of smallpox or measles.

Asymptomatic infections with SARS CoV were uncommon during the outbreak of SARS in 2003 (81, 86). Most persons at high risk through family or health care exposure either developed overt disease or did not seroconvert at all. This is in marked contrast to exposure to the precursor animal virus, where asymptomatic infection was common (45).

Quantitative studies on the viral load in the upper respiratory tracts and feces of infected patients revealed a progressive increase in the viral load, peaking around day 10 after the onset of disease symptoms (9, 15, 120). This explains the epidemiological observation that transmission mainly occurred after the fifth day of illness and was less common in the early stage of the illness (95, 128). This unusual feature of SARS allowed public health measures to be so dramatically successful in interrupting disease transmission. Although virus RNA was detectable by RT-PCR for many weeks into convalescence, virus isolation after the third week of illness was rare. There are no reports of transmission after 10 days of defervescence.

CLINICAL FEATURES

SARS typically presents as an illness with acute onset, fever, myalgia, malaise, and chills or rigor, with rhinorrhea and sore throat being less common features (references 4, 82, 119, 125, and 154; reviewed in reference 121). A dry cough is common, but shortness of breath, tachypnea, or pleurisy is prominent only later in the course of the illness. About one-third of patients improve, with defervescence and resolution of radiographic changes. Others progress to have increasing shortness of breath, tachypnea, oxygen desaturation, worsening of chest signs on physical examination, and onset of diarrhea. About 20 to 30% of all patients need observation in intensive care, and most of these require mechanical ventilation. Overall, the case fatality rate was 9.6%, and the terminal events were severe respiratory failure, multiple-organ failure, sepsis, and intercurrent medical illness, such as an acute myocardial infarction. In Hong Kong, mortality rates in patients with SARS aged 0 to 24, 25 to 44, 45 to 64, and >65 years were 0%, 6%, 15%, and 52%, respectively.

A watery diarrhea occurs in some patients, typically associated with clinical deterioration in the second week of the illness (17, 120). Other extrapulmonary findings include hepatic dysfunction (11) and central nervous system manifestations (76).

The initial chest radiograph was abnormal in 60 to 100% of the cases at initial presentation, depending on the duration of illness (Fig. 3). High-resolution computed tomography (CT) scanning allows detection of abnormalities in a proportion of those with initially normal chest radiographs. Typically, the chest radiograph shows ground-glass opacities and focal consolidation over the periphery and in the subpleural regions of the lower zones of the lung. Radiological shadows may be shifting, and both lungs may be progressively involved (Fig. 3) (112, 120). Pneumomediastinum without preceding positive-pressure ventilation or intubation is seen later in the disease.

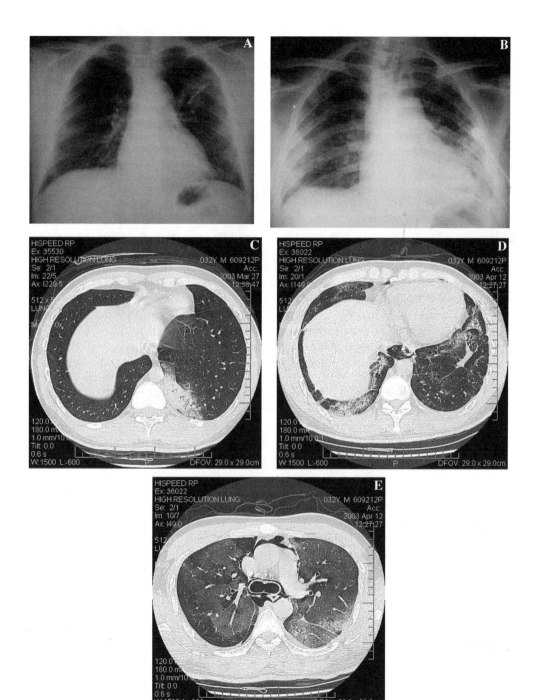

Figure 3. Chest radiographs (A and B) and high-resolution CT scans (C to E) from two SARS patients. (Courtesy of C. M. Chu. Reproduced with permission from reference 120.) (A) Chest radiograph of a man aged 34 years at day 7 of illness, with consolidation in the left upper and middle lobes. (B) By day 20, resolution of consolidation in the left upper and middle lobes and new widespread air space opacities were noted. Those in the left lung base were confluent. (C) High-resolution CT scan of a man aged 32 years who presented with fever, chills, rigor, and myalgia with a clear chest radiograph at admission, demonstrating peripheral subpleural consolidation in the medial basal segment of the left lower lobe. (D) At day 18, there was resolution of the original left lower lobe consolidation. (E) Disease was complicated by spontaneous pneumomediastinum.

Age, the presence of comorbidities, more extensive lung involvement and high neutrophil counts at presentation, increased lactic dehydrogenase levels, hyperuricemia, and acute renal failure are indicators of a poor prognosis (26, 58, 172). High viral loads in the nasopharynx and serum early in the illness are independent risk factors for mortality (24, 108). Similarly, the viral loads in the nasopharynx and serum between days 10 and 15 of clinical illness also correlated with the clinical outcome, including the need for mechanical ventilation and death (59).

Children have a much milder clinical course than adults (84). Few children with SARS required intensive care, mortality was exceedingly rare, and few children transmitted infection to others. Atypical presentations of SARS can occur in the elderly and in the immunocompromised. Patients may be afebrile and may present with nonspecific clinical symptoms, such as decreased appetite or a general deterioration in their clinical condition. Such cases have led to nosocomial disease outbreaks with devastating consequences (21). SARS in pregnancy is associated with an increased case fatality rate. However, transmission to the neonate has not been documented (184).

Lymphopenia involving both CD4 and CD8 T cells is a common finding during the acute phase of SARS and is associated with an adverse outcome (4, 82, 119, 125, 154, 163). The lymphopenia is rapidly reversed during convalescence. Some patients also have other hematological abnormalities, such as a low platelet count and activated plasma thromboplastin time. Alanine aminotransferase, creatine kinase, and lactic dehydrogenase may be increased.

Residual impairment of lung function persists in convalescence in over 20% of patients (117). Posttraumatic stress disorder and depression are common in patients with SARS and persist into convalescence (80).

Autopsy findings in patients who died within the first 10 days of illness revealed diffuse alveolar damage, desquamation of pneumocytes, an inflammatory infiltrate, edema, and hyaline membrane formation. Patients who died later in the illness had organizing diffuse alveolar damage, together with squamous metaplasia and multinucleate giant cells of either macrophage or epithelial cell origin (38, 70, 82, 111) (Color Plate 1 [see color insert]). Viral RNA was detectable by RT-PCR at a high viral load in the lung, bowel, and lymph node, but was also detectable in the spleen, liver, and kidney, correlating with the multiorgan involvement of the disease (36). Virus-infected cells have been identified by in situ hybridization techniques as primarily alveolar epithelial cells, although a few infected macrophages and bronchial epithelial cells have also been detected (107, 151). Viral antigen is detectable in lung biopsy or autopsy tissue of patients within the first 10 days of illness but rarely after that (111a). In the lungs, the infected cells demonstrated by immunohistochemistry are similar to those seen with in situ hybridization, that is, they are mainly flattened pneumocytes and less often macrophages. Unlike influenza, there is little histological evidence of bronchial epithelial cell necrosis. Laboratory infection of golden Syrian hamsters also shows a similar cellular pattern of infection, though hyaline membranes are not a conspicuous finding (130). The clinical features of SARS have also been reviewed elsewhere (23, 121).

VIROLOGICAL DIAGNOSIS

In the absence of an epidemiological history of exposure, clinical findings are not pathognomic of SARS (106). Therefore, a positive virological laboratory finding of SARS

CoV infection is required for confirmation of the diagnosis (reviewed in reference 124). Virus has been cultured from respiratory secretions, feces, and urine (9, 70, 119), while virus RNA has also been detected in serum (108). Thus, respiratory secretions, feces, and serum are suitable specimens for molecular detection of SARS CoV RNA. Specimens from the lower respiratory tract, such as endotracheal aspirates and bronchoalveolar lavage fluid, appear to have higher viral loads and to be more productive for virus detection, although collecting such specimens carries a risk of nosocomial transmission.

Molecular detection of viral RNA is in general far more sensitive than viral culture. In particular, relatively few isolates have been obtained from feces, although viral RNA is present at high titer. The viral load in respiratory secretions and feces by quantitative RT-PCR tests is low in the first few days and peaks at around day 10 of illness (9, 15, 120). As a consequence, first-generation RT-PCR tests had low sensitivity in the first 5 days of illness. Real-time PCR methods now provide improved sensitivity (>80%) in respiratory secretions and serum in the early stages of the disease (108, 123). However, a single negative test in the first 5 days of disease still does not provide reliable grounds for exclusion of a suspect case. Multiple tests of different specimens (e.g., respiratory and fecal) improves the diagnostic yield and certainty.

Viral-antigen detection methods (particularly directed at the nucleoprotein) have been developed and evaluated but remain much less sensitive than molecular detection methods.

In the absence of ongoing SARS CoV transmission, a positive detection of SARS CoV RNA by molecular methods needs to be treated with caution. The result must be confirmed by testing for a different region of the genome (e.g., the replicase and nucleoprotein genes) repeated on a new RNA extract from the suspect clinical specimen and, wherever possible, on an independent clinical specimen (http://www.who.int/csr/resources/publications/WHO_CDS_CSR_ARO_2004_1/en/index.html; 124).

Serological diagnosis using immunofluorescence or virus neutralization remains the gold standard for confirmation of a diagnosis of SARS CoV infection. However, seroconversion (including immunoglobulin M or immunoglobulin A) occurs during the second week of illness; therefore, serology can provide only a retrospective confirmation of diagnosis. Enzyme-linked immunosorbent assays using inactivated whole virus (70) or recombinant antigens (165) provide alternative methods amenable to a higher specimen throughput, but it is advisable that any positive results be confirmed using immunofluorescent or neutralization tests (124, 166).

When serological tests for coronaviruses are interpreted, especially in periods without a known outbreak, the potential for anamnestic rise in titers of preexisting antibodies to other coronaviruses must be kept in mind (10, 12).

IMMUNE RESPONSE AND PATHOGENESIS

Although critical clinical symptoms relate to the respiratory tract, SARS CoV results in a disseminated infection. Evidence of SARS CoV replication in the lungs and intestine is provided by detection of virus particles through electron microscopy, by virus isolation, and by the detection of viral antigens and nucleic acid through immunohistology and in situ hybridization (9, 33, 70, 87, 119). Viral RNA has also been detected by using RT-PCR in the lymph nodes, spleen, liver, heart, kidney, and skeletal muscle (36), and recently, virus particles have been reported by electron microscopy in lymphocytes (44). The viral load in the upper respiratory tract or in the serum in the first few days of illness is an independent predictor of the clinical outcome (24, 108). This suggests that the final outcome of the disease is determined early in the course of the illness. Thus, the dose of the infecting virus inoculum, the early innate defenses of the host, or both, are critical in determining the disease prognosis.

Genetic polymorphisms associated with susceptibility and disease severity have been identified. HLA-B*4601 was reported to be associated with both disease susceptibility and severity in a Chinese population in Taiwan (94), but this association was not found in Hong Kong Chinese patients (109). In contrast, among Hong Kong Chinese, HLA-B*0703 rather than HLA-B*4601 was found to be associated with SARS. A number of polymorphisms of the innate immune response have been studied. Genetic polymorphisms associated with low serum levels of mannose-binding lectin were associated with increased susceptibility to SARS (61). Furthermore, it was shown that mannose-binding lectin binds and neutralizes the SARS CoV. A report of the association of SARS infection with polymorphisms of the interferon-inducing gene *OAS-1* and the *MxA* gene is notable but requires confirmation by larger independent studies (48).

Neutralizing immune responses appear in the second week of illness, peak at around 20 to 30 days, and are sustained for over 18 months (113). The SARS CoV spike protein is necessary and sufficient for protection in animal (hamster) experimental models and is the predominant antigen inducing neutralizing antibodies (6). In immunized mice, adoptive-transfer and T-cell depletion studies suggested that protection was mediated predominantly by antibody (142, 177). The major neutralizing-antibody epitopes are located in the region within amino acids 441 to 700 of the spike protein (2, 98).

Many of the prototype SARS CoV isolates commonly used (e.g., HKU 39849, Urbani, and Tor2) derive from the global outbreak arising from the superspreading event at hotel M in Hong Kong and are genetically and antigenically very similar (46). Virus isolates from the earliest patients in the course of the outbreak or isolates of the animal precursor virus detected in civets are not available. Consequently, neutralization of these animal precursor-like viruses has been explored by generating lentivirus pseudotypes incorporating spike proteins representing the spike proteins of SARS CoV-like viruses detected in civets (SZ3 and SZ16), GD03 (a civet-like virus isolated from humans following the reemergence of SARS in December 2003), and the human SARS CoV strains (e.g., Urbani) isolated during the major SARS outbreak in mid-2003. The prototype Urbani virus, isolated from a patient from the major human outbreak in 2003, was neutralized efficiently with homologous antibody, as well as antibody to the animal-like SARS CoV GD03. Surprisingly, the animal precursor-like virus pseudotypes were refractory to neutralization with both homologous antibody and antibody to the prototype Urbani virus. Indeed, the antibody to the Urbani virus enhanced entry of the civet SARS CoVs SZ3 and SZ16 (176). The evasion of neutralization exhibited by the animal precursor-like SARS CoV was correlated with poor binding to the ACE2 receptor. Thus, it appears likely that the animal precursor SARS CoV uses an alternative receptor for viral entry and is possibly adapted to evade neutralization by host antibodies. This potentially has major implications for the efficacy of a vaccine based on generating neutralizing antibody to the SARS CoV spike protein. However, these findings are derived from pseudotyped virus, and it is important to confirm whether similar findings will be produced when these animal SARS-like coronaviruses are recreated using an infectious clone.

As well as being the receptor for SARS CoV, ACE2 is an enzyme involved in the renin-angiotensin system, and it may have a protective effect in acute lung injury (60, 71). It may play a role in the pathogenesis of SARS and other infectious agents associated with acute lung injury leading to acute respiratory distress syndrome. In mouse models, treatment with recombinant human ACE2 or with inhibitors of the renin-angiotensin system appears to mitigate the effects of acute lung injury. These may provide promising novel approaches for the management of acute respiratory distress syndrome (60, 71, 110).

There is more limited information on the T-cell responses in SARS. HLA-A2-restricted T-cell epitopes have been identified that are capable of eliciting a cytotoxic CD8 T-cell response in patients who have recovered from SARS (159). Both chemokines (interleukin 8 [IL-8], CCL2, and CXCL10) and proinflammatory cytokines (IL-1, IL-6, and IL-12) have been found to be elevated in patients with SARS (63, 162). Prolonged dysregulation of cytokine production has also been demonstrated by enzyme-linked immunospot assays in vitro (65). In comparative gene expression profile studies in human hepatoma and intestinal epithelilal cell lines in vitro, infection with SARS CoV showed marked upregulation of proinflammatory cytokine genes (30, 147).

The primary mechanism of pathogenesis in the lung is likely to be direct virus damage to primarily type 1 and, to a lesser extent, type 2 pneumocytes. The infiltration of macrophages into the lung is a prominent manifestation of the disease. Viral infection of monocyte-derived macrophages in vitro leads to the release of monocyte-attractant chemokines, such as CCL2 and CXCL10 (18), and patients with SARS also have high levels of these chemokines detectable in the serum. In contrast, SARS CoV infection of primary human macrophages, dendritic cells, and the transformed kidney epithelial cell line 293 failed to reveal evidence of induction of a type 1 interferon response (18, 79, 139). Furthermore, in contrast to patients with influenza virus infection, gene expression profiling of peripheral blood mononuclear cells from patients with SARS did not reveal induction of type 1 interferon responses (127). Therefore, it remains possible that a failure of the innate antiviral immune defenses of the host in the early stages of the disease may contribute to pathogenesis and may also explain the progressive increase in viral load peaking at day 10, the stage of illness when the adaptive immune responses become activated, presumably controlling further virus replication. On the other hand, mice that are resistant to the action of interferon because of defects in Stat-1 have a more severe and disseminated disease (56).

Diarrhea was another prominent manifestation in patients with SARS. There is evidence of viral replication in enterocytes of the gastrointestinal tract (87). However, there is minimal cellular infiltrate or disruption of the intestinal architecture. The reasons for this and the mechanism underlying the pathogenesis of diarrhea remain unclear. It may be relevant that some human intestinal epithelial cell lines induce antiapoptotic cellular responses and support the persistent replication of SARS CoV in vitro (29).

Necrosis and atrophy of the lymphoid tissue of lymph nodes and the white pulp of the spleen are observed at autopsy. B and T lymphocytes, including both CD4+ and CD8+ T-lymphocyte subsets, natural killer cells, and dendritic cells, appear to be decreased during the acute stage of SARS (32, 187). The mechanism underlying the lymphopenia seen in SARS remains obscure. Lymphocytes do not carry ACE2 on their surfaces (49) and appear to be refractory to virus infection (79); therefore, apoptosis of bystander uninfected lymphocytes, as happens with other viral infections, remains a possibility. However, one report suggests that virus particles can be detected by electron microscopy in a high proportion of lymphocytes from patients with SARS (44). If confirmed, this would provide an alternative explanation for the lymphopenia seen with SARS. Aspects of SARS pathogenesis have been recently reviewed (78).

ANIMAL MODELS

Experimental infections in relevant animal models are important for understanding pathogenesis and evaluating therapeutic and vaccine strategies. A number of species have been studied as potential animal models for SARS. These include cynomolgus and rhesus macaques (37, 101, 132), African green monkeys (7), ferrets (100), BALB/c mice (142), hamsters (130), and marmosets (41). All of these animals support viral replication, but only some of them develop pathological lesions (cynomolgus macaques, ferrets, hamsters, and marmosets), and even fewer have overt clinical disease (ferrets). While young adult BALB/c mice develop asymptomatic infection, older (12-month-old) mice develop significant pathology and clinical disease (129). Asymptomatic infection is sufficient to evaluate the protective effects of antivirals and vaccines, but significant pathology (and ideally disease) is a prerequisite for meaningful studies on pathogenesis. Furthermore, few animal models develop the gastrointestinal component of the disease or reproduce the progressive course of infection observed in humans (120). Therefore, conclusions on pathogenesis drawn from such animal models must be tempered with caution.

CLINICAL MANAGEMENT AND ANTIVIRALS

The clinical management of patients with SARS includes respiratory support with intensive care when appropriate, prevention of nosocomial transmission, and the possible use of antivirals and immunomodulators.

Infection of health care workers has been associated with failure to implement contact and droplet precautions, suggesting that this was a major source of transmission in health care settings (134). It is advisable to avoid aerosol-generating equipment (e.g., nebulizers) and procedures as far as possible. For example, oxygen is best administered by a low-flow nasal cannula rather than a high-flow face mask. Other modes of noninvasive ventilation, such as continuous positive airway pressure and bilevel positive airway pressure, carry risks of aerosolization and nosocomial spread and should be carried out by health care workers with appropriate personal protective equipment and within negative-pressure isolation rooms (19).

In vitro susceptibility tests have shown that beta interferon, alpha-n1 interferon, alpha-n3 interferon, and alpha interferon appear to have antiviral effects against SARS CoV (13, 28, 31, 53, 141, 146, 188). A number of other drugs have been reported to have antiviral activity against SARS CoV, including glycyrrhizin, baicalin, reserpine, niclosamide, chloroquine, and the human immunodeficiency virus protease inhibitors, such as nelfinavir (27, 51, 66, 68, 169, 170, 173, 175). There are conflicting reports on the effect of ribavirin in vitro, likely due to differences between the susceptibilities of different cell culture systems (31). Ribavirin appears to have reasonable levels of activity in vitro when tested on pig, human, and some monkey kidney cells but has poor activity in Vero-E6 cells. Moreover, ribavirin has been shown to be synergistic with the interferons (105, 146). Peptides designed to block the function of the heptad repeat region of the spike protein interfere with membrane fusion, blocking virus entry and thereby interfering with virus replication (5, 183, 191). Screening of combinatorial libraries has led to the discovery of inhibitors of the SARS CoV helicase, protease, and spike protein functions in mediating cell entry (66). ACE2 analogues have shown antiviral activity in vitro (152). Inhibition of SARS CoV replication has been achieved using sequence-specific small interfering RNA in cell cultures in vitro (50, 160, 186). The prophylactic and therapeutic efficacies of this strategy have been demonstrated in a primate model in vivo (88).

During the SARS outbreak in 2003, immunomodulators were used empirically with the intention of modulating the possible harmful effects of the inflammatory responses in the lung. These included corticosteroids, intravenous immunoglobulins, pentaglobulins (16, 55), anti-tumor necrosis factor, thymosin, and thalidomide. Corticosteroids, when used early in the course of the illness without an effective antiviral agent, may increase the plasma viral load (83). Long-term high-dose corticosteroids also may be associated with adverse effects, such as avascular necrosis of bone (43). Combinations of steroid with alfacon-1 (97) or with protease inhibitors and ribavirin (25) appeared to improve the clinical outcome compared to historical controls.

In summary, in the last 2 years, a number of drugs have been demonstrated to have antiviral effects in vitro, but in the absence of controlled clinical trials, their efficacy in treating SARS remains unclear. The observation that high viral load in both the first and second weeks of disease correlates with adverse clinical outcome (see above) suggests that there is a reasonable window of time during the first week of the illness during which an effective antiviral has the potential to provide clinical benefit. Given the absence of human SARS at present, experiments involving animal models are currently the only option available for assessing the efficacies of potential therapeutic interventions. For example, in the cynomolgus macaque animal model, pegylated alpha-2a interferon reduced viral shedding and lung pathology when used as prophylaxis and also had some effect when used as a treatment (47). Similarly, the prophylactic and therapeutic efficacies of small interfering RNA have been demonstrated in macaques (88).

PASSIVE AND ACTIVE IMMUNIZATION

SARS convalescent-phase plasma was used in therapy during the SARS outbreak; although there were no obvious adverse effects, the clinical benefit was unclear. In animal models, passive transfer of immune serum was sufficient to prevent infection (142). Humanized monoclonal antibodies to the SARS CoV spike protein have been developed and shown to be effective at inhibiting virus replication in vitro (42, 143, 144, 149, 153). Passive immunization of ferrets and mice with one of these monoclonal antibodies was shown to suppress viral replication in the lungs, but less so in the nasopharynx (149).

Natural infection with SARS CoV leads to a long-lasting neutralizing-antibody response (113), suggesting that active immunization may be a feasible proposition. There are no known instances of reexposure of individuals who have preexisting immunity to confirm whether this immune response is effective in protection. An attenuated parainfluenza virus type 3 vector was used to individually express the SARS CoV spike, envelope, membrane, and nucleocapsid proteins, and only the recombinants expressing the spike protein were able to induce neutralizing antibody and to protect hamsters from experimental challenge (6). African green monkeys immunized by the mucosal route with this parainfluenza-SARS CoV spike protein chimeric virus were also protected from challenge with experimental SARS CoV (7). Mice immunized with a SARS CoV spike DNA vaccine were protected from experimental challenge, and experiments using adoptive transfer and T-cell depletion confirmed that protection was mediated predominantly by antibody rather than T-cell immunity (142).

A number of vaccine strategies have been explored in search of a useful SARS CoV vaccine candidate. In addition to those mentioned above, approaches have included inactivated whole virus (52, 145, 148); DNA vaccines (142, 185); recombinant vaccinia- and baculovirus-expressed spike protein fragments (1, 2, 14); adenoviral vectors carrying spike, membrane, or nucleocapsid proteins (40); and vesicular stomatitis virus-vectored vaccines (67). Most of these recombinant-vaccine strategies have targeted the gene encoding the spike protein. There have also been attempts to develop DNA vaccines to the SARS CoV nucleocapsid linked to calreticulin (69). The vaccine generated humoral and T-cell immune responses in BALB/c mice and reduced the replication of vaccine virus carrying the SARS CoV nucleoprotein. Wild-type and SCID-PBL/hu mice immunized with a plasmid vector encoding SARS CoV nucleocapsid or carrying membrane genes developed specific T-cell responses to the respective antigen expressed on type 2 alveolar epithelial cells (114).

The DNA vaccines, parainfluenza virus chimeric vaccines, and modified vaccinia virus Ankara vaccines have been tested for efficacy in preventing reinfection after challenge in animal models (1, 2, 6, 7, 78). An inactivated whole-virus vaccine (Sinovac) has been tested in phase 1 clinical trials in human volunteers and is reportedly safe and immunogenic, although these findings have not yet been published in peer-reviewed scientific journals.

Prior experience with vaccines against coronaviruses in animal diseases has not met with unqualified success (133). One problem has been virus strain variation in field isolates, leading to variable vaccine efficacy. The experience with feline infectious peritonitis virus, where prior immunity and passive antibody can enhance disease, has been a cause of particular concern (115). Here, the virus replicates within macrophages, and antibody results in enhanced virus replication within feline macrophages in vitro. SARS CoV leads to abortive infection in human macrophages (18, 180), and addition of antibody does not convert this to a productive infection (J. S. M. Peiris, unpublished data). In animal models with SARS CoV infections, passive transfer of antibody was not associated with enhanced disease. However, in one study, ferrets immunized with modified vaccinia virus Ankara-based vectored SARS CoV vaccine developed increased liver dysfunction following challenge with live SARS CoV (161). The underlying mechanisms need to be investigated in greater detail.

In the absence of ongoing SARS CoV circulation in humans, the development and evaluation of vaccines for SARS is handicapped by the lack of a clear demand and application. Prophylactic strategies, whether passive antibody, active immunization, or antiviral drug based, are needed for laboratory workers and front-line health care workers in regions at risk for reemergence of SARS. They will clearly be critically important if SARS reemerges to cause a local or regional outbreak. There may also be a place for vaccination of animals reared in captivity for the live-game animal market trade.

CONCLUSIONS

SARS has dramatically illustrated the impact of an emerging infectious disease on a globalized world. In addition to its effect on health care systems around the world, the social, political, and economic impacts of SARS were substantial (3, 164). Aspects of its pathogenesis and transmission allowed the human disease outbreak to be quickly interrupted. It cannot be taken for granted that other emerging infections, such as pandemic influenza, can be similarly controlled by public health interventions. Pandemic influenza, although having an R_0 comparable to that of SARS (104), is transmitted early in the illness and therefore will probably not be as amenable to control through the public health measures of case detection and isolation alone (39).

As with many other new, emerging infections, SARS had zoonotic origins, highlighting the need for a better understanding of the virus ecology of animals, both domestic and wild. As many of these zoonoses do not cause disease in their natural hosts, surveillance must encompass viruses causing inapparent infections, as well as those causing overt disease. As relevant information is likely to involve multiple agencies, including those dealing with public health, veterinary medicine, and wildlife or the environment, there is a need for a coordinated strategy of surveillance and risk assessment (73). In the 2 years since SARS refocused attention on coronaviruses, a number of new human (156, 167) and animal (64, 122) coronaviruses have been recognized, suggesting that many human and animal viruses remain to be discovered.

The global response to SARS demonstrated that a rapid mobilization and coordination of relevant expertise is possible, when faced with a global emerging disease threat. It also highlighted the need for improved international regulations governing the reporting of and response to unusual infectious-disease syndromes. The new International Health Regulations, which were recently agreed upon by the World Health Assembly, are an important step in this direction (103).

REFERENCES

1. **Bisht, H., A. Roberts, L. Vogel, A. Bukreyev, P. L. Collins, B. R. Murphy, K. Subbarao, and B. Moss.** 2004. Severe acute respiratory syndrome coronavirus spike protein expressed by attenuated vaccinia virus protectively immunizes mice. *Proc. Natl. Acad. Sci. USA* **101:**6641–6646.
2. **Bisht, H., A. Roberts, L. Vogel, K. Subbarao, and B. Moss.** 2005. Neutralizing antibody and protective immunity to SARS coronavirus infection of mice induced by a soluble recombinant polypeptide containing an N-terminal segment of the spike glycoprotein. *Virology* **334:**160–165.
3. **Blendon, R. J., J. M. Benson, C. M. DesRoches, E. Raleigh, and K. Taylor-Clark.** 2004. The public's response to severe acute respiratory syndrome in Toronto and the United States. *Clin. Infect. Dis.* **38:**925–931.
4. **Booth, C. M., L. M. Matukas, G. A. Tomlinson, A. R. Rachlis, D. B. Rose, H. A. Dwosh, S. L. Walmsley, T. Mazzulli, M. Avendano, P. Derkach, I. E. Ephtimios, I. Kitai, B. D. Mederski, S. B. Shadowitz, W. L. Gold, L. A. Hawryluck, E. Rea, J. S. Chenkin, D. W. Cescon, S. M. Poutanen, and A. S. Detsky.** 2003. Clinical features and short-term outcomes of 144 patients with SARS in the greater Toronto area. *JAMA* **289:**2801–2809.
5. **Bosch, B. J., B. E. Martina, R. Van Der Zee, J. Lepault, B. J. Haijema, C. Versluis, A. J. Heck, R. De Groot, A. D. Osterhaus, and P. J. Rottier.** 2004. Severe acute respiratory syndrome coronavirus (SARS-CoV) infection inhibition using spike protein heptad repeat-derived peptides. *Proc. Natl. Acad. Sci. USA* **101:**8455–8460.
6. **Buchholz, U. J., A. Bukreyev, L. Yang, E. W. Lamirande, B. R. Murphy, K. Subbarao, and P. L. Collins.** 2004. Contributions of the structural proteins of severe acute respiratory syndrome coronavirus to protective immunity. *Proc. Natl. Acad. Sci. USA* **101:**9804–9809.
7. **Bukreyev, A., E. W. Lamirande, U. J. Buchholz, L. N. Vogel, W. R. Elkins, M. St. Claire, B. R. Murphy, K. Subbarao, and P. L. Collins.** 2004. Mucosal immunisation of African green monkeys (*Cercopithecus aethiops*) with an attenuated parainfluenza virus expressing the SARS coronavirus spike protein for the prevention of SARS. *Lancet* **363:**2122–2127.

8. **Centers for Disease Control and Prevention.** 2003. Update: outbreak of severe acute respiratory syndrome—worldwide. *Morb. Mortal. Wkly. Rep.* **52:**241–248.

9. **Chan, K. H., L. L. Poon, V. C. Cheng, Y. Guan, I. F. Hung, J. Kong, L. Y. Yam, W. H. Seto, K. Y. Yuen, and J. S. Peiris.** 2004. Detection of SARS coronavirus in patients with suspected SARS. *Emerg. Infect. Dis.* **10:**294–299.

10. **Chan, K. H., V. C. C. Cheng, P. C. Y. Woo, S. K. P. Lau, L. L. M. Poon, Y. Guan, W. H. Seto, K. Y. Yuen, and J. S. M. Peiris.** 2005. Serological response in patients with SARS coronavirus infection and cross reactivity with human coronaviruses 229E, OC43, and NL63. *Clin. Diagn. Lab. Immunol.* **12:**1317–1321.

10a. **Chan, V. S. F., K. Y. K. Chan, Y. Chen, L. L. M. Poon, A. N. Y. Cheung, B. Zheng, K. H. Chan, W. Mak, H. Y. S. Ngan, X. Y. S. Ngan, X. Xu, G. Screaton, P. K. H. Tam, J. M. Austyn, L. C. Chan, S. P. Yip, M. Peiris, U. S. Khoo, and C. L. Lin.** 2006. Homozygous L-SIGN *(CLEC4M)* plays a protective role in SARS coronavirus infection. *Nat. Genet.* **38:**38–46.

11. **Chau, T. N., K. C. Lee, H. Yao, T. Y. Tsang, T. C. Chow, Y. C. Yeung, K. W. Choi, Y. K. Tso, T. Lau, S. T. Lai, and C. L. Lai.** 2004. SARS-associated viral hepatitis caused by a novel coronavirus: report of three cases. *Hepatology* **39:**302–310.

12. **Che, X. Y., L. W. Qiu, Z. Y. Liao, Y. D. Wang, K. Wen, Y. X. Pan, W. Hao, Y. B. Mei, V. C. Cheng, and K. Y. Yuen.** 2005. Antigenic cross-reactivity between severe acute respiratory syndrome-associated coronavirus and human coronaviruses 229E and OC43. *J. Infect. Dis.* **191:**2033–2037.

13. **Chen, F., K. H. Chan, Y. Jiang, R. Y. Kao, H. T. Lu, K. W. Fan, V. C. Cheng, W. H. Tsui, I. F. Hung, T. S. Lee, Y. Guan, J. S. Peiris, and K. Y. Yuen.** 2004. In vitro susceptibility of 10 clinical isolates of SARS coronavirus to selected antiviral compounds. *J. Clin. Virol.* **31:**69–75.

14. **Chen, Z., L. Zhang, C. Qin, L. Ba, C. E. Yi, F. Zhang, Q. Wei, T. He, W. Yu, J. Yu, H. Gao, X. Tu, A. Gettie, M. Farzan, K. Y. Yuen, and D. D. Ho.** 2005. Recombinant modified vaccinia virus Ankara expressing the spike glycoprotein of severe acute respiratory syndrome coronavirus induces protective neutralizing antibodies primarily targeting the receptor binding region. *J. Virol.* **79:**2678–2688.

15. **Cheng, P. K., D. A. Wong, L. K. Tong, S. M. Ip, A. C. Lo, C. S. Lau, E. Y. Yeung, and W. W. Lim.** 2004. Viral shedding patterns of coronavirus in patients with probable severe acute respiratory syndrome. *Lancet* **363:**1699–1700.

16. **Cheng, V. C., B. S. Tang, A. K. Wu, C. M. Chu, and K. Y. Yuen.** 2004. Medical treatment of viral pneumonia including SARS in immunocompetent adults. *J. Infect.* **49:**262–273.

17. **Cheng, V. C., I. F. Hung, B. S. Tang, C. M. Chu, M. M. Wong, K. H. Chan, A. K. Wu, D. M. Tse, K. S. Chan, B. J. Zheng, J. S. Peiris, J. J. Sung, and K. Y. Yuen.** 2004. Viral replication in the nasopharynx is associated with diarrhea in patients with severe acute respiratory syndrome. *Clin. Infect. Dis.* **38:**467–475.

18. **Cheung, C. Y, L. L. M. Poon, I. H. Y. Ng, W. Luk, S. F. Sia, M. H. S. Wu, K. H. Chan, K. Y. Yuen, S. Gordon, Y. Guan, and J. S. M. Peiris.** 2005. Cytokine responses in severe acute respiratory syndrome coronavirus-infected macrophages in vitro: possible relevance to pathogenesis. *J. Virol.* **79:**7819–7826.

19. **Cheung, T. M., L. Y. Yam, L. K. So, A. C. Lau, E. Poon, B. M. Kong, and R. W. Yung.** 2004. Effectiveness of noninvasive positive pressure ventilation in the treatment of acute respiratory failure in severe acute respiratory syndrome. *Chest* **126:**845–850.

20. **Chinese SARS Molecular Epidemiology Consortium.** 2004. Molecular evolution of the SARS coronavirus during the course of the SARS epidemic in China. *Science* **303:**1666–1669.

21. **Chow, K. Y., C. E. Lee, M. L. Ling, D. M. Heng, and S. G. Yap.** 2004. Outbreak of severe acute respiratory syndrome in a tertiary hospital in Singapore, linked to an index patient with atypical presentation: epidemiological study. *Br. Med. J.* **328:**195.

22. **Christian, M. D., M. Loufty, L. C. McDonald, K. F. Martinez, M. Ofner, T. Wong, T. Wallington, W. L. Gold, B. Mederski, K. Green, D. E. Low, and the SARS Investigation Team.** 2004. Possible SARS coronavirus transmission during cardiopulmonary resuscitation. *Emerg. Infect. Dis.* **10:**287–293.

23. **Christian, M. D., S. M. Poutanen, M. R. Loufty, M. P. Mueller, and D. E. Low.** 2004. Severe acute respiratory syndrome. *Clin. Infect. Dis.* **38:**1420–1427.

24. **Chu, C.-M., L. L. M. Poon, V. C. C. Cheng, K.-S. Chan, I. F. N. Hung, M. M. L. Wong, K.-H. Chan, W.-S. Leung, B. S. F. Tang, V. L. Chan, W.-L. Ng, T.-C. Sim, P.-W. Ng, K.-I. Law, D. M. W. Tse, J. S. M. Peiris, and K.-Y. Yuen.** 2004. Initial viral load and the outcomes of SARS. *CMAJ* **171:**1349–1352.

25. **Chu, C. M., V. C. Cheng, I. F. Hung, M. M. Wong, K. H. Chan, K. S. Chan, R. Y. Kao, L. L. Poon, C. L. Wong, Y. Guan, J. S. Peiris, K. Y. Yuen, and the HKU/UCH SARS Study Group.** 2004. Role of lopinavir/ritonavir in the treatment of SARS: initial virological and clinical findings. *Thorax* **59:**252–256.

26. **Chu, K. H., W. K. Tsang, C. S. Tang, M. F. Lam, F. M. Lai, K. F. To, K. S. Fung, H. L. Tang, W. W. Yan, H. W. Chan, T. S. Lai, K. L. Tong, and K. N. Lai.** 2005. Acute renal impairment in coronavirus-associated severe acute respiratory syndrome. *Kidney Int.* **67:**698–705.

27. **Cinatl, J., B. Morgenstern, G. Bauer, P. Chandra, H. Rabenau, and H. W. Doerr.** 2003. Glycyrrhizin, an active component of liquorice roots, and replication of SARS-associated coronavirus. *Lancet* **361:** 2045–2046.

28. **Cinatl, J., B. Morgenstern, G. Bauer, P. Chandra, H. Rabenau, and H. W. Doerr.** 2003. Treatment of SARS with human interferons. *Lancet* **362:**293–294.

29. **Cinatl, J., Jr., G. Hoever, B. Morgenstern, W. Preiser, J. U. Vogel, W. K. Hofmann, G. Bauer, M. Michaelis, H. F. Rabenau, and H. W. Doerr.** 2004. Infection of cultured intestinal epithelial cells with severe acute respiratory syndrome coronavirus. *Cell Mol. Life Sci.* **61:**2100–2112.

30. **Cinatl, J., Jr., M. Michaelis, B. Morgenstern, and H. W. Doerr.** 2005. High-dose hydrocortisone reduces expression of the pro-inflammatory chemokines CXCL8 and CXCL10 in SARS coronavirus-infected intestinal cells. *Int. J. Mol. Med.* **15:**323–327.

31. **Cinatl, J., M. Michaelis, G. Hoever, W. Preiser, and H. W. Doerr.** 2005. Development of antiviral therapy for severe acute respiratory syndrome. *Antivir. Res.* **66:**81–97.

32. **Cui, W., Y. Fan, W. Wu, F. Zhang, J. Y. Wang, and A. P. Ni.** 2003. Expression of lymphocytes and lymphocyte subsets in patients with severe acute respiratory syndrome. *Clin. Infect. Dis.* **37:**857–859.

33. **Ding, Y., H. Wang, H. Shen, Z. Li, J. Geng, H. Han, J. Cai, X. Li, W. Kang, D. Weng, Y. Lu, D. Wu, L. He, and K. Yao.** 2003. The clinical pathology of severe acute respiratory syndrome (SARS): a report from China. *J. Pathol.* **200:**282–289.

34. **Drosten, C., S. Gunther, W. Preiser, S. van der Werf, H. R. Brodt, S. Becker, H. Rabenau, M. Panning, L. Kolesnikova, R. A. Fouchier, A. Berger, A. M. Burguiere, J. Cinatl, M. Eickmann, N. Escriou, K. Grywna, S. Kramme, J. C. Manuguerra, S. Muller, V. Rickerts, M. Sturmer, S. Vieth, H. D. Klenk, A. D. Osterhaus, H. Schmitz, and H. W. Doerr.** 2003. Identification of a novel coronavirus in patients with severe acute respiratory syndrome. *N. Engl. J. Med.* **348:**1967–1976.

35. **Duan, S. M., X. S. Zhao, R. F. Wen, J. J. Huang, G. H. Pi, S. X. Zhang, J. Han, S. L. Bi, L. Ruan, X. P. Dong, and the SARS Research Team.** 2003. Stability of SARS coronavirus in human specimens and environment and its sensitivity to heating and UV irradiation. *Biomed. Environ. Sci.* **16:**246–255.

36. **Farcas, G. A., S. M. Poutanen, T. Mazzulli, B. M. Willey, J. Butany, S. L. Asa, P. Faure, P. Akhavan, D. E. Low, and K. C. Kain.** 2005. Fatal severe acute respiratory syndrome is associated with multiorgan involvement by coronavirus. *J. Infect. Dis.* **191:**193–197.

37. **Fouchier, R. A., T. Kuiken, M. Schutten, G. van Amerongen, G. J. van Doornum, B. G. van den Hoogen, M. Peiris, W. Lim, K. Stohr, and A. D. Osterhaus.** 2003. Aetiology: Koch's postulates fulfilled for SARS virus. *Nature* **423:**240.

38. **Franks. T. J., P. Y. Chong, P. Chui, J. R. Galvin, R. M. Lourens, A. H. Reid, E. Selbs, C. P. McEvoy, C. D. Hayden, J. Fukuoka, J. K. Taubenberger, and W. D. Travis.** 2003. Lung pathology of severe acute respiratory syndrome (SARS): a study of 8 autopsy cases from Singapore. *Hum. Pathol.* **34:**743–748.

39. **Fraser, C., S Riley, R. M. Anderson, and N. M. Ferguson.** 2004. Factors that make an infectious disease outbreak controllable. *Proc. Natl. Acad. Sci. USA* **101:**6146–6151.

40. **Gao, W., A. Tamin, A. Soloff, L. D'Aiuto, E. Nwanegbo, P. D. Robbins, W. J. Bellini, S. Barratt-Boyes, and A. Gambotto.** 2003. Effects of a SARS-associated coronavirus vaccine in monkeys. *Lancet* **362:** 1895–1896.

41. **Greenough, T. C., A. Carville, J. Coderre, M. Somasundaran, J. L. Sullivan, K. Luzuriaga, and K. Mansfield.** 2005. Pneumonitis and multi-organ system disease in common marmosets (*Callithrix jacchus*) infected with the severe acute respiratory syndrome-associated coronavirus. *Am. J. Pathol.* **167:**455–463.

42. **Greenough, T. C., G. J. Babcock, A. Roberts, H. J. Hernandez, W. D. Thomas, Jr., J. A. Coccia, R. F. Graziano, M. Srinivasan, I. Lowy, R. W. Finberg, K. Subarao, L. Vogel, M. Somasundaran, K. Luzuriaga, J. L. Sullivan, and D. M. Ambrosino.** 2005. Development and characterization of a severe acute respiratory syndrome-associated coronavirus-neutralizing human monoclonal antibody that provides effective immunoprophylaxis in mice. *J. Infect. Dis.* **191:**507–514.

43. **Griffith, J. F., G. E. Antonio, S. M. Kumta, D. S. Cheong Hui, J. K. Tak Wong, G. M. Joynt, A. K. Lun Wu, A. Y. Kiu Cheung, K. H. Chiu, K. M. Chan, P. C. Leung, and A. T. Ahuja.** 2005. Osteonecrosis of hip and knee in patients with severe acute respiratory syndrome treated with steroids. *Radiology* **235:**168–175.

44. Gu, J., E. Gong, B. Zhang, J. Zheng, Z. Gao, Y. Zhong, W. Zou, J. Zhan, S. Wang, Z. Xie, H. Zhuang, B. Wu, H. Zhong, H. Shao, W. Fang, D. Gao, F. Pei, X. Li, Z. He, D. Xu, X. Shi, V. M. Anderson, and A. S. Leong. 2005. Multiple organ infection and the pathogenesis of SARS. *J. Exp. Med.* **202:**415–424.

45. Guan, Y., B. J. Zheng, Y. Q. He, X. L. Liu, Z. X. Zhuang, C. L. Cheung, S. W. Luo, P. H. Li, L. J. Zhang, Y. J. Guan, K. M. Butt, K. L. Wong, K. W. Chan, W. Lim, K. F. Shortridge, K. Y. Yuen, J. S. Peiris, and L. L. Poon. 2003. Isolation and characterization of viruses related to the SARS coronavirus from animals in southern China. *Science* **302:**276–278.

46. Guan, Y., J. S. Peiris, B. Zheng, L. L. Poon, K. H. Chan, F. Y. Zeng, C. W. Chan, M. N. Chan, J. D. Chen, K. Y. Chow, C. C. Hon, K. H. Hui, J. Li, V. Y. Li, Y. Wang, S. W. Leung, K. Y. Yuen, and F. C. Leung. 2004. Molecular epidemiology of the novel coronavirus that causes severe acute respiratory syndrome. *Lancet* **363:**99–104.

47. Haagmans, B. L., T. Kuiken, B. E. Martina, R. A. Fouchier, G. F. Rimmelzwaan, G. van Amerongen, D. van Riel, T. de Jong, S. Itamura, K. H. Chan, M. Tashiro, and A. D. Osterhaus. 2004. Pegylated interferon-alpha protects type 1 pneumocytes against SARS coronavirus infection in macaques. *Nat. Med.* **10:**290–293.

48. Hamano, E., M. Hijikata, S. Itoyama, T. Quy, N. C. Phi, H. T. Long, le D. Ha, V. V. Ban, I. Matsushita, H. Yanai, F. Kirikae, T. Kirikae, T. Kuratsuji, T. Sasazuki, and N. Keicho. 2005. Polymorphisms of interferon-inducible genes OAS-1 and MxA associated with SARS in the Vietnamese population. *Biochem. Biophys. Res. Commun.* **329:**1234–1239.

49. Hamming, I., W. Timens, M. L. Bulthuis, A. T. Lely, G. J. Navis, and H. van Goor. 2004. Tissue distribution of ACE2 protein, the functional receptor for SARS coronavirus. A first step in understanding SARS pathogenesis. *J. Pathol.* **203:**631–637.

50. He, M. L., B. Zheng, Y. Peng, J. S. Peiris, L. L. Poon, K. Y. Yuen, M. C. Lin, H. F. Kung, and Y. Guan. 2003. Inhibition of SARS-associated coronavirus infection and replication by RNA interference. *JAMA* **290:**2665–2666.

51. He, R., A. Adonov, M. Traykova-Adonova, J. Cao, T. Cutts, E. Grudesky, Y. Deschambaul, J. Berry, M. Drebot, and X. Li. 2004. Potent and selective inhibition of SARS coronavirus replication by aurintricarboxylic acid. *Biochem. Biophys. Res. Commun.* **320:**1199–1203.

52. He, Y., Y. Zhou, P. Siddiqui, and S. Jiang. 2004. Inactivated SARS-CoV vaccine elicits high titers of spike protein-specific antibodies that block receptor binding and virus entry. *Biochem. Biophys. Res. Commun.* **325:**445–452.

53. Hensley, L. E., L. E. Fritz, P. B. Jahrling, C. L. Karp, J. W. Huggins, and T. W. Geisbert. 2004. Interferon-beta 1a and SARS coronavirus replication. *Emerg. Infect. Dis.* **10:**317–319.

54. Heymann, D. 2005. SARS: a global perspective, p. 13–20. *In* M. Peiris, L. Anderson, A. Osterhaus, K. Stohr, and K. Y. Yuen (ed.), *Severe Acute Respiratory Syndrome*. Blackwell, Oxford, United Kingdom.

55. Ho, J. C., A. Y. Wu, B. Lam, G. C. Ooi, P. L. Khong, P. L. Ho, M. Chan-Yeung, N. S. Zhong, C. Ko, W. K. Lam, and K. W. Tsang. 2004. Pentaglobin in steroid-resistant severe acute respiratory syndrome. *Int. J. Tuberc. Lung. Dis.* **8:**1173–1179.

56. Hogan, R. J., G. Gao, T. Rowe, P. Bell, D. Flieder, J. Paragas, G. P. Kobinger, N. A. Wivel, R. G. Crystal, J. Boyer, H. Feldmann, T. G. Voss, and J. M. Wilson. 2004. Resolution of primary severe acute respiratory syndrome-associated coronavirus infection requires Stat1. *J. Virol.* **78:**11416–11421.

57. Holmes, K. V. 2001. Coronaviruses, p. 1187–1203. *In* D. M. Knipe and P. M. Howley (ed.), *Fields Virology*. Lippincott Williams & Wilkins, Philadelphia, Pa.

58. Hui, D. S., K. T. Wong, G. E. Antonio, N. Lee, A. Wu, V. Wong, W. Lau, J. C. Wu, L. S. Tam, L. M. Yu, G. M. Joynt, S. S. Chung, A. T. Ahuja, and J. J. Sung. 2004. Severe acute respiratory syndrome: correlation between clinical outcome and radiologic features. *Radiology* **233:**579–585.

59. Hung, I. F. N., V. C. C. Cheng, A. K. L. Wu, B. S. F. Tang, K. H. Chan, C. M. Chu, M. M. L. Wong, W. T. Hui, L. L. M. Poon, D. M. W. Tse, K. S. Chan, P. C. Y. Woo, S. K. P. Lau, J. S. M. Peiris, and K. Y. Yuen. 2004. Viral loads in clinical specimens and SARS manifestations. *Emerg. Infect. Dis.* **10:**1550–1557.

60. Imai, Y., K. Kuba, S. Rao, Y. Huan, F. Guo, B. Guan, P. Yang, R. Sarao, T. Wada, P. Leong, M. A. Crackower, A. Fukamizu, C. C. Hui, L. Hein, S. Uhlig, A. S. Slutsky, C. Jiang, and J. M. Penninger. 2005. Angiotensin-converting enzyme 2 protects from severe acute lung failure. *Nature* **436:**112–116.

61. Ip, W. K., K. H. Chan, H. K. Law, G. H. Tso, E. K. Kong, W. H. Wong, Y. F. To, R. W. Yung, E. Y. Chow, K. L. Au, E. Y. Chan, W. Lim, J. C. Jensenius, M. W. Turner, J. S. Peiris, and Y. L. Lau. 2005.

Mannose-binding lectin in severe acute respiratory syndrome coronavirus infection. *J. Infect. Dis.* **191:** 1697–1704.

62. Jeffers, S. A., S. M. Tusell, L. Gillim-Ross, E. M. Hemmila, J. E. Achenbach, G. J. Babcock, W. D. Thomas, Jr., L. B. Thackray, M. D. Young, R. J. Mason, D. M. Ambrosino, D. E. Wentworth, J. C. Demartini, and K. V. Holmes. 2004. CD209L (L-SIGN) is a receptor for severe acute respiratory syndrome coronavirus. *Proc. Natl. Acad. Sci. USA* **101:**15748–15753.

63. Jiang, Y., J. Xu, C. Zhou, Z. Wu, S. Zhong, J. Liu, W. Luo, T. Chen, Q. Qin, and P. Deng. 2005. Characterization of cytokine and chemokine profiles of severe acute respiratory syndrome. *Am. J. Respir. Crit. Care. Med.* **171:**850–857.

64. Jonassen, C. M., T. Kofstad, I.-L. Larsen, A. Lovland, K. Handeland, A. Follestadt, and A. Lillehaug. 2005. Molecular identification and characterization of novel coronaviruses infecting graylag geese *(Anser anser),* feral pigeons *(Columba livia)* and mallards *(Anas platyrhynchos). J. Gen. Virol.* **86:**1597–1607.

65. Jones, B. M., E. S. Ma, J. S. Peiris, P. C. Wong, J. C. Ho, B. Lam, K. N. Lai, and K. W. Tsang. 2004. Prolonged disturbances of in vitro cytokine production in patients with severe acute respiratory syndrome (SARS) treated with ribavirin and steroids. *Clin. Exp. Immunol.* **135:**467–473.

66. Kao, R. Y., W. H. W. Tsui, T. S. W. Lee, J. A. Tanner, R. M. Watt, J. D. Hung, L. H. Hu, G. H. Chen, Z. W. Chen, L. Q. Zhang, T. He, K. H. Chan, H. Tse, A. P. C. To, L. W. Y. Ng, B. C. W. Wong, H. W. Tsoi, D. Yang, D. D. Ho, and K. Y. Yuen. 2004. Identification of novel small molecule inhibitors of severe acute respiratory syndrome associated coronavirus by chemical genetics. *Chem. Biol.* **11:**1293–1299.

67. Kapadia, S. U., J. K. Rose, E. Lamirande, L. Vogel, K. Subbarao, and A. Roberts. 2005. Long-term protection from SARS coronavirus infection conferred by a single immunization with an attenuated VSV-based vaccine. *Virology* **340:**174–182.

68. Keyaerts, E., L. Vijgen, P. Maes, J. Neyts, and M. V. Ranst. 2004. In vitro inhibition of severe acute respiratory syndrome coronavirus by chloroquine. *Biochem. Biophys. Res. Commun.* **323:**264–268.

69. Kim, T. W., J. H. Lee, C. F. Hung, S. Peng, R. Roden, M. C. Wang, R. Viscidi, Y. C. Tsai, L. He, P. J. Chen, D. A. Boyd, and T. C. Wu. 2004. Generation and characterization of DNA vaccines targeting the nucleocapsid protein of severe acute respiratory syndrome coronavirus. *J. Virol.* **78:**4638–4645.

70. Ksiazek, T. G., D. Erdman, C. S. Goldsmith, S. R. Zaki, T. Peret, S. Emery, S. Tong, C. Urbani, J. A. Comer, W. Lim, P. E. Rollin, S. F. Dowell, A. E. Ling, C. D. Humphrey, W. J. Shieh, J. Guarner, C. D. Paddock, P. Rota, B. Fields, J. DeRisi, J. Y. Yang, N. Cox, J. M. Hughes, J. W. LeDuc, W. J. Bellini, L. J. Anderson, and the SARS Working Group. 2003. A novel coronavirus associated with severe acute respiratory syndrome. *N. Engl. J. Med.* **348:**1953–1966.

71. Kuba, K., Y. Imai, S. Rao, H. Gao, F. Guo, B. Guan, Y. Huan, P. Yang, Y. Zhang, W. Deng, L. Bao, B. Zhang, G. Liu, Z. Wang, M. Chappell, Y. Liu, D. Zheng, A. Leibbrandt, T. Wada, A. S. Slutsky, D. Liu, C. Qin, C. Jiang, and J. M. Penninger. 2005. A crucial role of angiotensin converting enzyme 2 (ACE2) in SARS coronavirus-induced lung injury. *Nat. Med.* **11:**875–879.

72. Kuiken, T., R. A. Fouchier, M. Schutten, G. F. Rimmelzwaan, G. van Amerongen, D. van Riel, J. D. Laman, T. de Jong, G. van Doornum, W. Lim, A. E. Ling, P. K. Chan, J. S. Tam, M. C. Zambon, R. Gopal, C. Drosten, S. van der Werf, N. Escriou, J. C. Manuguerra, K. Stohr, J. S. Peiris, and A. D. Osterhaus. 2003. Newly discovered coronavirus as the primary cause of severe acute respiratory syndrome. *Lancet* **362:**263–270.

73. Kuiken, T., F. A. Leighton, R. A. M. Fouchier, J. W. LeDuc, J. S. M. Peiris, A. Schudel, K. Stohr, and A. D. M. E. Osterhaus. 2005. Pathogen surveillance in animals. *Science* **309:**1680–1681.

74. Kung, N. Y., Y. Guan, N. R. Perkins, L. Bissett, T. Ellis, L. Sims, R. S. Morris, K. F. Shortridge, and J. S. Peiris. 2003. The impact of a monthly rest day on avian influenza virus isolation rates in retail live poultry markets in Hong Kong. *Avian. Dis.* **47**(Suppl. 3)**:**1037–1041.

75. Lau, J. T., X. Yang, P. C. Leung, L. Chan, E. Wong, C. Fong, and H. Y. Tsui. 2004. SARS in three categories of hospital workers, Hong Kong. *Emerg. Infect. Dis.* **10:**1399–1404.

76. Lau, K. K., W. C. Yu, C. M. Chu, S. T. Lau, B. Sheng, and K. Y. Yuen. 2004. Possible central nervous system infection by SARS coronavirus. *Emerg. Infect. Dis.* **10:**342–344.

77. Lau, S. K., P. C. Woo, K. S. Li, Y. Huang, H. W. Tsoi, B. H. Wong, S. S. Wong, S. Y. Leung, K. H. Chan, and K. Y. Yuen. 2005. Severe acute respiratory syndrome coronavirus-like virus in Chinese horseshoe bats. *Proc. Natl. Acad. Sci. USA* **102:**14040–14045.

78. **Lau, Y. L., and J. S. Peiris.** 2005. Pathogenesis of severe acute respiratory syndrome. *Curr. Opin. Immunol.* **17:**404–410.

79. **Law, H. K., C. Y. Cheung, H. Y. Ng, S. F. Sia, Y. O. Chan, W. Luk, J. M. Nicholls, J. S. Peiris, and Y. L. Lau.** 2005. Chemokine upregulation in SARS coronavirus infected human monocyte derived dendritic cells. *Blood* **106:**2366–2374.

80. **Lee, D. T., Y. K. Wing, H. C. Leung, J. J. Sung, Y. K. Ng, G. C. Yiu, R. Y. Chen, and H. F. Chiu.** 2004. Factors associated with psychosis among patients with severe acute respiratory syndrome: a case-control study. *Clin. Infect. Dis.* **39:**1247–1249.

81. **Lee, H. K., E. Y. Tso, T. N. Chau, O. T. Tsang, K. W. Choi, and T. S. Lai.** 2003. Asymptomatic severe acute respiratory syndrome-associated coronavirus infection. *Emerg. Infect. Dis.* **9:**1491–1492.

82. **Lee, N., D. Hui, A. Wu, P. Chan, P. Cameron, G. M. Joynt, A. Ahuja, M. Y. Yung, C. B. Leung, K. F. To, S. F. Lui, C. C. Szeto, S. Chung, and J. J. Sung.** 2003. A major outbreak of severe acute respiratory syndrome in Hong Kong. *N. Engl. J. Med.* **348:**1986–1994.

83. **Lee, N., K. C. Allen Chan, D. S. Hui, E. K. Ng, A. Wu, R. W. Chiu, V. W. Wong, P. K. Chan, K. T. Wong, E. Wong, C. S. Cockram, J. S. Tam, J. J. Sung, and Y. M. Lo.** 2004. Effects of early corticosteroid treatment on plasma SARS-associated coronavirus RNA concentrations in adult patients. *J. Clin. Virol.* **31:**304–309.

84. **Leung, C. W., Y. W. Kwan, P. W. Ko, S. S. Chiu, P. Y. Loung, N. C. Fong, L. P. Lee, Y. W. Hui, H. Law, W. H. Wong, K. H. Chan, J. S. Peiris, W. W. Lim, Y. L. Lau, and M. C. Chiu.** 2004. Severe acute respiratory syndrome among children. *Pediatrics* **113:**e535–e543. [Online.]

85. **Leung, G. M., A. J. Hedley, L. M. Ho, P. Chau, I. O. Wong, T. Q. Thach, A. C. Ghani, C. A. Donnelly, C. Fraser, S. Riley, N. M. Ferguson, R. M. Anderson, T. Tsang, P. Y. Leung, V. Wong, J. C. Chan, E. Tsui, S. V. Lo, and T. H. Lam.** 2004. The epidemiology of severe acute respiratory syndrome in the 2003 Hong Kong epidemic: an analysis of all 1755 patients. *Ann. Intern. Med.* **141:**662–673.

86. **Leung, G. M., P. H. Chung, T. Tsang, W. Lim, S. K. Chan, P. Chau, C. A. Donnelly, A. C. Ghani, C. Fraser, S. Riley, N. M. Ferguson, R. M. Anderson, Y. L. Law, T. Mok, T. Ng, A. Fu, P. Y. Leung, J. S. Peiris, T. H. Lam, and A. J. Hedley.** 2004. SARS-CoV antibody prevalence in all Hong Kong patient contacts. *Emerg. Infect. Dis.* **10:**1653–1656.

87. **Leung, W. K., K. F. To, P. K. Chan, H. L. Chan, A. K. Wu, N. Lee, K. Y. Yuen, and J. J. Sung.** 2003. Enteric involvement of severe acute respiratory syndrome-associated coronavirus infection. *Gastroenterology* **125:**1011–1017.

88. **Li, B. J., Q. Tang, D. Cheng, C. Qin, F. Y. Xie, Q. Wei, J. Xu, Y. Liu, B. J. Zheng, M. C. Woodle, N. Zhong, and P. Y. Lu.** 2005. Using siRNA in prophylactic and therapeutic regimens against SARS coronavirus in rhesus macaques. *Nat. Med.* doi:10.1038/nm1280. [Online.]

89. **Li, W., Z. Shi, M. Yu, W. Ren, C. Smith, J. H. Epstein, H. Wang, G. Crameri, Z. Hu, H. Zhang, J. Zhang, J. McEachern, H. Field, P. Daszak, B. T. Eaton, S. Zhang, and L. F. Wang.** 2005. Bats are natural reservoirs of SARS-like coronaviruses. *Science* **310:**676–679.

90. **Li, W., C. Zhang, J. Sui, J. H. Kuhn, M. J. Moore, S. Luo, S. K. Wong, I. C. Huang, K. Xu, N. Vasilieva, A. Murakami, Y. He, W. A. Marasco, Y. Guan, H. Choe, and M. Farzan.** 2005. Receptor and viral determinants of SARS-coronavirus adaptation to human ACE2. *EMBO J.* **24:**1634–1643.

91. **Li, W., M. J. Moore, N. Vasilieva, J. Sui, S. K. Wong, M. A. Berne, M. Somasundaran, J. L. Sullivan, K. Luzuriaga, T. C. Greenough, H. Choe, and M. Farzan.** 2003. Angiotensin-converting enzyme 2 is a functional receptor for the SARS coronavirus. *Nature* **426:**450–454.

92. **Liang, G., Q. Chen, J. Xu, Y. Liu, W. Lim, J. S. Peiris, L. J. Anderson, L. Ruan, H. Li, B. Kan, B. Di, P. Cheng, K. H. Chan, D. D. Erdman, S. Gu, X. Yan, W. Liang, D. Zhou, L. Haynes, S. Duan, X. Zhang, H. Zheng, Y. Gao, S. Tong, D. Li, L. Fang, P. Qin, W. Xu, and the SARS Diagnosis Working Group.** 2004. Laboratory diagnosis of four recent sporadic cases of community-acquired SARS, Guangdong Province, China. *Emerg. Infect. Dis.* **10:**1774–1781.

93. **Lim, P. L., A. Kurup, G. Gopalakrishna, K. P. Chan, C. W. Wong, L. C. Ng, S. Y. Se-Thoe, L. Oon, X. Bai, L. W. Stanton, Y. Ruan, L. D. Miller, V. B. Vega, L. James, P. L. Ooi, C. S. Kai, S. J. Olsen, B. Ang, and Y. S. Leo.** 2004. Laboratory-acquired severe acute respiratory syndrome. *N. Engl. J. Med.* **350:**1740–1745.

94. **Lin, M., H. K. Tseng, J. A. Trejaut, H. L. Lee, J. H. Loo, C. C. Chu, P. J. Chen, Y. W. Su, K. H. Lim, Z. U. Tsai, R. Y. Lin, R. S. Lin, and C. H. Huang.** 2003. Association of HLA class I with severe acute respiratory syndrome coronavirus infection. *BMC Med. Genet.* **4:**9.

95. Lipsitch, M., T. Cohen, B. Cooper, J. M. Robins, S. Ma, L. James, G. Gopalakrishna, S. K. Chew, C. C. Tan, M. H. Samore, D. Fisman, and M. Murray. 2003. Transmission dynamics and control of severe acute respiratory syndrome. *Science* **300:**1966–1970.

96. Loon, S. C., S. C. Teoh, L. L. Oon, S. Y. Se-Thoe, A. E. Ling, Y. S. Leo, and H. N. Leong. 2004. The severe acute respiratory syndrome coronavirus in tears. *Br. J. Ophthalmol.* **88:**861–863.

97. Loutfy, M. R., L. M. Blatt, K. A. Siminovitch, S. Ward, B. Wolff, H. Lho, D. H. Pham, H. Deif, E. A. LaMere, M. Chang, K. C. Kain, G. A. Farcas, P. Ferguson, M. Latchford, G. Levy, J. W. Dennis, E. K. Lai, and E. N. Fish. 2003. Interferon alfacon-1 plus corticosteroids in severe acute respiratory syndrome: a preliminary study. *JAMA* **290:**3222–3228.

98. Lu, L., I. Manopo, B. P. Leung, H. H. Chng, A. E. Ling, L. L. Chee, E. E. Ooi, S. W. Chan, and J. Kwang. 2004. Immunological characterization of the spike protein of the severe acute respiratory syndrome coronavirus. *J. Clin. Microbiol.* **42:**1570–1576.

99. Marra, M. A., S. J. Jones, C. R. Astell, R. A. Holt, A. Brooks-Wilson, Y. S. Butterfield, J. Khattra, J. K. Asano, S. A. Barber, S. Y. Chan, A. Cloutier, S. M. Coughlin, D. Freeman, N. Girn, O. L. Griffith, S. R. Leach, M. Mayo, H. McDonald, S. B. Montgomery, P. K. Pandoh, A. S. Petrescu, A. G. Robertson, J. E. Schein, A. Siddiqui, D. E. Smailus, J. M. Stott, G. S. Yang, F. Plummer, A. Andonov, H. Artsob, N. Bastien, K. Bernard, T. F. Booth, D. Bowness, M. Czub, M. Drebot, L. Fernando, R. Flick, M. Garbutt, M. Gray, A. Grolla, S. Jones, H. Feldmann, A. Meyers, A. Kabani, Y. Li, S. Normand, U. Stroher, G. A. Tipples, S. Tyler, R. Vogrig, D. Ward, B. Watson, R. C. Brunham, M. Krajden, M. Petric, D. M. Skowronski, C. Upton, and R. L. Roper. 2003. The genome sequence of the SARS-associated coronavirus. *Science* **300:**1399–1404.

100. Martina, B. E., B. L. Haagmans, T. Kuiken, R. A. Fouchier, G. F. Rimmelzwaan, G. Van Amerongen, J. S. Peiris, W. Lim, and A. D. Osterhaus. 2003. SARS virus infection of cats and ferrets. *Nature* **425:**915.

101. McAuliffe, J., L. Vogel, A. Roberts, G. Fahle, S. Fischer, W. J. Shieh, E. Butler, S. Zaki, M. St Claire, B. Murphy, and K. Subbarao. 2004. Replication of SARS coronavirus administered into the respiratory tract of African green, rhesus and cynomolgus monkeys. *Virology* **330:**8–15.

102. Merianos, A., R. Condon, H. Oshitani, D. Werker, and R. Andraghetti. 2005. Epidemiology and transmission of SARS, p.13–20. *In* M. Peiris, L. Anderson, A. Osterhaus, K. Stohr, and K.Y. Yuen (ed.), *Severe Acute Respiratory Syndrome*. Blackwell, Oxford, United Kingdom.

103. Merianos, A., and M. Peiris. 2005. International health regulations. *Lancet* **366:**1249–1251.

104. Mills, C. E., J. M. Robins, and M. Lipsitch. 2004. Transmissibility of 1918 pandemic influenza. *Nature* **432:**904–906.

105. Morgenstern, B., M. Michaelis, P. C. Baer, H. W. Doerr, and J. Cinatl, Jr. 2005. Ribavirin and interferon-beta synergistically inhibit SARS-associated coronavirus replication in animal and human cell lines. *Biochem. Biophys. Res. Commun.* **326:**905–908.

106. Muller, M. P., G. Tomlinson, T. J. Marrie, P. Tang, A. McGeer, D. E. Low, A. S. Detsky, and W. L. Gold. 2005. Can routine laboratory tests discriminate between severe acute respiratory syndrome and other causes of community-acquired pneumonia? *Clin. Infect. Dis.* **40:**1079–1086.

107. Nakajima, N., Y. Asahi-Ozaki, N. Nagata, Y. Sato, F. Dizon, F. J. Paladin, R. M. Olveda, T. Odagiri, M. Tashio, and T. Sata. 2003. SARS coronavirus-infected cells in lung detected by new in situ hybridization technique. *Jpn. J. Infect. Dis.* **56:**139–141.

108. Ng, E. K., D. S. Hui, K. C. Chan, E. C. Hung, R. W. Chiu, N. Lee, A. Wu, S. S. Chim, Y. K. Tong, J. J. Sung, J. S. Tam, and Y. M. Lo. 2003. Quantitative analysis and prognostic implication of SARS coronavirus RNA in the plasma and serum of patients with severe acute respiratory syndrome. *Clin. Chem.* **49:**1976–1980.

109. Ng, M. H., K. M. Lau, L. Li, S. H. Cheng, W. Y. Chan, P. K. Hui, B. Zee, C. B. Leung, and J. J. Sung. 2004. Association of human-leukocyte-antigen class I (B*0703) and class II (DRB1*0301) genotypes with susceptibility and resistance to the development of severe acute respiratory syndrome. *J. Infect. Dis.* **190:** 515–518.

110. Nicholls, J., and M. Peiris. 2005. Good ACE, bad ACE do battle in lung injury, SARS. *Nat. Med.* **11:**821–822.

111. Nicholls, J. M., L. L. Poon, K. C. Lee, W. F. Ng, S. T. Lai, C. Y. Leung, C. M. Chu, P. K. Hui, K. L. Mak, W. Lim, K. W. Yan, K. H. Chan, N. C. Tsang, Y. Guan, K. Y. Yuen, and J. S. Peiris. 2003. Lung pathology of fatal severe acute respiratory syndrome. *Lancet* **361:**1773–1778.

111a. **Nicholls, J. M., J. Butany, L. L. M. Poon, K. H. Chan, S. L. Beh, S. Poutanen, J. S. M. Peiris, and M. Wong.** 2006. Time course and cellular localization of SARS-CoV nucleoprotein and RNA in lungs from fatal cases of SARS. *PLoS Med.* **3:**e27.

112. **Nicolaou, S., N. A. Al-Nakshabandi, and N. L. Muller.** 2003. SARS: imaging of severe acute respiratory syndrome. *Am. J. Roentgenol.* **180:**1247–1249.

113. **Nie, Y., G. Wang, X. Shi, H. Zhang, Y. Qiu, Z. He, W. Wang, G. Lian, X. Yin, L. Du, L. Ren, J. Wang, X. He, T. Li, H. Deng, and M. Ding.** 2004. Neutralizing antibodies in patients with severe acute respiratory syndrome-associated coronavirus infection. *J. Infect. Dis.* **190:**1119–1126.

114. **Okada, M., Y. Takemoto, Y. Okuno, S. Hashimoto, S. Yoshida, Y. Fukunaga, T. Tanaka, Y. Kita, S. Kuwayama, Y. Muraki, N. Kanamaru, H. Takai, C. Okada, Y. Sakaguchi, I. Furukawa, K. Yamada, M. Matsumoto, T. Kase, D. E. Demello, J. S. Peiris, P. J. Chen, N. Yamamoto, Y. Yoshinaka, T. Nomura, I. Ishida, S. Morikawa, M. Tashiro, and M. Sakatani.** 2005. The development of vaccines against SARS coronavirus in mice and SCID-PBL/hu mice. *Vaccine* **23:**2269–2272.

115. **Olsen, C. W.** 1993. A review of feline infectious peritonitis virus: molecular biology, immunopathogenesis, clinical aspects, and vaccination. *Vet. Microbiol.* **36:**1–37.

116. **Olsen, S. J., H. L. Chang, T. Y. Cheung, A. F. Tang, T. L. Fisk, S. P. Ooi, H. W. Kuo, D. D. Jiang, K. T. Chen, J. Lando, K. H. Hsu, T. J. Chen, and S. F. Dowell.** 2003. Transmission of the severe acute respiratory syndrome on aircraft. *N. Engl. J. Med.* **349:**2416–2422.

117. **Ong, K. C., A. W. Ng, L. S. Lee, G. Kaw, S. K. Kwek, M. K. Leow, and A. Earnest.** 2004. Pulmonary function and exercise capacity in survivors of severe acute respiratory syndrome. *Eur. Respir. J.* **24:**436–442.

118. **Orellana, C.** 2004. Laboratory-acquired SARS raises worries on biosafety. *Lancet Infect. Dis.* **4:**64.

119. **Peiris, J. S., S. T. Lai, L. L. Poon, Y. Guan, L. Y. Yam, W. Lim, J. Nicholls, W. K. Yee, W. W. Yan, M. T. Cheung, V. C. Cheng, K. H. Chan, D. N. Tsang, R. W. Yung, T. K. Ng, K. Y. Yuen, and the SARS Study Group.** 2003. Coronavirus as a possible cause of severe acute respiratory syndrome. *Lancet* **361:**1319–1325.

120. **Peiris, J. S., C. M. Chu, V. C. Cheng, K. S. Chan, I. F. Hung, L. L. Poon, K. I. Law, B. S. Tang, T. Y. Hon, C. S. Chan, K. H. Chan, J. S. Ng, B. J. Zheng, W. L. Ng, R. W. Lai, Y. Guan, K. Y. Yuen, and the HKU/UCH SARS Study Group.** 2003. Clinical progression and viral load in a community outbreak of coronavirus-associated SARS pneumonia: a prospective study. *Lancet* **361:**1767–1772.

121. **Peiris, J. S. M., K. Y. Yuen, A. D. M. E. Osterhaus, and K. Stohr.** 2003. The severe acute respiratory syndrome. *N. Engl. J. Med.* **349:**2431–2441.

122. **Poon, L. L., D. K. Chu, K. H. Chan, O. K. Wong, T. M. Ellis, Y. H. Leung, S. K. Lau, P. C. Woo, K. Y. Suen, K. Y. Yuen, Y. Guan, and J. S. Peiris.** 2005. Identification of a novel coronavirus in bats. *J. Virol.* **79:**2001–2009.

123. **Poon, L. L., K. H. Chan, O. K. Wong, W. C. Yam, K. Y. Yuen, Y. Guan, Y. M. Lo, and J. S. Peiris.** 2003. Early diagnosis of SARS coronavirus infection by real time RT-PCR. *J. Clin. Virol.* **28:**233–238.

124. **Poon, L. L., Y. Guan, J. M. Nicholls, K. Y. Yuen, and J. S. Peiris.** 2004. The aetiology, origins, and diagnosis of severe acute respiratory syndrome. *Lancet Infect. Dis.* **4:**663–671.

125. **Poutanen, S. M., D. E. Low, B. Henry, S. Finkelstein, D. Rose, K. Green, R. Tellier, R. Draker, D. Adachi, M. Ayers, A. K. Chan, D. M. Skowronski, I. Salit, A. E. Simor, A. S. Slutsky, P. W. Doyle, M. Krajden, M. Petric, R. C. Brunham, A. J. McGeer, the National Microbiology Laboratory, Canada, and the Canadian Severe Acute Respiratory Syndrome Study Team.** 2003. Identification of severe acute respiratory syndrome in Canada. *N. Engl. J. Med.* **348:**1995–2005.

126. **Rabenau, H. F., J. Cinatl, B. Morgenstern, G. Bauer, W. Preiser, and H. W. Doerr.** 2005. Stability and inactivation of SARS coronavirus. *Med. Microbiol. Immunol.* **194:**1–6.

127. **Reghunathan, R., M. Jayapal, L. Y. Hsu, H. H. Chng, D. Tai, B. P. Leung, and A. J. Melendez.** 2005. Expression profile of immune response genes in patients with severe acute respiratory syndrome. *BMC Immunol.* **6:**2–12.

128. **Riley, S., C. Fraser, C. A. Donnelly, A. C. Ghani, L. J. Abu-Raddad, A. J. Hedley, G. M. Leung, L. M. Ho, T. H. Lam, T. Q. Thach, P. Chau, K. P. Chan, S. V. Lo, P. Y. Leung, T. Tsang, W. Ho, K. H. Lee, E. M. Lau, N. M Ferguson, and R. M. Anderson.** 2003. Transmission dynamics of the etiological agent of SARS in Hong Kong: impact of public health interventions. *Science* **300:**1961–1966.

129. **Roberts, A., C. Paddock, L. Vogel, E. Butler, S. Zaki, and K. Subbarao.** 2005. Aged BALB/c mice as a model for increased severity of severe acute respiratory syndrome in elderly humans. *J. Virol.* **79:**5833–5838.

130. Roberts, A., L. Vogel, J. Guarner, N. Hayes, B. Murphy, S. Zaki, and K. Subbarao. 2005. Severe acute respiratory syndrome coronavirus infection of golden Syrian hamsters. *J. Virol.* **79:**503–511.

131. Rota, P. A., M. S. Oberste, S. S. Monroe, W. A. Nix, R. Campagnoli, J. P. Icenogle, S. Penaranda, B. Bankamp, K. Maher, M. H. Chen, S. Tong, A. Tamin, L. Lowe, M. Frace, J. L. DeRisi, Q. Chen, D. Wang, D. D. Erdman, T. C. Peret, C. Burns, T. G. Ksiazek, P. E. Rollin, A. Sanchez, S. Liffick, B. Holloway, J. Limor, K. McCaustland, M. Olsen-Rasmussen, R. Fouchier, S. Gunther, A. D. Oster-haus, C. Drosten, M. A. Pallansch, L. J. Anderson, and W. J. Bellini. 2003. Characterization of a novel coronavirus associated with severe acute respiratory syndrome. *Science* **300:**1394–1399.

132. Rowe, T., G. Gao, R. J. Hogan, R. G. Crystal, T. G. Voss, R. L. Grant, P. Bell, G. P. Kobinger, N. A. Wivel, and J. M. Wilson. 2004. Macaque model for severe acute respiratory syndrome. *J. Virol.* **78:** 11401–11404.

133. Saif, L. 2005. Comparative biology of coronaviruses: lessons for SARS, p. 84–99. *In* M. Peiris, L. Anderson, A. Osterhaus, K. Stohr, and K.Y. Yuen (ed.), *Severe Acute Respiratory Syndrome.* Blackwell, Oxford, United Kingdom.

134. Seto, W. H., D. Tsang, R. W. Yung, T. Y. Ching, T. K. Ng, M. Ho, L. M. Ho, J. S. Peiris, and the Advisors of the Expert SARS Group of the Hospital Authority. 2003. Effectiveness of precautions against droplets and contact in prevention of nosocomial transmission of severe acute respiratory syndrome (SARS). *Lancet* **361:**1519–1520.

135. Shen, Z., F. Ning, W. Zhou, X. He, C. Lin, D. P. Chin, Z. Zhu, and A. Schuchat. 2004. Superspreading SARS events, Beijing, 2003. *Emerg. Infect. Dis.* **10:**256–260.

136. Simmons, G., J. D. Reeves, A. J. Rennekamp, S. M. Amberg, A. J. Piefer, and P. Bates. 2004. Characterization of severe acute respiratory syndrome-associated coronavirus (SARS-CoV) spike glycoprotein-mediated viral entry. *Proc. Natl. Acad. Sci. USA* **101:**4240–4245.

137. Snijder, E. J., P. J. Bredenbeek, J. C. Dobbe, V. Thiel, J. Ziebuhr, L. L. Poon, Y. Guan, M. Rozanov, W. J. Spaan, and A. E. Gorbalenya. 2003. Unique and conserved features of genome and proteome of SARS-coronavirus, an early split-off from the coronavirus group 2 lineage. *J. Mol. Biol.* **331:**991–1004.

138. Song, H. D., C. C. Tu, G. W. Zhang, S. Y. Wang, K. Zheng, L. C. Lei, Q. X. Chen, Y. W. Gao, H. Q. Zhou, H. Xiang, H. J. Zheng, S. W. Chern, F. Cheng, C. M. Pan, H. Xuan, S. J. Chen, H. M. Luo, D. H. Zhou, Y. F. Liu, J. F. He, P. Z. Qin, L. H. Li, Y. Q. Ren, W. J. Liang, Y. D. Yu, L. Anderson, M. Wang, R. H. Xu, X. W. Wu, H. Y. Zheng, J. D. Chen, G. Liang, Y. Gao, M. Liao, L. Fang, L. Y. Jiang, H. Li, F. Chen, B. Di, L. J. He, J. Y. Lin, S. Tong, X. Kong, L. Du, P. Hao, H. Tang, A. Bernini, X. J. Yu, O. Spiga, Z. M. Guo, H. Y. Pan, W. Z. He, J. C. Manuguerra, A. Fontanet, A. Danchin, N. Niccolai, Y. X. Li, C. I. Wu, and G. P. Zhao. 2005. Cross-host evolution of severe acute respiratory syndrome coronavirus in palm civet and human. *Proc. Natl. Acad. Sci. USA* **102:**2430–2435.

139. Spiegel, M., A. Pichlmair, L. Martinez-Sobrido, J. Cros, A. Garcia-Sastre, O. Haller, and F. Weber. 2005. Inhibition of beta interferon induction by severe acute respiratory syndrome coronavirus suggests a two-step model for activation of interferon regulatory factor 3. *J. Virol.* **79:**2079–2086.

140. Stadler, K., V. Masignani, M. Eickmann, S. Becker, S. Abrignani, H.-D. Klenk, and R. Rappuoli. 2003. Beginning to understand a new virus. *Nat. Rev. Microbiol.* **1:**209–218.

141. Stroher, U., A. DiCaro, Y. Li, J. E. Strong, F. Aoki, F. Plummer, S. M. Jones, and H. Feldmann. 2004. Severe acute respiratory syndrome-related coronavirus is inhibited by interferon-alpha. *J. Infect. Dis.* **189:**1164–1167.

142. Subbarao, K., J. McAuliffe, L. Vogel, G. Fahle, S. Fischer, K. Tatti, M. Packard, W. J. Shieh, S. Zaki, and B. Murphy. 2004. Prior infection and passive transfer of neutralizing antibody prevent replication of severe acute respiratory syndrome coronavirus in the respiratory tract of mice. *J. Virol.* **78:**3572–3577.

143. Sui, J., W. Li, A. Murakami, A. Tamin, L. J. Matthews, S. K. Wong, M. J. Moore, A. S. Tallarico, M. Olurinde, H. Choe, L. J. Anderson, W. J. Bellini, M. Farzan, and W. A. Marasco. 2004. Potent neutralization of severe acute respiratory syndrome (SARS) coronavirus by a human mAb to S1 protein that blocks receptor association. *Proc. Natl. Acad. Sci. USA* **101:**2536–2541.

144. Sui, J., W. Li, A. Roberts, L. J. Matthews, A. Murakami, L. Vogel, S. K. Wong, K. Subbarao, M. Farzan, and W. A. Marasco. 2005. Evaluation of human monoclonal antibody 80R for immunoprophylaxis of severe acute respiratory syndrome by an animal study, epitope mapping, and analysis of spike variants. *J. Virol.* **79:**5900–5906.

145. Takasuka, N., H. Fujii, Y. Takahashi, M. Kasai, S. Morikawa, S. Itamura, K. Ishii, M. Sakaguchi, K. Ohnishi, M. Ohshima, S. Hashimoto, T. Odagiri, M. Tashiro, H. Yoshikura, T. Takemori, and

Y. Tsunetsugu-Yokota. 2004. A subcutaneously injected UV-inactivated SARS coronavirus vaccine elicits systemic humoral immunity in mice. *Int. Immunol.* **16:**1423–1430.

146. Tan, E. L. C., E. E. Ooi, C. Y. Lin, H. C. Tan, A. E. Ling, B. Lim, and L. W. Stanton. 2004. Inhibition of SARS coronavirus infection in vitro with clinically approved antiviral drugs. *Emerg. Infect. Dis.* **10:**581–586.

147. Tang, B. S., K. H. Chan, V. C. Cheng, P. C. Woo, S. K. Lau, C. C. Lam, T. L. Chan, A. K. Wu, I. F. Hung, S. Y. Leung, and K. Y. Yuen. 2005. Comparative host gene transcription by microarray analysis early after infection of the Huh7 cell line by severe acute respiratory syndrome coronavirus and human coronavirus 229E. *J. Virol.* **79:**6180–6193.

148. Tang, L., Q. Zhu, E. Qin, M. Yu, Z. Ding, H. Shi, X. Cheng, C. Wang, G. Chang, Q. Zhu, F. Fang, H. Chang, S. Li, X. Zhang, X. Chen, J. Yu, J. Wang, and Z. Chen. 2004. Inactivated SARS-CoV vaccine prepared from whole virus induces a high level of neutralizing antibodies in BALB/c mice. *DNA Cell Biol.* **23:**391–394.

149. ter Meulen, J., A. B. Bakker, E. N. van den Brink, G. J. Weverling, B. E. Martina, B. L. Haagmans, T. Kuiken, J. de Kruif, W. Preiser, W. Spaan, H. R. Gelderblom, J. Goudsmit, A. D. Osterhaus. 2004. Human monoclonal antibody as prophylaxis for SARS coronavirus infection in ferrets. *Lancet* **363:** 2139–2141.

150. To, K. F., and A. W. Lo. 2004. Exploring the pathogenesis of severe acute respiratory syndrome (SARS): the tissue distribution of the coronavirus (SARS-CoV) and its putative receptor, angiotensin-converting enzyme 2 (ACE2). *J. Pathol.* **203:**740–743.

151. To, K. F., J. H. Tong, P. K. Chan, F. W. Au, S. S. Chim, K. C. Chan, J. L. Cheung, E. Y. Liu, G. M. Tse, A. W. Lo, Y. M. Lo, and H. K. Ng. 2004. Tissue and cellular tropism of the coronavirus associated with severe acute respiratory syndrome: an in-situ hybridization study of fatal cases. *J. Pathol.* **202:**157–163.

152. Towler, P., B. Staker, S. G. Prasad, S. Menon, J. Tang, T. Parsons, D. Ryan, M. Fisher, D. Williams, N. A. Dales, M. A. Patane, and M. W. Pantoliano. 2004. ACE2 X-ray structures reveal a large hinge-bending motion important for inhibitor binding and catalysis. *J. Biol. Chem.* **279:**17996–18007.

153. Traggiai, E., S. Becker, K. Subbarao, L. Kolesnikova, Y. Uematsu, M. R. Gismondo, B. R. Murphy, R. Rappuoli, and A. Lanzavecchia. 2004. An efficient method to make human monoclonal antibodies from memory B cells: potent neutralization of SARS coronavirus. *Nat. Med.* **10:**871–875.

154. Tsang, K. W., P. L. Ho, G. C. Ooi, W. K. Yee, T. Wang, M. Chan-Yeung, W. K. Lam, W. H. Seto, L. Y. Yam, T. M. Cheung, P. C. Wong, B. Lam, M. S. Ip, J. Chan, K. Y. Yuen, and K. N. Lai. 2003. A cluster of cases of severe acute respiratory syndrome in Hong Kong. *N. Engl. J. Med.* **348:**1977–1985.

155. Tu, C., G. Crameri, X. Kong, J. Chen, Y. Sun, M. Yu, H. Xiang, X. Xia, S. Liu, T. Ren, Y. Yu, B. T. Eaton, H. Xuan, and L. F. Wang. 2004. Antibodies to SARS coronavirus in civets. *Emerg. Infect. Dis.* **10:**2244–2248.

156. van der Hoek, L., K. Pyrc, M. F. Jebbink, W. Vermeulen-Oost, R. J. Berkhout, K. C. Wolthers, P. M. Wertheim-Van Dillen, J. Kaandorp, J. Spaargaren, and B. Berkhout. 2004. Identification of a new human coronavirus. *Nat. Med.* **10:**368–373.

157. Varia, M., S. Wilson, S. Sarwal, A. McGeer, E. Gournis, E. Galanis, B. Henry, and the Hospital Outbreak Investigation Team. 2003. Investigation of a nosocomial outbreak of severe acute respiratory syndrome (SARS) in Toronto, Canada. *CMAJ* **19:**285–292.

158. Wang, P., J. Chen, A. Zheng, Y. Nie, X. Shi, W. Wang, G. Wang, M. Luo, H. Liu, L. Tan, X. Song, Z. Wang, X. Yin, X. Qu, X. Wang, T. Qing, M. Ding, and H. Deng. 2004. Expression cloning of functional receptor used by SARS coronavirus. *Biochem. Biophys. Res. Commun.* **315:**439–444.

159. Wang, Y. D., W. Y. Sin, G. B. Xu, H. H. Yang, T. Y. Wong, X. W. Pang, X. Y. He, H. G. Zhang, J. N. Ng, C. S. Cheng, J. Yu, L. Meng, R. F. Yang, S. T. Lai, Z. H. Guo, Y. Xie, and W. F. Chen. 2004. T-cell epitopes in severe acute respiratory syndrome (SARS) coronavirus spike protein elicit a specific T-cell immune response in patients who recover from SARS. *J. Virol.* **78:**5612–5618.

160. Wang, Z., L. Ren, X. Zhao, T. Hung, A. Meng, J. Wang, and Y. G. Chen. 2004. Inhibition of severe acute respiratory syndrome virus replication by small interfering RNAs in mammalian cells. *J. Virol.* **78:** 7523–7527.

161. Weingartl, H., M. Czub, S. Czub, J. Neufeld, P. Marszal, J. Gren, G. Smith, S. Jones, R. Proulx, Y. Deschambault, E. Grudeski, A. Andonov, R. He, Y. Li, J. Copps, A. Grolla, D. Dick, J. Berry, S. Ganske, L. Manning, and J. Cao. 2004. Immunization with modified vaccinia virus Ankara-based recombinant vaccine against severe acute respiratory syndrome is associated with enhanced hepatitis in ferrets. *J. Virol.* **78:**12672–12676.

162. **Wong, C. K., C. W. Lam, A. K. Wu, W. K. Ip, N. L. Lee, I. H. Chan, L. C. Lit, D. S. Hui, M. H. Chan, S. S. Chung, and J. J. Sung.** 2004. Plasma inflammatory cytokines and chemokines in severe acute respiratory syndrome. *Clin. Exp. Immunol.* **136:**95–103.

163. **Wong, R. S., A. Wu, K. F. To, N. Lee, C. W. Lam, C. K. Wong, P. K. Chan, M. H. Ng, L. M. Yu, D. S. Hui, J. S. Tam, G. Cheng, and J. J. Sung.** 2003. Haematological manifestations in patients with severe acute respiratory syndrome: retrospective analysis. *BMJ* **326:**1358–1362.

164. **Wong, Y. C. R., and A. Siu.** 2005. Counting the economic cost of SARS, p. 213–230. *In* M. Peiris, L. Anderson, A. Osterhaus, K. Stohr, and K.Y. Yuen (ed.), *Severe Acute Respiratory Syndrome.* Blackwell, Oxford, United Kingdom.

165. **Woo, P. C., S. K. Lau, B. H. Wong, H. W. Tsoi, A. M. Fung, K. H. Chan, V. K. Tam, J. S. Peiris, and K. Y. Yuen.** 2004. Detection of specific antibodies to severe acute respiratory syndrome (SARS) coronavirus nucleocapsid protein for serodiagnosis of SARS coronavirus pneumonia. *J. Clin. Microbiol.* **42:**2306–2309.

166. **Woo, P. C., S. K. Lau, B. H. Wong, K. H. Chan, W. T. Hui, G. S. Kwan, J. S. Peiris, R. B. Couch, and K. Y. Yuen.** 2004. False-positive results in a recombinant severe acute respiratory syndrome-associated coronavirus (SARS-CoV) nucleocapsid enzyme-linked immunosorbent assay due to HCoV-OC43 and HCoV-229E rectified by Western blotting with recombinant SARS-CoV spike polypeptide. *J. Clin. Microbiol.* **42:**5885–5888.

167. **Woo, P. C., S. K. Lau, C. M. Chu, K. H. Chan, H. W. Tsoi, Y. Huang, B. H. Wong, R. W. Poon, J. J. Cai, W. K. Luk, L. L. Poon, S. S. Wong, Y. Guan, J. S. Peiris, and K. Y. Yuen.** 2005. Characterization and complete genome sequence of a novel coronavirus, coronavirus HKU1, from patients with pneumonia. *J. Virol.* **79:**884–895.

168. **World Health Organization.** 2003. A multicentre collaboration to investigate the cause of severe acute respiratory syndrome. *Lancet* **361:**1730–1733.

169. **Wu, C. J., J. T. Jan, C. M. Chen, H. P. Hsieh, D. R. Hwang, H. W. Liu, C. Y. Liu, H. W. Huang, S. C. Chen, C. F. Hong, R. K. Lin, Y. S. Chao, and J. T. Hsu.** 2004. Inhibition of severe acute respiratory syndrome coronavirus replication by niclosamide. *Antimicrob. Agents Chemother.* **48:**2693–2696.

170. **Wu, C. Y., J. T. Jan, S. H. Ma, C. J. Kuo, H. F. Juan, Y. S. Cheng, H. H. Hsu, H. C. Huang, D. Wu, A. Brik, F. S. Liang, R. S. Liu, J. M. Fang, S. T. Chen, P. H. Liang, and C. H. Wong.** 2004. Small molecules targeting severe acute respiratory syndrome human coronavirus. *Proc. Natl. Acad. Sci. USA* **101:**10012–10017.

171. **Wu, D., C. Tu, C. Xin, H. Xuan, Q. Meng, Y. Liu, Y. Yu, Y. Guan, Y. Jiang, X. Yin, G. Crameri, M. Wang, C. Li, S. Liu, M. Liao, L. Feng, H. Xiang, J. Sun, J. Chen, Y. Sun, S. Gu, N. Liu, D. Fu, B. T. Eaton, L. F. Wang, and X. Kong.** 2005. Civets are equally susceptible to experimental infection by two different severe acute respiratory syndrome coronavirus isolates. *J. Virol.* **79:**2620–2625.

172. **Wu, V. C., J. W. Huang, P. R. Hsueh, Y. F. Yang, H. B. Tsai, W. C. Kan, H. W. Chang, and K. D. Wu.** 2005. Renal hypouricemia is an ominous sign in patients with severe acute respiratory syndrome. *Am. J. Kidney Dis.* **45:**88–95.

173. **Xiong, B., C. S. Gui, X. Y. Xu, C. Luo, J. Chen, H. B. Luo, L. L. Chen, G. W. Li, T. Sun, C. Y. Yu, L. D. Yue, W. H. Duan, J. K. Shen, L. Qin, T. L. Shi, Y. X. Li, K. X. Chen, X. M. Luo, X. Shen, J. H. Shen, and H. L. Jiang.** 2003. A 3D model of SARS-CoV 3CL proteinase and its inhibitors design by virtual screening. *Acta Pharmacol. Sin.* **24:**497–504.

174. **Xu, R. H., J. F. He, M. R. Evans, G. W. Peng, H. E. Field, D. W. Yu, C. K. Lee, H. M. Luo, W. S. Lin, P. Lin, L. H. Li, W. J. Liang, J. Y. Lin, and A. Schnur.** 2004. Epidemiologic clues to SARS origin in China. *Emerg. Infect. Dis.* **10:**1030–1037.

175. **Yamamoto, N., R. Yang, Y. Yoshinaka, S. Amari, T. Nakano, J. Cinatl, H. Rabenau, H. W. Doerr, G. Hunsmann, A. Otaka, H. Tamamura, N. Fujii, and N. Yamamoto.** 2004. HIV protease inhibitor nelfinavir inhibits replication of SARS-associated coronavirus. *Biochem. Biophys. Res. Commun.* **318:**719–725.

176. **Yang, Z. Y., H. C. Werner, W. P. Kong, K. Leung, E. Traggiai, A. Lanzavecchia, and G. J. Nabel.** 2005. Evasion of antibody neutralization in emerging severe acute respiratory syndrome coronaviruses. *Proc. Natl. Acad. Sci. USA* **102:**797–801.

177. **Yang, Z. Y., W. P. Kong, Y. Huang, A. Roberts, B. R. Murphy, K. Subbarao, and G. J. Nabel.** 2004. A DNA vaccine induces SARS coronavirus neutralization and protective immunity in mice. *Nature* **428:**561–564.

178. **Yang, Z. Y., Y. Huang, L. Ganesh, K. Leung, W. P. Kong, O. Schwartz, K. Subbarao, and G. J. Nabel.** 2004. pH-dependent entry of severe acute respiratory syndrome coronavirus is mediated by the spike glycoprotein and enhanced by dendritic cell transfer through DC-SIGN. *J. Virol.* **78:**5642–5650.

179. **Yeh, S. H., H. Y. Wang, C. Y. Tsai, C. L. Kao, J. Y. Yang, H. W. Liu, I. J. Su, S. F. Tsai, D. S. Chen, P. J. Chen, and the National Taiwan University SARS Research Team.** 2004. Characterization of severe acute respiratory coronavirus genomes in Taiwan: molecular epidemiology and genome evolution. *Proc. Natl. Acad. Sci. USA* **101:**2542–2547.

180. **Yilla, M., B. H. Harcourt, C. J. Hickman, M. McGrew, A. Tamin, C. S. Goldsmith, W. J. Bellini, and L. J. Anderson.** 2005. SARS-coronavirus replication in human peripheral monocytes/macrophages. *Virus Res.* **107:**93–101.

181. **Yount, B., K. M. Curtis, E. A. Fritz, L. E. Hensley, P. B. Jahrling, E. Prentice, M. R. Denison, T. W. Geisbert, and R. S. Baric.** 2003. Reverse genetics with a full-length infectious cDNA of severe acute respiratory syndrome coronavirus. *Proc. Natl. Acad. Sci. USA* **100:**12995–13000.

182. **Yu, I. T., Y. Li, T. W. Wong, W. Tam, A. T. Chan, J. H. Lee, D. Y. Leung, and T. Ho.** 2004. Evidence of airborne transmission of the severe acute respiratory syndrome virus. *N. Engl. J. Med.* **350:**1731–1739.

183. **Yuan, K., L. Yi, J. Chen, X. Qu, T. Qing, X. Rao, P. Jiang, J. Hu, Z. Xiong, Y. Nie, X. Shi, W. Wang, C. Ling, X. Yin, K. Fan, L. Lai, M. Ding, and H. Deng.** 2004. Suppression of SARS-CoV entry by peptides corresponding to heptad regions on spike glycoprotein. *Biochem. Biophys. Res. Commun.* **319:** 746–752.

184. **Yudin, M. H., D. M. Steele, M. D. Sgro, S. E. Read, P. Kopplin, and K. A. Gough.** 2005. Severe acute respiratory syndrome in pregnancy. *Obstet. Gynecol.* **105:**124–127.

185. **Zeng, F., K. Y. Chow, C. C. Hon, K. M. Law, C. W. Yip, K. H. Chan, J. S. Peiris, and F. C. Leung.** 2004. Characterization of humoral responses in mice immunized with plasmid DNAs encoding SARS-CoV spike gene fragments. *Biochem. Biophys. Res. Commun.* **315:**1134–1139.

186. **Zhang, Y., T. Li, L. Fu, C. Yu, Y. Li, X. Xu, Y. Wang, H. Ning, S. Zhang, W. Chen, L. A. Babiuk, and Z. Chang.** 2004. Silencing SARS-CoV Spike protein expression in cultured cells by RNA interference. *FEBS Lett.* **560:**141–146.

187. **Zhang, Z., F. S. Wang, M. Zhao, J. C. Liu, D. P. Xu, L. Jin, J. M. Chen, M. Wang, and F. L. Chu.** 2004. Characterization of peripheral dendritic cell subsets and its implication in patients infected with severe acute respiratory syndrome. *Zhonghua Yi Xue Za Zhi* **84:**22–26.

188. **Zheng, B., M. L. He, K. L. Wong, C. T. Lum, L. L. Poon, Y. Peng, Y. Guan, M. C. Lin, and H. F. Kung.** 2004. Potent inhibition of SARS-associated coronavirus (SCOV) infection and replication by type I interferons (IFN-alpha/beta) but not by type II interferon (IFN-gamma). *J. Interferon Cytokine Res.* **24:**388–390.

189. **Zhong, N. S., and G. Q. Zeng.** 2003. Our strategies for fighting severe acute respiratory syndrome (SARS). *Am. J. Respir. Crit. Care. Med.* **168:**7–9.

190. **Zhong, N. S., B. J. Zheng, Y. M. Li, L. L. M. Poon, Z. H. Xie, K. H. Chan, P. H. Li, S. Y. Tan, Q. Chang, J. P. Xie, X. Q. Liu, J. Xu, D. X. Li, K. Y. Yuen, J. S. M. Peiris, and Y. Guan.** 2003. Epidemiology and cause of severe acute respiratory syndrome (SARS) in Guangdong, People's Republic of China, in February, 2003. *Lancet* **362:**1353–1358.

191. **Zhu, J., G. Xiao, Y. Xu, F. Yuan, C. Zheng, Y. Liu, H. Yan, D. K. Cole, J. I. Bell, Z. Rao, P. Tien, and G. F. Gao.** 2004. Following the rule: formation of the 6-helix bundle of the fusion core from severe acute respiratory syndrome coronavirus spike protein and identification of potent peptide inhibitors. *Biochem. Biophys. Res. Commun.* **319:**283–288.

Emerging Infections 7
Edited by W. M. Scheld, D. C. Hooper, and J. M. Hughes
© 2007 ASM Press, Washington, D.C.

Chapter 3

Human Metapneumovirus

Bernadette G. van den Hoogen, Albert D. M. E. Osterhaus, and Ron A. M. Fouchier

DISCOVERY OF A NEW PARAMYXOVIRUS

The subfamilies *Paramyxovirinae* and *Pneumovirinae* of the family *Paramyxoviridae* include several major pathogens of humans and animals. The *Pneumovirinae* are taxonomically divided into the genera *Pneumovirus* and *Metapneumovirus* (30). Human respiratory syncytial virus (RSV), the type species of the genus *Pneumovirus,* is the single most important cause of lower respiratory tract infections (RTIs) during infancy and early childhood worldwide (14). Avian pneumovirus (APV) is the etiological agent of an upper RTI of turkeys and, until 2001, was the sole member of the genus *Metapneumovirus* (9). The classification of the two genera is based primarily on their gene constellations: metapneumoviruses lack the nonstructural proteins NS1 and NS2, and the gene order is different from that of pneumoviruses (see below for gene identifications) (RSV, 3'-NS1-NS2-N-P-M-SH-G-F-M2-L-5'; APV, 3'-N-P-M-F-M2-SH-G-L-5') (47, 62, 95). Until 2001, metapneumoviruses had not been associated with infections or disease in mammals.

Acute respiratory infections are the most common illnesses experienced by people of all ages worldwide (55). In past decades, a wide variety of etiological agents of RTI were identified, but a significant proportion still cannot be attributed to known pathogens. In 2001, a previously unknown virus was isolated from 28 hospitalized children who suffered from severe RTIs that were epidemiologically unrelated (80). Electron microscopy analyses and classical virology studies revealed that this new virus belonged to the family *Paramyxoviridae,* and genetic analyses revealed sequence similarities with APV and a genomic organization identical to that of APV. Based on these similarities, the virus was classified as the first mammalian member of the genus *Metapneumovirus*; hence its name, human metapneumovirus (hMPV) (79, 80) (Fig. 1). Despite the homologies between APV and hMPV, the latter virus does not replicate in turkeys and chickens. Moreover, seroprevalence studies have demonstrated that hMPV has circulated for at least 50 years in the

Bernadette G. van den Hoogen, Albert D. M. E. Osterhaus, and Ron A. M. Fouchier • Department of Virology, Erasmus MC, Dr. Molewaterplein 50, 3015 GE Rotterdam, The Netherlands.

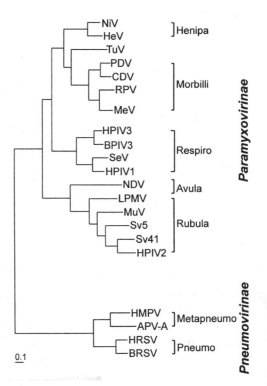

Figure 1. Phylogenetic analysis of the polymerase open reading frames of hMPV and selected paramyxoviruses. The tree was generated by maximum likelihood analyses using 100 bootstraps and three jumbles. The scale bars roughly represent 10% nucleotide changes between close relatives. NiV, Nipah virus; HeV, Hendra virus; TuV, Tupaia virus; PDV, phocine distemper virus; CDV, canine distemper virus; RPV, rinderpest virus; MeV, measles virus; SeV, Sendai virus; NDV, Newcastle disease virus; LPMV, porcine rubulavirus; MuV, mumps virus; Sv5, simian virus 5; Sv41, simian virus 41; APV-A, avian pneumovirus type A; B, bovine; H, human.

human population (80). It is thus likely that hMPV emerged in humans a long time ago after a zoonosis caused by APV and has since been endemic in humans.

GENETIC AND ANTIGENIC CHARACTERISTICS OF hMPV

The genome of hMPV consists of a single negative strand of RNA of approximately 13 kb that contains eight genes and codes for at least nine different proteins—the nucleoprotein (N), phosphoprotein (P), matrix protein (M), fusion protein (F), putative transcription elongation factor (M2.1), putative RNA synthesis regulatory factor (M2.2), small hydrophobic protein (SH), attachment glycoprotein (G), and large polymerase subunit (L)—in the order 3′-N-P-M-F-M2.1-M2.2-SH-G-L-5′ (79). When hMPV was first described as the causative agent of RTI in children, at least two lineages were identified, which have subsequently been reported to circulate around the globe (80).

Genetic analyses of the F and G genes of numerous hMPV isolates identified two main genetic lineages (A and B), each divided into two sublineages (A1, A2, B1, and B2). Whereas the F protein revealed approximately 95% amino acid sequence identity between viruses from the two lineages, the G protein showed only 30% identity (81). Sequences obtained for the complete genomes of viruses from the two lineages revealed overall 80 to 81% nucleotide sequence identity, with 92 to 93% identity between strains belonging to the same main lineage (81). The G and SH proteins are the most divergent between the two main lineages, and the G protein is even more divergent than between human RSV types A and B (Table 1).

Table 1. Percent amino acid sequence identities between the putative proteins of prototype viruses belonging to the different lineages of hMPV

Lineage	% Amino acid identity between putative proteins								
	N	P	M	F	M2.1	M2.2	SH	G	L
A1 vs A2	99	96	99	98	96	96	83	65	99
B1 vs B2	98	96	100	99	98	99	83	65	99
A vs B	96	86	97	94	95	98	60	30	94

Viruses from the four lineages have been detected worldwide, and some studies have indicated that there are differences in dominance between the lineages from year to year (1, 23, 49). Although these studies are limited, this could imply that the genetic lineages of the virus enable evasion of herd immunity. For the design of optimal diagnostic, therapeutic, and preventive strategies, it is important to determine whether the genetic diversity is related to antigenic diversity.

Virus neutralization assays using virus lineage-specific ferret antisera collected shortly after infection demonstrated a 12- to more than 100-fold difference in virus neutralization titers between viruses from the two main lineages (Table 2). Classical virology studies have used a definition of a homologous-to-heterologous virus neutralization titer of more than 16 as a definition of serotypes. On the basis of this definition, the large antigenic differences, and the high sequence divergence between the two main lineages, two serotypes (A and B) of hMPV were defined (81). In studies with sera collected after experimental infection of hamsters and nonhuman primates, large differences in virus-neutralizing antibody titers were not observed, but antibody titers against the homologous virus were somewhat higher than against the heterologous virus (74). Upon experimental infection, hamsters and nonhuman primates were protected from reinfection with either serotype when challenged 6 weeks after the primary infection (73, 77). This contrasts with a study of cynomolgus macaques challenged 3 to 8 months after the primary infection, which were not protected from either homologous or heterologous infection in the upper respiratory tract (unpublished data).

Seroprevalence studies among humans in different age categories have demonstrated that reinfections with hMPV occur frequently, and virus incidence studies have detected both homologous and heterologous reinfections; one heterologous reinfection was re-

Table 2. Virus-neutralizing antibody titers using ferret antisera obtained 21 days after infection with hMPV isolates belonging to different genetic hMPV lineages

Virus	Titer with ferret antisera raised against lineage:	
	A	B
Lineage A	256–768	6–32
Lineage B	12–64	256–512
A/B ratio	12–24	
B/A ratio		16–43

ported within 1 month after the primary infection in an otherwise healthy infant (15, 16, 46, 80). These reinfections in young children are no surprise, since it is well established that children mount a poor antibody response upon primary respiratory-virus infection (11). Seroprevalence studies have indicated that all children at the age of 5 years have antibodies to the virus. Despite this observation, severe hMPV infections are detected in the adult population (21, 80). These data suggest that reinfections can occur throughout life due to incomplete protective immune responses and/or acquisition of new genotypes.

At this time, little is known about the immunological response of young infants after an hMPV infection, i.e., whether they produce a neutralizing-antibody response or to what proteins these antibodies are directed. A potential future vaccine should provide long-term protection against both virus lineages and should aim to induce protection better than that induced by natural infection. The F protein could represent a good vaccine target protein, as it is the most conserved membrane protein between the different hMPV lineages (73, 81). In addition, it has been demonstrated in animal studies that the F protein is able to induce a highly cross-reactive and cross-protective immune response (73, 77, 78).

LABORATORY DIAGNOSIS OF hMPV INFECTIONS

Because hMPV replicates poorly in conventional cell cultures used for respiratory-virus diagnosis, the virus circulated unnoticed for quite some time. The virus is dependent on trypsin in cell culture medium and is highly sensitive to freeze-thawing. After the original isolation of hMPV on tertiary monkey kidney cells, several laboratories showed that LLC-MK_2 and Vero cell lines are permissive (13, 50). However, hMPV replicates inefficiently, and primary virus isolation often requires blind passages in these cell lines. Because cytopathic effects are difficult to observe, immunostaining is often necessary. Immunofluorescence staining of clinical specimens is a method commonly used in clinical virology laboratories for rapid diagnosis (31). These antigen detection assays have been described for the detection of hMPV, based on monoclonal antibodies against the hMPV fusion and matrix proteins (17, 24, 43, 60). It is anticipated that these monoclonal antibodies could be incorporated into antibody pools to screen for multiple respiratory viruses in shell vial centrifugation cultures.

The identification of the two genetic lineages of hMPV has implications for the development of both serological tests and reverse transcription (RT)-PCR assays. Serological tests based on prototype viruses from one lineage are less sensitive in detecting viruses with different antigenic properties, indicating that mixtures of antigens should be used in developing diagnostic tests. For instance, virus neutralization assays with a lineage A virus did not detect antibodies against the lineage B virus in nonhuman primates (74).

For seroprevalence studies, enzyme-linked immunosorbent assays have been developed, based on recombinant hMPV proteins (32, 46). It is important to note that, using a recombinant nucleoprotein of both lineages of hMPV, higher titers against the homologous virus than against the heterologous virus were detected (26).

For RT-PCR assays, it is important to design primers based on regions that are conserved between viruses of the four genetic lineages. Assays based on genetic information of one lineage are sometimes unable to detect the other lineages (1), but good PCR-based methods have been described recently (51). Finally, since the two lineages are highly variable, continuous monitoring of the circulating genotypes is required to keep the assays up to date.

CLINICAL IMPACT OF hMPV INFECTIONS

After the discovery of hMPV as an etiologic agent of RTI and the development of diagnostic assays, worldwide surveys were initiated to reveal the clinical impact of hMPV infections. These surveys demonstrated that the virus circulates on every continent and primarily among the pediatric population.

hMPV in Hospitalized Children

Several studies have confirmed the original observation that children younger than 5 years of age are most susceptible to hospitalization due to hMPV infection (22, 52, 59, 66, 83). In this population, hMPV is the second most commonly detected respiratory virus after RSV, accounting for approximately 5 to 25% of the reported RTIs (7, 56, 82). The incidence depends on a number of factors, such as the season, the collection and detection methods used, inclusion criteria for the cohorts, and whether other respiratory viruses were included in the surveys (Table 3).

Researchers at Vanderbilt University Medical Center have evaluated the role of hMPV in lower RTIs among otherwise healthy hospitalized children under the age of 5 prospectively over more than 20 years. hMPV was the causative agent in 12% of the lower RTIs (88). In addition, hMPV was detected in 5% of the children suffering from upper RTIs (92). In our study of hospitalized patients of all ages, we detected hMPV in 6.5% of the patients suffering from RTIs. Most of the hMPV infections were found in children younger than 5 years, and the peak ages for hMPV infections were between 6 and 9 months (82). An Italian study of hospitalized children during three consecutive winter seasons detected hMPV in 12.2, 9.9, and 26.1% of the samples in the respective years. The majority of the infections occurred in children during the first 3 months of life (23). During a 22-month surveillance of hospitalized patients at the St. Louis Children's Hospital, Agapov et al. detected hMPV in 5.4% of 3,740 specimens, with 58% of the positive samples obtained from children under the age of 2 years, 21% from children between 2 and 5 years old, and 21% from patients older than 5 years (1).

The combined results of the studies conducted among children indicate that the peak age for hMPV infection in otherwise healthy children, leading to severe disease requiring hospitalization, is between 6 and 12 months. In contrast, the peak age for RSV-induced severe disease is between 2 and 4 months (6, 56, 82, 88, 92) (Table 3).

hMPV in Elderly and Immunocompromised Individuals

Like RSV and influenza virus infections, hMPV infections also account for RTIs in the elderly and in patients with underlying disease or impaired immunity. In our study, most of the hMPV-positive patients between the ages of 5 and 65 years ($n = 13$) either had an underlying disease or received immunotherapy (82). Other studies of patients hospitalized for RTI reported that 25 to 50% of the hMPV-positive patients were suffering from underlying diseases. Numerous studies reported hMPV infection in patients with a specified underlying disease, such as lung transplant patients (41, 44), patients with hematologic malignancies and patients receiving hematopoietic stem cell transplantation (53, 89), and patients with asthma or preexisting lung diseases (27, 34, 65, 84, 87, 90). One study of the elderly indicated that hMPV caused more severe disease in frail elderly patients, such as nursing home residents, than in elderly or younger adults who were "fit" (21).

Table 3. Detection of hMPV in studies conducted on samples obtained in a variety of study groups, seasons, and locations

Reference[a]	Country	Study period	Study group	No.	No. (%) hMPV positive	Peak age	Peak period
Hospital							
56	United States	August 2000–September 2001	<5 yr; RTI	668	26 (3.9)	11.5 mo	March–April
82	The Netherlands	October 2000–March 2002	All ages; RTI	681	47 (7)	4–6 mo	December–January
19	United States	November 2001–October 2002	<5 yr; RTI	668	54 (8.1)	7.5 mo	March
22	France	November 2001–February 2002	Children; RTI	337	26 (6.6)	3 mo–12 yr	December–January
59	Hong Kong	August 2001–March 2002	<18 yr; RTI	587	32 (5.5)	3–72 mo	Respiratory infection season
7	France	September 2001–June 2002	<2 yr; bronchiolitis	94	6 (6.4)	2–6 mo	January
52	Italy	January 2000–May 2002	<2 yr; RTI			7.8 mo	Respiratory infection season
		2000		19	7 (37)		
		2001		41	3 (7)		
		2002		30	13 (43)		
83	Germany	January–May 2002	<2 yr; RTI	63	11 (17.5)		January–April
23	Italy	2001–2004	Children; RTI				
		2001–2002		261	11 (4.2)		
		2002–2003		241	8 (3.3)		
		2003–2004		306	31 (10.1)		

16	Japan	October 2002–May 2003	<12 yr; RTI	353	31 (8.8)	1–3 yr	March–April
88	United States	1982–2002	<5 yr; upper RTI	2,384	118 (5)	20 mo	December–May
92	United States	1976–2002	<5 yr; lower RTI	408	49 (12)	11.6 mo	December–April
36	United Kingdom	2001–2003	Adults; RTI	373	20 (5.4)		
General community							
54	United States	October 2000–August 2002	<18 yr; RTI	868	54 (6.2)	3–24 mo	January–February
75	United Kingdom	October 2000–March 2001	All ages; ILI	405	9 (2.2)	0–>65 yr	December
67	Japan	Winter 2002–2003	All ages; ILI	1,498	84 (5.6)	3 adults; 2 elderly	
20	United States	January–April 2004	>18 yr; RTI	146	5 (3.4)		
			>18 yr; healthy	158	0		
48	United States	January–March 2002	>18 yr; RTI	266	4 (2)	41.8 yr	
36	United Kingdom	November 2001–February 2002	>18 yr; RTI	219	28 (12.8)	>66 yr	
		November 2002–February 2003		216	16 (7.4)		
8	Canada	2001	All ages; RTI	1,125	41 (3.6)	9 mo	January–March
64	Canada	2002–2003	<17 yr; RTI	1,079	42 (3.9)		January–April
85	Denmark	November 1999–May 2000	<15 yr; ARTI[b]	374	11 (2.9)	1–6 mo	February–March

[a]See references for study groups.
[b]ARTI, acute respiratory tract illness.

These combined studies have demonstrated that hMPV has a major role in causing severe RTI in immunocompromised individuals and in patients with impaired immunity or underlying disease, as has been shown for RSV and influenza virus.

Although hospitalized adults suffering from severe RTI due to hMPV infection are in most cases patients with underlying disease or with impaired immunity, healthy adults are also at risk for severe disease resulting in hospitalization. Kaye et al. reported the presence of hMPV in 5.4% of adults hospitalized for severe RTI, with positive samples across all age groups, with the exception of those aged 45 to 54 years (36).

hMPV in the General Community

In the general community, both young adults and the elderly suffer from hMPV infections that lead to medically attended illnesses, with incidence rates ranging from 1 to 9%. However, frail elderly people with hMPV infections appear to seek medical attention more frequently (1, 8, 16, 19–21, 36, 48, 54, 64). In the United Kingdom, 1.3% of patients presenting to family physicians with influenza-like illnesses (ILI) were positive for hMPV (75). This study did not include all RTIs but was limited to samples from patients with ILI who were negative for other viruses. A study evaluating 167 adult volunteers younger than 40 years of age during home visits for respiratory disease detected hMPV in 6.6% of the patients (21). It is important to note that hMPV is rarely detected in patients hospitalized for other diseases or in patients seeing a physician for complaints other than RTI, indicating that asymptomatic or subclinical infections are rare (80, 82, 86).

Seasonality of hMPV Infections

Whereas some of the respiratory viruses, such as parainfluenza viruses and rhinoviruses, may circulate throughout the year, others, such as RSV and influenza viruses, circulate mainly during the winter season in temperate regions and in the late-spring-summer season in subtropical areas.

Year-round surveillance studies have demonstrated that hMPV infections occur mainly during the winter in temperate regions and in the late spring and summer in the subtropics, similar to RSV and influenza viruses (52, 57, 59, 82). In some studies, the peak of hMPV epidemics coincides with that of RSV or influenza virus (8, 64), while in other studies, hMPV epidemics occur somewhat later (1, 19, 42, 54, 82).

In most epidemiological studies, RSV is the most common cause of bronchiolitis in the first half of the winter RSV epidemics, while in the second half, hMPV and RSV may occur with equal frequency. When hMPV epidemics start after the RSV season, hMPV is often the primary cause of bronchiolitis among pediatric patients (88).

Although hMPV epidemics peak in the winter, the virus has been detected throughout the year, including the summer months. This is in contrast to RSV and influenza virus, whose epidemics are generally restricted to the winter (8, 16, 19, 64, 82, 88, 92).

hMPV causes yearly epidemics of RTI; however, the incidences vary from year to year or between locations, as is seen for RSV epidemics (23, 49, 52, 67). For example, in a 25-year surveillance of patients with lower RTIs, Williams et al. reported incidences varying from 0 to 31% in a given year (88, 92).

Nosocomial Infections

Transmission of nosocomial respiratory viruses is usually seasonal, with the peak incidence occurring in the winter months, mirroring the disease activity in the community. Pediatric units and wards with elderly and immunosuppressed individuals are particularly prone to seasonal introductions and nosocomial spread of viral infection. hMPV is the second most commonly detected pathogen after RSV in pediatric wards and has been detected as frequently as RSV in immunocompromised individuals, and it is thus no surprise that nosocomial hMPV infections have been reported (8, 18). In a study by Williams et al., nosocomial infections were reported for 45% of the infections (89). These findings should influence the protocols for prevention of nosocomial infections followed in many health care facilities for children with RTIs, such as patient isolation and cohort criteria. Finally, it indicates that timely diagnosis of hMPV is crucial to prevent nosocomial infections.

CLINICAL MANIFESTATIONS OF hMPV INFECTIONS

A wide spectrum of clinical symptoms associated with hMPV infection has been reported in patients of all ages, ranging from mild upper RTI to severe lower RTI requiring hospitalization (82, 88, 92). Clinical symptoms in hMPV-infected children have included fever, nonproductive cough, rhinorrhea, wheezing, and dyspnea. The resulting diagnoses may range from rhinopharyngitis to bronchiolitis and/or pneumonia and asthma-associated illnesses. In addition, diarrhea, vomiting, rash, febrile seizures, feeding difficulties, conjunctivitis, and, in a high percentage of the patients, otitis media have been reported. Although hMPV-related diseases range from mild to severe in young infants, virus infections in immunocompromised individuals or patients with underlying disease, such as asthma, can be extremely severe, and a number of deaths related to hMPV infection in such patients have been reported (8, 18, 58, 59). hMPV was also detected as the only pathogen in postmortem samples from the brain and lungs of a patient with fatal encephalitis (69). This result, in addition to the development of febrile seizures and convulsions reported in hMPV-infected children (35, 59, 76), suggests that a clinical study of central nervous system complications, such as febrile seizures, meningitis, and encephalopathy, is warranted.

The wide spectrum of hMPV-induced illnesses reported thus far is similar to those caused by RSV and influenza virus infections. When comparing the clinical symptoms associated with hMPV infections with those associated with RSV infections, most studies have not found statistically significant differences, although hMPV infections may tend to be slightly milder than RSV infections (18, 57, 82, 83, 85). For example, when we compared the clinical symptoms of 25 hMPV-infected children with those of age-matched RSV-infected children, we could not discriminate between clinical symptoms caused by RSV and those caused by hMPV, although dyspnea, hypoxemia, and feeding difficulties were found more often in RSV-infected individuals than in hMPV-infected patients. In addition, hMPV patients had 38% of all recorded symptoms compared to 50% for the RSV-infected children, indicating that hMPV infections may be slightly milder than RSV infections. However, some studies have observed that hMPV is associated with pneumonia and/or lower RTI more frequently than RSV (5, 52) and hMPV infection has been associated with several cases of severe pneumonitis leading to death (59).

In the general population, the virus has been associated with influenza-like illnesses and colds in healthy adults (67, 75). Falsey et al. observed a higher rate of influenza-like illnesses among young adults, although older adults experienced more dyspnea and wheezing, and those with cardiopulmonary conditions were ill for nearly twice as long as younger adults (21).

Association of hMPV with Asthma

The role of viral respiratory tract infections in acute and chronic asthma has been the subject of much debate and research. Viruses such as RSV and rhinoviruses, in particular, have been suggested as the principal triggers of asthma exacerbation in older children and adults, and after the discovery of hMPV, several studies have indicated an association between hMPV infection and asthma (34, 56, 65, 84, 85, 87, 90, 92). For instance, von Linstow et al. reported a diagnosis of asthmatic bronchitis in 66.7% of hMPV-infected patients and in 10.6% of RSV-infected children (85). Williams et al. demonstrated a significant association between hMPV infection and wheezing in children younger than 3 years, especially during the midwinter months (90). In contrast, in children 3 years of age and older, no significant association was detected, but instead, rhinovirus was detected most often. These researchers showed that hMPV is also associated with acute asthma exacerbation in adults (88). In contrast, other studies have found asthma to be more frequently associated with rhinoviruses than with hMPV (33, 63). Studies aiming at the identification of an association between RSV and/or hMPV and asthma are problematic, since asthma is a difficult clinical diagnosis in children younger than 2 years of age, the population most at risk of severe infection. Although hMPV is frequently detected in patients with asthma exacerbations, and one of the profound clinical signs of hMPV infection is wheezing, it is not yet clear whether the virus is associated with the induction of asthma.

Coinfection with hMPV and Other Respiratory Viruses

Many respiratory viruses share seasonality and susceptible populations; therefore, it is not surprising that coinfections with RSV, parainfluenza virus, and influenza virus are detected at a high frequency in various sample sets. However, it is uncertain whether coinfections predispose for more severe disease. A few reports have suggested that hMPV-RSV coinfections occur frequently and cause more severe disease than infection with either virus alone (25, 38, 71). Other studies did not detect high frequencies of hMPV-RSV coinfections, or if they did, did not report disease features other than those seen in patients with a single virus infection (7, 19, 45, 94). Care should be taken with the diagnosis of coinfections. Sensitive RT-PCR assays may enable the detection of viral genomes during two consecutive infections, which may be mistaken for double infections.

Based on the detection of hMPV in severe acute respiratory syndrome (SARS) patients in different parts of the world, hMPV has also been suggested to play a role in SARS. However, a novel coronavirus was isolated from far more SARS patients and was identified as the primary causative agent. In addition, studies of macaques have revealed that hMPV did not cause the lesions associated with SARS, whereas the SARS coronavirus did. This same study showed that in cynomolgus macaques, the disease caused by the SARS coronavirus was not enhanced upon subsequent inoculation with hMPV (39).

Although the role of double infections with hMPV remains elusive, it is certain that hMPV infection alone can cause severe disease, just as RSV can.

It is currently not known whether a significant association exists between hMPV infection and bacterial infections. hMPV-induced lower RTI is associated with a high frequency of otitis media requiring antibiotics in children, suggesting an association between hMPV and bacterial infection, but the true extent of this association remains to be elucidated (70, 76, 92).

ANIMAL MODELS TO STUDY hMPV INFECTIONS

To study host responses and the virological, immunological, and pathological features of hMPV infections, several animal models are available. Ferrets, guinea pigs, hamsters, and rabbits are used to produce virus-specific antibodies to the virus (17, 50, 74, 80, 81). Syrian golden hamsters are the most commonly used small-animal model in infection experiments, since the virus replicates in the respiratory tracts of these animals to reasonable titers, and the animals develop a virus-specific antibody response (50, 91). The results obtained in mouse and cotton rat models are contradictory. Some groups reported the permissiveness of BALB/c mice and/or cotton rats (12, 28, 91, 93), whereas others did not detect virus replication in these animals (50, 91) or detected viral genomes for more than 60 days after experimental infection of mice (2, 3). These discrepancies may reflect the use of different virus strains, animals, or infection methods.

For a number of studies, it is necessary to use nonhuman primates. Both cynomolgus macaques and African green monkeys support virus replication in the respiratory tract, and these infections result in the induction of virus-specific immune responses (40, 50, 74).

DEVELOPMENT OF ANTIBODY THERAPY AND VACCINATION

The clinical impact of hMPV in the pediatric and elderly populations has resulted in efforts to generate (live attenuated) hMPV vaccines, as well as neutralizing hMPV monoclonal antibodies, by a number of research institutions worldwide. For the pneumoviruses, such as RSV and hMPV, the F and G proteins are the main targets for the neutralizing and protective antibody response, with the F protein being one of the most conserved proteins and G the most variable. Recently, reverse-genetics techniques have been designed to recover infectious virus from cDNA clones of hMPV (4, 29). These reverse-genetics systems provide a powerful tool for the generation of vaccine candidates, including live attenuated vaccines, because point mutations, deletions, and insertions can be engineered to suit specific needs. For instance, these techniques are now used to develop live attenuated vaccines by deleting nonessential genes, such as M2, G, or SH, and such viruses have been found to induce protective antibodies in animals (4, 68).

By using reverse genetics, it is possible to combat RTI in humans by construction of chimeric viruses between hMPV and other human respiratory pathogens, such as RSV and parainfluenza virus. For instance, a chimeric virus has been constructed based on the backbone of parainfluenza virus type 3 (PIV-3) by inserting the immunogenic F protein of hMPV. This virus was found to induce protective antibody titers against PIV-3 and both hMPV types, and after vaccination, nonhuman primates were protected from infection with both viruses upon challenge (77, 78). Another example of such a chimeric virus involved the insertion of the N and/or P protein of APV in the backbone of hMPV. These viruses were slightly attenuated in hamsters and African green monkeys and induced neutralizing serum antibodies, and the animals were protected against hMPV infection (61).

hMPV vaccine development might encounter problems similar to those of RSV vaccine development; the use of formalin-inactivated RSV vaccines and the enhanced disease observed upon subsequent natural infection have been major complications of RSV vaccine development (37). For RSV, these problems have led to the exploration of different vaccine candidates, such as subunit vaccines based on the RSV F and/or G protein (reviewed in reference 10). These subunit products are not particularly immunogenic in young infants; however, they are suitable for immunization of previously infected patients who are at high risk of severe disease, or the elderly. Similar approaches may be developed for hMPV.

For RSV, the prophylactic use of a virus-neutralizing monoclonal antibody preparation directed against the F protein has been shown to decrease the severity of lower respiratory tract diseases (72). It is anticipated that similar reagents targeting the conserved F protein of hMPV will become available for prophylactic treatment of hMPV infections.

CONCLUSIONS

Epidemiological studies for the detection of etiologic agents of RTI detect a causative agent in 50 to 85% of the specimens, primarily depending on the skills of the laboratory involved. Studies so far have shown that with the discovery of hMPV, a substantial proportion of unknown causes of RTI have been resolved. It is highly likely that other unknown agents are responsible for a proportion of the remaining unidentified samples.

At this time, at least two circulating serotypes of hMPV have been identified, and this variability must be taken into account in the development of diagnostic tests and possibly in the development of intervention strategies and vaccines.

hMPV accounts for approximately 5 to 15% of RTIs in hospitalized children, with high incidences during epidemics in the winter months in moderate climate zones and late spring-early summer in the subtropics. Only RSV, and occasionally influenza virus, was detected more frequently in the studies that included surveys for other respiratory viruses. Very young children (under the age of 2), people with underlying disease, the immunocompromised, and the fragile elderly are most at risk for hMPV infections; thus, the virus shares its susceptible population with RSV (Fig. 2). Surveillance in the general community showed that 1 to 9% of the samples from individuals seeing physicians for RTIs were positive for hMPV, and serological studies indicate that hMPV may cause a self-limiting "common

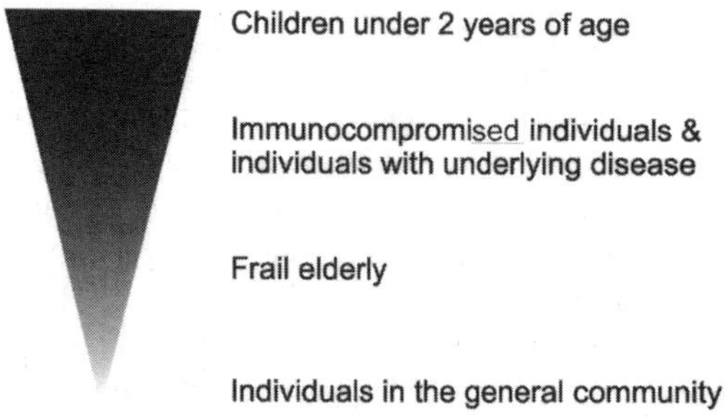

Children under 2 years of age

Immunocompromised individuals & individuals with underlying disease

Frail elderly

Individuals in the general community

Figure 2. Risk populations for hMPV-induced severe disease.

cold" among adults. The spectrum of clinical symptoms observed in hMPV-infected individuals is comparable to that in RSV-infected individuals, ranging from common-cold-like symptoms in the general community to severe pneumonia in hospitalized patients. At present, RSV and hMPV infections cannot be discriminated on the basis of clinical signs.

Although it has become clear that young children and patients with underlying disease or impaired immunity are most at risk for severe hMPV infections, limited data are available on the clinical impact of hMPV in the elderly. Prospective and retrospective studies must be conducted to obtain a better understanding of the clinical impact of hMPV infections in the elderly.

In addition, the preliminary results on the association between asthma and hMPV infections and the possible consequences of coinfection of hMPV and RSV (and other respiratory viruses) for the severity of disease warrant further research. Only limited data are available on the host response against hMPV. For evaluation of the host response to future vaccines, immune-pathology studies must reveal more information on the host response.

REFERENCES

1. **Agapov, E., K. C. Sumino, M. Gaudreault-Keener, G. A. Storch, and M. J. Holtzman.** 2006. Genetic variability of human metapneumovirus infection: evidence of a shift in viral genotype without a change in illness. *J. Infect. Dis.* **193:**396–403.
2. **Alvarez, R., K. S. Harrod, W. J. Shieh, S. Zaki, and R. A. Tripp.** 2004. Human metapneumovirus persists in BALB/c mice despite the presence of neutralizing antibodies. *J. Virol.* **78:**14003–14011.
3. **Alvarez, R., and R. A. Tripp.** 2005. The immune response to human metapneumovirus is associated with aberrant immunity and impaired virus clearance in BALB/c mice. *J. Virol.* **79:**5971–5978.
4. **Biacchesi, S., M. H. Skiadopoulos, K. C. Tran, B. R. Murphy, P. L. Collins, and U. J. Buchholz.** 2004. Recovery of human metapneumovirus from cDNA: optimization of growth in vitro and expression of additional genes. *Virology* **321:**247–259.
5. **Boivin, G., Y. Abed, G. Pelletier, L. Ruel, D. Moisan, S. Cote, T. C. Peret, D. D. Erdman, and L. J. Anderson.** 2002. Virological features and clinical manifestations associated with human metapneumovirus: a new paramyxovirus responsible for acute respiratory-tract infections in all age groups. *J. Infect. Dis.* **186:**1330–1334.
6. **Bosis, S., S. Esposito, H. G. Niesters, P. Crovari, A. D. Osterhaus, and N. Principi.** 2005. Impact of human metapneumovirus in childhood: comparison with respiratory syncytial virus and influenza viruses. *J. Med. Virol.* **75:**101–104.
7. **Bouscambert-Duchamp, M., B. Lina, A. Trompette, H. Moret, J. Motte, and L. Andreoletti.** 2005. Detection of human metapneumovirus RNA sequences in nasopharyngeal aspirates of young French children with acute bronchiolitis by real-time reverse transcriptase PCR and phylogenetic analysis. *J. Clin. Microbiol.* **43:**1411–1414.
8. **Chano, F., C. Rousseau, C. Laferriere, M. Couillard, and H. Charest.** 2005. Epidemiological survey of human metapneumovirus infection in a large pediatric tertiary care center. *J. Clin. Microbiol.* **43:**5520–5525.
9. **Cook, J. K.** 2000. Avian rhinotracheitis. *Rev. Sci. Technol.* **19:**602–613.
10. **Crowe, J. E. J.** 2001. Respiratory syncytial virus vaccine development. *Vaccine* **20**(Suppl. 1)**:**S32–S37.
11. **Crowe, J. E. J., and J. V. Williams.** 2003. Immunology of viral respiratory tract infection in infancy. *Paediatr. Respir. Rev.* **4:**112–119.
12. **Darniot, M., T. Petrella, S. Aho, P. Pothier, and C. Manoha.** 2005. Immune response and alteration of pulmonary function after primary human metapneumovirus (hMPV) infection of BALB/c mice. *Vaccine* **23:**4473–4480.
13. **Deffrasnes, C., S. Cote, and G. Boivin.** 2005. Analysis of replication kinetics of the human metapneumovirus in different cell lines by real-time PCR. *J. Clin. Microbiol.* **43:**488–490.
14. **Domachowske, J. B., and H. F. Rosenberg.** 1999. Respiratory syncytial virus infection: immune response, immunopathogenesis, and treatment. *Clin. Microbiol. Rev.* **12:**298–309.

15. **Ebihara, T., R. Endo, N. Ishiguro, T. Nakayama, H. Sawada, and H. Kikuta.** 2004. Early reinfection with human metapneumovirus in an infant. *J. Clin. Microbiol.* **42:**5944–5946.

16. **Ebihara, T., R. Endo, H. Kikuta, N. Ishiguro, H. Ishiko, M. Hara, Y. Takahashi, and K. Kobayashi.** 2004. Human metapneumovirus infection in Japanese children. *J. Clin. Microbiol.* **42:**126–132.

17. **Ebihara, T., R. Endo, X. Ma, N. Ishiguro, and H. Kikuta.** 2005. Detection of human metapneumovirus antigens in nasopharyngeal secretions by an immunofluorescent-antibody test. *J. Clin. Microbiol.* **43:**1138–1141.

18. **Esper, F., D. Boucher, C. Weibel, R. A. Martinello, and J. S. Kahn.** 2003. Human metapneumovirus infection in the United States: clinical manifestations associated with a newly emerging respiratory infection in children. *Pediatrics* **111:**1407–1410.

19. **Esper, F., R. A. Martinello, D. Boucher, C. Weibel, D. Ferguson, M. L. Landry, and J. S. Kahn.** 2004. A 1-year experience with human metapneumovirus in children aged <5 years. *J. Infect. Dis.* **189:**1388–1396.

20. **Falsey, A. R., M. C. Criddle, and E. E. Walsh.** 2006. Detection of respiratory syncytial virus and human metapneumovirus by reverse transcription polymerase chain reaction in adults with and without respiratory illness. *J. Clin. Virol.* **35:**46–50.

21. **Falsey, A. R., D. Erdman, L. J. Anderson, and E. E. Walsh.** 2003. Human metapneumovirus infections in young and elderly adults. *J. Infect. Dis.* **187:**785–790.

22. **Freymouth, F., A. Vabret, L. Legrand, N. Eterradossi, F. Lafay-Delaire, J. Brouard, and B. Guillois.** 2003. Presence of the new human metapneumovirus in French children with bronchiolitis. *Pediatr. Infect. Dis. J.* **22:**92–94.

23. **Gerna, G., G. Campanini, F. Rovida, A. Sarasini, D. Lilleri, S. Paolucci, A. Marchi, F. Baldanti, and M. G. Revello.** 2005. Changing circulation rate of human metapneumovirus strains and types among hospitalized pediatric patients during three consecutive winter-spring seasons. *Arch. Virol.* **150:**2365–2375.

24. **Gerna, G., A. Sarasini, E. Percivalle, E. Genini, G. Campanini, and R. M. Grazia.** 2006. Simultaneous detection and typing of human metapneumovirus strains in nasopharyngeal secretions and cell cultures by monoclonal antibodies. *J. Clin. Virol.* **35:**113–116.

25. **Greensill, J., P. S. McNamara, W. Dove, B. Flanagan, R. L. Smyth, and C. A. Hart.** 2003. Human metapneumovirus in severe respiratory syncytial virus bronchiolitis. *Emerg. Infect. Dis.* **9:**372–375.

26. **Hamelin, M. E., and G. Boivin.** 2005. Development and validation of an enzyme-linked immunosorbent assay for human metapneumovirus serology based on a recombinant viral protein. *Clin. Diagn. Lab. Immunol.* **12:**249–253.

27. **Hamelin, M. E., S. Cote, J. Laforge, N. Lampron, J. Bourbeau, K. Weiss, R. Gilca, G. DeSerres, and G. Boivin.** 2005. Human metapneumovirus infection in adults with community-acquired pneumonia and exacerbation of chronic obstructive pulmonary disease. *Clin. Infect. Dis.* **41:**498–502.

28. **Hamelin, M. E., K. Yim, K. H. Kuhn, R. P. Cragin, M. Boukhvalova, J. C. Blanco, G. A. Prince, and G. Boivin.** 2005. Pathogenesis of human metapneumovirus lung infection in BALB/c mice and cotton rats. *J. Virol.* **79:**8894–8903.

29. **Herfst, S., M. de Graaf, J. H. Schickli, R. S. Tang, J. Kaur, C. F. Yang, R. R. Spaete, A. A. Haller, B. G. van den Hoogen, A. D. Osterhaus, and R. A. Fouchier.** 2004. Recovery of human metapneumovirus genetic lineages A and B from cloned cDNA. *J. Virol.* **78:**8264–8270.

30. **International Committee on Taxonomy of Viruses.** 2000. *Virus Taxonomy: Seventh Report of the International Committee on Taxonomy of Viruses.* Academic Press, San Diego, Calif.

31. **Irmen, K. E., and J. J. Kelleher.** 2000. Use of monoclonal antibodies for rapid diagnosis of respiratory viruses in a community hospital. *Clin. Diagn. Lab. Immunol.* **7:**396–403.

32. **Ishiguro, N., T. Ebihara, R. Endo, X. Ma, R. Shirotsuki, S. Ochiai, H. Ishiko, and H. Kikuta.** 2005. Immunofluorescence assay for detection of human metapneumovirus-specific antibodies by use of baculovirus-expressed fusion protein. *Clin. Diagn. Lab. Immunol.* **12:**202–205.

33. **Jartti, T., P. Lehtinen, T. Vuorinen, R. Osterback, B. G. van den Hoogen, A. D. Osterhaus, and O. Ruuskanen.** 2004. Respiratory picornaviruses and respiratory syncytial virus as causative agents of acute expiratory wheezing in children. *Emerg. Infect. Dis.* **10:**1095–1101.

34. **Jartti, T., B. van den Hoogen, R. P. Garofalo, A. D. Osterhaus, and O. Ruuskanen.** 2002. Metapneumovirus and acute wheezing in children. *Lancet* **360:**1393–1394.

35. **Kashiwa, H., H. Shimozono, and S. Takao.** 2004. Clinical pictures of children with human metapneumovirus infection: comparison with respiratory syncytial virus infection. *Jpn. J. Infect. Dis.* **57:**80–82.

36. **Kaye, M., S. Skidmore, H. Osman, M. Weinbren, and R. Warren.** 3 January 2006. Surveillance of respiratory virus infections in adult hospital admissions using rapid methods. *Epidemiol. Infect.* [Online.] doi: 10.1017/S0950268805005364.

37. **Kim, H. W., J. G. Canchola, C. D. Brandt, G. Pyles, R. M. Chanock, K. Jensen, and R. H. Parrott.** 1969. Respiratory syncytial virus disease in infants despite prior administration of antigenic inactivated vaccine. *Am. J. Epidemiol.* **89:**422–434.

38. **Konig, B., W. Konig, R. Arnold, H. Werchau, G. Ihorst, and J. Forster.** 2004. Prospective study of human metapneumovirus infection in children less than 3 years of age. *J. Clin. Microbiol.* **42:**4632–4635.

39. **Kuiken, T., R. A. Fouchier, M. Schutten, G. F. Rimmelzwaan, G. van Amerongen, D. van Riel, J. D. Laman, T. de Jong, G. van Doornum, W. Lim, A. E. Ling, P. K. Chan, J. S. Tam, M. C. Zambon, R. Gopal, C. Drosten, S. van der Werf, N. Escriou, J. C. Manuguerra, K. Stohr, J. S. Peiris, and A. D. Osterhaus.** 2003. Newly discovered coronavirus as the primary cause of severe acute respiratory syndrome. *Lancet* **362:**263–270.

40. **Kuiken, T., B. G. van den Hoogen, D. A. van Riel, J. D. Laman, G. van Amerongen, L. Sprong, R. A. Fouchier, and A. D. Osterhaus.** 2004. Experimental human metapneumovirus infection of cynomolgus macaques (*Macaca fascicularis*) results in virus replication in ciliated epithelial cells and pneumocytes with associated lesions throughout the respiratory tract. *Am. J. Pathol.* **164:**1893–1900.

41. **Kumar, D., D. Erdman, S. Keshavjee, T. Peret, R. Tellier, D. Hadjiliadis, G. Johnson, M. Ayers, D. Siegal, and A. Humar.** 2005. Clinical impact of community-acquired respiratory viruses on bronchiolitis obliterans after lung transplant. *Am. J. Transplant.* **5:**2031–2036.

42. **Laham, F. R., V. Israele, J. M. Casellas, A. M. Garcia, C. M. Lac Prugent, S. J. Hoffman, D. Hauer, B. Thumar, M. I. Name, A. Pascual, N. Taratutto, M. T. Ishida, M. Balduzzi, M. Maccarone, S. Jackli, R. Passarino, R. A. Gaivironsky, R. A. Karron, N. R. Polack, and F. P. Polack.** 2004. Differential production of inflammatory cytokines in primary infection with human metapneumovirus and with other common respiratory viruses of infancy. *J. Infect. Dis.* **189:**2047–2056.

43. **Landry, M. L., D. Ferguson, S. Cohen, T. C. Peret, and D. D. Erdman.** 2005. Detection of human metapneumovirus in clinical samples by immunofluorescence staining of shell vial centrifugation cultures prepared from three different cell lines. *J. Clin. Microbiol.* **43:**1950–1952.

44. **Larcher, C., C. Geltner, H. Fischer, D. Nachbaur, L. C. Muller, and H. P. Huemer.** 2005. Human metapneumovirus infection in lung transplant recipients: clinical presentation and epidemiology. *J. Heart Lung Transplant.* **24:**1891–1901.

45. **Lazar, I., C. Weibel, J. Dziura, D. Ferguson, M. L. Landry, and J. S. Kahn.** 2004. Human metapneumovirus and severity of respiratory syncytial virus disease. *Emerg. Infect. Dis.* **10:**1318–1320.

46. **Leung, J., F. Esper, C. Weibel, and J. S. Kahn.** 2005. Seroepidemiology of human metapneumovirus (hMPV) on the basis of a novel enzyme-linked immunosorbent assay utilizing hMPV fusion protein expressed in recombinant vesicular stomatitis virus. *J. Clin. Microbiol.* **43:**1213–1219.

47. **Ling, R., A. J. Easton, and C. R. Pringle.** 1992. Sequence analysis of the 22K, SH and G genes of turkey rhinotracheitis virus and their intergenic regions reveals a gene order different from that of other pneumoviruses. *J. Gen. Virol.* **73:**1709–1715.

48. **Louie, J. K., J. K. Hacker, R. Gonzales, J. Mark, J. H. Maselli, S. Yagi, and W. L. Drew.** 2005. Characterization of viral agents causing acute respiratory infection in a San Francisco University Medical Center Clinic during the influenza season. *Clin. Infect. Dis.* **41:**822–828.

49. **Ludewick, H. P., Y. Abed, N. van Niekerk, G. Boivin, K. P. Klugman, and S. A. Madhi.** 2005. Human metapneumovirus genetic variability, South Africa. *Emerg. Infect. Dis.* **11:**1074–1078.

50. **MacPhail, M., J. H. Schickli, R. S. Tang, J. Kaur, C. Robinson, R. A. Fouchier, A. D. Osterhaus, R. R. Spaete, and A. A. Haller.** 2004. Identification of small-animal and primate models for evaluation of vaccine candidates for human metapneumovirus (hMPV) and implications for hMPV vaccine design. *J. Gen. Virol.* **85:**1655–1663.

51. **Maertzdorf, J., C. K. Wang, J. B. Brown, J. D. Quinto, M. Chu, M. de Graaf, B. G. van den Hoogen, R. Spaete, A. D. Osterhaus, and R. A. Fouchier.** 2004. Real-time reverse transcriptase PCR assay for detection of human metapneumoviruses from all known genetic lineages. *J. Clin. Microbiol.* **42:**981–986.

52. **Maggi, F., M. Pifferi, M. Vatteroni, C. Fornai, E. Tempestini, S. Anzilotti, L. Lanini, E. Andreoli, V. Ragazzo, M. Pistello, S. Specter, and M. Bendinelli.** 2003. Human metapneumovirus associated with respiratory tract infections in a 3-year study of nasal swabs from infants in Italy. *J. Clin. Microbiol.* **41:**2987–2991.

53. **Martino, R., R. P. Porras, N. Rabella, J. V. Williams, E. Ramila, N. Margall, R. Labeaga, J. E. Crowe, Jr., P. Coll, and J. Sierra.** 2005. Prospective study of the incidence, clinical features, and outcome of symptomatic upper and lower respiratory tract infections by respiratory viruses in adult recipients of hematopoietic stem cell transplants for hematologic malignancies. *Biol. Blood Marrow Transplant.* **11:** 781–796.

54. **McAdam, A. J., M. E. Hasenbein, H. A. Feldman, S. E. Cole, J. T. Offermann, A. M. Riley, and T. A. Lieu.** 2004. Human metapneumovirus in children tested at a tertiary-care hospital. *J. Infect. Dis.* **190:**20–26.

55. **Monto, A. S.** 2002. Epidemiology of viral respiratory infections. *Am. J. Med.* **112**(Suppl. 6A)**:**4S–12S.

56. **Mullins, J. A., D. D. Erdman, G. A. Weinberg, K. Edwards, C. B. Hall, F. J. Walker, M. Iwane, and L. J. Anderson.** 2004. Human metapneumovirus infection among children hospitalized with acute respiratory illness. *Emerg. Infect. Dis.* **10:**700–705.

57. **Nissen, M. D., D. J. Siebert, I. M. Mackay, T. P. Sloots, and S. J. Withers.** 2002. Evidence of human metapneumovirus in Australian children. *Med. J. Aust.* **176:**188.

58. **Noyola, D. E., A. G. Alpuche-Solis, A. Herrera-Diaz, R. E. Soria-Guerra, J. Sanchez-Alvarado, and R. Lopez-Revilla.** 2005. Human metapneumovirus infections in Mexico: epidemiological and clinical characteristics. *J. Med. Microbiol.* **54:**969–974.

59. **Peiris, J. S., W. H. Tang, K. H. Chan, P. L. Khong, Y. Guan, Y. L. Lau, and S. S. Chiu.** 2003. Children with respiratory disease associated with metapneumovirus in Hong Kong. *Emerg. Infect. Dis.* **9:**628–633.

60. **Percivalle, E., A. Sarasini, L. Visai, M. G. Revello, and G. Gerna.** 2005. Rapid detection of human metapneumovirus strains in nasopharyngeal aspirates and shell vial cultures by monoclonal antibodies. *J. Clin. Microbiol.* **43:**3443–3446.

61. **Pham, Q. N., S. Biacchesi, M. H. Skiadopoulos, B. R. Murphy, P. L. Collins, and U. J. Buchholz.** 2005. Chimeric recombinant human metapneumoviruses with the nucleoprotein or phosphoprotein open reading frame replaced by that of avian metapneumovirus exhibit improved growth in vitro and attenuation in vivo. *J. Virol.* **79:**15114–15122.

62. **Randhawa, J. S., A. C. Marriott, C. R. Pringle, and A. J. Easton.** 1997. Rescue of synthetic minireplicons establishes the absence of the NS1 and NS2 genes from avian pneumovirus. *J. Virol.* **71:**9849–9854.

63. **Rawlinson, W. D., Z. Waliuzzaman, I. W. Carter, Y. C. Belessis, K. M. Gilbert, and J. R. Morton.** 2003. Asthma exacerbations in children associated with rhinovirus but not human metapneumovirus infection. *J. Infect. Dis.* **187:**1314–1318.

64. **Robinson, J. L., B. E. Lee, N. Bastien, and Y. Li.** 2005. Seasonality and clinical features of human metapneumovirus infection in children in Northern Alberta. *J. Med. Virol.* **76:**98–105.

65. **Rohde, G., I. Borg, U. Arinir, J. Kronsbein, R. Rausse, T. T. Bauer, A. Bufe, and G. Schultze-Werninghaus.** 2005. Relevance of human metapneumovirus in exacerbations of COPD. *Respir. Res.* **6:**150.

66. **Samransamruajkit, R., W. Thanasugarn, N. Prapphal, A. Theamboonlers, and Y. Poovorawan.** 2006. Human metapneumovirus in infants and young children in Thailand with lower respiratory tract infections; molecular characteristics and clinical presentations. *J Infect.* **52:**254–263.

67. **Sasaki, A., H. Suzuki, R. Saito, M. Sato, I. Sato, Y. Sano, and M. Uchiyama.** 2005. Prevalence of human metapneumovirus and influenza virus infections among Japanese children during two successive winters. *Pediatr. Infect. Dis. J.* **24:**905–908.

68. **Schickli, J. H., J. Kaur, N. Ulbrandt, R. R. Spaete, and R. S. Tang.** 2005. An S101P substitution in the putative cleavage motif of the human metapneumovirus fusion protein is a major determinant for trypsin-independent growth in Vero cells and does not alter tissue tropism in hamsters. *J. Virol.* **79:**10678–10689.

69. **Schildgen, O., T. Glatzel, T. Geikowski, B. Scheibner, B. Matz, L. Bindl, M. Born, S. Viazov, A. Wilkesmann, G. Knopfle, M. Roggendorf, and A. Simon.** 2005. Human metapneumovirus RNA in encephalitis patient. *Emerg. Infect. Dis.* **11:**467–470.

70. **Schildgen, O., and A. Simon.** 2005. Induction of acute otitis media by human metapneumovirus. *Pediatr. Infect. Dis. J.* **24:**1126.

71. **Semple, M. G., A. Cowell, W. Dove, J. Greensill, P. S. McNamara, C. Halfhide, P. Shears, R. L. Smyth, and C. A. Hart.** 2005. Dual infection of infants by human metapneumovirus and human respiratory syncytial virus is strongly associated with severe bronchiolitis. *J. Infect. Dis.* **191:**382–386.

72. **Simoes, E. A.** 1999. Respiratory syncytial virus infection. *Lancet* **354:**847–852.

73. **Skiadopoulos, M. H., S. Biacchesi, U. J. Buchholz, E. Amaro-Carambot, S. R. Surman, P. L. Collins, and B. R. Murphy.** 2006. Individual contributions of the human metapneumovirus F, G, and SH surface glycoproteins to the induction of neutralizing antibodies and protective immunity. *Virology* **345:**492–501.

74. **Skiadopoulos, M. H., S. Biacchesi, U. J. Buchholz, J. M. Riggs, S. R. Surman, E. Amaro-Carambot, J. M. McAuliffe, W. R. Elkins, M. St. Claire, P. L. Collins, and B. R. Murphy.** 2004. The two major human metapneumovirus genetic lineages are highly related antigenically, and the fusion (F) protein is a major contributor to this antigenic relatedness. *J. Virol.* **78:**6927–6937.

75. **Stockton, J., I. Stephenson, D. Fleming, and M. Zambon.** 2002. Human metapneumovirus as a cause of community-acquired respiratory illness. *Emerg. Infect. Dis.* **8:**897–901.

76. **Suzuki, A., O. Watanabe, M. Okamoto, H. Endo, H. Yano, M. Suetake, and H. Nishimura.** 2005. Detection of human metapneumovirus from children with acute otitis media. *Pediatr. Infect. Dis. J.* **24:** 655–657.

77. **Tang, R. S., K. Mahmood, M. MacPhail, J. M. Guzzetta, A. A. Haller, H. Liu, J. Kaur, H. A. Lawlor, E. A. Stillman, J. H. Schickli, R. A. Fouchier, A. D. Osterhaus, and R. R. Spaete.** 2005. A host-range restricted parainfluenza virus type 3 (PIV3) expressing the human metapneumovirus (hMPV) fusion protein elicits protective immunity in African green monkeys. *Vaccine* **23:**1657–1667.

78. **Tang, R. S., J. H. Schickli, M. MacPhail, F. Fernandes, L. Bicha, J. Spaete, R. A. Fouchier, A. D. Osterhaus, R. Spaete, and A. A. Haller.** 2003. Effects of human metapneumovirus and respiratory syncytial virus antigen insertion in two 3′ proximal genome positions of bovine/human parainfluenza virus type 3 on virus replication and immunogenicity. *J. Virol.* **77:**10819–10828.

79. **van den Hoogen, B. G., T. M. Bestebroer, A. D. Osterhaus, and R. A. Fouchier.** 2002. Analysis of the genomic sequence of a human metapneumovirus. *Virology* **295:**119–132.

80. **van den Hoogen, B. G., J. C. de Jong, J. Groen, T. Kuiken, R. de Groot, R. A. Fouchier, and A. D. Osterhaus.** 2001. A newly discovered human pneumovirus isolated from young children with respiratory tract disease. *Nat. Med.* **7:**719–724.

81. **van den Hoogen, B. G., S. Herfst, L. Sprong, P. A. Cane, E. Forleo-Neto, R. L. de Swart, A. D. Osterhaus, and R. A. Fouchier.** 2004. Antigenic and genetic variability of human metapneumoviruses. *Emerg. Infect. Dis.* **10:**658–666.

82. **van den Hoogen, B. G., G. J. van Doornum, J. C. Fockens, J. J. Cornelissen, W. E. Beyer, R. R. Groot, A. D. Osterhaus, and R. A. Fouchier.** 2003. Prevalence and clinical symptoms of human metapneumovirus infection in hospitalized patients. *J. Infect. Dis.* **188:**1571–1577.

83. **Viazov, S., F. Ratjen, R. Scheidhauer, M. Fiedler, and M. Roggendorf.** 2003. High prevalence of human metapneumovirus infection in young children and genetic heterogeneity of the viral isolates. *J. Clin. Microbiol.* **41:**3043–3045.

84. **Vicente, D., M. Montes, G. Cilla, and E. Perez-Trallero.** 2004. Human metapneumovirus and chronic obstructive pulmonary disease. *Emerg. Infect. Dis.* **10:**1338–1339.

85. **von Linstow, M. L., L. H. Henrik, J. Eugen-Olsen, A. Koch, W. T. Nordmann, A. M. Meyer, H. Westh, B. Lundgren, M. Melbye, and B. Hogh.** 2004. Human metapneumovirus and respiratory syncytial virus in hospitalized Danish children with acute respiratory tract infection. *Scand. J. Infect. Dis.* **36:**578–584.

86. **Wilbrink, B., B. G. van den Hoogen, D. Dekker, H. Boswijk, H. van der Nat, and M. L. A. Heijnen.** 2002. Humaan metapneumovirus, een nieuw ontdekt virus; voorkomen in de ARI-EL studie. *Infectieziekten Bull.* **9:**360–361.

87. **Williams, J. V., J. E. Crowe, Jr., R. Enriquez, P. Minton, R. S. Peebles, Jr., R. G. Hamilton, S. Higgins, M. Griffin, and T. V. Hartert.** 2005. Human metapneumovirus infection plays an etiologic role in acute asthma exacerbations requiring hospitalization in adults. *J. Infect. Dis.* **192:**1149–1153.

88. **Williams, J. V., P. A. Harris, S. J. Tollefson, L. L. Halburnt-Rush, J. M. Pingsterhaus, K. M. Edwards, P. F. Wright, and J. E. Crowe, Jr.** 2004. Human metapneumovirus and lower respiratory tract disease in otherwise healthy infants and children. *N. Engl. J. Med.* **350:**443–450.

89. **Williams, J. V., R. Martino, N. Rabella, M. Otegui, R. Parody, J. M. Heck, and J. E. Crowe, Jr.** 2005. A prospective study comparing human metapneumovirus with other respiratory viruses in adults with hematologic malignancies and respiratory tract infections. *J. Infect. Dis.* **192:**1061–1065.

90. **Williams, J. V., S. J. Tollefson, P. W. Heymann, H. T. Carper, J. Patrie, and J. E. Crowe.** 2005. Human metapneumovirus infection in children hospitalized for wheezing. *J. Allergy Clin. Immunol.* **115:**1311–1312.

91. **Williams, J. V., S. J. Tollefson, J. E. Johnson, and J. E. Crowe, Jr.** 2005. The cotton rat (*Sigmodon hispidus*) is a permissive small animal model of human metapneumovirus infection, pathogenesis, and protective immunity. *J. Virol.* **79:**10944–10951.

92. **Williams, J. V., C. K. Wang, C. F. Yang, S. J. Tollefson, F. S. House, J. M. Heck, M. Chu, J. B. Brown, L. D. Lintao, J. D. Quinto, D. Chu, R. R. Spaete, K. M. Edwards, P. F. Wright, and J. E. Crowe, Jr.**

2006. The role of human metapneumovirus in upper respiratory tract infections in children: a 20-year experience. *J. Infect. Dis.* **193:**387–395.

93. **Wyde, P. R., S. N. Chetty, A. M. Jewell, S. L. Schoonover, and P. A. Piedra.** 2005. Development of a cotton rat-human metapneumovirus (hMPV) model for identifying and evaluating potential hMPV antivirals and vaccines. *Antivir. Res.* **66:**57–66.

94. **Xepapadaki, P., S. Psarras, A. Bossios, M. Tsolia, D. Gourgiotis, G. Liapi-Adamidou, A. G. Constantopoulos, D. Kafetzis, and N. G. Papadopoulos.** 2004. Human metapneumovirus as a causative agent of acute bronchiolitis in infants. *J. Clin. Virol.* **30:**267–270.

95. **Yu, Q., P. J. Davis, J. Li, and D. Cavanagh.** 1992. Cloning and sequencing of the matrix protein (M) gene of turkey rhinotracheitis virus reveal a gene order different from that of respiratory syncytial virus. *Virology* **186:**426–434.

Emerging Infections 7
Edited by W. M. Scheld, D. C. Hooper, and J. M. Hughes
© 2007 ASM Press, Washington, D.C.

Chapter 4

Changing Patterns of Respiratory Viral Infections in Transplant Recipients

Michael G. Ison and Jay A. Fishman

Advances in the care of immunocompromised hosts have been driven by the development of a variety of increasingly potent immunosuppressive agents for use in solid-organ and hematopoietic stem cell transplant recipients. With the intensification of immunosuppressive and chemotherapeutic regimens, infections have replaced graft rejection and graft failure as the main complications of these therapies. Renal-transplant recipients, for example, can expect to have an 89 to 96% 1-year graft survival and 66 to 79% 5-year graft survival (82). Routine prophylaxis with trimethoprim-sulfamethoxazole and antiviral agents has reduced the incidence of *Pneumocystis* pneumonia, nocardiosis, and respiratory, urinary, and gastrointestinal infections due to susceptible pathogens and cytomegalovirus (CMV) infection (24, 97). Other infectious diseases, notably those caused by the respiratory viruses, are increasingly recognized as important in transplant recipients. A group of newer pathogens that may merit consideration in the differential diagnosis of immunocompromised hosts with infectious syndromes has been described recently.

EPIDEMIOLOGY OF RESPIRATORY VIRAL INFECTIONS

General Principles

The incidence of respiratory viral infection is poorly defined. There have been few prospective studies of respiratory viral infection using the most sensitive assays available for viral detection. In addition, most studies have been limited to selected populations, usually stem cell transplant recipients or lung transplant recipients. The estimated incidence rates of respiratory viral infections are listed in Table 1. The frequency of asymptomatic infections is under investigation but is generally thought to exceed the rate of symptomatic disease. For example, in a recent study of CMV infection in solid-organ

Michael G. Ison • Transplant Infectious Diseases Service, Northwestern University Feinberg School of Medicine, 676 North St. Clair Street, Suite 200, Chicago, IL 60611.   ***Jay A. Fishman*** • Transplant Infectious Disease and Compromised Host Program, Infectious Diseases Division, Massachusetts General Hospital, Harvard Medical School, Boston, MA 02114.

Table 1. Estimated annual incidences of respiratory viral infections in transplant recipients[a]

Virus	Incidence (%)	
	Stem cell transplant	Solid-organ transplant
Influenza virus	11–23	10
Respiratory syncytial virus	35–49	12–38
Parainfluenza virus	9–30	8–43
Adenovirus	6	24
Rhinovirus	18–24	18
Multiple pathogens		14

[a]Source: references 47 and 48.

transplant recipients, adenovirus DNA was detected in 19 of 263 patients (7.2%), with viremia in 6.5 to 8.3% of liver, kidney, and heart recipients. Of viremic patients, 79% had few or no symptoms of infection. Only 21% had either gastrointestinal or respiratory complaints (46). Data from retrospective studies allow some generalizations about respiratory viral infections in transplant recipients.

1. The seasonal variability of each respiratory virus in immunocompromised hosts reflects that seen in the general community. As a result, influenza virus, respiratory syncytial virus (RSV), and human metapneumovirus (hMPV) generally cause disease from November through April in the Northern Hemisphere; rhinovirus typically circulates in the fall and spring; and adenovirus and parainfluenza virus circulate throughout the year (47, 48). Some cases may be observed earlier in immunocompromised hosts than in the general community as harbingers of an impending outbreak.
2. Respiratory viruses cause more severe disease with more frequent complications in immunocompromised individuals (47, 48). The true incidence of asymptomatic respiratory viral infection is unknown. Atypical presentations are common (e.g., adenovirus myocarditis) and may go unrecognized. Infections limited to the upper respiratory tract are rarely fatal, with higher mortality when infections progress to the lower respiratory tract, particularly in allogeneic stem cell transplant recipients (47, 48). Progression to lower respiratory tract disease occurs in 7 to 50% of stem cell transplant recipients and approximately 13% of solid-organ recipients infected with influenza virus (47, 48, 67). Lower respiratory tract disease may occur in the presence of negative screening assays for respiratory viruses (e.g., nasal swabs for antigen detection) (Fig. 1). In solid-organ transplant recipients, risk factors for progressive disease include early posttransplantation infection (during the period of most intensive immune suppression), high doses of corticosteroids, anti-lymphocyte antisera for immune suppression, and age of ≤1 year for solid-organ recipients (13). In allogeneic stem cell recipients, early posttransplantation

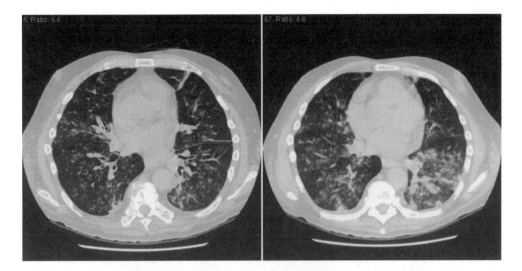

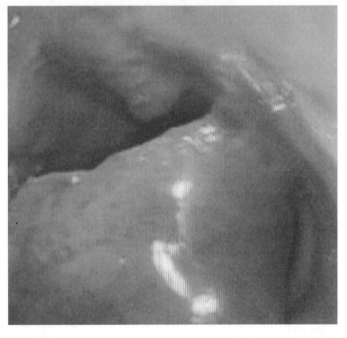

Figure 1. Adenovirus pneumonia in a hematopoietic stem cell transplant recipient. Nasal swabs and sputum were negative for adenovirus. (Top) Chest computed tomography scans reveal patchy consolidation and diffuse tree-in-bud opacities consistent with diffuse pneumonia. (Bottom) Severe bronchitis with pseudomembrane formation was observed on bronchoscopic examination with direct fluorescence of respiratory specimens positive for adenovirus serotype 4. Blood cultures and blood PCR were also positive for adenovirus.

infections, graft-versus-host disease, and lymphopenia have been associated with poor outcome from viral infections (65). Mortality in
influenza may be reduced if potent antiviral therapy is given early in
the course of disease, but prospective randomized trials are needed
(50, 57, 66, 79).

3. "Indirect effects" of viral infection in transplant recipients may include graft rejection or graft-versus-host disease, allograft injury,
and susceptibility to other opportunistic infections. Respiratory viral
infections, for example, are associated with a 2.1-fold-increased risk
of subsequent development of *Aspergillus* infections (72). Respiratory viral infections are a risk factor for graft rejection, particularly
chronic graft rejection in lung transplant recipients (4, 12, 26, 52,
109, 110). Respiratory viral infections of the lower respiratory tract,
but not the upper respiratory tract, predispose to bronchiolitis obliterans syndrome (BOS) in lung transplant patients (relative risk, 2.3;
95% confidence interval, 1.1 to 4.9) (4). There is a seasonal trend in
BOS that peaks shortly after the peak of winter respiratory viral infections, which suggests a link between respiratory viral infections
and BOS (47, 48). In a rat lung transplant model of Sendai virus infection, a virus related to parainfluenza virus, a link between lower
respiratory tract disease and development of BOS has been demonstrated (113). The pathogenesis of virally mediated rejection has not
been defined but may be related to direct damage to the tissue, enhanced immune reactivity (e.g., upregulation of histocompatibility
antigens), or the production of proinflammatory cytokines during infection (109).

4. The kinetics of infection are altered in the absence of normal immune function. Replication of respiratory viruses is more prolonged
in transplant recipients (47, 48). Viral shedding during influenza
virus infection lasts for 3 to 5 days in healthy, immunocompetent
adults, while shedding persists for 9 days in over 50% of allogeneic
stem cell transplant recipients, and shedding for several months has
been described (G. Nichols, personal communication). Prolonged
shedding carries increased risk for viral transmission, particularly
with viruses that produce limited symptoms during shedding, such as
rhinovirus (108). Further, prolongation of viral replication during
therapy risks the emergence of resistance to antiviral agents. Emergence of resistance to adamantane derivatives and, to a lesser extent,
neuraminidase inhibitors occurs more frequently in immunocompromised individuals than in healthy hosts (20, 31).

Diagnosis of Respiratory Viral Infections

The availability of molecular assays and viral-antigen detection testing has dramatically altered the clinical approach to respiratory viral infection. Viral culture remains necessary for susceptibility testing, viral typing, and identification of new pathogens.

However, laboratories are increasingly utilizing rapid testing methods for identification of respiratory viruses. The sensitivity of these assays is limited compared with that of molecular assays. In the absence of viral cultures, the risk exists that newer pathogens may go uninvestigated and undetected unless they present with unusual virulence or epidemiology compared with more common pathogens.

The yields of viral cultures by either cell culture or more rapid shell vial techniques are heavily influenced by specimen type, handling, storage of the source materials, target cells used, viral strain, and methods used for virus isolation. Recovery of virus may take days to weeks, and the data may be available too late for clinical utility.

Rapid antigen detection methods have been developed for RSV, influenza A and B viruses, and adenovirus. These tests have the advantage of being technically simple and rapid (results are provided within 15 to 30 minutes) but are of relatively low sensitivity, particularly in immunocompromised adults (21, 49). In immunocompetent patients, the sensitivity of the RSV rapid tests is greater in children than in adults (59 to 97% versus 0 to 25%) (80). The sensitivity of a rapid RSV antigen test (the Becton Dickinson Directogen kit) was compared to that of routine culture in 372 patients, including 398 nasal washes/throat swabs, 67 endotracheal aspirates, and 74 bronchoalveolar lavage (BAL) samples tested. Fifty-six samples had positive cultures for RSV, but only 19 (34%) of the culture-positive samples had positive rapid antigen test results. Compared to culture, the sensitivity of the antigen test was greatest for BAL samples (89%) and endotracheal aspirates (71%) but was exceptionally low (15%) for the nasal washes/throat swabs; specificity was greater than 97% for all sources (21). None of the influenza rapid antigen tests have been studied with immunocompromised hosts. For immunocompetent adults, the sensitivities have ranged widely (0 to 89%) (77, 85, 99, 115). Data on the sensitivity and specificity of adenovirus rapid testing are limited for compromised hosts. For all of the rapid tests, a negative test of the upper respiratory tract from an immunocompromised patient does not rule out the presence of disease; BAL fluid typically has the highest yield (Fig. 1).

Direct detection of viral antigens in respiratory tract specimens using monoclonal antibodies may have increased sensitivity compared with the rapid, commercially available methods. These assays appear to have diagnostic accuracies similar to that of PCR, but assays are available for only a limited number of pathogens. Direct fluorescent antibody assays may require more technician time and reagents than rapid antigen detection tests and generally cannot be done at the point of care (90).

PCR-based assays allow the rapid diagnosis of multiple agents simultaneously. Multiplex reverse transcription-PCR-enzyme hybridization assays (Hexaplex Plus) allow simultaneous detection of parainfluenza virus, influenza virus, respiratory syncytial virus, human metapneumovirus, and adenovirus with a sensitivity that may exceed that of culture or immunofluorescence test results for immunocompromised patients (62). The advantages of PCR over other methods for immunocompromised patients have been demonstrated in a number of recent studies (87, 90, 106–108).

Emerging Respiratory Viral Infections

Against the background of significant morbidity due to common community-acquired respiratory viruses in immunocompromised hosts, some newer pathogens have been described.

SARS

Severe acute respiratory syndrome (SARS) is discussed in detail in chapter 2. The possibility that immune status plays a pivotal role in the transmission of SARS was suggested by the identification of individuals who appeared to be "super spreaders" of infection. These individuals infected a number of secondary individuals, more than the average of 2.7 secondary cases. Corticosteroid treatment was associated with higher subsequent plasma viral loads, consistent with observations in patients with other respiratory viral infections. In the few transplant recipients infected with the SARS coronavirus, disease progression was more rapid than in healthy hosts. A 74-year-old male liver transplant recipient presented with asymmetric patchy pulmonary infiltrates, hypoxemia, and lymphopenia and died from progressive multiorgan system failure 18 days into his illness. A 57-year-old man 4 months after double lung transplantation developed fever, diarrhea, and dyspnea with pulmonary infiltrates and BAL positive for SARS coronavirus by PCR. This patient was the source of infection for numerous contacts (as a "super spreader"), including three health care workers. Of note, the viral loads in lung and heart tissues from this patient were at least 10,000-fold greater than those in the Toronto SARS cohort in general (A. Humar, personal communication). These observations suggest that viral loads may be higher and disease more aggressive in immunocompromised individuals than in healthy hosts.

Human Metapneumovirus

Until recently, the only known metapneumoviruses (see chapter 3) affected birds and were not associated with infections or disease in humans. van den Hoogen et al. identified a virus, termed hMPV, from 28 children with acute respiratory illnesses similar to those caused by RSV over a 20-year period in The Netherlands (103). Subsequently, hMPV has been recognized as a significant respiratory pathogen, particularly in children, throughout the world (34, 104). Unlike the SARS coronavirus, recent studies suggest that hMPV has been an unrecognized pathogen for as long as serologic samples have been available (103). There are two serospecific genotypes of hMPV found worldwide; the clinical diseases caused by these viruses are indistinguishable.

The virus produces a cytopathic effect indistinguishable from that of RSV in cell culture but takes up to 14 days to grow. The preferred method for the diagnosis of hMPV infection is by PCR (15, 16, 22, 68, 70). Serologic diagnosis may also be performed but is not useful acutely for diagnosis in immunocompromised hosts (35).

Clinically, hMPV infections have an epidemiology and presentation similar to those of RSV. Most children are exposed to hMPV during the first decade of life, with reinfection occurring throughout life. It is not known whether these recurrent infections represent incomplete protective immunity or acquisition of new viral genotypes. The peak incidence of disease is from December through May, although infection can occur throughout the year (112). The incidence of disease among hospitalized immunocompetent adults and children has generally been reported to be in the 5 to 10% range (34), although higher incidences have been demonstrated in single studies (71). Several transplant patients have had documented infections with hMPV.

Most infected young children present with nonspecific cough, coryza, and rhinitis. Over half present with fever, wheezing, and abnormal tympanic membranes, and over 40% have bronchiolitis or pneumonitis. Older children and adults often present with exacerbation of underlying reactive airway disease or an influenza-like illness (6, 23, 34,

69, 94, 104, 105, 112). The presence of other respiratory viral copathogens, particularly RSV, appears to predispose to lower respiratory tract disease and a more severe clinical course (30). Coinfection with RSV is associated with a 10-fold increase in the relative risk of admission to a pediatric intensive-care unit for mechanical ventilation compared to infection with hMPV alone (94). Proinflammatory cytokine levels are lower in hMPV infection than in RSV infections, despite the clinical similarities between the two diseases (54).

In immunocompromised hosts, the incidence of hMPV-related pneumonia is unknown. In some cases, it is associated with progressive infection indistinguishable from that of RSV, requiring mechanical ventilation and, uncommonly, causing death (6, 10, 60, 83).

Therapeutic options for hMPV infection are under investigation. Pooled immunoglobulin, but not palivizumab, appeared to neutralize hMPV in vitro but has not been studied in vivo (116). Ribavirin and a sulfated sialyl lipid (NMSO3) inhibit hMPV replication in vitro with 50% effective concentrations of 74 ± 35 µM and 4 ± 2 µg/ml, respectively (116, 118). A new animal model of hMPV pneumonia will allow testing of antiviral agents in vivo (117).

Adenovirus

Adenovirus has been identified as an increasingly important pathogen in immunocompromised hosts. Adenovirus infections are detected throughout the year, and most (65%) are diagnosed during the first 100 days posttransplantation (median time to diagnosis, 62 days). The incidence of adenoviral infection is between 3 and 29% in hematopoietic stem cell transplant (HSCT) recipients and 5 to 10% in solid-organ recipients (73, 76). High viral loads in symptomatic patients may be predictive of progression to disseminated disease (18). Lymphopenia is also a poor prognostic sign; adenovirus-specific CD4 T-cell responses and neutralizing-antibody titers increase with clearance of virus from the blood (39, 40). Studies have correlated a decline in viral load with clinical improvement, whether as the result of antivirals or of the host's immune response (39, 55, 59). The role of asymptomatic viremia or tissue infections remains unclear.

In the HSCT population, hemorrhagic cystitis is the most frequent manifestation of adenovirus infection; adenovirus type 11 is most frequently associated with hemorrhagic cystitis (1). Adenovirus is rarely recovered (3%) from the urine of asymptomatic HSCT patients compared to BK and JC polyomaviruses, which are frequently shed without pathology (30%). Of those patients without hemorrhagic cystitis, 19 to 24% had upper respiratory infections (median time to onset, 44 days posttransplantation; range, −2 to 179 days), 10 to 21% had enteritis (median onset, 37 days posttransplantation; range, −2 to 168 days), 18% had pneumonia, 9% had disseminated disease without pneumonia, and 5% had disseminated disease with pneumonia (56, 91). Diarrhea and fever were the most common manifestations of gastrointestinal involvement. Hepatitis (16% with serotype 1), pneumonitis (15% with serotype 7), and central nervous system (10% serotype 2) involvement (confusion and seizures) may occur. The mortality for symptomatic patients is 26 to 54%, and patients with disseminated disease and/or pneumonia have significant mortality (50 to 80%) (56, 91). Fatal outcomes may be more common with concurrent infection due to CMV, aspergillosis, and mixed bacteria. Severe disease is more common in those with acute graft-versus-host disease and donor adenovirus seropositivity. Antilymphocyte globulin conditioning was associated with earlier onset of disease (56, 91). Adenoviral infections may be complicated by graft failure or delayed engraftment and concurrent fungal infections in HSCT recipients (3, 33, 44).

In solid-organ transplant recipients, adenoviral disease may reflect either the absence of preformed immunity (in pediatric recipients), transmission with the transplanted organ, or reactivation of persistent, endogenous latent virus in adults. Adenoviral disease is best described in pediatric liver transplant recipients but is also described in individuals following kidney, small bowel, lung, and heart transplantation (2, 5, 53, 73, 76, 92, 95). Most studies have suggested a high risk of severe invasive disease in solid-organ recipients, with a high mortality. However, depending on the sensitivity of the assays used, asymptomatic viremia has also been observed.

In the liver transplant recipient population, adenovirus follows hepatitis C virus, hepatitis B virus, and CMV in frequency as a cause of posttransplantation hepatitis. One to 10% of pediatric liver transplant recipients develop adenovirus infection, while 5.8% of adult liver transplant recipients develop infection. Hepatitis is associated with viremia in most cases and may cause disseminated disease and death. Adenovirus infection is described in pediatric liver (4.1%) and intestinal (20.8%) transplant recipients, often by PCR testing of biopsy samples. In lung transplant recipients, adenovirus pneumonia generally occurs early after transplantation and is often fatal (81).

In lung and heart transplantation, adenovirus infection is associated with graft rejection and accelerated graft atherogenesis. In two series, adenovirus infection (by tissue PCR) was associated with apparent graft rejection, graft loss, and coronary vasculopathy (93, 95). In lung recipients, adenovirus infection is common and has been associated with graft failure and chronic rejection/bronchiolitis obliterans (8).

Therapeutic options for management of adenoviral infections are limited. Ribavirin, ganciclovir, and cidofovir have demonstrated variable activities against adenovirus (Table 2). Cidofovir is the most active agent but carries significant risk of nephrotoxicity in populations that have a high rate of preexisting renal dysfunction. In vitro testing of ribavirin has failed to document consistent antiviral activity (84); some activity against subgroup C adenovirus (serogroups 1, 2, 5, and 6) has been demonstrated, with 50% inhibitory concentrations (IC_{50}s) ranging from 20 to 136 μM (78). Recent studies of ribavirin have not supported clinical efficacy (55). Patients who do not receive ganciclovir to prevent cytomegalovirus infection in HSCT recipients have a higher risk of developing

Table 2. Available agents with activity against adenovirus

Compound (reference)[b]	Availability	IC_{50}[a] (μM)	Achievable concn
Ribavirin (84)	Commercial	12–>1,000	10.75–18 μg/liter
Cidofovir (17)	Commercial	8.5–100	7.3–19.6 μg/ml
Lipid esters of cidofovir (37)	Investigational	0.5–20	
HPMPA (37)	Investigational	0.5–22	
MMF	Commercial		3.7–24.1 μg/ml
Ganciclovir (96, 101)	Commercial	4.5–33	5.5–9 μg/ml
ddC (75)[c]	Commercial	0.05–0.83	7.6–25.2 ng/ml
Vidarabine (111)	Commercial	175–>700	

[a]IC_{50}s were determined using different viral serotypes, cell types, and techniques and may not be directly comparable.
[b]These compounds are FDA approved for other indications but are not FDA approved for adenovirus infections.
[c]ddC, dideoxycytosine.

adenoviral disease (odds ratio, 3.4; 95% confidence interval, 2.1 to 5.6; $P < 0.0001$) than those who receive prophylaxis (9). A prospective study of valganciclovir versus oral ganciclovir in solid-organ recipients found no apparent benefit against adenoviral disease (7.2% of the patients developed adenoviremia) (46).

Cidofovir is active against all tested serogroups of adenovirus, with in vitro IC_{50}s of 17 to 81 μM in Hep-2 cell lines (78). Animal models have likewise demonstrated efficacy against adenovirus keratoconjunctivitis (17, 27, 28, 42, 51, 88, 89). However, clinical responses to cidofovir (5 mg/kg of body weight every 1 to 2 weeks typically, with adequate hydration and probenecid) are highly variable, with survival rates of 50 to 80% (7, 11, 38, 58, 64, 86). Longer-term therapy with low-dose cidofovir (1 mg/kg three times a week) may minimize nephrotoxicity but requires up to 8 months for virus suppression (43). The absence of an early response to therapy appears to be a poor prognostic factor. Cidofovir is associated with significant nephrotoxicity (Fanconi-like tubular toxicity with heavy proteinuria) and hematologic toxicity (especially neutropenia). Lipid esters of cidofovir have been created and, in animal models, are orally bioavailable and associated with less toxicity and are significantly more active against virus in vitro (37). A compound related to cidofovir, HPMPA, and its lipid esters have also been tested and have significant activity in vitro, as well (50% effective concentration, 0.04 to 2.2 μM) (37). These new compounds are entering human trials.

Alternative therapies have been used in some patients with invasive adenovirus disease. Donor lymphocyte infusion has been attempted in some patients, with reports of clinical improvement (14, 45). Pooled intravenous immune globulins have been anecdotally associated with improvement in a few cases (19, 25).

Avian Influenza

Influenza remains an important cause of respiratory infection in healthy and immunocompromised individuals. Pandemics, which result from the introduction of a novel type A virus, have occurred three times over the past century, with consequent increased morbidity and mortality. It has been estimated that the next pandemic in the United States will result in 89,000 to 207,000 excess deaths, 314,000 to 734,000 excess hospitalizations, and 18 to 42 million excess clinic visits (74). Influenza A/H5N1 virus (see chapter 1), prevalent in wild birds and domesticated pigs in Asia, is commonly referred to as avian influenza and has caused intermittent outbreaks in humans. Avian influenza viruses are typically strains of low pathogenicity that are associated with mild or asymptomatic disease in migratory birds and waterfowl. Influenza A/H5N1 virus was first recognized as a human pathogen in 1997, when 18 patients became ill with a purely avian virus, A/H5N1, with six deaths in Hong Kong. Outbreaks were limited by widespread culling of chickens and waterfowl and apparently inefficient human-to-human spread of the virus (100). The virus has continued to mutate; the Z strain of A/H5N1 has emerged as the dominant strain in at least nine countries in Asia (61). As of April 2005, there had been 121 cases of avian influenza in humans (41), including at least one case of probable human-to-human transmission, and 79 deaths (102, 114).

It is unknown whether additional morbidity will be seen in immunocompromised hosts due to avian influenza. For influenza, transplant recipients generally have a more severe course with greater morbidity and mortality (47, 48). Vaccination is only partially protective in most immunocompromised individuals. HSCT recipients have a significantly lower response rate to influenza vaccination, with nearly no response in the first 6 to 12 months after transplantation (47, 48). Vaccination is recommended annually, as much of the burden of influenza is related to secondary superinfections, graft rejection (in lung transplant recipients), or graft-versus-host disease (in HSCT recipients).

Vaccines against H5N1 viruses are not yet available (63, 98). Neuraminidase inhibitors (oseltamivir and zanamivir) are active against all recognized strains of influenza A and B viruses, including avian influenza virus (29, 32). M2 protein inhibitors (amantadine and rimantadine) are active only against most influenza A virus strains, but not against avian H5N1 strains (29). Recent data from HSCT recipients has demonstrated that the neuraminidase inhibitors are both safe to use and effective in reducing progression to lower respiratory tract disease and death (50, 57, 66, 79). The efficacy of the neuraminidase inhibitors in solid-organ transplant recipients has not been studied. Although the neuraminidase inhibitors are very effective at preventing influenza virus infections in the immunocompetent patient (36), there are no published data on the safety and efficacy of these agents in immunocompromised patients.

CONCLUSIONS

Over the past 5 years, two new respiratory viruses that are clinically important to transplant recipients have been described: SARS coronavirus and human metapneumovirus. The clinical manifestations of these infections in the immunocompromised host include greater likelihood of progression to invasive disease and death, reflecting more persistent replication and viremia with higher viral loads. Prospective studies of therapeutic interventions are needed. Recent data on adenovirus infections suggest that asymptomatic viremia is common in immunocompromised individuals. The impacts of such infections remain undefined but appear to reflect that of cytomegalovirus infection, with indirect manifestations including acute and chronic graft rejection and graft loss and bacterial, viral, and fungal superinfections. Newer antiviral therapies are needed, given the toxicities of currently available agents. Reversal of immune suppression is an important component of therapy in the immunocompromised host. Assays that measure host immunity to common viruses in these populations are needed. Influenza remains a significant cause of morbidity and mortality in transplant recipients. Avian influenza has the potential to cause the next pandemic of infection. Neuraminidase inhibitors are safe and effective in HSCT recipients; therapeutic and prophylactic studies are needed in solid-organ recipients. Early treatment using neuraminidase inhibitors may prove useful against avian influenza; however, the optimal deployment (dose and duration) of these agents remains to be defined for immunocompromised hosts.

REFERENCES

1. **Akiyama, H., T. Kurosu, C. Sakashita, T. Inoue, S. Mori, K. Ohashi, S. Tanikawa, H. Sakamaki, Y. Onozawa, Q. Chen, H. Zheng, and T. Kitamura.** 2001. Adenovirus is a key pathogen in hemorrhagic cystitis associated with bone marrow transplantation. *Clin. Infect. Dis.* **32:**1325–1330.
2. **Ardehali, H., K. Volmar, C. Roberts, M. Forman, and L. C. Becker.** 2001. Fatal disseminated adenoviral infection in a renal transplant patient. *Transplantation* **71:**998–999.
3. **Baldwin, A., H. Kingman, M. Darville, A. B. Foot, D. Grier, J. M. Cornish, N. Goulden, A. Oakhill, D. H. Pamphilon, C. G. Steward, and D. I. Marks.** 2000. Outcome and clinical course of 100 patients with adenovirus infection following bone marrow transplantation. *Bone Marrow Transplant.* **26:**1333–1338.

4. **Billings, J. L., M. I. Hertz, K. Savik, and C. H. Wendt.** 2002. Respiratory viruses and chronic rejection in lung transplant recipients. *J. Heart Lung Transplant.* **21:**559–566.

5. **Blohme, I., G. Nyberg, S. Jeansson, and C. Svalander.** 1992. Adenovirus infection in a renal transplant patient. *Transplant. Proc.* **24:**295.

6. **Boivin, G., Y. Abed, G. Pelletier, L. Ruel, D. Moisan, S. Cote, T. C. Peret, D. D. Erdman, and L. J. Anderson.** 2002. Virological features and clinical manifestations associated with human metapneumovirus: a new paramyxovirus responsible for acute respiratory-tract infections in all age groups. *J. Infect. Dis.* **186:** 1330–1334.

7. **Bordigoni, P., A. S. Carret, V. Venard, F. Witz, and A. Le Faou.** 2001. Treatment of adenovirus infections in patients undergoing allogeneic hematopoietic stem cell transplantation. *Clin. Infect. Dis.* **32:**1290–1297.

8. **Bridges, N. D., T. L. Spray, M. H. Collins, N. E. Bowles, and J. A. Towbin.** 1998. Adenovirus infection in the lung results in graft failure after lung transplantation. *J. Thorac. Cardiovasc. Surg.* **116:**617–623.

9. **Bruno, B., T. Gooley, R. C. Hackman, C. Davis, L. Corey, and M. Boeckh.** 2003. Adenovirus infection in hematopoietic stem cell transplantation: effect of ganciclovir and impact on survival. *Biol. Blood Marrow Transplant.* **9:**341–352.

10. **Cane, P. A., B. G. van den Hoogen, S. Chakrabarti, C. D. Fegan, and A. D. Osterhaus.** 2003. Human metapneumovirus in a haematopoietic stem cell transplant recipient with fatal lower respiratory tract disease. *Bone Marrow Transplant.* **31:**309–310.

11. **Carter, B. A., S. J. Karpen, R. E. Quiros-Tejeira, I. F. Chang, B. S. Clark, G. J. Demmler, H. E. Heslop, J. D. Scott, P. Seu, and J. A. Goss.** 2002. Intravenous cidofovir therapy for disseminated adenovirus in a pediatric liver transplant recipient. *Transplantation* **74:**1050–1052.

12. **Chakinala, M. M., and M. J. Walter.** 2004. Community acquired respiratory viral infections after lung transplantation: clinical features and long-term consequences. *Semin. Thorac. Cardiovasc. Surg.* **16:**342–349.

13. **Chakrabarti, S., K. E. Collingham, T. Marshall, K. Holder, T. Gentle, G. Hale, C. D. Fegan, and D. W. Milligan.** 2001. Respiratory virus infections in adult T cell-depleted transplant recipients: the role of cellular immunity. *Transplantation* **72:**1460–1463.

14. **Chakrabarti, S., V. Mautner, H. Osman, K. E. Collingham, C. D. Fegan, P. E. Klapper, P. A. Moss, and D. W. Milligan.** 2002. Adenovirus infections following allogeneic stem cell transplantation: incidence and outcome in relation to graft manipulation, immunosuppression, and immune recovery. *Blood* **100:** 1619–1627.

15. **Cote, S., Y. Abed, and G. Boivin.** 2003. Comparative evaluation of real-time PCR assays for detection of the human metapneumovirus. *J. Clin. Microbiol.* **41:**3631–3635.

16. **Deffrasnes, C., S. Cote, and G. Boivin.** 2005. Analysis of replication kinetics of the human metapneumovirus in different cell lines by real-time PCR. *J. Clin. Microbiol.* **43:**488–490.

17. **de Oliveira, C. B., D. Stevenson, L. LaBree, P. J. McDonnell, and M. D. Trousdale.** 1996. Evaluation of cidofovir (HPMPC, GS-504) against adenovirus type 5 infection in vitro and in a New Zealand rabbit ocular model. *Antivir. Res.* **31:**165–172.

18. **Echavarria, M., M. Forman, M. J. van Tol, J. M. Vossen, P. Charache, and A. C. Kroes.** 2001. Prediction of severe disseminated adenovirus infection by serum PCR. *Lancet* **358:**384–385.

19. **Emovon, O. E., A. Lin, D. N. Howell, F. Afzal, M. Baillie, J. Rogers, P. K. Baliga, K. Chavin, V. Nickeleit, P. R. Rajagapalan, and S. Self.** 2003. Refractory adenovirus infection after simultaneous kidney-pancreas transplantation: successful treatment with intravenous ribavirin and pooled human intravenous immunoglobulin. *Nephrol. Dial. Transplant.* **18:**2436–2438.

20. **Englund, J. A., R. E. Champlin, P. R. Wyde, H. Kantarjian, R. L. Atmar, J. Tarrand, H. Yousuf, H. Regnery, A. I. Klimov, N. J. Cox, and E. Whimbey.** 1998. Common emergence of amantadine- and rimantadine-resistant influenza A viruses in symptomatic immunocompromised adults. *Clin. Infect. Dis.* **26:**1418–1424.

21. **Englund, J. A., P. A. Piedra, A. Jewell, K. Patel, B. B. Baxter, and E. Whimbey.** 1996. Rapid diagnosis of respiratory syncytial virus infections in immunocompromised adults. *J. Clin. Microbiol.* **34:**1649–1653.

22. **Esper, F., D. Boucher, C. Weibel, R. A. Martinello, and J. S. Kahn.** 2003. Human metapneumovirus infection in the United States: clinical manifestations associated with a newly emerging respiratory infection in children. *Pediatrics* **111:**1407–1410.

23. **Falsey, A. R., D. Erdman, L. J. Anderson, and E. E. Walsh.** 2003. Human metapneumovirus infections in young and elderly adults. *J. Infect. Dis.* **187:**785–790.

24. **Fishman, J. A.** 2001. Prevention of infections caused by *Pneumocystis carinii* in transplant recipients. *Clin. Infect. Dis.* **33:**1397–1405.

25. Flomenberg, P., J. Babbitt, W. R. Drobyski, R. C. Ash, D. R. Carrigan, G. V. Sedmak, T. McAuliffe, B. Camitta, M. M. Horowitz, and N. Bunin. 1994. Increasing incidence of adenovirus disease in bone marrow transplant recipients. *J. Infect. Dis.* **169**:775–781.

26. Garantziotis, S., D. N. Howell, H. P. McAdams, R. D. Davis, N. G. Henshaw, and S. M. Palmer. 2001. Influenza pneumonia in lung transplant recipients: clinical features and association with bronchiolitis obliterans syndrome. *Chest* **119**:1277–1280.

27. Gordon, Y. J., T. P. Araullo-nCruz, Y. F. Johnson, E. G. Romanowski, and P. R. Kinchington. 1996. Isolation of human adenovirus type 5 variants resistant to the antiviral cidofovir. *Investig. Ophthalmol. Vis. Sci.* **37**:2774–2778.

28. Gordon, Y. J., L. Naesens, E. DeClercq, P. C. Maudgal, and M. Veckeneer. 1996. Treatment of adenoviral conjunctivitis with topical cidofovir. *Cornea* **15**:546.

29. Govorkova, E. A., I. A. Leneva, O. G. Goloubeva, K. Bush, and R. G. Webster. 2001. Comparison of efficacies of RWJ-270201, zanamivir, and oseltamivir against H5N1, H9N2, and other avian influenza viruses. *Antimicrob. Agents Chemother.* **45**:2723–2732.

30. Greensill, J., P. S. McNamara, W. Dove, B. Flanagan, R. L. Smyth, and C. A. Hart. 2003. Human metapneumovirus in severe respiratory syncytial virus bronchiolitis. *Emerg. Infect. Dis.* **9**:372–375.

31. Gubareva, L. V. 2004. Molecular mechanisms of influenza virus resistance to neuraminidase inhibitors. *Virus Res.* **103**:199–203.

32. Gubareva, L. V., L. Kaiser, and F. G. Hayden. 2000. Influenza virus neuraminidase inhibitors. *Lancet* **355**:827–835.

33. Hale, G. A., H. E. Heslop, R. A. Krance, M. A. Brenner, D. Jayawardene, D. K. Srivastava, and C. C. Patrick. 1999. Adenovirus infection after pediatric bone marrow transplantation. *Bone Marrow Transplant.* **23**:277–282.

34. Hamelin, M. E., Y. Abed, and G. Boivin. 2004. Human metapneumovirus: a new player among respiratory viruses. *Clin. Infect. Dis.* **38**:983–990.

35. Hamelin, M. E., and G. Boivin. 2005. Development and validation of an enzyme-linked immunosorbent assay for human metapneumovirus serology based on a recombinant viral protein. *Clin. Diagn. Lab. Immunol.* **12**:249–253.

36. Harper, S. A., K. Fukuda, T. M. Uyeki, N. J. Cox, C. B. Bridges, and Centers for Disease Control and Prevention Advisory Committee on Immunization. 2004. Prevention and control of influenza: recommendations of the Advisory Committee on Immunization Practices (ACIP). *Morb. Mortal. Wkly. Rep. Recomm. Rep.* **53**:1–40. (Erratum, **53**:743.)

37. Hartline, C. B., K. M. Gustin, W. B. Wan, S. L. Ciesla, J. R. Beadle, K. Y. Hostetler, and E. R. Kern. 2005. Ether lipid-ester prodrugs of acyclic nucleoside phosphonates: activity against adenovirus replication in vitro. *J. Infect. Dis.* **191**:396–399.

38. Hatakeyama, N., N. Suzuki, T. Kudoh, T. Hori, N. Mizue, and H. Tsutsumi. 2003. Successful cidofovir treatment of adenovirus-associated hemorrhagic cystitis and renal dysfunction after allogeneic bone marrow transplant. *Pediatr. Infect. Dis. J.* **22**:928–929.

39. Heemskerk, B., A. C. Lankester, T. van Vreeswijk, M. F. Beersma, E. C. Claas, L. A. Veltrop-Duits, A. C. Kroes, J. M. Vossen, M. W. Schilham, and M. J. van Tol. 2005. Immune reconstitution and clearance of human adenovirus viremia in pediatric stem-cell recipients. *J. Infect. Dis.* **191**:520–530.

40. Heemskerk, B., L. A. Veltrop-Duits, T. van Vreeswijk, M. M. ten Dam, S. Heidt, R. E. Toes, M. J. van Tol, and M. W. Schilham. 2003. Extensive cross-reactivity of CD4+ adenovirus-specific T cells: implications for immunotherapy and gene therapy. *J. Virol.* **77**:6562–6566.

41. Hien, T. T., N. T. Liem, N. T. Dung, L. T. San, P. P. Mai, N. V. Chau, P. T. Suu, V. C. Dong, L. T. Q. Mai, N. T. Thi, D. B. Khoa, L. P. Phat, N. T. Truong, H. T. Long, C. V. Tung, L. T. Giang, N. D. Tho, L. H. Nga, N. T. K. Tien, L. H. San, L. V. Tuan, C. Dolecek, T. T. Thanh, M. de Jong, C. Schultsz, P. Cheng, W. Lim, P. Horby, the World Health Organization International Avian Influenza Investigative Team, and J. Farrar. 2004. Avian influenza A (H5N1) in 10 patients in Vietnam. *N. Engl. J. Med.* **350**:1179–1188.

42. Hillenkamp, J., T. Reinhard, R. S. Ross, D. Bohringer, O. Cartsburg, M. Roggendorf, E. De Clercq, E. Godehardt, and R. Sundmacher. 2001. Topical treatment of acute adenoviral keratoconjunctivitis with 0.2% cidofovir and 1% cyclosporine: a controlled clinical pilot study. *Arch. Ophthalmol.* **119**:1487–1491.

43. Hoffman, J. A., A. J. Shah, L. A. Ross, and N. Kapoor. 2001. Adenoviral infections and a prospective trial of cidofovir in pediatric hematopoietic stem cell transplantation. *Biol. Blood Marrow Transplant.* **7**:388–394.

44. **Howard, D. S., I. G. Phillips, D. E. Reece, R. K. Munn, J. Henslee-Downey, M. Pittard, M. Barker, and C. Pomeroy.** 1999. Adenovirus infections in hematopoietic stem cell transplant recipients. *Clin. Infect. Dis.* **29:**1494–1501.

45. **Hromas, R., C. Clark, C. Blanke, G. Tricot, K. Cornetta, A. Hedderman, and E. R. Broun.** 1994. Failure of ribavirin to clear adenovirus infections in T cell-depleted allogeneic bone marrow transplantation. *Bone Marrow Transplant.* **14:**663–664.

46. **Humar, A., G. Moussa, T. Mazzulli, R. Razonable, C. Paya, E. Covington, E. Alecock, and the PV 16000 Study Group.** 2004. Presented at the American Transplant Congress, Boston, Mass.

47. **Ison, M. G.** 2005. Respiratory viral infections in transplant recipients. *Curr. Opin. Organ Transplant.* **10:**312–319.

48. **Ison, M. G., and F. G. Hayden.** 2002. Viral infections in immunocompromised patients: what's new with respiratory viruses? *Curr. Opin. Infect. Dis.* **15:**355–367.

49. **Ison, M. G., J. Mills, P. Openshaw, M. Zambon, A. Osterhaus, and F. Hayden.** 2002. Current research on respiratory viral infections: fifth international symposium. *Antivir. Res.* **55:**227–278.

50. **Johny, A. A., A. Clark, N. Price, D. Carrington, A. Oakhill, and D. I. Marks.** 2002. The use of zanamivir to treat influenza A and B infection after allogeneic stem cell transplantation. *Bone Marrow Transplant.* **29:**113–115.

51. **Kaneko, H., S. Mori, O. Suzuki, T. Iida, S. Shigeta, M. Abe, S. Ohno, K. Aoki, and T. Suzutani.** 2004. The cotton rat model for adenovirus ocular infection: antiviral activity of cidofovir. *Antivir. Res.* **61:**63–66.

52. **Khalifah, A. P., R. R. Hachem, M. M. Chakinala, K. B. Schechtman, G. A. Patterson, D. P. Schuster, T. Mohanakumar, E. P. Trulock, and M. J. Walter.** 2004. Respiratory viral infections are a distinct risk for bronchiolitis obliterans syndrome and death. *Am. J. Respir. Crit. Care Med.* **170:**181–187.

53. **Koneru, B., R. Jaffe, C. O. Esquivel, R. Kunz, S. Todo, S. Iwatsuki, and T. E. Starzl.** 1987. Adenoviral infections in pediatric liver transplant recipients. *JAMA* **258:**489–492.

54. **Laham, F. R., V. Israele, J. M. Casellas, A. M. Garcia, C. M. Lac Prugent, S. J. Hoffman, D. Hauer, B. Thumar, M. I. Name, A. Pascual, N. Taratutto, M. T. Ishida, M. Balduzzi, M. Maccarone, S. Jackli, R. Passarino, R. A. Gaivironsky, R. A. Karron, N. R. Polack, and F. P. Polack.** 2004. Differential production of inflammatory cytokines in primary infection with human metapneumovirus and with other common respiratory viruses of infancy. *J. Infect. Dis.* **189:**2047–2056.

55. **Lankester, A. C., B. Heemskerk, E. C. Claas, M. W. Schilham, M. F. Beersma, R. G. Bredius, M. J. van Tol, and A. C. Kroes.** 2004. Effect of ribavirin on the plasma viral DNA load in patients with disseminating adenovirus infection. *Clin. Infect. Dis.* **38:**1521–1525.

56. **La Rosa, A. M., R. E. Champlin, N. Mirza, J. Gajewski, S. Giralt, K. V. Rolston, I. Raad, K. Jacobson, D. Kontoyiannis, L. Elting, and E. Whimbey.** 2001. Adenovirus infections in adult recipients of blood and marrow transplants. *Clin. Infect. Dis.* **32:**871–876.

57. **La Rosa, A. M., S. Malik, J. A. Englund, R. Couch, I. I. Raad, K. V. Rolston, K. L. Jacobson, D. P. Kontoyiannis, and E. Whimbey.** 2001. Presented at the 39th annual meeting of the Infectious Diseases Society of America, San Francisco, Calif.

58. **Legrand, F., D. Berrebi, N. Houhou, F. Freymuth, A. Faye, M. Duval, J. F. Mougenot, M. Peuchmaur, and E. Vilmer.** 2001. Early diagnosis of adenovirus infection and treatment with cidofovir after bone marrow transplantation in children. *Bone Marrow Transplant.* **27:**621–626.

59. **Leruez-Ville, M., V. Minard, F. Lacaille, A. Buzyn, E. Abachin, S. Blanche, F. Freymuth, and C. Rouzioux.** 2004. Real-time blood plasma polymerase chain reaction for management of disseminated adenovirus infection. *Clin. Infect. Dis.* **38:**45–52.

60. **Levin, M. D., and G. J. van Doornum.** 2004. An immunocompromised host with bilateral pulmonary infiltrates. *Neth. J. Med.* **62:**197, 210.

61. **Li, K. S., Y. Guan, J. Wang, G. J. Smith, K. M. Xu, L. Duan, A. P. Rahardjo, P. Puthavathana, C. Buranathai, T. D. Nguyen, A. T. Estoepangestie, A. Chaisingh, P. Auewarakul, H. T. Long, N. T. Hanh, R. J. Webby, L. L. Poon, H. Chen, K. F. Shortridge, K. Y. Yuen, R. G. Webster, and J. S. Peiris.** 2004. Genesis of a highly pathogenic and potentially pandemic H5N1 influenza virus in eastern Asia. *Nature* **430:**209–213.

62. **Liolios, L., A. Jenney, D. Spelman, T. Kotsimbos, M. Catton, and S. Wesselingh.** 2001. Comparison of a multiplex reverse transcription-PCR-enzyme hybridization assay with conventional viral culture and immunofluorescence techniques for the detection of seven viral respiratory pathogens. *J. Clin. Microbiol.* **39:**2779–2783.

63. **Lipatov, A. S., R. J. Webby, E. A. Govorkova, S. Krauss, and R. G. Webster.** 2005. Efficacy of H5 influenza vaccines produced by reverse genetics in a lethal mouse model. *J. Infect. Dis.* **191:**1216–1220.

64. Ljungman, P., P. Ribaud, M. Eyrich, S. Matthes-Martin, H. Einsele, M. Bleakley, M. Machaczka, M. Bierings, A. Bosi, N. Gratecos, C. Cordonnier, and the Infectious Diseases Working Party of the European Group for Blood and Marrow Transplantation. 2003. Cidofovir for adenovirus infections after allogeneic hematopoietic stem cell transplantation: a survey by the Infectious Diseases Working Party of the European Group for Blood and Marrow Transplantation. *Bone Marrow Transplant.* **31:**481–486.

65. Ljungman, P., K. N. Ward, B. N. Crooks, A. Parker, R. Martino, P. J. Shaw, L. Brinch, M. Brune, R. De La Camara, A. Dekker, K. Pauksen, N. Russell, A. P. Schwarer, and C. Cordonnier. 2001. Respiratory virus infections after stem cell transplantation: a prospective study from the Infectious Diseases Working Party of the European Group for Blood and Marrow Transplantation. *Bone Marrow Transplant.* **28:**479–484.

66. Machado, C. M., L. S. Boas, A. V. Mendes, I. F. da Rocha, D. Sturaro, F. L. Dulley, and C. S. Pannuti. 2004. Use of oseltamivir to control influenza complications after bone marrow transplantation. *Bone Marrow Transplant.* **34:**111–114.

67. Machado, C. M., L. S. Boas, A. V. Mendes, M. F. Santos, I. F. da Rocha, D. Sturaro, F. L. Dulley, and C. S. Pannuti. 2003. Low mortality rates related to respiratory virus infections after bone marrow transplantation. *Bone Marrow Transplant.* **31:**695–700.

68. Mackay, I. M., K. C. Jacob, D. Woolhouse, K. Waller, M. W. Syrmis, D. M. Whiley, D. J. Siebert, M. Nissen, and T. P. Sloots. 2003. Molecular assays for detection of human metapneumovirus. *J. Clin. Microbiol.* **41:**100–105.

69. Madhi, S. A., H. Ludewick, Y. Abed, K. P. Klugman, and G. Boivin. 2003. Human metapneumovirus-associated lower respiratory tract infections among hospitalized human immunodeficiency virus type 1 (HIV-1)-infected and HIV-1-uninfected African infants. *Clin. Infect. Dis.* **37:**1705–1710.

70. Maertzdorf, J., C. K. Wang, J. B. Brown, J. D. Quinto, M. Chu, M. de Graaf, B. G. van den Hoogen, R. Spaete, A. D. Osterhaus, and R. A. Fouchier. 2004. Real–time reverse transcriptase PCR assay for detection of human metapneumoviruses from all known genetic lineages. *J. Clin. Microbiol.* **42:**981–986.

71. Maggi, F., M. Pifferi, M. Vatteroni, C. Fornai, E. Tempestini, S. Anzilotti, L. Lanini, E. Andreoli, V. Ragazzo, M. Pistello, S. Specter, and M. Bendinelli. 2003. Human metapneumovirus associated with respiratory tract infections in a 3-year study of nasal swabs from infants in Italy. *J. Clin. Microbiol.* **41:**2987–2991.

72. Marr, K. A., R. A. Carter, M. Boeckh, P. Martin, and L. Corey. 2002. Invasive aspergillosis in allogeneic stem cell transplant recipients: changes in epidemiology and risk factors. *Blood* **100:**4358–4366.

73. McGrath, D., M. E. Falagas, R. Freeman, R. Rohrer, R. Fairchild, C. Colbach, and D. R. Snydman. 1998. Adenovirus infection in adult orthotopic liver transplant recipients: incidence and clinical significance. *J. Infect. Dis.* **177:**459–462.

74. Meltzer, M. I., N. J. Cox, and K. Fukuda. 1999. The economic impact of pandemic influenza in the United States: priorities for intervention. *Emerg. Infect. Dis.* **5:**659–671.

75. Mentel, R., M. Kinder, U. Wegner, M. von Janta-Lipinski, and E. Matthes. 1997. Inhibitory activity of 3'-fluoro-2' deoxythymidine and related nucleoside analogues against adenoviruses in vitro. *Antivir. Res.* **34:**113–119.

76. Michaels, M. G., M. Green, E. R. Wald, and T. E. Starzl. 1992. Adenovirus infection in pediatric liver transplant recipients. *J. Infect. Dis.* **165:**170–174.

77. Monto, A., M. Herlocker, J. Rotthoff, and S. Bidol. 2001. Presented at the 39th annual meeting of the Infectious Diseases Society of America, San Francisco, Calif.

78. Morfin, F., S. Dupuis-Girod, S. Mundweiler, D. Falcon, D. Carrington, P. Sedlacek, M. Bierings, P. Cetkovsky, A. C. Kroes, M. J. van Tol, and D. Thouvenot. 2005. In vitro susceptibility of adenovirus to antiviral drugs is species-dependent. *Antivir. Ther.* **10:**225–229.

79. Nichols, W. G., K. A. Guthrie, L. Corey, and M. Boeckh. 2004. Influenza infections after hematopoietic stem cell transplantation: risk factors, mortality, and the effect of antiviral therapy. *Clin. Infect. Dis.* **39:**1300–1306.

80. Ohm-Smith, M. J., P. S. Nassos, and B. L. Haller. 2004. Evaluation of the Binax NOW, BD Directigen, and BD Directigen EZ assays for detection of respiratory syncytial virus. *J. Clin. Microbiol.* **42:**2996–2999.

81. Ohori, N. P., M. G. Michaels, R. Jaffe, P. Williams, and S. A. Yousem. 1995. Adenovirus pneumonia in lung transplant recipients. *Hum. Pathol.* **26:**1073–1079.

82. Organ Procurement and Transplantation Network/Scientific Registry of Transplant Recipients. 2004. Unadjusted graft and patient survival at 3 months, 1 year, 3 years, 5 years, and 10 years: standard errors of the survival rates, Table 1.13. *In OPTN/SRTR 2004 Annual Report: Summary Tables, Transplant Data 1993–2002.* http://www.ustransplant.org/annual_reports/archives/2004.

83. **Pelletier, G., P. Dery, Y. Abed, and G. Boivin.** 2002. Respiratory tract reinfections by the new human metapneumovirus in an immunocompromised child. *Emerg. Infect. Dis.* **8:**976–978.

84. **Potter, C. W., J. P. Phair, L. Vodinelich, R. Fenton, and R. Jennings.** 1976. Antiviral, immunosuppressive and antitumour effects of ribavirin. *Nature* **259:**496–497.

85. **Rawlinson, W. D., Z. M. Waliuzzaman, M. Fennell, J. R. Appleman, C. D. Shimasaki, and I. W. Carter.** 2004. New point of care test is highly specific but less sensitive for influenza virus A and B in children and adults. *J. Med. Virol.* **74:**127–131.

86. **Ribaud, P., C. Scieux, F. Freymuth, F. Morinet, and E. Gluckman.** 1999. Successful treatment of adenovirus disease with intravenous cidofovir in an unrelated stem-cell transplant recipient. *Clin. Infect. Dis.* **28:**690–691.

87. **Roghmann, M., K. Ball, D. Erdman, J. Lovchik, L. J. Anderson, and R. Edelman.** 2003. Active surveillance for respiratory virus infections in adults who have undergone bone marrow and peripheral blood stem cell transplantation. *Bone Marrow Transplant.* **32:**1085–1088.

88. **Romanowski, E. G., Y. J. Gordon, T. Araullo-Cruz, K. A. Yates, and P. R. Kinchington.** 2001. The antiviral resistance and replication of cidofovir-resistant adenovirus variants in the New Zealand White rabbit ocular model. *Investig. Ophthalmol. Vis. Sci.* **42:**1812–1815.

89. **Romanowski, E. G., K. A. Yates, and Y. J. Gordon.** 2001. Antiviral prophylaxis with twice daily topical cidofovir protects against challenge in the adenovirus type 5/New Zealand rabbit ocular model. *Antivir. Res.* **52:**275–280.

90. **Rovida, F., E. Percivalle, M. Zavattoni, M. Torsellini, A. Sarasini, G. Campanini, S. Paolucci, F. Baldanti, M. G. Revello, and G. Gerna.** 2005. Monoclonal antibodies versus reverse transcription-PCR for detection of respiratory viruses in a patient population with respiratory tract infections admitted to hospital. *J. Med. Virol.* **75:**336–347.

91. **Runde, V., S. Ross, R. Trenschel, E. Lagemann, O. Basu, K. Renzing-Kohler, U. W. Schaefer, M. Roggendorf, and E. Holler.** 2001. Adenoviral infection after allogeneic stem cell transplantation (SCT): report on 130 patients from a single SCT unit involved in a prospective multicenter surveillance study. *Bone Marrow Transplant.* **28:**51–57.

92. **Saad, R. S., A. J. Demetris, R. G. Lee, S. Kusne, and P. S. Randhawa.** 1997. Adenovirus hepatitis in the adult allograft liver. *Transplantation* **64:**1483–1485.

93. **Schowengerdt, K. O., J. Ni, S. W. Denfield, R. J. Gajarski, B. Radovancevic, H. O. Frazier, G. J. Demmler, D. Kearney, J. T. Bricker, and J. A. Towbin.** 1996. Diagnosis, surveillance, and epidemiologic evaluation of viral infections in pediatric cardiac transplant recipients with the use of the polymerase chain reaction. *J. Heart Lung Transplant.* **15:**111–123.

94. **Semple, M. G., A. Cowell, W. Dove, J. Greensill, P. S. McNamara, C. Halfhide, P. Shears, R. L. Smyth, and C. A. Hart.** 2005. Dual infection of infants by human metapneumovirus and human respiratory syncytial virus is strongly associated with severe bronchiolitis. *J. Infect. Dis.* **191:**382–386.

95. **Shirali, G. S., J. Ni, R. E. Chinnock, J. K. Johnston, G. L. Rosenthal, N. E. Bowles, and J. A. Towbin.** 2001. Association of viral genome with graft loss in children after cardiac transplantation. *N. Engl. J. Med.* **344:**1498–1503.

96. **Smith, K. O., K. S. Galloway, W. L. Kennell, K. K. Ogilvie, and B. K. Radatus.** 1982. A new nucleoside analog, 9-[[2-hydroxy-1-(hydroxymethyl)ethoxy]methyl]guanine, highly active in vitro against herpes simplex virus types 1 and 2. *Antimicrob. Agents Chemother.* **22:**55–61.

97. **Snydman, D. R.** 2005. Counterpoint: prevention of cytomegalovirus (CMV) infection and CMV disease in recipients of solid organ transplants: the case for prophylaxis. *Clin. Infect. Dis.* **40:**709–712.

98. **Stephenson, I., R. Bugarini, K. G. Nicholson, A. Podda, J. M. Wood, M. C. Zambon, and J. M. Katz.** 2005. Cross-reactivity to highly pathogenic avian influenza H5N1 viruses after vaccination with nonadjuvanted and MF59-adjuvanted influenza A/Duck/Singapore/97 (H5N3) vaccine: a potential priming strategy. *J. Infect. Dis.* **191:**1210–1215.

99. **Storch, G. A.** 2003. Rapid diagnostic tests for influenza. *Curr. Opin. Pediatr.* **15:**77–84.

100. **Trampuz, A., R. M. Prabhu, T. F. Smith, and L. M. Baddour.** 2004. Avian influenza: a new pandemic threat? *Mayo Clin. Proc.* **79:**523–530.

101. **Trousdale, M. D., P. L. Goldschmidt, and R. Nobrega.** 1994. Activity of ganciclovir against human adenovirus type-5 infection in cell culture and cotton rat eyes. *Cornea* **13:**435–439.

102. **Ungchusak, K., P. Auewarakul, S. F. Dowell, R. Kitphati, W. Auwanit, P. Puthavathana, M. Uiprasertkul, K. Boonnak, C. Pittayawonganon, N. J. Cox, S. R. Zaki, P. Thawatsupha, M. Chittaganpitch,**

R. Khontong, J. M. Simmerman, and S. Chunsutthiwat. 2005. Probable person-to-person transmission of avian influenza A (H5N1). *N. Engl. J. Med.* **352:**333–340.

103. van den Hoogen, B. G., J. C. de Jong, J. Groen, T. Kuiken, R. de Groot, R. A. Fouchier, and A. D. Osterhaus. 2001. A newly discovered human pneumovirus isolated from young children with respiratory tract disease. *Nat. Med.* **7:**719–724.

104. van den Hoogen, B. G., D. M. Osterhaus, and R. A. Fouchier. 2004. Clinical impact and diagnosis of human metapneumovirus infection. *Pediatr. Infect. Dis. J.* **23:**S25–S32.

105. van den Hoogen, B. G., G. J. van Doornum, J. C. Fockens, J. J. Cornelissen, W. E. Beyer, R. de Groot, A. D. Osterhaus, and R. A. Fouchier. 2003. Prevalence and clinical symptoms of human metapneumovirus infection in hospitalized patients. *J. Infect. Dis.* **188:**1571–1577.

106. van Elden, L. J., M. G. van Kraaij, M. Nijhuis, K. A. Hendriksen, A. W. Dekker, M. Rozenberg-Arska, and A. M. van Loon. 2002. Polymerase chain reaction is more sensitive than viral culture and antigen testing for the detection of respiratory viruses in adults with hematological cancer and pneumonia. *Clin. Infect. Dis.* **34:**177–183.

107. van Elden, L. J., A. M. van Loon, A. van der Beek, K. A. Hendriksen, A. I. Hoepelman, M. G. van Kraaij, P. Schipper, and M. Nijhuis. 2003. Applicability of a real-time quantitative PCR assay for diagnosis of respiratory syncytial virus infection in immunocompromised adults. *J. Clin. Microbiol.* **41:** 4378–4381.

108. van Kraaij, M. G., L. J. van Elden, A. M. van Loon, K. A. Hendriksen, L. Laterveer, A. W. Dekker, and M. Nijhuis. 2005. Frequent detection of respiratory viruses in adult recipients of stem cell transplants with the use of real–time polymerase chain reaction, compared with viral culture. *Clin. Infect. Dis.* **40:** 662–669.

109. Vilchez, R. A., J. Dauber, and S. Kusne. 2003. Infectious etiology of bronchiolitis obliterans: the respiratory viruses connection—myth or reality? *Am. J. Transplant.* **3:**245–249.

110. Vilchez, R. A., K. McCurry, J. Dauber, A. Lacono, B. Griffith, J. Fung, and S. Kusne. 2002. Influenza virus infection in adult solid organ transplant recipients. *Am. J. Transplant.* **2:**287–291.

111. Waring, G. E., P. R. Laibson, J. E. Satz, and N. H. Joseph. 1976. Use of vidarabine in epidemic keratoconjunctivitis due to adenovirus types 3, 7, 8, and 19. *Am. J. Ophthalmol.* **82:**781–785.

112. Williams, J. V., P. A. Harris, S. J. Tollefson, L. L. Halburnt-Rush, J. M. Pingsterhaus, K. M. Edwards, P. F. Wright, and J. E. Crowe, Jr. 2004. Human metapneumovirus and lower respiratory tract disease in otherwise healthy infants and children. *N. Engl. J. Med.* **350:**443–450.

113. Winter, J. B., A. S. Gouw, M. Groen, C. Wildevuur, and J. Prop. 1994. Respiratory viral infections aggravate airway damage caused by chronic rejection in rat lung allografts. *Transplantation* **57:**418–422.

114. World Health Organization. 2005. Cumulative number of confirmed human cases of avian influenza A/(H5N1) since 28 January 2004. [Online.] http://www.who.int/csr/disease/avian_influenza/country/cases_table_2005_04_04/en/.

115. Wunderli, W., Y. Thomas, D. A. Muller, M. Dick, and L. Kaiser. 2003. Rapid antigen testing for the surveillance of influenza epidemics. *Clin. Microbiol. Infect.* **9:**295–300.

116. Wyde, P. R., S. N. Chetty, A. M. Jewell, G. Boivin, and P. A. Piedra. 2003. Comparison of the inhibition of human metapneumovirus and respiratory syncytial virus by ribavirin and immune serum globulin in vitro. *Antivir. Res.* **60:**51–59.

117. Wyde, P. R., S. N. Chetty, A. M. Jewell, S. L. Schoonover, and P. A. Piedra. 2005. Development of a cotton rat-human metapneumovirus (hMPV) model for identifying and evaluating potential hMPV antivirals and vaccines. *Antivir. Res.* **66:**57–66.

118. Wyde, P. R., E. H. Moylett, S. N. Chetty, A. Jewell, T. L. Bowlin, and P. A. Piedra. 2004. Comparison of the inhibition of human metapneumovirus and respiratory syncytial virus by NMSO3 in tissue culture assays. *Antivir. Res.* **63:**51–59.

Emerging Infections 7
Edited by W. M. Scheld, D. C. Hooper, and J. M. Hughes
© 2007 ASM Press, Washington, D.C.

Chapter 5

Monkeypox Virus: Insights on Its Emergence in Human Populations

Inger Damon

Human monkeypox, a zoonotic disease of western and central Africa that was comprehensively reviewed in *Emerging Infections 4* (4), demonstrated its ability to emerge in geographically distinctive human and other animal populations in the United States in 2003. This chapter focuses on epidemiologic, ecologic, and biologic observations made since publication of *Emerging Infections 4* which enhance our understanding of this zoonotic disease and the pathogen that causes it.

BACKGROUND: SUMMARY OF EPIDEMIOLOGIC, CLINICAL, LABORATORY, AND ECOLOGY STUDIES PRIOR TO 2003

Monkeypox virus was first identified in 1958 and was so named because the disease manifests as a smallpox-like rash illness in nonhuman primates. Initially detected in an Asiatic-primate colony in Denmark, in the subsequent 10 years the virus was identified as a cause of 10 outbreaks in primate colonies and in zoo animals; the origin of the Rotterdam zoo outbreak was traced to an anteater that had close contact with primates from Malaysia (2, 3). The majority of primates implicated as the index cases had origins in Malaysia or the Philippines (a long-tailed macaque [*Macaca philippinensis*, currently *Macaca fascicularis*] or *Macaca irus* [currently *Macaca fascicularis*] in five outbreaks, including the Rotterdam Zoo), India (rhesus monkeys [*Macaca mulatta*] in two outbreaks), unknown areas (in two outbreaks), and Sierra Leone (a chimpanzee [*Pan troglodytes*] in one outbreak). Additional species of nonhuman primates, including orangutans (*Pongo pygmaeus*), were subsequently infected. During this period, no human illnesses were observed in animal handlers or other humans in contact with the animals. Serosurveillance of primate populations, conducted within 5 to 10 years after the outbreaks in Malaysia (2), revealed only nonsignificant evidence of orthopoxvirus-neutralizing activity in a minority of the indigenous *M. irus* primate population sampled. Similar studies, of varying magnitudes, revealed no orthopoxvirus seroreactivity in other nonhuman primates sampled from

Inger Damon • Poxvirus Program, Centers for Disease Control and Prevention, Atlanta, GA 30329-4018.

India, Chad, Upper Volta, Mali, and Kenya (2). Thus, the origin of the infections in the index animals is uncertain; it appears that they were not the disease reservoir.

The virus was biologically characterized as an orthopoxvirus distinct from variola virus (the causative agent of smallpox) and other previously characterized orthopoxviruses. Both genome restriction fragment maps and the observance of pocks on the chorioallantoic membrane differentiated the virus from other orthopoxviruses; the latter method was more commonly used as a clinical laboratory diagnostic test (12, 14). Other methods that distinguished the virus were a ceiling growth temperature of 39°C and various tests on small animals. Currently, many laboratories perform nucleic acid testing—usually PCR, followed by restriction endonuclease digestion—or sequencing to provide laboratory evidence of viral infection (41, 45). Development of a serologic test that is both sensitive and specific for monkeypox has been problematic, given the close antigenic similarity between the orthopoxviruses and the lack of available animal species type-specific secondary antibody reagents. Recent efforts, using a strategy primarily directed at serologic recognition of the monkeypox B21 protein, hold promise (19). This gene product, absent in vaccinia virus and present in other orthopoxviruses, may permit the discrimination of a monkeypox serologic response, at least from that of previous vaccination. Additional advances in serologic testing are described below.

Identification of human infections in western and central Africa was first made in 1970. The human disease was identified as a vesiculopustular rash illness which resembled smallpox. Given that smallpox had been eliminated in that region of the world, the discovery of this human illness resembling smallpox prompted additional investigations. Subsequent studies of outbreaks, passive surveillance, and active surveillance compiled a literature on the clinical disease, focusing mostly on disease in the Congo basin country of Zaire, now the Democratic Republic of the Congo (DRC), although a number of case series on the disease in West African countries were also published (7, 8, 17, 28). Outbreaks of disease were reported to have varying case fatality rates up to 15%, prompting an active surveillance program in the DRC. Observations derived from the active surveillance program in the DRC from 1981 to 1986 characterized the disease in humans as similar to discrete ordinary smallpox, with lymphadenopathy as the clinical feature that distinguished monkeypox from smallpox (28). Human-to-human transmission of monkeypox was less than that of smallpox. The secondary attack rate in unvaccinated contacts of monkeypox patients was calculated to be 9.3%, versus 37 to 88% for smallpox (26, 27). Prior smallpox vaccination (3 to 19 years previously) appeared to be 85% protective in preventing disease acquisition in contacts (23, 27) and also ameliorated disease severity (23, 28). Overall, the majority of cases identified acquired the disease from a presumed animal exposure(s); only 28% of cases were ascribed to person-to-person transmission (23–25). A case fatality rate of ~10% was observed in unvaccinated persons; the majority of fatalities and the severest disease manifestations were observed in children under the age of 5 (23, 28). Serosurveys suggested that subclinical infection may have occurred in up to 28% of close contacts of monkeypox patients in some communities (23, 27), which may have contributed to the rarity of sustained generations of human-to-human transmission in household and other close-contact situations (22).

As the majority of patients were believed to have acquired the disease through animal exposures (23), case control studies were attempted to determine the source of infection.

These were not feasible, as the population appeared to have multiple daily contacts with the same animals in settlements, forests, or cleared agricultural areas (23). Among primary case patients, recent close contact, via hunting, skinning, killing, cooking, or playing with carcasses, was identified with *Cercopithecus, Colobus,* and *Cercocebus* primates; *Cricetomys* terrestrial rodents; and *Funisciurus* and *Heliosciurus* squirrel species. Ecologic studies, usually using convenient samples of animals collected in areas surrounding human patients in West Africa and central Africa, demonstrated orthopoxvirus- and sometimes monkeypox virus-specific seroprevalence in various members of these species, but it was not reported for *Cricetomys* species (5, 31–33). This work has been comprehensively reviewed (23). Virus was found in only one euthanized, moribund squirrel of the species *Funisciurus anerythrus* (30). The prevailing hypothesis was that squirrel species were the likely reservoir of the disease. Near the end of the 1980s, disease surveillance waned after modeling studies based on the epidemiologic observations of secondary-attack rates from human-to-human exposure suggested that a limited number of transmission events were feasible even with low population immunity provided by waning immunization rates in the populations of central Africa. The virus had not, therefore, adapted to survive solely through human infection and would not manifest with the same human-to-human transmission dynamics as smallpox (15). This work also led to recommendations not to continue routine smallpox vaccination.

A reemergence of the disease was noted in 1996 in the DRC; a salient observation from a series of investigations was that more cases were derived from secondary human-to-human contact (88%) than were seen in the 1981 to 1986 investigations (28%). This was, in part, attributed to a larger population of humans fully susceptible to the disease because of the cessation of routine smallpox vaccination in 1980 after smallpox eradication. Another observation was that the disease epidemiology showed more cases in the older-child/young-adult population (21). Disease mortality (1%) was observed to be lower than previously seen from 1981 to 1986; this may have been due to a smaller demographic of very young children (0 to 4 years of age) being infected or due to technical limitations in the investigations. The ongoing civil strife precluded systematic collection of rash specimens for virologic analysis during active disease. Of those who had rash samples collected in the initial two investigations, 5 of 20 (25%) were determined to be chicken pox cases and 15 of 20 (75%) were monkeypox; in 2 of these cases, coinfection with monkeypox and chicken pox was detected. Serologic data were obtained on the majority of the cases identified. Both varicella virus and orthopoxvirus seroreactivities were detected in a significant number of patients, making retrospective epidemiologic analysis difficult.

Whereas previous ecologic serosurveys of animal populations had implicated tree squirrels as having significant orthopoxvirus seroreactivity, these investigations were the first to show orthopoxvirus seroprevalence in terrestrial rodents (*Cricetomys emini*) and in one domestic pig (*Sus scrofa*) sampled (21).

The concerns about increased transmissibility of disease between humans and increased disease incidence raised by these limited investigations led to the issuance of the 1999 WHO Monkeypox Technical Advisory Group recommendations regarding the need for ongoing monkeypox surveillance and infrastructure rebuilding (4). Although a limited number of outbreaks have been characterized in the DRC since the report's release in 1999 (40), only recently has a fully resourced program been established (42). The disease appears to be endemic in the Sankuro region of the DRC, but its current epidemiology and ecology await characterization.

NEW INSIGHTS ON ECOLOGY AND EPIDEMIOLOGY OF MONKEYPOX FROM THE 2003 OUTBREAKS IN THE UNITED STATES AND THE REPUBLIC OF THE CONGO

In 2003, two concurrent outbreaks of disease, one in the United States and one in the Republic of the Congo, permitted additional analyses and studies which have substantially amplified our understanding of monkeypox viruses and their pathogeneses in various animal species, which in turn will allow the design of public health control measures. Reports of human disease in 2003 were the first in these two countries.

Discovery of Human Monkeypox and Clinical Description in the United States

Human disease was initially reported as an outbreak of febrile, vesiculopustular rash illness among persons in the midwestern United States in contact with ill prairie dogs. Many of the initial 11 human case patients reported being bitten or scratched by their prairie dogs, and pustular lesions were apparent at these sites, in addition to disseminated lesions (44). No fatalities were reported (although 6 of the 11 patients had never been vaccinated, and 1 was a child less than 5 years old), and disease severity as assessed by the rash burden also appeared to be minimal; most cases were reported to manifest 1 to 50 generalized rash lesions. Also, no human-to-human transmission was described (44). The distributor of the prairie dogs had been involved in the disposition of an ill giant Gambian rat (*Cricetomys* species). Preliminary genetic analysis of the virus isolated from one human and the prairie dog suggested that the virus segregated with isolates previously obtained from the early primate colony outbreaks or humans in West Africa and was distinct from those isolates obtained from the DRC.

The initial suggestions that clinical presentations of human monkeypox in the United States were less severe than what had previously been reported in central Africa in the 1981 to 1986 surveillance program held true at the end of the outbreak. The predominant signs and symptoms of illness appeared similar to what had been described in central Africa. Rash, fever, chills, adenopathy, headache, and myalgias were seen in the majority of patients (20). However, among the 37 laboratory-confirmed cases, there were no deaths (39). The rash burden, a historic indicator of disease severity, was moderate. Studies based on chart review (20) or standardized questionnaire analysis (39) demonstrated that between 80 and 89% of U.S. cases had <100 rash lesions. In contrast to the African literature, previous vaccination did not appear to ameliorate disease presentation, nor did age. Of those with confirmed disease, analysis of clinical observations based on chart review (20) revealed no differences in frequency or duration of fever, severe rash, or hospitalization between those previously vaccinated and those who had never been vaccinated, nor were there differences in these factors on comparison of pediatric to adult patients. Pediatric patients were, however, more likely to be admitted to the intensive-care unit. In the United States, the two severe cases described in the literature, one with encephalitis and the other with pronounced retropharyngeal lymphadenopathy and abscess, occurred in pediatric patients (1, 46). Blood chemistries and hematologic studies were evaluated, when available, in a subgroup of those patients with medical charts. A median twofold elevation in transaminases was seen in at least 50% of those tested during illness, suggestive of hepatic involvement (20).

Subclinical disease was suggested by a serostudy of persons associated with the outbreak (19); three persons, previously vaccinated against smallpox and without symptoms of fever or rash, were monkeypox seroreactive in an assay designed to discriminate monkeypox seroreactivity from smallpox vaccine (vaccinia) seroreactivity. Another study, which evaluated anti-orthopoxvirus immunoglobulin M (IgM) responses in individuals associated with the outbreak, may also provide some evidence of subclinical infection (29); at least two individuals with anti-orthopoxvirus IgM-reactive sera were deemed noncase patients during the outbreak because of a lack of clinical findings to fit the case definition. Studies that carefully evaluate different types of virus exposures may be valuable in determining the relative effects of age, vaccination, exposure dosage, and exposure route on the development of illness.

Epidemiology: Studies on Transmission

In the health care setting, even suboptimal compliance with personal protective measures in a partially vaccinated cohort appeared to be protective against both infection and illness. No health care workers associated with three cases in an Indiana hospital acquired monkeypox disease or appeared to have been subclinically infected. Of those participating in a study, only 29% reported strict adherence at all times with barrier and respiratory personal-protection precautions, and 70% reported one or more lapses. Whereas noncompliance with mask or N-95 respirator use was reported in 75 or 81% of one or more patient encounters, glove use (16) lapsed in only 39% of participant patient encounters. The median duration of encounters (defined by proximity within 2 m) was 10 min and ranged from 1 to 68 min. Interestingly, during the 4 days of hospitalization prior to diagnosis—by analogy to smallpox, a period when infection risk may have been high (6)—compliance with barrier and respiratory precautions was low; 25% reported being compliant with all precautions prior to diagnosis, and 63% reported compliance after disease diagnosis. Overall, 54% of those participating had received smallpox vaccination in the past.

In contrast, probable and confirmed cases of monkeypox within a household day care setting were associated with the extent of exposure to two monkeypox-infected prairie dogs (34). No percutaneous exposures were reported, but there was a significant association between illness acquisition and the extent of time in direct contact or association with the prairie dogs; household members with extensive exposure to the animals were more likely than those with moderate exposure from veterinary care of the animals or contact in the day care setting to be a probable or confirmed case patient. No cases were identified in members of kindergarten classes who merely visited the child care facility. These studies, and the investigations of the overall outbreak (10), suggested that human disease resulted from prairie dog exposure.

Animals Susceptible to Monkeypox Disease: Africa and North America

The origin of monkeypox virus in the United States was traced to a consignment of animals imported from the West African country of Ghana, destined for the exotic pet trade, which arrived in Texas in April 2003 (9, 10). Interestingly, monkeypox disease of humans or animals has never been reported from Ghana, although it has been reported from other West African countries. Distribution of animals from the shipment to areas across the United States resulted in detection of virus in African animals found dead on, or shortly after, arrival in the United States. Gambian rats (*Cricetomys* sp.) and rope squirrels (*Funisciurus* spp.) separated from the shipment immediately on arrival in the United States, discovered moribund and later dead in Texas and New Jersey, respectively, were found positive for monkeypox virus. As the animal distribution was traced across the United States, African dormice (*Graphiurus* spp.) were also found moribund, and on autopsy they were positive for the presence of monkeypox virus. This information substantially increased our knowledge of African species capable of being symptomatically infected with monkeypox virus.

Black-tailed prairie dogs (*Cynomys ludovicianus*) appear to have been infected at a central pet distributorship (10). Epidemiologic findings, described above, from both the overall outbreak (9, 10) and specific situations (34) led to the hypothesis that prairie dogs were responsible for transmitting the disease to humans. This is supported by pathologic analysis of deceased prairie dogs (18, 36) associated with the outbreak, which found evidence of virus in the eyelid, tongue, respiratory system, skin, and other organs that might be implicated in contact or respiratory transmission of virus. Additional studies using monkeypox virus to experimentally challenge both prairie dogs and another North American ground squirrel species demonstrated that these non-African native species are quite susceptible to monkeypox virus, are able to shed virus in mucosal secretions, and may provide additional models of systemic orthopoxvirus disease (47, 48) and transmission.

Public Health Control Measures

Recent observations have suggested that at least one of the African genera, *Cricetomys*, implicated in importation of monkeypox into the United States has sustained a population within a region of the United States (the Florida Keys) (43) and could emerge in a wider geographic distribution. As a result of the recognition of the monkeypox outbreak and its being traced back to the original importation of African rodents, and arguably most important in the resolution of the U.S. outbreak, the Centers for Disease Control and Prevention and the Food and Drug Administration issued *Federal Register* 42 CFR 71.56 banning importation of African rodents, as well as movement of prairie dogs. Other control measures included recommendations for utilization of vaccinated personnel and education in the use of personal protective equipment and measures (http://www.cdc.gov/ncidod/monkeypox/infectioncontrol.htm).

Discovery of Monkeypox in the Republic of the Congo

Simultaneous with the U.S. outbreak, human disease in the Republic of the Congo in central Africa was discovered. An outbreak in Impfondo, separated from the DRC by the Ubangi River, proceeded through six uninterrupted chains of human-to-human transmission, resulting in seven generations of human disease. This is the longest laboratory-verified outbreak of monkeypox from interhuman transmission. It is important to note that the virus appeared to be transmitted more efficiently between humans than had been previously described in the DRC. Time intervals between disease acquisitions from humans were shorter than those described previously in the DRC (23, 37). Overall, the outbreak comprised 11 probable and confirmed cases and 1 suspect case, with a case fatality rate of 10%. The rash burden was objectively described as severe (>200 lesions) in one-third of the cases for which data were available (37).

Comparison of Human Monkeypox Cases in the United States and Africa: Evidence for Two Clades of Virus with Different Clinical and Epidemiologic Properties

Recognition of the decreased severity of human monkeypox illness in the United States, previous genetic evidence suggesting genetic differences between viruses from West Africa and those from central Africa (Fig. 1), and the rarity of cases reported from West Africa led to more in-depth comparative analysis of differences between illnesses described in Africa and the United States. Not enough cases have been identified in West Africa to use that group in the comparison. However, detailed comparison of the clinical and epidemiologic characteristics of the U.S. cases (virus imported from West Africa) with DRC cases from 1981 to 1986 demonstrated significant differences in human disease manifestations (39); pronounced rash and more severe illness were seen in the Congo basin cases. When age and vaccination status were controlled for, disease severity remained

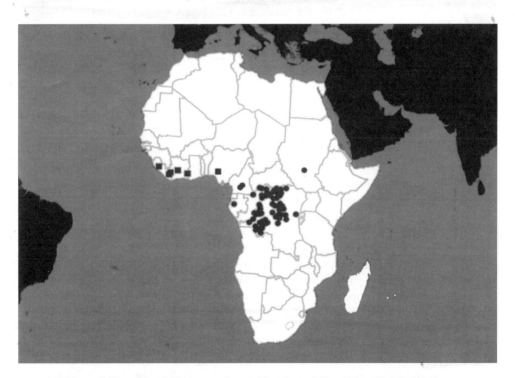

Figure 1. The squares indicate georeferenced locations of West African clade human isolates of monkeypox virus. The circles indicate georeferenced locations of Congo basin isolates of monkeypox virus.

more extreme in the Congo basin than in the U.S. case patients. Monkeypox-related mortality and human-to-human transmission were seen only in the Congo basin, both in the DRC 1981 to 1986 case patients and in the more recent Republic of the Congo case patients.

Objective evidence of different disease pathogeneses was observed. Viremia, as ascertained by PCR of whole-blood specimen clinical samples, appeared to be more prolonged and of greater magnitude in samples from the Republic of the Congo than in those from the United States in the small number of specimens tested. The different disease presentations could be due to different routes and or dosages of viral exposure, perhaps related to the animal species responsible for transmission, or potentially due to differences in the health infrastructures. However, the viral-clade differences between the U.S./West African isolates and the Congo basin isolates suggested by limited genomic analyses (13, 14, 44) led to more thorough analysis of monkeypox virus isolates.

Complete genome sequencing of the U.S. isolate, West African isolates, and Congo basin isolates, including that from the Republic of the Congo, allowed more extensive viral-genome comparison and permitted prediction of viral open reading frames that may be involved in the differences in human pathogenesis (11, 39). Complete genome sequencing clearly identified two significantly different clades by parsimony and maximum likelihood analyses (Fig. 2). At least five open reading frames whose orthologs in other orthopoxviruses have been shown to promote viral persistence and/or to evade immune recognition and clearance discriminate viruses from West Africa and those from the Congo basin. These clade-specific orthologs may modulate viral pathogenesis or host response, perhaps playing roles in the observed differential clearance of virus from the blood of individuals infected with these strains. Animal models are supportive of greater pathogenicity associated with the Congo basin isolates; nonhuman primates infected with virus isolates from either of the two clades manifest more severe disease, and greater mortality, when infected with a Congo basin isolate (11).

DIAGNOSTICS

Advances in diagnostic capacity have also been achieved in the past decade. Increasingly, PCR assays have been used to provide evidence of virus in clinical specimens. The use of real-time PCR has increased the throughput of specimens testing, as well as shortened the time to acquisition of results. A number of real-time PCR assay methods were available to be used for monkeypox detection during the recent outbreaks (35, 38). Although historic serology-specific assays for orthopoxviruses have been technically time-consuming and reagent and technician dependent, recent reports hold promise for monkeypox species-specific serologic assays (19). These assays await further validation to assess potential cross-recognition of orthopoxviruses which express B21R homolog proteins, as well as their sensitivities in early infection. The use of IgM capture PCR orthopoxvirus assays has advanced our capability to detect recent orthopoxvirus infections (29), as well as to detect evidence of viral infection of the central nervous system (46). Although they are not species specific, in the appropriate epidemiologic setting, the assays have provided meaningful information to assess the extent of an outbreak (37). The development of diagnostics suitable for use in remote field settings will further advance our ability to understand the burden of this disease.

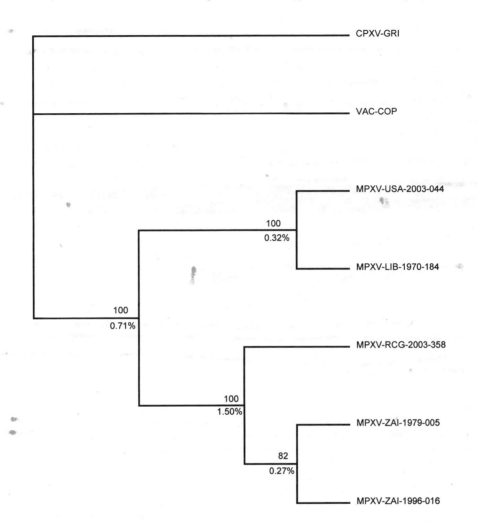

Figure 2. Phylogeny of monkeypox viruses (adapted from reference 39). The phylogeny was based on the whole-genome alignments of five monkeypox virus (MPXV) genomes, rooted with the cowpox virus (CPXV) strain Grishak-90 (CPXV-GRI) and vaccinia virus Copenhagen (VAC-COP). MPXV-USA 2003-044 and MPXV-LIB-1970-184 are of U.S. origin imported from Ghana (isolated in 2003) and Liberia (isolated in 1970); MPXV-RCG-2003-358 is a 2003 isolate from the Republic of the Congo; MPXV-ZAI-1979-005 and MPXV-ZAI-1996-016 are isolates from the DRC obtained in 1979 and 1996.

FUTURE STUDIES

There are a number of outstanding questions that need to be addressed in investigations of monkeypox. The implications of two clades of monkeypox virus are significant when thinking about reservoir species, ecology, human pathogenesis, and potential interventions.

The explanation for the efficient interhuman transmission seen in the Republic of the Congo is unclear. Although considerable potential genetic differences between clades clearly exist, it is difficult to determine if this is representative of a trend in the adaptation of Congo basin monkeypox virus to humans. In addition, we do not know what genetic elements of the virus are most likely responsible for efficient interhuman transmission. Are there aspects of the epidemiology that account for the dynamics of the Republic of the Congo outbreak? The outbreak predominantly affected a community of persons associated with or living near a hospital facility. Hospitals were associated with interhuman transmission of a related orthopoxvirus infection, smallpox.

The true burden of disease with human monkeypox illness or infection remains unclear. Recognition of the illness in the Republic of the Congo was facilitated by increased education regarding vesiculopustular illness suspicious for smallpox, as well as the availability of a physician(s) familiar with smallpox. In western Africa, only rare cases of monkeypox illness have been reported, and none in the past 20 years. Human monkeypox has never been reported in Ghana, yet that was the origin of the virus in the U.S. outbreak. Studies have suggested that inapparent or subclinical infection can occur. Careful epidemiologic case control studies will be required, in concert with ecologic investigations, to assess the extents of ongoing epizootic activity and the extents of disease severity in different regions.

What are the reservoir hosts of monkeypox virus? Investigation of the U.S. outbreak demonstrated a number of additional African species that were susceptible to monkeypox. The taxonomy and distribution within these genera are complex and are still being fully elucidated. In the U.S. outbreak, however, there has been no convincing evidence that any of these African species transmitted the virus directly to humans. Instead, prairie dogs, a non-African species, were associated with transmission of monkeypox virus to humans, resulting in illness. The factors which make prairie dogs such susceptible hosts, as well as the host potential for other North American species, are ill defined. Are there similar factors at work in West Africa and the Congo basin, i.e., are there distinct reservoir hosts and transmitting hosts? If these hypotheses are correct, studying both the reservoir and potential amplifying/transmitting species will be critical to effective public health approaches to education regarding control of the virus and the disease it causes. Alternatively, are there practices which result in human exposure to large doses of virus, resulting in illness versus infection? Overall, what are the different factors which support the maintenance of two clades of monkeypox virus, in addition to their initial emergence?

These issues are of public health importance, both in control of the disease in areas where the virus appears to be endemic and in understanding and preventing the spread of the virus through the increased globalization of human activities and commerce. Understanding the burden of disease and the dynamics of primary (animal-to-human) and secondary (human-to-human) transmission will guide future control efforts. Specifically, as vaccinia virus-based vaccines under study for smallpox, with fewer reactogenic properties, are developed and evaluated, they may be tools to help prevent human monkeypox. Also, development of antivirals with antiorthopoxvirus properties will most likely be orthopoxvirus generic and may also have potential benefit; a number of compounds that have been developed for smallpox treatment through bioterrorism response research programs may be of benefit.

CONCLUSIONS

Monkeypox virus continues to emerge in new populations; recent reports from Sudan indicate that the virus has the capacity to cause human illness in yet another ecologically distinct environment. Better understanding of the ecological, clinical, and epidemiologic impacts of the virus ~~will require enhancements in international surveillance, laboratory capacity, and research efforts~~. The observation of two clades of virus, with apparent differences in human clinical and epidemiologic properties, may correlate with differences in natural histories of reservoir species. A more in-depth understanding of these aspects of this emerging virus will aid public health interventions and control efforts.

REFERENCES

1. **Anderson, M. G., L. D. Frenkel, S. Homann, and J. Guffey.** 2003. A case of severe monkeypox virus disease in an American child: emerging infections and changing professional values. *Pediatr. Infect. Dis. J.* **22:**1093–1096.
2. **Arita, I., R. Gispen, S. S. Kalter, L. T. Wah, S. S. Marennikova, R. Netter, and I. Tagaya.** 1972. Outbreaks of monkeypox and serological surveys in nonhuman primates. *Bull. W. H. O.* **46:**625–631.
3. **Arita, I., and D. A. Henderson.** 1968. Smallpox and monkeypox in non-human primates. *Bull. W. H. O.* **39:**277–283.
4. **Breman, J. G.** 2000. Monkeypox: an emerging infection for humans?, p. 45–67. *In* W. M. Scheld, W. A. Craig, and J. M. Hughes (ed.), *Emerging Infections 4.* ASM Press, Washington, D.C.
5. **Breman, J. G., J. Bernadou, and J. H. Nakano.** 1977. Poxvirus in West African nonhuman primates: serological survey results. *Bull. W. H. O.* **55:**605–612.
6. **Breman, J. G., and D. A. Henderson.** 2002. Diagnosis and management of smallpox. *N. Engl. J. Med.* **346:**1300–1308.
7. **Breman, J. G., R. Kalisa, M. V. Steniowski, E. Zanotto, A. I. Gromyko, and I. Arita.** 1980. Human monkeypox, 1970–79. *Bull. W. H. O.* **58:**165–182.
8. **Breman, J. G., J. H. Nakano, E. Coffi, H. Godfrey, and J. C. Gautun.** 1977. Human poxvirus disease after smallpox eradication. *Am. J. Trop. Med. Hyg.* **26:**273–281.
9. **Centers for Disease Control and Prevention.** 2003. Update: multistate outbreak of monkeypox—Illinois, Indiana, Kansas, Missouri, Ohio, and Wisconsin, 2003. *Morb. Mortal. Wkly. Rep.* **52:**616–618.
10. **Centers for Disease Control and Prevention.** 2003. Update: multistate outbreak of monkeypox—Illinois, Indiana, Kansas, Missouri, Ohio, and Wisconsin, 2003. *Morb. Mortal. Wkly. Rep.* **52:**642–646.
11. **Chen, N., G. Li, M. K. Liszewski, J. P. Atkinson, P. B. Jahrling, Z. Feng, J. Schriewer, C. Buck, C. Wang, E. J. Lefkowitz, J. J. Esposito, T. Harms, I. K. Damon, R. L. Roper, C. Upton, and R. M. Buller.** 2005. Virulence differences between monkeypox virus isolates from West Africa and the Congo basin. *Virology* **340:**46–63.
12. **Cho, C. T., and H. A. Wenner.** 1973. Monkeypox virus. *Bacteriol. Rev.* **37:**1–18.
13. **Douglass, N. J., M. Richardson, and K. R. Dumbell.** 1994. Evidence for recent genetic variation in monkeypox viruses. *J. Gen. Virol.* **75:**1303–1309.
14. **Esposito, J. J., and J. C. Knight.** 1985. Orthopoxvirus DNA: a comparison of restriction profiles and maps. *Virology* **143:**230–251.
15. **Fine, P. E., Z. Jezek, B. Grab, and H. Dixon.** 1988. The transmission potential of monkeypox virus in human populations. *Int. J. Epidemiol.* **17:**643–650.
16. **Fleischauer, A. T., J. C. Kile, M. Davidson, M. Fischer, K. L. Karem, R. Teclaw, H. Messersmith, P. Pontones, B. A. Beard, Z. H. Braden, J. Cono, J. J. Sejvar, A. S. Khan, I. Damon, and M. J. Kuehnert.** 2005. Evaluation of human-to-human transmission of monkeypox from infected patients to health care workers. *Clin. Infect. Dis.* **40:**689–694.
17. **Foster, S. O., E. W. Brink, D. L. Hutchins, J. M. Pifer, B. Lourie, C. R. Moser, E. C. Cummings, O. E. Kuteyi, R. E. Eke, J. B. Titus, E. A. Smith, J. W. Hicks, and W. H. Foege.** 1972. Human monkeypox. *Bull. W. H. O.* **46:**569–576.
18. **Guarner, J., B. J. Johnson, C. D. Paddock, W. J. Shieh, C. S. Goldsmith, M. G. Reynolds, I. K. Damon, R. L. Regnery, and S. R. Zaki.** 2004. Monkeypox transmission and pathogenesis in prairie dogs. *Emerg. Infect. Dis.* **10:**426–431.
19. **Hammarlund, E., M. W. Lewis, S. V. Carter, I. Amanna, S. G. Hansen, L. I. Strelow, S. W. Wong, P. Yoshihara, J. M. Hanifin, and M. K. Slifka.** 2005. Multiple diagnostic techniques identify previously vaccinated individuals with protective immunity against monkeypox. *Nat. Med.* **11:**1005–1011.

20. **Huhn, G. D., A. M. Bauer, K. Yorita, M. B. Graham, J. Sejvar, A. Likos, I. K. Damon, M. G. Reynolds, and M. J. Kuehnert.** 2005. Clinical characteristics of human monkeypox, and risk factors for severe disease. *Clin. Infect. Dis.* **41:**1742–1751.

21. **Hutin, Y. J., R. J. Williams, P. Malfait, R. Pebody, V. N. Loparev, S. L. Ropp, M. Rodriguez, J. C. Knight, F. K. Tshioko, A. S. Khan, M. V. Szczeniowski, and J. J. Esposito.** 2001. Outbreak of human monkeypox, Democratic Republic of Congo, 1996 to 1997. *Emerg. Infect. Dis.* **7:**434–438.

22. **Jezek, Z., I. Arita, M. Mutombo, C. Dunn, J. H. Nakano, and M. Szczeniowski.** 1986. Four generations of probable person-to-person transmission of human monkeypox. *Am. J. Epidemiol.* **123:**1004–1012.

23. **Jezek, Z., and F. Fenner.** 1988. *Human Monkeypox*, p. 1–140. Karger, New York, N.Y.

24. **Jezek, Z., B. Grab, K. M. Paluku, and M. V. Szczeniowski.** 1988. Human monkeypox: disease pattern, incidence and attack rates in a rural area of northern Zaire. *Trop. Geogr. Med.* **40:**73–83.

25. **Jezek, Z., B. Grab, M. Szczeniowski, K. M. Paluku, and M. Mutombo.** 1988. Clinico-epidemiological features of monkeypox patients with an animal or human source of infection. *Bull. W. H. O.* **66:**459–464.

26. **Jezek, Z., B. Grab, M. V. Szczeniowski, K. M. Paluku, and M. Mutombo.** 1988. Human monkeypox: secondary attack rates. *Bull. W. H. O.* **66:**465–470.

27. **Jezek, Z., S. S. Marennikova, M. Mutombo, J. H. Nakano, K. M. Paluku, and M. Szczeniowski.** 1986. Human monkeypox: a study of 2,510 contacts of 214 patients. *J. Infect. Dis.* **154:**551–555.

28. **Jezek, Z., M. Szczeniowski, K. M. Paluku, and M. Mutombo.** 1987. Human monkeypox: clinical features of 282 patients. *J. Infect. Dis.* **156:**293–298.

29. **Karem, K. L., M. Reynolds, Z. Braden, G. Lou, N. Bernard, J. Patton, and I. K. Damon.** 2005. Characterization of acute-phase humoral immunity to monkeypox: use of immunoglobulin M enzyme-linked immunosorbent assay for detection of monkeypox infection during the 2003 North American outbreak. *Clin. Diagn. Lab. Immunol.* **12:**867–872.

30. **Khodakevich, L., Z. Jezek, and K. Kinzanzka.** 1986. Isolation of monkeypox virus from wild squirrel infected in nature. *Lancet* **i:**98–99.

31. **Khodakevich, L., Z. Jezek, and D. Messinger.** 1988. Monkeypox virus: ecology and public health significance. *Bull. W. H. O.* **66:**747–752.

32. **Khodakevich, L., M. Szczeniowski, Nambu-ma-Disu, Z. Jezek, S. Marennikova, J. Nakano, and D. Messinger.** 1987. The role of squirrels in sustaining monkeypox virus transmission. *Trop. Geogr. Med.* **39:**115–122.

33. **Khodakevich, L., M. Szczeniowski, Nambu-ma-Disu, Z. Jezek, S. Marennikova, J. Nakano, and F. Meier.** 1987. Monkeypox virus in relation to the ecological features surrounding human settlements in Bumba zone, Zaire. *Trop. Geogr. Med.* **39:**56–63.

34. **Kile, J. C., A. T. Fleischauer, B. Beard, M. J. Kuehnert, R. S. Kanwal, P. Pontones, H. J. Messersmith, R. Teclaw, K. L. Karem, Z. H. Braden, I. Damon, A. S. Khan, and M. Fischer.** 2005. Transmission of monkeypox among persons exposed to infected prairie dogs in Indiana in 2003. *Arch. Pediatr. Adolesc. Med.* **159:**1022–1025.

35. **Kulesh, D. A., B. M. Loveless, D. Norwood, J. Garrison, C. A. Whitehouse, C. Hartmann, E. Mucker, D. Miller, L. P. Wasieloski, Jr., J. Huggins, G. Huhn, L. L. Miser, C. Imig, M. Martinez, T. Larsen, C. A. Rossi, and G. V. Ludwig.** 2004. Monkeypox virus detection in rodents using real-time 3′-minor groove binder TaqMan assays on the Roche LightCycler. *Lab. Investig.* **84:**1200–1208.

36. **Langohr, I. M., G. W. Stevenson, H. L. Thacker, and R. L. Regnery.** 2004. Extensive lesions of monkeypox in a prairie dog (*Cynomys* sp.). *Vet. Pathol.* **41:**702–707.

37. **Learned, L. A., M. G. Reynolds, D. W. Wassa, Y. Li, V. A. Olson, K. Karem, L. L. Stempora, Z. H. Braden, R. Kline, A. Likos, F. Libama, H. Moudzeo, J. D. Bolanda, P. Tarangonia, P. Boumandoki, P. Formenty, J. M. Harvey, and I. K. Damon.** 2005. Extended interhuman transmission of monkeypox in a hospital community in the Republic of the Congo, 2003. *Am. J. Trop. Med. Hyg.* **73:**428–434.

38. **Li, Y., V. A. Olson, T. Laue, M. T. Laker, and I. Damon.** 2006. Detection of *Monkeypox virus* with real-time PCR assays. *J. Clin. Virol.* **36:**194–203.

39. **Likos, A. M., S. A. Sammons, V. A. Olson, A. M. Frace, Y. Li, M. Olsen-Rasmussen, W. Davidson, R. Galloway, M. L. Khristova, M. G. Reynolds, H. Zhao, D. S. Carroll, A. Curns, P. Formenty, J. J. Esposito, R. L. Regnery, and I. K. Damon.** 2005. A tale of two clades: monkeypox viruses. *J. Gen. Virol.* **86:**2661–2672.

40. **Meyer, H., M. Perrichot, M. Stemmler, P. Emmerich, H. Schmitz, F. Varaine, R. Shungu, F. Tshioko, and P. Formenty.** 2002. Outbreaks of disease suspected of being due to human monkeypox virus infection in the Democratic Republic of Congo in 2001. *J. Clin. Microbiol.* **40:**2919–2921.

41. **Meyer, H., S. L. Ropp, and J. J. Esposito.** 1997. Gene for A-type inclusion body protein is useful for a polymerase chain reaction assay to differentiate orthopoxviruses. *J. Virol. Methods* **64:**217–221.
42. **Nalca, A., A. W. Rimoin, S. Bavari, and C. A. Whitehouse.** 2005. Reemergence of monkeypox: prevalence, diagnostics, and countermeasures. *Clin. Infect. Dis.* **41:**1765–1771.
43. **Peterson, A. T., M. Papes, M. R. Reynolds, N. D. Perry, B. Hanson, R. L. Regnery, C. L. Hutson, I. K. Damon, and D. S. Carroll.** 2006. Native-range ecology and invasive potential of *Cricetomys* in North America. *J. Mammal.* **87:**427–433.
44. **Reed, K. D., J. W. Melski, M. B. Graham, R. L. Regnery, M. J. Sotir, M. V. Wegner, J. J. Kazmierczak, E. J. Stratman, Y. Li, J. A. Fairley, G. R. Swain, V. A. Olson, E. K. Sargent, S. C. Kehl, M. A. Frace, R. Kline, S. L. Foldy, J. P. Davis, and I. K. Damon.** 2004. The detection of monkeypox in humans in the Western Hemisphere. *N. Engl. J. Med.* **350:**342–350.
45. **Ropp, S. L., Q. Jin, J. C. Knight, R. F. Massung, and J. J. Esposito.** 1995. PCR strategy for identification and differentiation of smallpox and other orthopoxviruses. *J. Clin. Microbiol.* **33:**2069–2076.
46. **Sejvar, J. J., Y. Chowdary, M. Schomogyi, J. Stevens, J. Patel, K. Karem, M. Fischer, M. J. Kuehnert, S. R. Zaki, C. D. Paddock, J. Guarner, W. J. Shieh, J. L. Patton, N. Bernard, Y. Li, V. A. Olson, R. L. Kline, V. N. Loparev, D. S. Schmid, B. Beard, R. R. Regnery, and I. K. Damon.** 2004. Human monkeypox infection: a family cluster in the Midwestern United States. *J. Infect. Dis.* **190:**1833–1840.
47. **Tesh, R. B., D. M. Watts, E. Sbrana, M. Siirin, V. L. Popov, and S. Y. Xiao.** 2004. Experimental infection of ground squirrels *(Spermophilus tridecemlineatus)* with monkeypox virus. *Emerg. Infect. Dis.* **10:**1563–1567.
48. **Xiao, S. Y., E. Sbrana, D. M. Watts, M. Siirin, A. P. da Rosa, and R. B. Tesh.** 2005. Experimental infection of prairie dogs with monkeypox virus. *Emerg. Infect. Dis.* **11:**539–545.

Emerging Infections 7
Edited by W. M. Scheld, D. C. Hooper, and J. M. Hughes
© 2005 ASM Press, Washington, D.C.

Chapter 6

West Nile Virus

Lyle R. Petersen

For more than 60 years after its initial isolation from the blood of a febrile woman in the West Nile district of Uganda in 1937 (136), West Nile virus (WNV) remained an occasional cause of febrile illness in Africa, the Middle East, parts of Europe and the former Soviet Union, South Asia, and Australia. It emerged from obscurity in the late 1990s after large outbreaks of unusual severity in Romania (143) and Russia (120). After its recognition in New York City in 1999 (111), the virus has spread rapidly in North America, producing outbreaks of severe neuroinvasive disease of unprecedented size.

This chapter highlights many aspects of this emerging pathogen, including its epidemiology in the Americas, new clinical syndromes, new modes of transmission and their impacts on public health, and progress in the development of therapeutics and vaccines. Virology, entomology, ecology, and pathogenesis are discussed only to the extent required to provide background for the main topics.

BACKGROUND

WNV is a member of the Japanese encephalitis virus (JEV) serocomplex, which contains four other medically important flaviviruses: JEV, St. Louis encephalitis virus (SLEV), Murray Valley encephalitis virus, and Kunjin virus. Before the emergence of WNV in the Americas, each of these flaviviral encephalitis viruses had a relatively unique geographic distribution (Fig. 1).

Strains of WNV can be divided into two genetic lineages (1 and 2) by phylogenetic analysis of the complete genome sequence or of the E protein gene sequence (92, 93). Major human outbreaks of WNV infection have been associated only with lineage 1 WNVs. Lineage 2 WNVs apparently maintain themselves in enzootic cycles only, primarily in Africa. Kunjin virus in Australia is now recognized as a subtype lineage 1 WNV.

Birds are the primary amplifying hosts, and the virus is maintained in a bird-mosquito-bird cycle primarily involving *Culex* sp. mosquitoes (71) (Fig. 2). Wild birds develop prolonged high levels of viremia and serve as amplifying hosts (86). Passerine

---

Lyle R. Petersen • Division of Vector-Borne Infectious Diseases, National Center for Infectious Diseases, Centers for Disease Control and Prevention, Fort Collins, CO 80522.

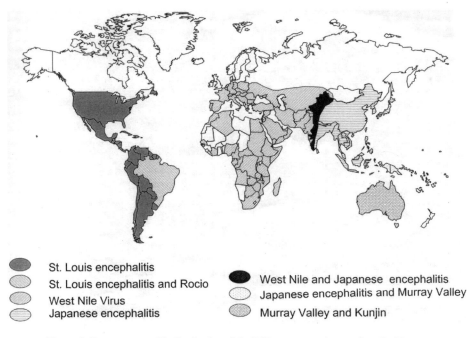

St. Louis encephalitis
St. Louis encephalitis and Rocio
West Nile Virus
Japanese encephalitis

West Nile and Japanese encephalitis
Japanese encephalitis and Murray Valley
Murray Valley and Kunjin

Figure 1. Known geographic distribution of the JEV serogroup viruses of medical importance before 1999. The distribution of WNV in the United States from 1999 through 2005 is shown in Color Plate 2.

birds develop high levels of viremia, are abundant, and become infected in high numbers during epizootics, suggesting that they may be the principal amplifying hosts for WNV (86, 87). Humans and other mammals, such as horses, do not develop a high-titer viremia and thus are thought to be incidental hosts who play a minor role in the transmission cycle.

Culex sp. mosquitoes are important for their role in allowing the virus to overwinter in temperate climates, where they hibernate as adult mosquitoes (109). The amplification cycle begins when infected overwintering mosquitoes emerge in the spring and infect birds. Amplification within the bird-mosquito-bird cycle continues until late summer and fall, when *Culex* mosquitoes begin diapause (a reduction of physiologic activity in which development is arrested) and rarely blood feed. The major mosquito vector in Africa and the Middle East is *Culex univittatus,* with *Culex picilipes, Culex neavei, Culex decens, Aedes albocephalus,* or *Mimomyia* spp. important in some areas (71). In Europe, *Culex pipiens, Culex modestus,* and *Coquillettidia richiardii* are important. In Asia, *Culex tritaeniorhynchus, Culex vishnui,* and *Culex quinquefasciatus* predominate (71). In North America, as of February 2006, surveillance had identified 58 mosquito species infected with WNV (118). WNV and SLEV appear to share the same maintenance and amplification vectors: *C. pipiens* (the northern house mosquito) and *Culex restuans* in the northeastern United States and Canada, *C. quinquefasciatus* (the southern house mosquito) in the southern United States, and *Culex tarsalis* in the western United States and Canada. *Culex nigripalpus* may prove important in Florida. It is unknown to what extent other mosquito species transmit WNV to humans.

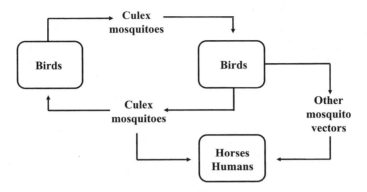

Figure 2. WNV transmission cycle. In North America, *C. pipiens, C. restuans, C. quin-quefasciatus,* and *C. tarsalis* are the main maintenance and amplification vectors. *Culex salinarius* and some mosquitoes of the genera *Aedes* and *Ochlerotatus* may be important vectors to humans in some areas.

EPIDEMIOLOGY

Emergence of Outbreaks of Unusual Virulence

Until the mid-1990s, WNV outbreaks were almost always associated with mild human illness (62, 76, 97, 110). The first recorded instance of severe neurological disease during an outbreak occurred in Israeli nursing homes in 1957 (139). Further evidence that WNV could produce severe neurological disease was obtained in the early 1950s during experiments with WNV as an experimental cancer therapy. In those studies, 11% of the study subjects developed encephalitis, sometimes accompanied by paralysis, involuntary twitching, and cogwheel rigidity (138). Nevertheless, severe neurological disease during outbreaks remained uncommon until the outbreaks in Algeria in 1994 (95), Romania in 1996 (143), Tunisia in 1997 (109), Russia in 1999 (120), the United States in 1999 to 2005 (118), Israel in 2000 (37), Sudan in 2002 (46), and Canada in 2003 and 2004. These outbreaks were caused by new, closely related lineage 1 variants of apparently increased virulence (18).

Emergence and Spread in North America

The virus' first detection in North America occurred during a human outbreak of meningitis and encephalitis and an accompanying epizootic in birds in 1999 in the New York City area (111). Sequencing of the original North American WNV isolate (NY99) implicated the Middle East as the likely source of the WNV that entered the New York City area (92, 93). This genotypic link was further confirmed by the similar phenotypic characteristics of the NY99 WNV and a strain of WNV isolated from storks in Israel. Both NY99 and Israeli strains of WNV killed birds. Since birds are the primary amplifying hosts for WNV, the high mortality in certain birds from these WNV strains was unusual. No other outbreaks of WNV have been associated with high bird mortality.

Mortality has been recorded in more than 280 native and captive bird species in North America (118). The NY99 strain of WNV appears to be lethal to most birds of the family

Corvidae (crows, ravens, and jays) (18, 87). The substantial crow and blue jay mortality in the United States and Canada has served as the foundation for the ecological WNV surveillance based on reporting dead birds to public health officials. The high American crow mortality rate for the NY99 WNV strain compared to two other lineage 1 WNV strains (Kunjin and a strain isolated in Kenya [KEN-3829]) has been confirmed in the laboratory (18).

As WNV has spread westward across the United States, its genome has remained remarkably stable, with minor temporal and regional variations observed. These variations usually represent less than 0.5% of the genomic sequence and result in only a few amino acid changes in any given isolate (10, 16, 43, 44, 51, 63). Nevertheless, certain variants have emerged and replaced previously circulating variants (45).

By 2003, ecologic surveillance documented the spread of the virus to the Pacific Coast (Color Plate 2 [see color insert]). From 1999 through 2001, only 149 cases of human disease were reported (Table 1) (25, 29, 99, 111, 118). However, in 2002, a multistate outbreak throughout the Midwest resulted in more than 4,000 reported cases, 2,946 of which involved reported neuroinvasive disease (Table 1 and Color Plate 2) (113). This outbreak was epidemiologically similar to a 1975 outbreak of SLEV infection, which involved approximately 2,000 persons (39). In 2003, nearly 10,000 cases were reported; 2,866 of them involved neuroinvasive disease. Wider availability of commercial WNV antibody detection assays resulted in increased diagnosis and reporting of patients with West Nile (WN) fever in 2003; however, the similar numbers of neuroinvasive-disease cases reported in 2002 and 2003 indicated that the two outbreaks were of similar magnitudes (Table 1) (118). The incidences of WNV neuroinvasive disease were lower in 2004 and 2005 than in the two previous years (Table 1).

Serological surveys indicate that even in areas experiencing outbreaks, less than 5% of the population has been exposed to the virus (26, 108, 143). Based on the 6,849 reported cases of WNV neuroinvasive disease from 1999 through 2004 and the estimated proportions of infected persons who develop WNV neuroinvasive disease, approximately 1 million persons have become infected with WNV in the United States, and approximately 190,000 of them have become ill (118). Through 2005, more than 780 deaths have been reported, with a fatality rate of approximately 10% among persons with neuroinvasive disease (113, 118).

Table 1. Reported numbers of cases of WNV infection, neuroinvasive disease, and death, United States, 1999 to 2005

Yr	Total no. of cases	No. of neuroinvasive cases	No. of fatalities
1999	62	54	7
2000	21	19	2
2001	66	64	9
2002	4,156	2,946	284
2003	9,862	2,866	264
2004	2,539	1,148	100
2005	3,000	1,294	114
Total	19,706	8,391	780

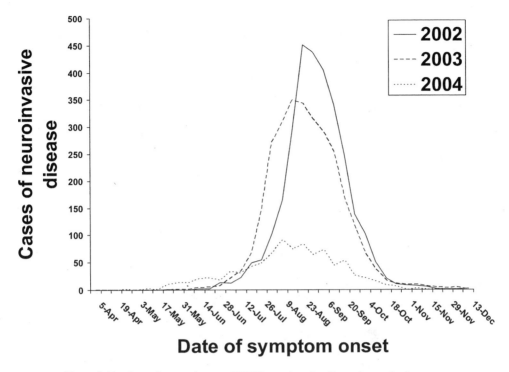

Figure 3. Numbers of reported cases of WNV neuroinvasive disease by week of symptom onset, 2002 to 2004.

In North America, human WNV infection incidence increases in early summer and peaks in August or early September (Fig. 3). However, an outbreak in Phoenix, Arizona, in 2004 began in May and peaked in late June and early July.

The first cases of human WNV disease in Canada occurred in 2002, with 426 illnesses and 20 deaths reported in Quebec and Ontario. In 2003, 1,494 cases were reported, 217 of which involved neuroinvasive disease and 10 of which were fatal. In 2004, only 26 cases were reported, 13 of which involved neuroinvasive disease and none of which were fatal. In 2005, 229 cases were reported, 49 of which involved neuroinvasive disease and 12 of which were fatal.

WNV in Latin America and the Caribbean

WNV was first detected south of the United States in 2001, when a resident of the Cayman Islands developed WNV encephalitis (29). Subsequently, serologic studies of birds and horses suggested that WNV has circulated in Colombia (101), Cuba (50), the Dominican Republic (88), Jamaica (49), Guadeloupe (94, 125), El Salvador (40), and Puerto Rico (50) and widely in Mexico (15, 53, 56, 96, 100). However, virus isolations have been infrequent and documented avian and equine morbidity and mortality from WNV in those areas are scant.

In 2002, WNV was isolated from a dead common raven in Tabasco State, Mexico (53), and in 2003, it was detected by genetic sequencing of cerebellar tissue from a dead horse from Nuevo Leon State, Mexico (16). In Guadeloupe, paired samples from horses sampled at an approximate 1-year interval indicated that 47% had developed neutralizing antibodies; however, clinical illness was not observed, and IgM antibodies were not detected (125).

The discrepancy between the serologic evidence indicating widespread WNV circulation in the Caribbean, Central America, and Mexico and the lack of substantial avian, equine, or human morbidity remains a mystery. Possible causes include false-positive serologic test results due to circulation of other flaviviruses, circulation of attenuated WNV strains, protection from serious infection because of previous flavivirus exposure, and suboptimal disease surveillance.

Risk Factors for Neuroinvasive Disease and Death

Serologic surveys in Romania (143) and New York City (108), as well as blood donor WNV screening data (84), indicate that WNV infection incidence is constant across all age groups during outbreaks. Surveillance data from the United States indicate that age is the most important host risk factor for development of neuroinvasive disease after infection, with the incidence of neuroinvasive disease approximately 30 times higher for persons 80 to 90 years old than for children younger than 10 years old (113).

Advanced age is the most important risk factor for death. Surveillance data indicate that case fatality rates for persons with WNV neuroinvasive disease increase from 1% among persons under 40 years of age to 36% among persons 90 years old and older (113). During outbreaks, hospitalized persons older than 70 years of age had case fatality rates of 15% in Romania (143) and 29% in Israel (37). Encephalitis with severe muscle weakness and change in the level of consciousness were also prominent clinical risk factors predicting fatal outcome (37, 111). Diabetes mellitus was an independent risk factor for death during the 1999 New York City outbreak (111). The incidence of neuroinvasive disease and the probability of death after acquiring neuroinvasive disease are slightly higher in men than women (113).

Organ transplant recipients are at extreme risk of developing neuroinvasive disease after WNV infection. A seroprevalence study carried out in patients of Canadian outpatient transplant clinics following a WNV epidemic in 2002 indicated that approximately 40% developed neuroinvasive disease following infection (90), a rate approximately 40 times that of the population at large (91). Individual case reports or small case series have described WNV neuroinvasive disease in kidney, pancreas, liver, lung, heart, bone marrow, and stem cell transplant recipients, as well as patients with hematologic malignancies. The risk of death among persons with WNV infection who have underlying immunodeficiencies is unknown and cannot be ascertained from these individual case reports. In a series of 11 transplant patients with WNV neuroinvasive disease, two died and three developed significant residual neurological deficits (85). Only one person with WNV encephalitis and human immunodeficiency virus infection has been reported (141).

Nonmosquito Transmission Routes

Epidemiologic investigations during recent epidemics have documented transmission by blood transfusion (115) and organ transplantation (36, 72). Intrauterine transmission, breast milk transmission, and dialysis-related transmission have been suspected. Human laboratory-acquired WNV infections by the percutaneous route (28) and suspected aerosol transmission in the laboratory (112) have been reported.

Blood transfusion-related transmission was considered a theoretical possibility because most persons with WNV infection have a short period of viremia but remain asymptomatic. The risk of WNV transmission from blood products obtained from donors living in the epicenter of the 1999 New York City outbreak was estimated at 1.8 per 10,000 units, although no instances of transfusion transmission were documented at that time (13). Transfusion-associated WNV transmission was proven during the 2002 U.S. WNV epidemic, when 23 transfusion recipients became infected after receipt of platelets, red blood cells, or plasma from 16 viremic blood donors (115). The 15 recipients who developed WNV-related illness became ill 2 to 21 (median, 10) days after transfusion. The implicated blood donations had low virus titers (0.8 to 75.1 PFU per ml), and all lacked WNV IgM antibodies at the time of donation. Mathematical models indicated that the mean risk of transfusion-associated WNV transmission during the 2002 epidemic ranged from 2.1 to 4.7 per 10,000 donors in high-incidence states (14).

Two instances of WNV transmission via organ transplantation have been documented (36, 72). In one instance, an organ donor had become infected from a contaminated blood transfusion 1 day before the organs were harvested. Retrospectively tested blood samples from the day of organ harvest identified WNV RNA. Both recipients of the donor's kidneys and the recipient of the donor's heart developed WNV encephalitis; the recipient of the donor's liver developed WN fever. Symptoms began 7 to 17 days after transplantation. The second instance involved a donor with a febrile illness approximately a week before organ harvest. Blood samples obtained the day before organ harvest showed WNV-specific IgG and IgM antibodies but were negative for WNV RNA. The liver and lung recipients developed WNV encephalitis 13 and 17 days after transplantation; a kidney recipient remained asymptomatic, but the serum was positive for WNV RNA; and another kidney recipient did not have serological evidence of WNV infection.

One possible WNV transmission via human breast milk has been reported (27). The mother was infected with WNV from a contaminated blood transfusion 1 day after delivery and developed WNV meningitis 11 days later. The infant was breast fed starting 1 day after delivery; WNV nucleic acid and WNV-specific IgM and IgG antibodies were detected in a sample of breast milk 16 days after delivery. The infant remained asymptomatic, but a serum sample obtained 25 days after delivery showed WNV-specific IgM antibodies.

Dialysis-related WNV transmission has also been suspected (32). Two persons developed symptomatic WNV infection 8 and 19 days after receiving dialysis on the same dialysis machine. A third person who received dialysis between these two patients on the same machine remained asymptomatic but had WNV IgG and neutralizing antibodies in serum 42 days after dialysis. An outbreak of WNV infection occurred among turkey farm workers; however, the means of transmission in that setting is unknown (30). One instance of WNV infection following conjunctival exposure has been reported (57).

CLINICAL SYNDROMES

Serological surveys following contemporary outbreaks indicate that about a fifth of human WNV infections result in clinical illness without neuroinvasive disease and 1 in

150 results in neuroinvasive disease (meningitis, encephalitis, or acute flaccid paralysis) (108, 143).

WN Fever

The term West Nile fever was coined by Goldblum when he investigated clinical illnesses during an Israeli outbreak in 1952 (62). He described the illness as one of sudden onset, characterized by malaise, general weakness, a chilly sensation with fever, drowsiness, severe frontal headache, aching of the eyes when moved, and pains mostly in the chest and lumbar regions, with a few patients having gastrointestinal disturbances, anorexia, nausea, and dryness of the throat. He noted that the acute illness lasted 3 to 6 days, but convalescence was slow, lasting 1 to 2 weeks and accompanied by general fatigue. This and subsequent investigations suggest that the typical incubation period is approximately 2 to 14 days.

WN fever has been reported in all age groups; the median age of persons reported with WN fever during the 2002 U.S. epidemic was 49 years (113). WN fever is considerably underreported, and age-specific incidence data and clinical descriptions of illness are subject to considerable bias. One contemporary study based on statewide WNV virus surveillance in Illinois found that approximately one-third of the reported patients with WN fever were hospitalized, and those hospitalized were older than those not hospitalized (mean, 65 years versus 46 years of age) (144). As described in earlier outbreaks of WN fever, fever, headache, fatigue, myalgias, and gastrointestinal complaints were prominent symptoms (Table 2). The Illinois study reaffirmed early observations that complete recovery from WN fever is typical, but some symptoms, particularly fatigue, and disability may be prolonged in some patients (144).

The rash associated with WN fever is morbilliform, maculopapular, and nonpruritic, and it predominates over the torso and extremities, sparing the palms and soles (6, 55). The rash often appears several days after symptom onset and may coincide with convalescence from initial symptoms. The rash may occur less commonly in patients with neuroinvasive disease, which may explain why it is reported less frequently in contemporary than in early outbreaks of WN fever (Table 2) (97).

Neuroinvasive Disease

U.S. surveillance data indicate that WNV neuroinvasive-disease incidence increases with age (113). WNV meningitis makes up the largest percentage of neuroinvasive-disease cases in younger age groups, while the proportion of encephalitis increases in older age groups. During the 2002 U.S. epidemic, the median ages of persons reported with WNV meningitis and encephalitis were 46 and 64 years, respectively (113).

WNV meningitis is clinically similar to other viral meningitides. Affected persons experience the abrupt onset of fever, headache, and meningeal signs, including nuchal rigidity, the presence of Kernig's and/or Brudzinski's signs, and photophobia or phonophobia. The associated headache may be severe, requiring hospitalization for pain control; associated gastrointestinal disturbance may result in dehydration, exacerbating head pain and systemic symptoms (132). WNV meningitis is generally associated with a favorable outcome, though similar to WN fever; some patients experience persistent headache, fatigue, and myalgias (132). During the 2002 U.S. epidemic, 2% of reported cases of meningitis from WNV were fatal (113).

Table 2. Symptoms reported among patients with WNV infection by location, year, and hospitalization status

Symptom[a]	% of patients with symptom					
	New York City (1999), hospitalized (n = 59)	Romania (1996), hospitalized (n = 393)	Israel, hospitalized		Illinois (2002)	
			2000 (n = 233)	1953 (n = 50)	Hospitalized (n = 30)	Outpatient (n = 68)
Fever	90	91	98	100	93	76
Fatigue				"Nearly all"	90	99
Weakness	56				70	57
Nausea	53			25		
Vomiting	51	53	31	10	43	21
Headache	47	77	58	80	50	81
Change in mental status	46	34[b]	40[b]			
Diarrhea	27		19	30	33	24
Rash	19		21	"About half"	23	72
Cough	19			8		
Stiff neck	19	57	29		43[c]	60[c]
Myalgia	17		15	25	50	68
Arthralgia	15				27	41
Lymphadenopathy	2		10	90		

[a]Symptoms reported among hospitalized patients with neuroinvasive disease during outbreaks in New York (1999) (111), Romania (1996) (143), and Israel (2000) (37); among hospitalized patients with WN fever (1953) (97); and among hospitalized and nonhospitalized patients with WN fever in Illinois (2002) (144). Some listed symptoms were not reported in all studies.
[b]Reported as confusion.
[c]Reported as stiff neck or neck pain.

WNV encephalitis may range in severity from a mild, self-limited confusional state to severe encephalopathy, coma, and death. Several neurological syndromes, primarily extrapyramidal disorders, have been observed in patients with WNV encephalitis (20, 116, 131, 132). Patients with WNV encephalitis frequently develop a coarse tremor, particularly in the upper extremities. The tremor tends to be postural and may have a kinetic component (20, 52, 131, 132). Myoclonus, predominantly of the upper extremities and facial muscles, may occur and also may have a kinesigenic component. Features of parkinsonism, including hypomimia, bradykinesia, and postural instability, may be seen and can be associated with falls and functional difficulties (127, 132). Similar to other causes of secondary tremor, a resting tremor is frequently absent. Cerebellar ataxia, with associated truncal instability and gait disturbance leading to falls, has been described (20, 78, 131). Opsoclonus-myoclonus has been reported (82, 131). These abnormal movements usually follow the onset of mental status changes and typically resolve over time; however, primary tremor and parkinsonism may persist in patients recovering from severe encephalitis (116, 132). Seizures are uncommon in patients with WNV encephalitis.

The development of these movement disorders is due to specific neurotropism of WNV for regions of the brain involved with control of movement. At a cellular level, it appears that WNV has a predilection for neurons in the central nervous system (48), with the most consistent involvement appearing in the brainstem (particularly the medulla and pons), the deep gray matter nuclei (particularly the substantia nigra of the basal ganglia and the thalami), and the cerebellum (17, 65, 80).

Few data exist regarding the long-term neurologic and functional outcomes of WNV encephalitis. As with many other viral encephalitides, initial severe neurologic illness does not necessarily correlate with eventual outcome, and some patients with initial severe encephalopathy with associated coma may experience dramatic recovery and minimal sequelae (132). However, others experience persistent neurologic dysfunction, including persistent movement disorders, headaches, fatigue, and cognitive complaints. Large hospital-based series suggest that patients with severe WNV encephalitis frequently require assistance with daily activities following acute-care discharge (52, 116). Patients may frequently self-report substantial functional and cognitive difficulties for up to a year following acute infection, and only 37% of patients in the 1999 New York City outbreak achieved full recovery at 1 year (83). Cognitive disturbances following WNV encephalitis have not been well characterized; however, difficulties with attention and concentration, as well as neuropsychiatric problems, including apathy and depression, have been described (83, 132).

Fatality rates range from 10% to 20% among patients with severe neuroinvasive disease (113, 116), and mortality is higher among the elderly and those with immunocompromising conditions. An Israeli study of hospitalized patients indicated a 12% 2-year mortality, with age, male sex, diabetes mellitus, and dementia as adverse prognostic indicators (64).

Acute weakness associated with WNV infection has been variably attributed to myelitis, Guillain-Barré syndrome, or radiculopathy. However, most cases of paralysis from WNV infection result from viral involvement of and damage to the lower motor neurons of the spinal cord (anterior horn cells), resulting in acute flaccid paralysis (133). The peak incidence occurs among persons aged 35 to 65 years (133). WNV poliomyelitis generally develops soon after illness onset, usually within the first 24 to 48 h. Limb paralysis generally develops rapidly and may be abrupt, occasionally raising clinical concern for stroke. The weakness is usually asymmetric and often results in monoplegia. Patients with severe and extensive spinal cord involvement will develop a more symmetric dense quadriplegia. Central facial weakness, frequently bilateral, can also be seen (73, 133). While sensory loss or numbness is generally absent, patients will often experience intense pain in the affected limbs just before or during the onset of weakness (133).

Diffuse involvement by WNV of the lower brainstem and high cervical spinal cord may result in diaphragmatic and intercostal muscle paralysis and subsequent neuromuscular respiratory failure requiring emergent endotracheal intubation (12, 48, 133). Respiratory involvement in WNV poliomyelitis is associated with high morbidity and mortality, and among survivors, prolonged ventilatory support may be required (12, 54, 98, 129, 133). Inability to be weaned off ventilatory support, and withdrawal of this support, may be a frequent cause of death among persons with respiratory involvement. Patients developing early dysarthria and dysphagia are at greater risk for subsequent respiratory failure.

WNV infection may cause other forms of acute weakness, including brachial plexopathy (4, 133), as well as radiculopathy and a predominantly demyelinating peripheral neuropathy similar to Guillain-Barré syndrome (3, 114, 133), but these are infrequent and may be recognized by their clinical and electrophysiologic features. The weakness associated with the Guillain-Barré-like syndrome is usually symmetric and ascending in nature and is associated with sensory and autonomic dysfunction. Additionally, cerebrospinal fluid examination will generally show albuminocytologic dissociation (elevated protein in the absence of pleocytosis), and electrodiagnostics will be consistent with a predominantly demyelinating polyneuropathy.

The long-term functional outcome in patients with WNV poliomyelitis has not yet been fully characterized; however, data indicate that recovery of limb strength is generally incomplete, often resulting in profound residual deficits (20, 24, 98, 133). However, some persons experience total or near-total recovery of strength, particularly those with milder initial weakness. Surviving motor unit numbers estimated by motor unit number estimation may have prognostic significance (24). Quadriplegia and respiratory failure are associated with high morbidity and mortality, and recovery is slow and almost invariably incomplete (12, 133).

Other Clinical Manifestations

Ocular manifestations are frequent, but usually of minor significance (61). A prospective study of ocular changes among consecutively enrolled patients presenting to a hospital with WNV infection during an outbreak in Tunisia indicated that 80% had multifocal chorioretinitis with mild vitreous inflammatory reaction on presentation or during follow-up (81). Other common findings included intraretinal hemorrhages in 72%, white-centered retinal hemorrhages in 24%, focal retinal vascular sheathing in 10%, and retinal vascular leakage in 17%.

An inflammatory vitritis has occurred concomitantly with the chorioretinitis and may be significant enough to obscure the optic disc. Symptomatic persons describe gradual visual blurring and loss, floaters, and flashes. Although experience with management is limited, improvement both in symptoms and in underlying chorioretinal lesions has been observed following treatment with intraocular corticosteroids (1). Retinal occlusive vasculitis without chorioretinal findings, anterior uveitis, and optic neuritis have also been reported.

Rhabdomyolysis (73, 89, 105), hepatitis, and pancreatitis have been reported (48, 117, 145). Myocarditis has been seen histopathologically in WNV infection (130), but clinical correlation with cardiac dysfunction in humans remains to be demonstrated. One case of stiff-person syndrome, a rare autoimmune disorder associated with antibodies against glutamic acid decarboxylase, has been reported following WNV infection (69). One person with central diabetes insipidus complicating WNV encephalitis has been reported (134).

THERAPEUTICS AND PREVENTION

Therapeutics

No specific, proven treatment exists for WNV infection. The fact that WN viremia in humans is short-lived and is usually cleared by the time of clinical presentation presents a substantial theoretical obstacle for specific antiviral therapies. However, studies with monkeys and humans indicate that WNV may persist in the central nervous system or other organs for prolonged periods (123, 138). The variability in clinical outcome of WNV infection complicates interpretation of nonrandomized clinical trials.

The antiviral agent ribavirin has had demonstrated in vitro activity against WNV infection (5, 75), but therapeutic efficacy has not yet been demonstrated in animal models. Ribavirin was used in an uncontrolled, nonblinded fashion in patients with WNV neuroinvasive disease in Israel in 2000, where it was found to be ineffective and potentially detrimental (37). Ribavirin increased mortality in Syrian golden hamsters when administered 2 days after WNV inoculation (106).

Interferon reduced viremia and slightly improved mortality in Syrian golden hamsters when administered 2 days after WNV inoculation and before the development of symptoms (106). No synergistic effect was noted with coadministration of ribavirin. Placebo-controlled trials of alpha-2a interferon in the treatment of the closely related flavivirus JEV failed to demonstrate a beneficial effect (137). Case reports of patients with WNV encephalitis have suggested a possible clinical benefit of alpha-2b interferon (77, 131). Nevertheless, two patients receiving alpha-2b interferon and ribavirin for hepatitis C infection developed WN fever after mosquito exposure (70).

Animal models have suggested the efficacy of high-titer WNV-specific intravenous immune globulin, particularly when administered before or shortly after WNV challenge (2, 11, 23, 47, 135, 142). Several patients with underlying immunodeficiencies who were treated with intravenous immune globulin have been reported with various outcomes (66, 68, 135).

Controlled trials of third-generation antisense compounds are under way. The use of angiotensin receptor blockers in the United States as definitive therapy for WNV infection has not been assessed in a controlled fashion (107). Improvement in clinical condition following administration of high-dose steroids was noted in one patient with encephalitis and acute flaccid paralysis (124).

WNV Screening of Transfused Blood and Transplanted Organs

Since 2003, all blood donations in the United States and Canada have been screened using WNV nucleic acid amplification tests. These tests are conducted on minipools of samples from 6 or 16 blood donations, depending on the test format (34). Screening has identified more than 1,000 viremic blood donors in the United States since 2003 (21, 118, 140). As expected, screening yields have been extremely temporally and geographically variable, with up to 1 in 200 donations proven viremic in some areas experiencing epidemics (21, 84, 140). Viremia levels were very low, and retrospective studies have indicated that between one-third and one-half of viremic donations are not identified by minipool screening (22, 119). However, most donations with viremia detectable only on individual-donation testing have demonstrable IgM antibodies. All 30 of the documented transfusion-associated transmissions from 2002 to 2005 were caused by IgM-negative donations, while recipients of IgM-positive viremic donations have failed to become infected (33, 34, 115, 118). To further minimize the risk of transfusion transmission, in 2003, blood centers began implementing algorithms to switch to single-donation screening in areas experiencing outbreaks. The estimated effectiveness in eliminating the residual risk of transfusion transmission by using various criteria to switch from minipool screening to single-unit testing ranged from 57 to 100% (41).

Mosquito Control

Reduction of vector populations by public mosquito control programs is another mainstay of WNV prevention in North America. These programs emphasize an integrated pest management approach, which combines surveillance, source reduction, larvicide

(*Bacillus thuringiensis* subsp. *israelensis, Bacillus sphaericus,* or methoprene), adulticide (organophosphates or pyrethroids), and other biological control, as well as public relations and education (128). Evaluation of the effectiveness of these programs on reducing the incidence of human WNV infection is complicated by the focal and sporadic nature of epidemics.

Ultra-low-volume application of adulticides is used during epidemics or when surveillance indicators suggest an impending epidemic; however, concern over environmental effects or adverse impact on public health makes their use controversial in many communities. Acute illness following application of adulticides is rare (31, 79), and pesticide exposures of the population at large during vector control operations are extremely low (35). Studies have shown that adulticide applications must cover a large geographic area and must involve multiple treatments; otherwise, vector mosquito populations will quickly rebound (7, 103, 126).

Human Personal Protection

Avoidance of exposure to mosquitoes by avoidance of outdoor activities at dawn and dusk when mosquito activity is high, wearing protective clothing during periods of likely exposure, and using repellants are recommended. However, evaluation of the effectiveness of repellents in community settings has been complicated by difficulties in quantifying mosquito exposure in relation to repellent use. Repellents containing DEET (*N,N*-diethyl-*meta*-toluamide or *N,N*-diethyl-3-methylbenzamide) have been used by the general public in the United States since 1957. DEET is available in many products, and its duration of mosquito-repellent action is related to its concentration, with concentrations above 50% providing no added benefit (19). DEET has an outstanding safety profile, and most data relating to its toxic effects concern inappropriate use, such as ingestion of the chemical (58). DEET has proven safe for children and pregnant women.

Other repellents available in the United States, such as picaridin [1-methyl-propyl 2-(2-hydroxyethyl)-1-piperidinecarboxylate] and oil of lemon eucalyptus (*p*-menthane-3,8-diol) have efficacies similar to that of DEET (9, 38, 59, 60). Until these products are available in higher concentration in the United States, their use should be limited to shorter outdoor exposures. Many other products are marketed for use on skin, but they have an unacceptably short duration of action, are ineffective, or have insufficient data from which to determine efficacy. Permethrin is an effective repellent approved for use on clothing or fabrics, but not on skin.

Vaccines

Three equine WNV vaccines have been licensed in the United States. A formalin-inactivated whole-virus WNV vaccine became available in 2001 in the United States and was fully licensed in 2003 (67). More recently, a recombinant canarypox virus vaccine expressing the PrM/E proteins of a 1999 WNV isolate has been licensed (102). A DNA vaccine containing the PrM/E genes of WNV has been shown to protect against mosquito-borne challenge with WNV in mice and horses and was licensed for equines in 2005 (42). More than 23,000 cases of WNV disease in equines were reported from 1999 through 2005 in the United States. Incidence peaked in 2002 and subsequently decreased after the first WNV equine vaccine became available.

Three candidate human WNV vaccines are in human clinical trials. The most advanced in development is a chimeric virus containing the nonstructural genes of the live attenuated yellow fever virus 17D vaccine virus backbone and the PrM/E genes of WNV (8). A candidate chimeric vaccine using an attenuated dengue virus type 4 backbone has also been developed (121, 122). Phase one clinical trials for a DNA vaccine are under way. Controversy exists as to whether vaccination with a related flavivirus can protect against WNV disease (104); however, previous vaccination with a related flavivirus failed to prevent WN fever in one population (74). Modeling has suggested that universal vaccination would not be cost-effective should a human vaccine become available (146).

CONCLUSIONS

Epidemics of unusual severity began appearing in the mid-1990s, caused by new viral variants of unusual virulence. The virus was then apparently imported into the New York City area, where an avian epizootic and a human outbreak of encephalitis and meningitis signaled its emergence in the Western Hemisphere. Within 4 years, the virus spread from coast to coast, causing the largest outbreaks of arboviral encephalitis ever recorded in North America. New clinical syndromes and new modes of transmission were identified, including transmission by transfused blood. This led to universal WNV screening of donated blood in the United States and Canada. Because WNV infects many species of birds and mosquitoes and infection produces very high-titer viremias in birds, the potential for continued epizootics is great and human outbreaks of various magnitudes are likely for years to come in North America.

REFERENCES

1. **Adelman, R. A., J. H. Membreno, N. A. Afshari, and K. M. Stoessel.** 2003. West Nile virus chorioretinitis. *Retina* **23:**100–101.
2. **Agrawal, A. G., and L. R. Petersen.** 2003. Human immunoglobulin as a treatment for West Nile virus infection. *J. Infect. Dis.* **188:**1–4.
3. **Ahmed, S., R. Libman, K. Wesson, F. Ahmed, and K. Einberg.** 2000. Guillain-Barre syndrome: an unusual presentation of West Nile virus infection. *Neurology* **55:**144–146.
4. **Almhanna, K., N. Palanichamy, M. Sharma, R. Hobbs, and A. Sil.** 2003. Unilateral brachial plexopathy associated with West Nile virus meningoencephalitis. *Clin. Infect. Dis.* **36:**1629–1630.
5. **Anderson, J. F., and J. J. Rahal.** 2002. Efficacy of interferon alpha-2b and ribavirin against West Nile virus in vitro. *Emerg. Infect. Dis.* **8:**107–108.
6. **Anderson, R. C., K. B. Horn, M. P. Hoang, E. Gottlieb, and B. Bennin.** 2004. Punctate exanthem of West Nile Virus infection: report of 3 cases. *J. Am. Acad. Dermatol.* **51:**820–823.
7. **Andis, M. D., S. R. Sackett, M. K. Carroll, and E. S. Bordes.** 1987. Strategies for the emergency control of arboviral epidemics in New Orleans. *J. Am. Mosq. Control. Assoc.* **3:**125–130.
8. **Arroyo, J., C. Miller, J. Catalan, G. A. Myers, M. S. Ratterree, D. W. Trent, and T. P. Monath.** 2004. ChimeriVax-West Nile virus live-attenuated vaccine: preclinical evaluation of safety, immunogenicity, and efficacy. *J. Virol.* **78:**12497–12507.
9. **Barnard, D. R., and R. Xue.** 2004. Laboratory evaluation of mosquito repellents against *Aedes albopictus*, *Culex nigripalpus*, and *Ocheleratatus triseriatus* (Diptera: Culicidae). *J. Med. Entomol.* **41:**726–730.
10. **Beasley, D. W., C. T. Davis, H. Guzman, D. L. Vanlandingham, A. P. Travassos da Rosa, R. E. Parsons, S. Higgs, R. B. Tesh, and A. D. Barrett.** 2003. Limited evolution of West Nile virus has occurred during its southwesterly spread in the United States. *Virology* **309:**190–195.

11. **Ben-Nathan, D., S. Lustig, G. Tam, S. Robinzon, S. Segal, and B. Rager-Zisman.** 2003. Prophylactic and therapeutic efficacy of human intravenous immunoglobulin in treating West Nile virus infection in mice. *J. Infect. Dis.* **188:**5–12.

12. **Betensley, A. D., S. H. Jaffery, H. Collins, N. Sripathi, and F. Alabi.** 2004. Bilateral diaphragmatic paralysis and related respiratory complications in a patient with West Nile virus infection. *Thorax* **59:**268–269.

13. **Biggerstaff, B. J., and L. R. Petersen.** 2002. Estimated risk of West Nile virus transmission through blood transfusion during an epidemic in Queens, New York City. *Transfusion* **42:**1019–1026.

14. **Biggerstaff, B. J., and L. R. Petersen.** 2003. Estimated risk of transmission of the West Nile virus through blood transfusion in the US, 2002. *Transfusion* **43:**1007–1017.

15. **Blitvich, B. J., I. Fernandez-Salas, J. F. Contreras-Cordero, N. L. Marlenee, J. I. Gonzalez-Rojas, N. Komar, D. J. Gubler, C. H. Calisher, and B. J. Beaty.** 2003. Serologic evidence of West Nile virus infection in horses, Coahuila State, Mexico. *Emerg. Infect. Dis.* **9:**853–856.

16. **Blitvich, B. J., I. Fernandez-Salas, J. F. Contreras-Cordero, M. A. Lorono-Pino, N. L. Marlenee, F. J. Diaz, J. I. Gonzalez-Rojas, N. Obregon-Martinez, J. A. Chiu-Garcia, W. C. T. Black, and B. J. Beaty.** 2004. Phylogenetic analysis of West Nile virus, Nuevo Leon State, Mexico. *Emerg. Infect. Dis.* **10:**1314–1317.

17. **Bosanko, C. M., J. Gilroy, A. M. Wang, W. Sanders, M. Dulai, J. Wilson, and K. Blum.** 2003. West Nile virus encephalitis involving the substantia nigra: neuroimaging and pathologic findings with literature review. *Arch. Neurol.* **60:**1448–1452.

18. **Brault, A. C., S. A. Langevin, R. A. Bowen, N. A. Panella, B. J. Biggerstaff, B. R. Miller, and N. Komar.** 2004. Differential virulence of West Nile strains for American crows. *Emerg. Infect. Dis.* **10:**2161–2168.

19. **Buescher, M. D., L. C. Rutledge, R. A. Wirtz, and J. H. Nelson.** 1983. The dose-persistence relationship of DEET against *Aedes aegypti. Mosq. News* **43:**364–366.

20. **Burton, J. M., R. Z. Kern, W. Halliday, D. Mikulis, J. Brunton, M. Fearon, C. Pepperell, and C. Jaigobin.** 2004. Neurological manifestations of West Nile virus infection. *Can. J. Neurol. Sci.* **31:**185–193.

21. **Busch, M. P., S. Caglioti, E. F. Robertson, J. D. McAuley, L. H. Tobler, H. Kamel, J. M. Linnen, V. Shyamala, P. Tomasulo, and S. H. Kleinman.** 2005. Screening the blood supply for West Nile virus RNA by nucleic acid amplification testing. *N. Engl. J. Med.* **353:**460–467.

22. **Busch, M. P., L. H. Tobler, J. Saldanha, S. Caglioti, V. Shyamala, J. M. Linnen, J. Gallarda, B. Phelps, R. I. Smith, M. Drebot, and S. H. Kleinman.** 2005. Analytical and clinical sensitivity of West Nile virus RNA screening and supplemental assays available in 2003. *Transfusion* **45:**492–499.

23. **Camenga, D. L., N. Nathanson, and G. A. Cole.** 1974. Cyclophosphamide-potentiated West Nile viral encephalitis: relative influence of cellular and humoral factors. *J. Infect. Dis.* **130:**634–641.

24. **Cao, N. J., C. Ranganathan, W. J. Kupsky, and J. Li.** 2005. Recovery and prognosticators of paralysis in West Nile virus infection. *J. Neurol. Sci.* **236:**73-80.

25. **Centers for Disease Control and Prevention.** 2000. Update: West Nile virus activity—Eastern United States, 2000. *Morb. Mortal. Wkly. Rep.* **49:**1044–1047.

26. **Centers for Disease Control and Prevention.** 2001. Serosurveys for West Nile virus infection—New York and Connecticut counties, 2000. *Morb. Mortal. Wkly. Rep.* **50:**37–39.

27. **Centers for Disease Control and Prevention.** 2002. Possible West Nile virus transmission to an infant through breast-feeding—Michigan, 2002. *Morb. Mortal. Wkly. Rep.* **51:**877–878.

28. **Centers for Disease Control and Prevention.** 2002. Laboratory-acquired West Nile virus infections—United States, 2002. *Morb. Mortal. Wkly. Rep.* **51:**1133–1135.

29. **Centers for Disease Control and Prevention.** 2002. West Nile Virus activity—United States, 2001. *Morb. Mortal. Wkly. Rep.* **51:**497–501.

30. **Centers for Disease Control and Prevention.** 2003. West Nile virus infection among turkey breeder farm workers—Wisconsin, 2002. *Morb. Mortal. Wkly. Rep.* **52:**1017–1019.

31. **Centers for Disease Control and Prevention.** 2003. Surveillance for acute insecticide-related illness associated with mosquito-control efforts—nine states, 1999–2002. *Morb. Mortal. Wkly. Rep.* **52:**629–634.

32. **Centers for Disease Control and Prevention.** 2004. Possible dialysis-related West Nile virus transmission—Georgia, 2003. *Morb. Mortal. Wkly. Rep.* **53:**738–739.

33. **Centers for Disease Control and Prevention.** 2004. Transfusion-associated transmission of West Nile virus—Arizona, 2004. *Morb. Mortal. Wkly. Rep.* **53:**842–844.

34. **Centers for Disease Control and Prevention.** 2004. Update: West Nile virus screening of blood donations and transfusion-associated transmission—United States, 2003. *Morb. Mortal. Wkly. Rep.* **53:**281–284.

35. **Centers for Disease Control and Prevention.** 2005. Human exposure to mosquito-control pesticides—Mississippi, North Carolina, and Virginia, 2002 and 2003. *Morb. Mortal. Wkly. Rep.* **54:**529–532.

36. **Centers for Disease Control and Prevention.** 2005. West Nile virus infections in organ transplant recipients—New York and Pennsylvania, August-September, 2005. *Morb. Mortal. Wkly. Rep.* **54:**1021–1023.

37. **Chowers, M. Y., R. Lang, F. Nassar, D. Ben-David, M. Giladi, E. Rubinshtein, A. Itzhaki, J. Mishal, Y. Siegman-Igra, R. Kitzes, N. Pick, Z. Landau, D. Wolf, H. Bin, E. Mendelson, S. D. Pitlik, and M. Weinberger.** 2001. Clinical characteristics of the West Nile fever outbreak, Israel, 2000. *Emerg. Infect. Dis.* **7:**675–678.

38. **Costantini, C., A. Badolo, and E. Ilboudo-Sanogo.** 2004. Field evaluation of the efficacy and persistence of insect repellents DEET, IR3535, and KBR 3023 against *Anopheles gambiae* complex and other Afrotropical vector mosquitoes. *Trans. R. Soc. Trop. Med. Hyg.* **98:**644–652.

39. **Creech, W. B.** 1977. St. Louis encephalitis in the United States, 1975. *J. Infect. Dis.* **135:**1014–1016.

40. **Cruz, L., V. M. Cardenas, M. Abarca, T. Rodriguez, R. F. Reyna, M. V. Serpas, R. E. Fontaine, D. W. Beasley, A. P. Da Rosa, S. C. Weaver, R. B. Tesh, A. M. Powers, and G. Suarez-Rangel.** 2005. Short report: serological evidence of West Nile virus activity in El Salvador. *Am. J. Trop. Med. Hyg.* **72:**612–615.

41. **Custer, B., P. A. Tomasulo, E. L. Murphy, S. Caglioti, D. Harpool, P. McEvoy, and M. P. Busch.** 2004. Triggers for switching from minipool testing by nucleic acid technology to individual-donation nucleic acid testing for West Nile virus: analysis of 2003 data to inform 2004 decision making. *Transfusion* **44:**1547–1554.

42. **Davis, B. S., G. J. Chang, B. Cropp, J. T. Roehrig, D. A. Martin, C. J. Mitchell, R. Bowen, and M. L. Bunning.** 2001. West Nile virus recombinant DNA vaccine protects mouse and horse from virus challenge and expresses in vitro a noninfectious recombinant antigen that can be used in enzyme-linked immunosorbent assays. *J. Virol.* **75:**4040–4047.

43. **Davis, C. T., D. W. Beasley, H. Guzman, R. Raj, M. D'Anton, R. J. Novak, T. R. Unnasch, R. B. Tesh, and A. D. Barrett.** 2003. Genetic variation among temporally and geographically distinct West Nile virus isolates, United States, 2001, 2002. *Emerg. Infect. Dis.* **9:**1423–1429.

44. **Davis, C. T., D. W. Beasley, H. Guzman, M. Siirin, R. Parsons, R. Tesh, and A. D. Barrett.** 2004. Emergence of attenuated West Nile virus variants in Texas. *Virology* **330:**342–350.

45. **Davis, C. T., G. D. Ebel, R. S. Lanciotti, A. C. Brault, H. Guzman, M. Siirin, A. Lambert, R. E. Parsons, D. W. Beasley, R. J. Novak, D. Elizondo-Quiroga, E. N. Green, D. S. Young, L. M. Stark, M. A. Drebot, H. Artsob, R. B. Tesh, L. D. Kramer, and A. D. Barrett.** 2005. Phylogenetic analysis of North American West Nile virus isolates, 2001–2004: evidence for the emergence of a dominant genotype. *Virology* **342:**252–265.

46. **Depoortere, E., J. Kavle, K. Keus, H. Zeller, S. Murri, and D. Legros.** 2004. Outbreak of West Nile virus causing severe neurological involvement in children, Nuba Mountains, Sudan, 2002. *Trop. Med. Int. Health* **9:**730–736.

47. **Diamond, M. S., E. M. Sitati, L. D. Friend, S. Higgs, B. Shrestha, and M. Engle.** 2003. A critical role for induced IgM in the protection against West Nile virus infection. *J. Exp. Med.* **198:**1853–1862.

48. **Doron, S. I., J. F. Dashe, L. S. Adelman, W. F. Brown, B. G. Werner, and S. Hadley.** 2003. Histopathologically proven poliomyelitis with quadriplegia and loss of brainstem function due to West Nile virus infection. *Clin. Infect. Dis.* **37:**e74–e77. [Online.]

49. **Dupuis, A. P., II, P. P. Marra, and L. D. Kramer.** 2003. Serologic evidence of West Nile virus transmission, Jamaica, West Indies. *Emerg. Infect. Dis.* **9:**860–863.

50. **Dupuis, A. P., II, P. P. Marra, R. Reitsma, M. J. Jones, K. L. Louie, and L. D. Kramer.** 2005. Serologic evidence for West Nile virus transmission in Puerto Rico and Cuba. *Am. J. Trop. Med. Hyg.* **73:**474–476.

51. **Ebel, G. D., J. Carricaburu, D. Young, K. A. Bernard, and L. D. Kramer.** 2004. Genetic and phenotypic variation of West Nile virus in New York, 2000–2003. *Am. J. Trop. Med. Hyg.* **71:**493–500.

52. **Emig, M., and D. J. Apple.** 2004. Severe West Nile virus disease in healthy adults. *Clin. Infect. Dis.* **38:**289–292.

53. **Estrada-Franco, J. G., R. Navarro-Lopez, D. W. Beasley, L. Coffey, A. S. Carrara, A. Travassos da Rosa, T. Clements, E. Wang, G. V. Ludwig, A. C. Cortes, P. P. Ramirez, R. B. Tesh, A. D. Barrett, and S. C. Weaver.** 2003. West Nile virus in Mexico: evidence of widespread circulation since July 2002. *Emerg. Infect. Dis.* **9:**1604–1607.

54. **Fan, E., D. M. Needham, J. Brunton, R. Z. Kern, and T. E. Stewart.** 2004. West Nile virus infection in the intensive care unit: a case series and literature review. *Can. Respir. J.* **11:**354–358.

55. **Ferguson, D. D., K. Gershman, A. LeBailly, and L. R. Petersen.** 2005. Characteristics of the rash associated with West Nile virus fever. *Clin. Infect. Dis.* **41:**1204–1207.

56. **Fernandez-Salas, I., J. F. Contreras-Cordero, B. J. Blitvich, J. I. Gonzalez-Rojas, A. Cavazos-Alvarez, N. L. Marlenee, A. Elizondo-Quiroga, M. A. Lorono-Pino, D. J. Gubler, B. C. Cropp, C. H. Calisher, and B. J. Beaty.** 2003. Serologic evidence of West Nile Virus infection in birds, Tamaulipas State, Mexico. *Vector Borne Zoonotic Dis.* **3:**209–213.

57. **Fonseca, K., G. D. Prince, J. Bratvold, J. D. Fox, M. Pybus, J. K. Preksaitis, and P. Tilley.** 2005. West Nile virus infection and conjunctival exposure. *Emerg. Infect. Dis.* **11:**1648–1649.

58. **Fradin, M. S.** 1998. Mosquitoes and mosquito repellents: a clinician's guide. *Ann. Intern. Med.* **128:**931–940.

59. **Frances, S. P., N. Van Dung, N. W. Beebe, and M. Debboun.** 2002. Field evaluation of repellent formulations against daytime and nighttime biting mosquitoes in a tropical rainforest in northern Australia. *J. Med. Entomol.* **39:**541–544.

60. **Frances, S. P., D. G. Waterson, N. W. Beebe, and R. D. Cooper.** 2004. Field evaluation of repellent formulations containing DEET and picaridin against mosquitoes in Northern Territory, Australia. *J. Med. Entomol.* **41:**414–417.

61. **Garg, S., and L. M. Jampol.** 2005. Systemic and intraocular manifestations of West Nile virus infection. *Surv. Ophthalmol.* **50:**3–13.

62. **Goldblum, N., V. V. Sterk, and B. Paderski.** 1954. West Nile fever; the clinical features of the disease and the isolation of West Nile virus from the blood of nine human cases. *Am. J. Hyg.* **59:**89–103.

63. **Granwehr, B. P., L. Li, C. T. Davis, D. W. Beasley, and A. D. Barrett.** 2004. Characterization of a West Nile virus isolate from a human on the Gulf Coast of Texas. *J. Clin. Microbiol.* **42:**5375–5377.

64. **Green, M. S., M. Weinberger, J. Ben-Ezer, H. Bin, E. Mendelson, D. Gandacu, Z. Kaufman, R. Dichtiar, A. Sobel, D. Cohen, and M. Y. Chowers.** 2005. Long-term death rates, West Nile virus epidemic, Israel, 2000. *Emerg. Infect. Dis.* **11:**1754–1757.

65. **Guarner, J., W. J. Shieh, S. Hunter, C. D. Paddock, T. Morken, G. L. Campbell, A. A. Marfin, and S. R. Zaki.** 2004. Clinicopathologic study and laboratory diagnosis of 23 cases with West Nile virus encephalomyelitis. *Hum. Pathol.* **35:**983–990.

66. **Haley, M., A. S. Retter, D. Fowler, J. Gea-Banacloche, and N. P. O'Grady.** 2003. The role for intravenous immunoglobulin in the treatment of West Nile virus encephalitis. *Clin. Infect. Dis.* **37:**e88–e90. [Online.]

67. **Hall, R. A., and A. A. Khromykh.** 2004. West Nile virus vaccines. *Exp. Opin. Biol. Ther.* **4:**1295–1305.

68. **Hamdan, A., P. Green, E. Mendelson, M. R. Kramer, S. Pitlik, and M. Weinberger.** 2002. Possible benefit of intravenous immunoglobulin therapy in a lung transplant recipient with West Nile virus encephalitis. *Transplant Infect. Dis.* **4:**160–162.

69. **Hassin-Baer, S., E. D. Kirson, L. Shulman, A. S. Buchman, H. Bin, M. Hindiyeh, L. Markevich, and E. Mendelson.** 2004. Stiff-person syndrome following West Nile fever. *Arch. Neurol.* **61:**938–941.

70. **Hrnicek, M. J., and M. E. Mailliard.** 2004. Acute West Nile virus in two patients receiving interferon and ribavirin for chronic hepatitis C. *Am. J. Gastroenterol.* **99:**957.

71. **Hubalek, Z., and J. Halouzka.** 1999. West Nile fever—a reemerging mosquito-borne viral disease in Europe. *Emerg. Infect. Dis.* **5:**643–650.

72. **Iwamoto, M., D. B. Jernigan, A. Guasch, M. J. Trepka, C. G. Blackmore, W. C. Hellinger, S. M. Pham, S. Zaki, R. S. Lanciotti, S. E. Lance-Parker, C. A. DiazGranados, A. G. Winquist, C. A. Perlino, S. Wiersma, K. L. Hillyer, J. L. Goodman, A. A. Marfin, M. E. Chamberland, and L. R. Petersen.** 2003. Transmission of West Nile virus from an organ donor to four transplant recipients. *N. Engl. J. Med.* **348:**2196–2203.

73. **Jeha, L. E., C. A. Sila, R. J. Lederman, R. A. Prayson, C. M. Isada, and S. M. Gordon.** 2003. West Nile virus infection: a new acute paralytic illness. *Neurology* **61:**55–59.

74. **Johnson, B. W., O. Kosoy, D. A. Martin, A. J. Noga, B. J. Russell, A. A. Johnson, and L. R. Petersen.** 2005. West Nile virus infection and serologic response among persons previously vaccinated against yellow fever and Japanese encephalitis viruses. *Vector Borne Zoonotic Dis.* **5:**137–145.

75. **Jordan, I., T. Briese, N. Fischer, J. Y. Lau, and W. I. Lipkin.** 2000. Ribavirin inhibits West Nile virus replication and cytopathic effect in neural cells. *J. Infect. Dis.* **182:**1214–1217.

76. **Jupp, P. G.** 2001. The ecology of West Nile virus in South Africa and the occurrence of outbreaks in humans. *Ann. N. Y. Acad. Sci.* **951:**143–152.

77. **Kalil, A. C., M. P. Devetten, S. Singh, B. Lesiak, D. P. Poage, K. Bargenquast, P. Fayad, and A. G. Freifeld.** 2005. Use of interferon-alpha in patients with West Nile encephalitis: report of 2 cases. *Clin. Infect. Dis.* **40:**764–766.

78. **Kanagarajan, K., S. Ganesh, M. Alakhras, E. S. Go, R. A. Recco, and M. M. Zaman.** 2003. West Nile virus infection presenting as cerebellar ataxia and fever: case report. *South. Med. J.* **96:**600–601.

79. **Karpati, A. M., M. C. Perrin, T. Matte, J. Leighton, J. Schwartz, and R. G. Barr.** 2004. Pesticide spraying for West Nile virus control and emergency department asthma visits in New York City, 2000. *Environ. Health Perspect.* **112:**1183–1187.

80. **Kelley, T. W., R. A. Prayson, A. I. Ruiz, C. M. Isada, and S. M. Gordon.** 2003. The neuropathology of West Nile virus meningoencephalitis. A report of two cases and review of the literature. *Am. J. Clin. Pathol.* **119:**749–753.

81. **Khairallah, M., S. Ben Yahia, A. Ladjimi, H. Zeghidi, F. Ben Romdhane, L. Besbes, S. Zaouali, and R. Messaoud.** 2004. Chorioretinal involvement in patients with West Nile virus infection. *Ophthalmology* **111:**2065–2070.

82. **Khosla, J.** 2004. West Nile encephalitis presenting as opsoclonus-myoclonus-cerebellar ataxia. *Ann. Neurol.* **56:**S70.

83. **Klee, A. L., B. Maidin, B. Edwin, I. Poshni, F. Mostashari, A. Fine, M. Layton, and D. Nash.** 2004. Long-term prognosis for clinical West Nile virus infection. *Emerg. Infect. Dis.* **10:**1405–1411.

84. **Kleinman, S., S. A. Glynn, M. Busch, D. Todd, L. Powell, L. Pietrelli, G. Nemo, G. Schreiber, C. Bianco, and L. Katz.** 2005. The 2003 West Nile virus United States epidemic: the America's Blood Centers experience. *Transfusion* **45:**469–479.

85. **Kleinschmidt-DeMasters, B. K., B. A. Marder, M. E. Levi, S. P. Laird, J. T. McNutt, E. J. Escott, G. T. Everson, and K. L. Tyler.** 2004. Naturally acquired West Nile virus encephalomyelitis in transplant recipients: clinical, laboratory, diagnostic, and neuropathological features. *Arch. Neurol.* **61:**1210–1220.

86. **Komar, N.** 2003. West Nile virus: epidemiology and ecology in North America. *Adv. Virus Res.* **61:**185–234.

87. **Komar, N., S. Langevin, S. Hinten, N. Nemeth, E. Edwards, D. Hettler, B. Davis, R. Bowen, and M. Bunning.** 2003. Experimental infection of North American birds with the New York 1999 strain of West Nile virus. *Emerg. Infect. Dis.* **9:**311–322.

88. **Komar, O., M. B. Robbins, K. Klenk, B. J. Blitvich, N. L. Marlenee, K. L. Burkhalter, D. J. Gubler, G. Gonzalvez, C. J. Pena, A. T. Peterson, and N. Komar.** 2003. West Nile virus transmission in resident birds, Dominican Republic. *Emerg. Infect. Dis.* **9:**1299–1302.

89. **Kulstad, E. B., and M. D. Wichter.** 2003. West Nile encephalitis presenting as a stroke. *Ann. Emerg. Med.* **41:**283.

90. **Kumar, D., M. A. Drebot, S. J. Wong, G. Lim, H. Artsob, P. Buck, and A. Humar.** 2004. A seroprevalence study of West Nile virus infection in solid organ transplant recipients. *Am. J. Transplant.* **4:**1883–1888.

91. **Kumar, D., G. V. Prasad, J. Zaltzman, G. A. Levy, and A. Humar.** 2004. Community-acquired West Nile virus infection in solid-organ transplant recipients. *Transplantation* **77:**399–402.

92. **Lanciotti, R. S., J. T. Roehrig, V. Deubel, J. Smith, M. Parker, K. Steele, B. Crise, K. E. Volpe, M. B. Crabtree, J. H. Scherret, R. A. Hall, J. S. MacKenzie, C. B. Cropp, B. Panigrahy, E. Ostlund, B. Schmitt, M. Malkinson, C. Banet, J. Weissman, N. Komar, H. M. Savage, W. Stone, T. McNamara, and D. J. Gubler.** 1999. Origin of the West Nile virus responsible for an outbreak of encephalitis in the northeastern United States. *Science* **286:**2333–2337.

93. **Lanciotti, R. S., G. D. Ebel, V. Deubel, A. J. Kerst, S. Murri, R. Meyer, M. Bowen, N. McKinney, W. E. Morrill, M. B. Crabtree, L. D. Kramer, and J. T. Roehrig.** 2002. Complete genome sequences and phylogenetic analysis of West Nile virus strains isolated from the United States, Europe, and the Middle East. *Virology* **298:**96–105.

94. **Lefrancois, T., B. J. Blitvich, J. Pradel, S. Molia, N. Vachiery, G. Pallavicini, N. L. Marlenee, S. Zientara, M. Petitclerc, and D. Martinez.** 2005. West Nile virus surveillance, Guadeloupe, 2003–2004. *Emerg. Infect. Dis.* **11:**1100–1103.

95. **Le Guenno, B., A. Bougermouh, T. Azzam, and R. Bouakaz.** 1996. West Nile: a deadly virus? *Lancet* **348:**1315.

96. **Lorono-Pino, M. A., B. J. Blitvich, J. A. Farfan-Ale, F. I. Puerto, J. M. Blanco, N. L. Marlenee, E. P. Rosado-Paredes, J. E. Garcia-Rejon, D. J. Gubler, C. H. Calisher, and B. J. Beaty.** 2003. Serologic evidence of West Nile virus infection in horses, Yucatan State, Mexico. *Emerg. Infect. Dis.* **9:**857–859.

97. **Marberg, K., N. Goldblum, V. V. Sterk, W. Jasinska-Klingberg, and M. A. Klingberg.** 1956. The natural history of West Nile fever. I. Clinical observations during an epidemic in Israel. *Am. J. Hyg.* **64:**259–269.

98. **Marciniak, C., S. Sorosky, and C. Hynes.** 2004. Acute flaccid paralysis associated with West Nile virus: motor and functional improvement in 4 patients. *Arch. Phys. Med. Rehabil.* **85:**1933–1938.

99. **Marfin, A. A., L. R. Petersen, M. Eidson, J. Miller, J. Hadler, C. Farello, B. Werner, G. L. Campbell, M. Layton, P. Smith, E. Bresnitz, M. Cartter, J. Scaletta, G. Obiri, M. Bunning, R. C. Craven, J. T. Roehrig, K. G. Julian, S. R. Hinten, D. J. Gubler, and the ArboNET Cooperative Surveillance Group.** 2001. Widespread West Nile virus activity, eastern United States, 2000. *Emerg. Infect. Dis.* **7:**730–735.

100. **Marlenee, N. L., M. A. Lorono-Pino, B. J. Beaty, and B. J. Blitvich.** 2004. Detection of antibodies to West Nile and Saint Louis encephalitis viruses in horses. *Salud Publica Mexico* **46:**373–375.

101. **Mattar, S., E. Edwards, J. Laguado, M. Gonzales, J. Alvarez, and N. Komar.** 2005. West Nile virus antibodies in Colombian horses. *Emerg. Infect. Dis.* **11:**1496–1497.

102. **Minke, J. M., L. Siger, K. Karaca, L. Austgen, P. Gordy, R. Bowen, R. W. Renshaw, S. Loosmore, J. C. Audonnet, and B. Nordgren.** 2004. Recombinant canarypoxvirus vaccine carrying the *prM/E* genes of West Nile virus protects horses against a West Nile virus-mosquito challenge. *Arch. Virol. Suppl.* **18:**221–230.

103. **Mitchell, C. J., J. W. Kilpatrick, R. O. Hayes, and H. W. Curry.** 1970. Effects of ultra-low volume applications of malathion in Hale County, Texas. II. Mosquito populations in treated and untreated areas. *J. Med. Entomol.* **7:**85–91.

104. **Monath, T. P.** 2002. Jennerian vaccination against West Nile virus. *Am. J. Trop. Med. Hyg.* **66:**113–114.

105. **Montgomery, S. P., C. C. Chow, S. W. Smith, A. A. Marfin, D. R. O'Leary, and G. L. Campbell.** 2005. Rhabdomyolysis in patients with west Nile encephalitis and meningitis. *Vector Borne Zoonotic Dis.* **5:**252–257.

106. **Morrey, J. D., C. W. Day, J. G. Julander, L. M. Blatt, D. F. Smee, and R. W. Sidwell.** 2004. Effect of interferon-alpha and interferon-inducers on West Nile virus in mouse and hamster animal models. *Antivir. Chem. Chemother.* **15:**101–109.

107. **Moskowitz, D. W., and F. E. Johnson.** 2004. The central role of angiotensin I-converting enzyme in vertebrate pathophysiology. *Curr. Top. Med. Chem.* **4:**1433–1454.

108. **Mostashari, F., M. L. Bunning, P. T. Kitsutani, D. A. Singer, D. Nash, M. J. Cooper, N. Katz, K. A. Liljebjelke, B. J. Biggerstaff, A. D. Fine, M. C. Layton, S. M. Mullin, A. J. Johnson, D. A. Martin, E. B. Hayes, and G. L. Campbell.** 2001. Epidemic West Nile encephalitis, New York, 1999: results of a household-based seroepidemiological survey. *Lancet* **358:**261–264.

109. **Murgue, B., S. Murri, H. Triki, V. Deubel, and H. G. Zeller.** 2001. West Nile in the Mediterranean basin: 1950–2000. *Ann. N. Y. Acad. Sci.* **951:**117–126.

110. **Murgue, B., H. Zeller, and V. Deubel.** 2002. The ecology and epidemiology of West Nile virus in Africa, Europe and Asia. *Curr. Top. Microbiol. Immunol.* **267:**195–221.

111. **Nash, D., F. Mostashari, A. Fine, J. Miller, D. O'Leary, K. Murray, A. Huang, A. Rosenberg, A. Greenberg, M. Sherman, S. Wong, and M. Layton.** 2001. The outbreak of West Nile virus infection in the New York City area in 1999. *N. Engl. J. Med.* **344:**1807–1814.

112. **Nir, Y. D.** 1959. Airborne West Nile virus infection. *Am. J. Trop. Med. Hyg.* **8:**537–539.

113. **O'Leary, D. R., A. A. Marfin, S. P. Montgomery, A. M. Kipp, J. A. Lehman, B. J. Biggerstaff, V. L. Elko, P. D. Collins, J. E. Jones, and G. L. Campbell.** 2004. The epidemic of West Nile virus in the United States, 2002. *Vector Borne Zoonotic Dis.* **4:**61–70.

114. **Park, M., J. S. Hui, and R. E. Bartt.** 2003. Acute anterior radiculitis associated with West Nile virus infection. *J. Neurol. Neurosurg. Psychiatry* **74:**823–825.

115. **Pealer, L. N., A. A. Marfin, L. R. Petersen, R. S. Lanciotti, P. L. Page, S. L. Stramer, M. G. Stobierski, K. Signs, B. Newman, H. Kapoor, J. L. Goodman, and M. E. Chamberland.** 2003. Transmission of West Nile virus through blood transfusion in the United States in 2002. *N. Engl. J. Med.* **349:**1236–1245.

116. **Pepperell, C., N. Rau, S. Krajden, R. Kern, A. Humar, B. Mederski, A. Simor, D. E. Low, A. McGeer, T. Mazzulli, J. Burton, C. Jaigobin, M. Fearon, H. Artsob, M. A. Drebot, W. Halliday, and J. Brunton.** 2003. West Nile virus infection in 2002: morbidity and mortality among patients admitted to hospital in southcentral Ontario. *Can. Med. Assoc. J.* **168:**1399–1405.

117. **Perelman, A., and J. Stern.** 1974. Acute pancreatitis in West Nile fever. *Am. J. Trop. Med. Hyg.* **23:** 1150–1152.

118. **Petersen, L. R., and E. B. Hayes.** 2004. Westward ho?—the spread of West Nile virus. *N. Engl. J. Med.* **351:**2257–2259.

119. **Petersen, L. R., and J. S. Epstein.** 2005. Problem solved? West Nile virus and transfusion safety. *N. Engl. J. Med.* **353:**516–517.

120. **Platonov, A. E., G. A. Shipulin, O. Y. Shipulina, E. N. Tyutyunnik, T. I. Frolochkina, R. S. Lanciotti, S. Yazyshina, O. V. Platonova, I. L. Obukhov, A. N. Zhukov, Y. Y. Vengerov, and V. I. Pokrovskii.** 2001. Outbreak of West Nile virus infection, Volgograd Region, Russia, 1999. *Emerg. Infect. Dis.* **7:** 128–132.

121. **Pletnev, A. G., R. Putnak, J. Speicher, E. J. Wagar, and D. W. Vaughn.** 2002. West Nile virus/dengue type 4 virus chimeras that are reduced in neurovirulence and peripheral virulence without loss of immunogenicity or protective efficacy. *Proc. Natl. Acad. Sci. USA* **99:**3036–3041.

122. **Pletnev, A. G., M. S. Claire, R. Elkins, J. Speicher, B. R. Murphy, and R. M. Chanock.** 2003. Molecularly engineered live-attenuated chimeric West Nile/dengue virus vaccines protect rhesus monkeys from West Nile virus. *Virology* **314:**190–195.

123. **Pogodina, V. V., M. P. Frolova, G. V. Malenko, G. I. Fokina, G. V. Koreshkova, L. L. Kiseleva, N. G. Bochkova, and N. M. Ralph.** 1983. Study on West Nile virus persistence in monkeys. *Arch. Virol.* **75:** 71–86.

124. **Pyrgos, V., and F. Younus.** 2004. High-dose steroids in the management of acute flaccid paralysis due to West Nile virus infection. *Scand. J. Infect. Dis.* **36:**509–512.

125. **Quirin, R., M. Salas, S. Zientara, H. Zeller, J. Labie, S. Murri, T. Lefrancois, M. Petitclerc, and D. Martinez.** 2004. West Nile virus, Guadeloupe. *Emerg. Infect. Dis.* **10:**706–708.

126. **Reisen, W. K., G. Yoshimura, W. C. Reeves, M. M. Milby, and R. P. Meyer.** 1984. The impact of aerial applications of ultra-low volume adulticides on *Culex tarsalis* populations (Diptera: Culicidae) in Kern County, California, USA, 1982. *J. Med. Entomol.* **21:**573–585.

127. **Robinson, R. L., S. Shahida, N. Madan, S. Rao, and N. Khardori.** 2003. Transient parkinsonism in West Nile virus encephalitis. *Am. J. Med.* **115:**252–253.

128. **Rose, R. I.** 2001. Pesticides and public health: integrated methods of mosquito management. *Emerg. Infect. Dis.* **7:**17–23.

129. **Saad, M., S. Youssef, D. Kirschke, M. Shubair, D. Haddadin, J. Myers, and J. Moorman.** 2005. Acute flaccid paralysis: the spectrum of a newly recognized complication of West Nile virus infection. *J. Infect.* **51:**120–127.

130. **Sampson, B. A., C. Ambrosi, A. Charlot, K. Reiber, J. F. Veress, and V. Armbrustmacher.** 2000. The pathology of human West Nile virus infection. *Hum. Pathol.* **31:**527–531.

131. **Sayao, A. L., O. Suchowersky, A. Al-Khathaami, B. Klassen, N. R. Katz, R. Sevick, P. Tilley, J. Fox, and D. Patry.** 2004. Calgary experience with West Nile virus neurological syndrome during the late summer of 2003. *Can. J. Neurol. Sci.* **31:**194–203.

132. **Sejvar, J. J., M. B. Haddad, B. C. Tierney, G. L. Campbell, A. A. Marfin, J. A. Van Gerpen, A. Fleischauer, A. A. Leis, D. S. Stokic, and L. R. Petersen.** 2003. Neurologic manifestations and outcome of West Nile virus infection. *JAMA* **290:**511–515.

133. **Sejvar, J. J., A. V. Bode, A. A. Marfin, G. L. Campbell, D. Ewing, M. Mazowiecki, P. V. Pavot, J. Schmitt, J. Pape, B. J. Biggerstaff, and L. R. Petersen.** 2005. West Nile virus-associated flaccid paralysis. *Emerg. Infect. Dis.* **11:**1021–1027.

134. **Sherman-Weber, S., and P. Axelrod.** 2004. Central diabetes insipidus complicating West Nile encephalitis. *Clin. Infect. Dis.* **38:**1042–1043.

135. **Shimoni, Z., M. J. Niven, S. Pitlick, and S. Bulvik.** 2001. Treatment of West Nile virus encephalitis with intravenous immunoglobulin. *Emerg. Infect. Dis.* **7:**759.

136. **Smithburn, K. C., T. P. Hughes, A. W. Burke, and J. H. Paul.** 1940. A neurotropic virus isolated from the blood of a native of Uganda. *Am. J. Trop. Med. Hyg.* **20:**470–492.

137. **Solomon, T., N. M. Dung, B. Wills, R. Kneen, M. Gainsborough, T. V. Diet, T. T. Thuy, H. T. Loan, V. C. Khanh, D. W. Vaughn, N. J. White, and J. J. Farrar.** 2003. Interferon alfa-2a in Japanese encephalitis: a randomised double-blind placebo-controlled trial. *Lancet* **361:**821–826.

138. **Southam, C. M., and A. E. Moore.** 1954. Induced virus infections in man by the Egypt isolates of West Nile virus. *Am. J. Trop. Med. Hyg.* **3:**19–50.

139. **Spigland, I., W. Jasinska-Klingberg, E. Hofshi, and N. Goldblum.** 1958. Clinical and laboratory observations in an outbreak of West Nile fever in Israel in 1957. *Harefuah* **54:**275–280.

140. **Stramer, S. L., C. T. Fang, G. A. Foster, A. G. Wagner, J. P. Brodsky, and R. Y. Dodd.** 2005. West Nile virus among blood donors in the United States, 2003 and 2004. *N. Engl. J. Med.* **353:**451–459.

141. **Szilak, I., and G. Y. Minamoto.** 2000. West Nile viral encephalitis in an HIV-positive woman in New York. *N. Engl. J. Med.* **342:**59–60.

142. **Tesh, R. B., J. Arroyo, A. P. Travassos Da Rosa, H. Guzman, S. Y. Xiao, and T. P. Monath.** 2002. Efficacy of killed virus vaccine, live attenuated chimeric virus vaccine, and passive immunization for prevention of West Nile virus encephalitis in hamster model. *Emerg. Infect. Dis.* **8:**1392–1397.

143. **Tsai, T. F., F. Popovici, C. Cernescu, G. L. Campbell, and N. I. Nedelcu.** 1998. West Nile encephalitis epidemic in southeastern Romania. *Lancet* **352:**767–771.

144. **Watson, J. T., P. E. Pertel, R. C. Jones, A. M. Siston, W. S. Paul, C. C. Austin, and S. I. Gerber.** 2004. Clinical characteristics and functional outcomes of West Nile fever. *Ann. Intern. Med.* **141:**360–365.

145. **Yim, R., K. M. Posfay-Barbe, D. Nolt, G. Fatula, and E. R. Wald.** 2004. Spectrum of clinical manifestations of West Nile virus infection in children. *Pediatrics* **114:**1673–1675.

146. **Zohrabian, A., E. B. Hayes, and L. R. Petersen.** 2006. Cost-effectiveness of West Nile virus vaccination. *Emerg. Infect. Dis.* **12:**375–380.

Emerging Infections 7
Edited by W. M. Scheld, D. C. Hooper, and J. M. Hughes
© 2007 ASM Press, Washington, D.C.

Chapter 7

Chandipura Encephalitis: a Newly Recognized Disease of Public Health Importance in India

Akhilesh Chandra Mishra

DISCOVERY OF CHANDIPURA VIRUS IN 1965

An outbreak of febrile illness was reported in Nagpur, Maharashtra State, India, from April to June 1965 (24). Chikungunya virus was recognized as the main etiological agent, though dengue 4 virus was also active during the period. During investigations conducted by the National Institute of Virology (NIV) (then known as the Virus Research Center), the serum samples collected from two febrile patients, negative for dengue and Chikungunya viruses, inoculated into BS-C-1 cells produced cytopathic effects (CPE). One of the two samples also produced mortality in infant mice after intracerebral inoculation. The filterable agent recovered was identified as a new virus that was named Chandipura (CHP) virus after the locality from which the clinical samples were collected (2). Studies were undertaken on a large number of sera collected earlier, and it was concluded that the virus was widely prevalent in many parts of India in both humans and a variety of animals. Propagation and transmission studies were undertaken in many cell cultures, domestic animals, monkeys, laboratory animals, and mosquitoes. However, involvement of this virus with the disease outbreak could not be determined.

Subsequently, CHP virus was isolated from the serum of a patient with a case of acute encephalopathy during an outbreak of viral encephalitis in Raipur and Jabalpur, Madhya Pradesh, India, in 1980 (25). The authors stated that though the clinical features resembled those of Reye's syndrome, there was an association of this virus with the acute fatal illness.

DISCOVERY OF CHP ENCEPHALITIS IN 2003

The year 2003 may be marked as the year of the discovery of CHP encephalitis. A large outbreak of acute encephalitis involving 329 children, with 183 deaths (case fatality rate [CFR], 55.6%), was reported between June and August 2003 from many districts of Andhra Pradesh State. The multiple lines of evidence together strongly implicated CHP virus as the etiological agent associated with this outbreak of acute encephalitis (22).

Akhilesh Chandra Mishra • National Institute of Virology, 20-A Dr. Ambedkar Road, Pune-411 001, India.

Simultaneously, another encephalitis outbreak was reported from June to August 2003 in 15 districts (11 in Vidarbha and 4 in Marathwada) of Maharashtra involving about 400 encephalitis cases with 115 deaths. The presence of anti-CHP virus immunoglobulin M (IgM) antibodies (Abs) in about 20% of the cases and the absence of other known causes of encephalitis indicated that the CHP virus was the most important etiological agent in this outbreak (National Institute of Virology, unpublished data).

Thus, about 40 years after the discovery of the CHP virus in 1965, an acute encephalitis disease with very high mortality was clearly attributed to the virus. Confirmation of acute encephalitis involving 24 children from Vadodara district, Gujarat State, from May to July 2004 as CHP encephalitis (3) further established the disease potential of the virus.

HISTORICAL PERSPECTIVE ON THE DISEASE

Until recently, Japanese encephalitis (JE) was recognized as the only encephalitis having outbreak potential in India (23). However, several encephalitis outbreaks over the years had remained undiagnosed. One of the earliest documented outbreaks was in Jamshedpur, Bihar State (15), in 1954. Khan provided an excellent account of the clinical features of this outbreak, and the features of one of the groups were very similar to those of CHP encephalitis.

The clinical features described for the viral encephalitis outbreak in Raipur and Jabalpur in 1980 (25) exactly match the typical case definition of Chandipura encephalitis. It is noteworthy that CHP virus was isolated from the serum of a patient with a fatal case of acute encephalitis, and clear seroconversion was noted in one patient during this outbreak.

Similar outbreaks, not confirmed as JE, reported from various parts of the country, such as Nagpur in Maharashtra, Muzaffarpur in Bihar, Warangal in Andhra Pradesh, and Vadodara in Gujarat, had remained mystery diseases or were labeled as Nagpur fever, Reye's syndrome (11), unusual measles (26, 30), etc., without proper verification of the etiological agent. Thus, there is evidence that this disease might have been in existence for at least the last 50 years. Undoubtedly, the virus has now attained the status of an important emerging pathogen of public health significance.

In this chapter, I briefly describe the outbreaks that have led to the identification of this disease and also provide a brief description of the classical, as well as modern, virological techniques used. Other important studies that have been undertaken on the virus and disease are also summarized.

OUTBREAK INVESTIGATIONS

Andhra Pradesh, 2003

An outbreak of acute encephalitis of unknown origin with a high CFR (183 of 329 cases) was reported in children from 11 districts of Andhra Pradesh, India, during 2003 (22). Clinical samples tested negative for IgM antibodies to Japanese encephalitis, West Nile, dengue, and measles viruses and for RNAs of coronaviruses, paramyxoviruses, enteroviruses, and influenza viruses. Six virus strains were isolated from different clinical samples originating from encephalitis case patients. The isolates were identified as rhabdoviruses by electron microscopy and confirmed as CHP virus by complement fixation and neutralization tests. CHP virus RNA was detected in the clinical samples from nine case patients, five of which were sequenced. The results showed 96.7 to 97.5% identity with the reference strain of 1965.

CHP virus antigen and RNA were detected in the brain tissue of a deceased child by immunofluorescent-antibody testing and PCR, respectively. Serological tests confirmed the presence of neutralizing antibodies (N Abs) and IgG and IgM antibodies to CHP virus in the patients. CHP virus-reactive IgM positivity was significantly higher in samples collected after 4 days of illness (69%) than in those collected before 4 days (13.3%). A similar trend was observed for neutralizing antibodies (Table 1). These findings suggested that CHP virus was the causative agent of the acute encephalitis outbreak in Andhra Pradesh in 2003.

Maharashtra, 2003

The Maharashtra public health department reported a total of 393 encephalitis cases, with 115 deaths, involving 15 districts from June to August 2003. Clinical samples from 202 case patients were received at the National Institute of Virology. All cases were in the pediatric age group, below 15 years of age. Usually, a single case was recorded in each village, with no clustering. Sera from three of these case patients were positive for JE IgM Abs and one for dengue virus IgM Abs. CHP virus IgM Abs were detected in 26% of the encephalitis cases from six districts (Table 2).

Analysis of the data based on the number of days postonset (DPO) was interesting. The percentage of cases positive for CHP virus IgM Abs in samples collected after 4 DPO (11/28; 52.3%) was significantly higher than in those collected before 4 DPO (10/114; 8.8%). This antibody pattern was highly suggestive of the involvement of CHP virus as the main etiological agent in the outbreak. IgM Abs were also detected in some fever case patients and contacts, which suggests a wider spectrum of CHP virus infection, characteristic of arthropod-borne viruses.

Isolation of the virus was not attempted. However, the brain tissues obtained by biopsy from one encephalitis case patient were found to be positive for CHP virus by immunofluorescence testing.

Table 1. Relationship of anti-CHP virus antibodies to number of DPO of sample collection in Andhra Pradesh, 2003

Antibody status	Encephalitis cases[a]		Fever cases without encephalitis[a]	Contacts without disease[a]
	DPO 0–4	DPO >4		
IgM+ IgG−	2/30	4/16	1/5	1/10
IgM+ IgG+	1/30	7/16	2/5	1/10
IgM− IgG+	0/30	1/16	0/5	2/10
IgM− IgG−	27/30	4/16	2/5	5/10
N Ab	2/29	15/18	2/5	7/10
Total no. of cases reported	30	18	5	10

[a]Number of samples positive/total number tested.

Table 2. Encephalitis cases showing CHP virus IgM antibodies in
different districts of Maharashtra, 2003

District	Deaths/no. of cases (CFR [%])	No. of encephalitis case patients antibody positive/no. tested (%)
Bhandara	16/30 (53)	6/31 (19)
Chandrapur	21/52 (40)	3/26 (12)
Gondia	6/14 (43)	3/12 (25)
Nagpur	29/123 (24)	11/67 (16)
Wardha	9/29 (31)	10/35 (29)
Nanded	13/43 (30)	8/20 (40)
Total	94/291 (32)	22/191 (26)

Vadodara District, Gujarat, 2004

An outbreak of acute encephalitis was reported among the tribes from the Vadodara district of Gujarat during June and July 2004 (3). A total of 23 cases with 16 deaths were reported (CFR, ~70%). About 80% of the deaths occurred within 24 h of hospitalization. The cases were restricted to rural areas, with no clustering, and usually only one case per village was observed. All case patients were less than 16 years of age; the male-to-female ratio was 1.5 to 1. Twenty-two blood samples, eight cerebrospinal fluid (CSF) samples, 14 throat swabs, and 11 urine samples were collected from 22 case patients with acute encephalitis; two blood samples from two patients were also collected during the convalescent phase.

Sera tested for IgM antibodies against JE, West Nile, Chandipura, and dengue viruses gave negative results. However, a second sample (a convalescent sample) from one case patient, the first sample from whom was negative, became positive for IgM and IgG antibodies to Chandipura virus, suggesting seroconversion. In reverse transcription-PCR, 9/21 serum samples were positive for CHP virus RNA. The presence of CHP virus RNA in 41% of case patients and of seroconversion in one of the patients was suggestive of CHP virus etiology. The virus was also isolated from a serum sample from a patient with a fatal case, in RD and PS cell lines, and in infant mice.

CLINICAL CHARACTERISTICS

The general clinical features of CHP encephalitis include high-grade fever of short duration, vomiting, altered sensorium, generalized convulsions, and decerebrate posture, leading to grade IV coma, acute encephalitis/encephalopathy, and death within a few to 48 hours of hospitalization. The CSF is usually under pressure, pleocytosis is absent, and neurological sequelae are rare in children who recover.

In the Andhra Pradesh outbreak (22), the typical clinical manifestations in the confirmed CHP encephalitis group ($n = 28$) included rapid onset of fever (100%), followed by vomiting (53.6%), altered sensorium (89.3%), convulsions (82.1%), diarrhea (17.9%), neurological deficit (14.3%), and meningeal irritation (7.2%). Though a specific analysis of the clinical features of cases in Maharashtra was not available, the general clinical features observed were consistent with those in the outbreak in Andhra Pradesh.

In Vadodara, Gujarat, detailed clinical findings for 20 patients were available for analysis. The presenting manifestations were fever (100%), altered sensorium (100%), convulsions (90%), vomiting (70%), diarrhea (50%), chills preceding fever (20%), and cough (20%). The full clinical spectrum of the disease is not clear. Preliminary data suggest a range from subclinical infection with mild- to high-grade fever to acute encephalitis.

CHP VIRUS

CHP virus belongs to the family *Rhabdoviridae,* genus *Vesiculovirus*. It is characterized by bullet-shaped particles (Fig. 1) 150 to 165 nm long and 50 to 60 nm wide showing distinct surface projections 9 to 11 nm in length and a stain-filled canal at the base of the virus particle (22). The 11-kb-long genomic RNA, encapsidated by nucleocapsid protein, serves as the template for both replication and transcription (16). Transcription of this genome by virus-encoded RNA polymerase produces five different structural proteins, the nucleocapsid protein (N), the phosphoprotein (P), the matrix protein (M),

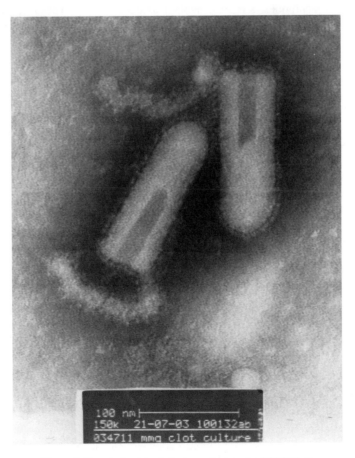

Figure 1. Negatively stained electron micrograph of CHP virus.

the glycoprotein (G), and the large protein (L), in sequential order and in decreasing amounts (20).

Dragunova and Závada (5) demonstrated that vesicular stomatitis virus type Indiana and CHP virus show a low-level but distinct cross-neutralization.

Temperature-Sensitive Mutants

Analysis and characterization of 50 different temperature-sensitive mutants of CHP virus resulted in the identification of six complementation groups. The intragroup complementation observed among the CHP virus temperature-sensitive mutants suggested that the functional form of at least one of the virion proteins is a multimer (7, 8).

ASSAY SYSTEMS AND DEVELOPMENT OF DIAGNOSTIC TESTS

Following the discovery of CHP virus, serological tests were developed for detection of anti-CHP virus antibodies. While revisiting CHP encephalitis etiology during the current outbreaks, we used conventional methods standardized several decades earlier and also employed newer techniques, a requirement of modern science. The different techniques employed are described below.

Virus Isolation

The cell lines Vero, BHK-21, RD, and PS and cell cultures from, e.g., bonnet monkey and langur kidneys, chicken embryos, and shrew tumor cells support growth of the virus and exhibit CPE (2, 22). The virus also multiplies in *Aedes albopictus, Aedes aegypti, Aedes vittatus, Aedes novalbopictus, Aedes w-albus,* and *Aedes krombeini* cell cultures without CPE (17). Infant mice are highly susceptible and very useful for primary isolation, as well as for propagation of the virus (22). Embryonated chicken eggs are also highly susceptible and are a good source for a high titer of the virus (18, 32).

Complement Fixation Test

Complement fixation tests for CHP virus were standardized using hyperimmune CHP virus antiserum raised against a prototype CHP virus strain, 653514 (CHPI-653514).

Genome Detection

Based on the G-gene sequence of an Indian CHP virus isolate (GenBank accession number J04350), the diagnostic PCR was standardized. The following primers were used in nested format for diagnosis: CHAND-G-F2, 5′-GTC TTG TGG TTA TGC TTC TGT-3′; CHAND-G-R5, 5′-TTC CGT TCC GAC CGC AAT AACT-3′, and CHAND-G-F5, 5′-GAG AAT GCG ACC AGT CTT AT-3′; and CHAND-G-R6, 5′-TGC AAG TTC GAG CAC CTT CCAT-3′ (3).

Immunofluorescence Assay

Infected cells or tissues spread on glass slides were air dried, fixed with acetone, and immunolabeled with mouse anti-Chandipura virus hyperimmune serum and anti-mouse fluorescein isothiocyanate conjugate by a standard procedure, along with an appropriate control. Green fluorescence indicated the presence of CHP virus antigen in cells or tissues (22).

ELISA

IgM and IgG capture enzyme-linked immunosorbent assays (ELISAs) were quickly developed and standardized for detection of antibodies against CHP virus. IgM or IgG from patients' sera were captured on anti-human IgM- or IgG-coated wells, respectively. Sucrose acetone-extracted mouse brain CHP virus was the source of the antigen. Captured antigen was detected using the IgG fraction of polyclonal anti-CHP virus mouse serum conjugated with biotin, followed by avidin-horseradish peroxidase. o-Phenylenediamine–hydrogen peroxide was added for color development. Negative controls included age-matched sera from apparently healthy children from an unaffected area and sera and CSF from flavivirus encephalitis pediatric case patients. The cutoff value was determined as the mean optical density for negative controls ± 3 standard deviations (22).

Neutralization Test

PS and Vero cells were used to standardize neutralization tests with 100 50% tissue culture infective doses of CHP virus (2). The virus N Ab titer was assigned as the reciprocal of the antibody dilution capable of neutralizing the virus. Hyperimmune serum raised in mice against the standard strain of CHP virus served as a positive control and was used for identification of the virus isolate. This is a very versatile test and is very useful for both seroprevalence studies and identification of the virus.

VIRUS ISOLATIONS FROM HUMAN PATIENTS

The first isolate of CHP virus was obtained from the sera of two febrile case patients from Nagpur in 1965 (2) by inoculation in BS-C-1 cells. Subsequent isolation was from the serum of a patient with a case of acute encephalopathy from Jabalpur, Madhya Pradesh, in 1980 by inoculation in infant mice (25).

In the Andhra Pradesh outbreak, 3 of 22 throat swabs (the first in MDCK cells; the second in RD, Vero, and MDCK cells; the third in Vero and RD cells), 1 brain aspirate in RD and Vero cell cultures, and 2 of 10 blood clots in peripheral blood mononuclear cell coculture were positive for virus isolations. In five of six cases yielding virus isolates, samples were collected within 4 DPO, and in the remaining case, at 4 DPO. In a fever case, 1 of 8 throat swabs also yielded the virus in the RD cell line. Isolates from one serum were obtained from Vadodara, Gujarat, by inoculations both in mice and in the RD and PS cell lines.

ANTIGEN AND VIRAL RNA DETECTIONS IN HUMAN CASES

From Andhra Pradesh, 4 of 21 throat swabs, 1 of 7 CSF samples, 5 of 25 sera, and 1 brain aspirate were found to be positive for CHP virus RNA by PCR tests. Serum samples from 9 of 21 encephalitis cases from Vadodara were positive for viral RNA. Brain tissues, one each obtained from Andhra Pradesh and Nanded, Maharashtra, showed viral antigen by immunofluorescence assay, providing direct evidence for the presence of the virus in the brains of deceased patients.

VIRUS ISOLATION FROM ANIMALS

One isolate of the virus was obtained from a hedgehog *(Alterix spiculus)* in Nigeria (14). Forty-five animal sera, collected during the Andhra Pradesh outbreak and tested by reverse transcription-PCR, were negative.

VIRUS ISOLATION AND RNA DETECTION FROM SAND FLIES AND MOSQUITOES

In India, the virus was isolated from one pool of 253 female *Phlebotomus* sand flies collected from Aurangabad, Maharashtra, in June 1969 by inoculation in infant mice (4). In Senegal, West Africa, one isolate was obtained from a pool of sand flies collected in 1992 (6, 29). One pool of sand flies collected from Andhra Pradesh in 2003 was found to be positive for CHP virus RNA (9).

Thirty-four pools, comprising 1,182 female *Aedes aegypti* mosquitoes tested from the locality where the virus was first isolated in 1965, were negative for the virus (2). Large numbers of mosquitoes collected from Andhra Pradesh and many other parts of India have been processed for virus isolation in infant mice without any isolations.

SEROPREVALENCE

Humans

Neutralizing antibodies have been detected in humans from many parts of India (2). A retrospective serologic investigation of sera in populations from different regions of India collected between 1955 and 1965 demonstrated prevalences of N Abs of 10% to 89% in different places (Table 3). During the Andhra Pradesh outbreak of 2003, N Abs were detected in 17 of 47 (36.2%) children in the encephalitis group, 2 of 5 children in the fever without encephalitis group, and 7 of 10 (70%) healthy contacts, which also included adults (Table 1). In Maharashtra (2003), 114 of 177 (64%) children during an encephalitis outbreak were found to be positive for CHP virus N Abs.

Animals

In India, CHP virus N Abs have been detected in camels (1/50), horses (13/40), cows (11/18), buffaloes (2/8), sheep (4/14), goats (6/19), and rhesus monkeys (7/43) but were not detected in any of 69 samples from bonnet monkeys. All of these samples were collected from 1955 to 1960, which suggests that the virus has been present in the area since at least 1955 (24). A seroepidemiological study of arboviruses in wild toque macaques *(Macaca sinica)* in Sri Lanka also showed a low seroprevalence (2/115) for this virus (19). N Abs were detected in about 19% of the sera collected in Andhra Pradesh and in about 49% of the sera collected in Maharashtra (Table 4).

Detection of anti-CHP virus antibodies in pigs and in the small number of dogs tested was an important observation, and the roles of these animals need to be elucidated further.

Table 3. Neutralization test results for human sera collected between
1955 and 1966 from different parts of India

Locality	State	No. positive/no. tested (% positive)
Kashmir	·Jammu and Kashmir	0/62 (0)
Delhi	Delhi	41/74 (57.7)
Lucknow	Uttar Pradesh	25/28 (89.3)
Bahadarpur	Gujarat	10/28 (35.7)
Banni	Gujarat	62/74 (83.8)
Bhuj area	Gujarat	10/91 (11.0)
Daulatpura	Gujarat	29/43 (67.4)
Nagpur	Maharashtra	146/202 (72.3)
Ramtek	Maharashtra	47/60 (78.3)
Bangalore	Mysore (Karnataka)	16/106 (15.1)
Visakhapatnam	Andhra Pradesh	23/33 (69.7)
Sagar	Mysore (Karnataka)	8/71 (11.3)
Vellore area	Madras (Tamil Nadu)	22/42 (52.4)
Madras	Madras (Tamil Nadu)	38/59 (64.4)
Kottayam	Kerala	4/70 (5.7)
Calcutta	West Bengal	5/73 (6.8)
NEFA[a]	NEFA (Arunachal Pradesh)	0/118 (0)

[a]NEFA, North East Frontier.

Table 4. N Abs for CHP virus in different animals
collected in 2003 and 2004

Animal	No. positive/no. tested (% positive)	
	Andhra Pradesh	Maharashtra
Pig	15/49 (28.6)	15/29 (51.7)
Cattle	4/28 (14.3)	2/3
Buffalo	5/28 (17.9)	1/6
Goat	4/43 (9.3)	
Sheep	2/26 (7.7)	
Dog	3/6 (50)	1/1
Total	33/180 (19.3)	19/39 (48.7)

EXPERIMENTAL INFECTION IN ANIMALS

Bhatt and Rodrigues (2) reported that the virus was lethal to both infant and adult animals by the intracerebral route. A low-grade viremia of short duration was observed in adult mice inoculated intraperitoneally and in a langur monkey inoculated subcutaneously. Serum samples from experimentally infected langur and bonnet monkeys showed the presence of neutralizing antibodies.

Sokhei and Obukhova (27) also reported that CHP virus was highly pathogenic for mice of different ages by various routes of inoculation. Wilks and House (32) demonstrated that virus inoculations increased neutralizing Abs in domestic animals, like ponies, sheep, goats, and pigs, that already had low levels of neutralizing Abs prior to virus inoculation. Lethal infections were produced in 1-day-old mice and hamsters by both intracranial and peritoneal routes of inoculation and by allantoic inoculation of embryonated chicken eggs (18). Adult mice, guinea pigs, and rabbits produced serum Abs but lacked clinical symptoms and signs (13).

At the NIV, guinea pigs and monkeys have been found suitable for preparation of high-titer immune sera. Recent studies on pathogenesis in mice showed that all mice up to the age of 2 weeks are killed after intracranial, intraperitoneal, and subcutaneous inoculations of the virus. Between 2 and 3 weeks, they become refractory to infection, and only about 50% mortality occurs. However, beyond 3 weeks, they become totally refractory, and all mice survive. Hemiplagia and retarded growth have been observed in some mice following virus inoculation (12). Urine retention in many infant mice observed at the NIV was a characteristic and significant observation, and the cause needs to be understood.

TRANSMISSION OF CHP VIRUS BY SAND FLIES AND MOSQUITOES

Ramchandra Rao et al. (21) reported successful transmission of CHP virus by four species of mosquitoes: *Aedes aegypti, A. albopictus, Anopheles stephensi,* and *Culex tritaeniorhynchus. Culex quinquefaciatus* picked up the virus but was not able to transmit it under similar conditions.

Ilkal et al. (10) compared the susceptibilities of *C. tritaeniorhynchus, Culex bitaeniorhynchus, C. quinquefaciatus,* and *A. aegypti* after parenteral inoculation of mosquitoes. All of the species supported virus growth and transmitted the virus to susceptible hosts. *A. aegypti* was found to be the most susceptible, and it was suggested that this species could be used as a substitute for laboratory mice for isolation and propagation of the virus.

Tesh and Modi (28) reported the multiplication of CHP virus in sand flies (*Phlebotomus papatasi*) following intrathoracic inoculation. These infected sand flies transmitted the virus to newborn mice by biting. Eight percent of the progeny of experimentally infected female parents were infected with CHP virus.

PHYLOGENETIC ANALYSIS

Based on the sequence of a conserved, small fragment of the G gene, the available CHP virus isolates were compared (Fig. 2). Broadly, the 20 isolates formed four groups. The first group included the 1965 isolate, two sandfly isolates from Andhra Pradesh (2003 and 2004), and three isolates from Andhra Pradesh (2003). The second group included four isolates from Andhra Pradesh and four isolates from Vadodara (2004). Five isolates from Vadodara constituted the third group, while one isolate from Vadodara was the sole member of the fourth group.

The percent nucleotide identities (PNI) within groups were 97.3 ± 0.45 (group 1), 99.04 ± 0.34 (group 2), and 98.8 ± 0.57 (group 3). Between groups, groups 1 and 4 showed the maximum difference (91.86 PNI), whereas groups 1 and 2 exhibited the minimum difference (96.94 PNI). The data show that, during outbreaks of the disease, multiple strains circulate. Sequence analysis of a hypervariable region will further clarify this issue.

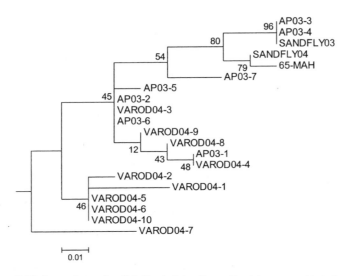

Figure 2. Phylogenetic tree for all Indian isolates. Percent bootstrap support is indicated by each node. AP, Andhra Pradesh; MAH, Maharashtra.

G-, N-, AND P-GENE-BASED ANALYSES OF CHP VIRUSES ISOLATED IN ANDHRA PRADESH

To understand the association of mutations in the CHP virus genome with pathogenesis, five cell culture isolates representing one patient with a fatal case of encephalitis, two recovered encephalitis case patients, and two fever case patients were examined (1). The G, N, and P genes were PCR amplified and sequenced. G gene-based phylogenetic analysis (Fig. 3a) showed that the brain-derived isolate (from the fatal case) clustered with the 1965 isolate. The other four isolates grouped together with PNI, with the 1965 isolate varying from 95.6% to 97.6%; similar tree topologies were obtained for P- and N-gene-based phylogenetic analyses (Fig. 3b and c).

Comparison of partial G-gene sequences from clinical samples ($n = 3$) with the corresponding cell line isolates documented that, though sequences derived from different clinical samples exhibited unique mutations, except for one substitution in isolate CIN0331M (A1167C), no changes were noted.

Comparison of the deduced amino acid sequences of the G protein (responsible for virus entry into cells and induction of neutralizing antibodies) documented seven differences between the epidemic isolates and the 1965 isolate (Fig. 4). None of them were in the transmembrane region sequence, the intracytoplasmic region sequence, or the signal sequence. Importantly, additional amino acid substitutions were recorded for the brain-derived isolate. These included Ile16Val, i.e., the signal sequence, and Arg502Lys, i.e., the transmembrane region sequence.

Both the N (mainly associated with cytotoxic T-lymphocyte responses) and P (associated with RNA polymerase) proteins were highly conserved, with only one amino acid substitution at positions 37 and 64. The importance of the amino acid substitutions in these proteins in the pathogenesis of CHP virus infection remains to be determined. In this connection, it is noteworthy that, as modeled by Walker and Kongsuwan (31), the major antigenic sites for

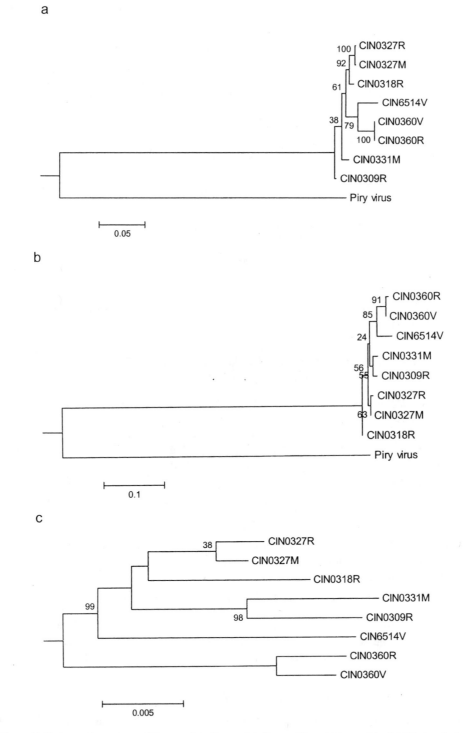

a

100 CIN0327R
92 CIN0327M
61 CIN0318R
CIN6514V
38 79 CIN0360V
100 CIN0360R
CIN0331M
CIN0309R
Piry virus

0.05

b

91 CIN0360R
85 CIN0360V
24 CIN6514V
CIN0331M
56 55 CIN0309R
CIN0327R
63 CIN0327M
CIN0318R
Piry virus

0.1

c

38 CIN0327R
CIN0327M
CIN0318R
CIN0331M
99 98 CIN0309R
CIN6514V
CIN0360R
CIN0360V

0.005

Figure 3. Phylogenetic analyses of the complete G gene (a), P gene (b), and N gene (c) of CHP virus isolates. Percent bootstrap support is indicated by the value at each node. For G- and P-gene-based analyses, Piry virus (accession number D26175) was used as an outgroup. For the N gene, an unrooted tree was constructed, as the sequence for Piry virus was not available.

vesicular stomatitis virus New Jersey neutralization escape mutations (epitopes VII and VI) correspond to the CHP virus G domain exhibiting multiple amino acid changes (Thr219Ala-Gly222Ala and Arg264Lys-His269Pro, respectively).

POSSIBLE INVOLVEMENT OF INTERLEUKIN 2 (IL-2) AND TUMOR NECROSIS FACTOR ALPHA (TNF-α) IN RECOVERY

As cytokines play an important role in the progression and clearance of disease, to assess the role of cytokines in the pathogenesis of CHP virus infection, 14 children with encephalitis admitted to a tertiary-care hospital and five age-matched apparently healthy control children were studied. Blood was collected ≤4 (group A) and >4 (group B) DPO.

The concentrations of IL-2, gamma interferon (IFN-γ), IL-6, and TNF-α in mitogen-stimulated peripheral blood mononuclear cell supernatants of patients and controls were assessed by ELISA. TNF-α levels were significantly higher in group B than in controls (555.47 ± 468.55 versus $113.4. \pm 132.7$; $P < 0.05$). IL-2 levels in group B were significantly higher than in group A (282.73 ± 307.64 versus 47.32 ± 41.36; $P < 0.05$) and controls (282.73 ± 307.64 versus <7.8; $P < 0.05$). No significant changes were observed in the levels of IL-6 and IFN-γ between the groups. Significant elevation of TNF-α and IL-2 in the later stage of the disease suggests the possibility that they had antiviral activity. Further studies are urgently required.

THE HLA-A28 ALLELE AMONG CHP ENCEPHALITIS PATIENTS FROM ANDHRA PRADESH

In order to assess the association of class I HLA alleles with CHP encephalitis, the HLA A, B, and Cw allele distribution was determined among 14 children with clinically and serologically confirmed CHP encephalitis, and the results were compared with those for 385 ethnically matched, apparently healthy individuals.

Genomic DNA was extracted from frozen peripheral blood mononuclear cells. For HLA A, B, and C typing, a PCR–single-strand polymorphism molecular method was followed. To overcome chance deviation in the frequency of the HLA allele, the P value was corrected by the use of the Bonferroni inequality method. The HLA A28 and A3 alleles were more commonly observed among CHP virus-infected individuals than in controls. In fact, A28 was significantly increased among CHP virus-infected children compared with controls ($P < 0.0001$), suggesting the involvement of HLA class I alleles in genetic susceptibility to CHP virus-associated encephalitis. Further molecular subtyping of the A28 gene would help in understanding the influence of haplotype association and other intervening genes within the major histocompatibility complex.

OTHER STUDIES

CHP virus has been widely used in many laboratories for various virological studies because of its ability to grow very rapidly (in a few hours) in a variety of cell cultures and mice. Studies on basic virology, protein structure, transport mechanisms, etc., have been done in several laboratories. There is an urgent need to develop rapid diagnostic methods

```
CIN036514V  ---------V  LLISFITPLY  SYLSIAFPEN  TKLDWKPVTK  NTRYCPMGGE    [ 50]
CIN0360V    ----------  .....V..S.  .S.......S  ..........  ..........    [ 50]
CIN0360R    ----------  .....V..S.  .S.......S  ..........  ..........    [ 50]
CIN0327M    ---------.  .......S.  .S.......  ..........R  ..........    [ 50]
CIN0327R    ---------.  .......S.  .S.......  ..........R  ..........    [ 50]
CIN0331M    ----------  .......S.  .S.......  ..........  ..........    [ 50]
CIN0318R    ----------  .......S.  .S.......  ..........  ..........    [ 50]
CIN0309R    MTSSVTISV.  .......S.  .S.......  ..........  ..........    [ 50]
```

Signal sequence

```
CIN036514V  WFLEPGLQEE  SFLSSTPIGA  TPSKSDGFLC  HAAKWVTTCD  FRWYGPKYIT    [100]
CIN0360V    ..........  ..........  ..........  ..........  ..........    [100]
CIN0360R    ..........  ..........  ..........  ..........  ..........    [100]
CIN0327M    ..........  ..........  ..........  ..........  ..........    [100]
CIN0327R    ..........  ..........  ..........  ..........  ..........    [100]
CIN0331M    ..........  ..........  ..........  ..........  ..........    [100]
CIN0318R    ..........  ..........  ..........  ..........  ..........    [100]
CIN0309R    ..........  ..........  ..........  ..........  ..........    [100]

CIN036514V  HSIHNIKPTR  SDCDTALASY  KSGTLVSPGF  PPESCGYASV  TDSEFLVIMI    [150]
CIN0360V    ..........  ..........  ..........  ..........  ..........    [150]
CIN0360R    ..........  ..........  ..........  ..........  ..........    [150]
CIN0327M    ..........  ..........  ..........  ..........  ..........    [150]
CIN0327R    ..........  ..........  ..........  ..........  ..........    [150]
CIN0331M    ..........  ..........  .........?  ..........  ..........    [150]
CIN0318R    ..........  ..........  ..........  ..........  ..........    [150]
CIN0309R    ..........  ..........  ..........  ..........  ..........    [150]

CIN036514V  TPHHVGVDDY  RGHWVDPLFV  GGECDQSYCD  TIHNSSVWIP  ADQTKKNICG    [200]
CIN0360V    ..........  ..........  ..........  ..........  ..........    [200]
CIN0360R    ..........  ..........  ..........  ..........  ..........    [200]
CIN0327M    ..........  ..........  ..........  ..........  ..........    [200]
CIN0327R    ..........  ..........  ..........  ..........  ..........    [200]
CIN0331M    ..........  ..........  ..........  ..........  ..........    [200]
CIN0318R    ..........  ..........  ..........  ..........  ..........    [200]
CIN0309R    ..........  ..........  ..........  ..........  ..........    [200]

CIN036514V  QSFTPLTVTV  AYDKTKEITA  GGIVFKSKYH  SHMEGARTCR  LSYCGRNGIK    [250]
CIN0360V    ..........  ......VA.  .A.......  ..........  ..........    [250]
CIN0360R    ..........  ......VA.  .A.......  ..........  ..........    [250]
CIN0327M    ..........  .......A.  .A.......  ..........  ..........    [250]
CIN0327R    ..........  .......A.  .A.......  ..........  ..........    [250]
CIN0331M    ..........  .......A.  .A.......  ..........  ..........    [250]
CIN0318R    ..........  .......A.  .A.......  ..........  ..........    [250]
CIN0309R    ..........  ..V.....A.  .A.......  ..........  ..........    [250]

CIN036514V  FPNGEWVSLD  VKTRIQEKHL  LPLFKECPTG  TEVRSTLQSD  GAQVLTSEIQ    [300]
CIN0360V    ..........  ...K....P.  ........A.  ..........  ..........    [300]
CIN0360R    ..........  ...K....P.  ........A.  ..........  ..........    [300]
CIN0327M    ..........  ...K....P.  ........A.  ..........  ..........    [300]
CIN0327R    ..........  ...K....P.  ........A.  ..........  ..........    [300]
CIN0331M    ..........  ...K....P.  ........A.  ..........  ..........    [300]
CIN0318R    ..........  ...K....P.  ........A.  ..........  ..........    [300]
CIN0309R    ..........  ...K....P.  ........A.  ..........  ..........    [300]
```

Figure 4. Alignment of the deduced amino acid sequences of the G proteins of different isolates of CHP virus. The solid bars represent the signal sequence (amino acids 1 to 18), transmembrane region sequence (amino acids 482 to 502), and intracytoplasmic region sequence (amino acids 503 to 530). Dashes indicate no data, and dots indicate the same amino acid as above.

```
CIN036514V  RILDYSLCQN  TWDKVERKEP  LSPLDLSYLA  SKSPGKGLAY  TVINGTLSFA   [350]
CIN0360V    ..........  ..........  ..........  ..........  ..........   [350]
CIN0360R    ..........  ..........  ..........  ..........  ..........   [350]
CIN0327M    ..........  ..........  ..........  ..........  ..........   [350]
CIN0327R    ..........  ..........  ..........  ..........  ..........   [350]
CIN0331M    ..........  ..........  ..........  ..........  ..........   [350]
CIN0318R    ..........  ..........  ..........  ..........  ..........   [350]
CIN0309R    ..........  ..........  ..........  ..........  ..........   [350]

CIN036514V  HTRYVRMWID  GPVLKEPKGK  RESPSGISSD  IWTQWFKYGD  MEIGPNGLLK   [400]
CIN0360V    ..........  ..........  ..........  ..........  ..........   [400]
CIN0360R    ..........  ..........  ..........  ..........  ..........   [400]
CIN0327M    ..........  ......M...  ..........  ..........  ..........   [400]
CIN0327R    ..........  ......M...  ..........  ..........  ..........   [400]
CIN0331M    ..........  ......M...  ..........  ..........  ..........   [400]
CIN0318R    ..........  ......M...  ..........  ..........  ..........   [400]
CIN0309R    ..........  ......M...  ..........  ..........  ..........   [400]

CIN036514V  TAGGYKFPWH  LIGMGIVDNE  LHELSEANPL  DHPQLPHAQS  IADDSEEIFF   [450]
CIN0360V    ..........  ..........  ..........  ..........  ..........   [450]
CIN0360R    ..........  ..........  ..........  ..........  ..........   [450]
CIN0327M    ..........  ..........  ...V......  ..........  ..........   [450]
CIN0327R    ..........  ..........  ...V......  ..........  ..........   [450]
CIN0331M    ..........  ..........  ..........  ..........  ..........   [450]
CIN0318R    ..........  ..........  ..........  ..........  ..........   [450]
CIN0309R    ..........  ..........  ..........  ..........  ..........   [450]

CIN036514V  GDTGVSKNPV  ELVTGWFTSW  KESLAAGVVL  ILVVVLIYGV  LRCFPVLCTTCR [502]
CIN0360V    ..........  ..........  ..........  ..........  .........K   [502]
CIN0360R    ..........  ..........  ..........  ..........  .........K   [502]
CIN0327M    ..........  ..........  ..........  ..........  ..........   [502]
CIN0327R    ..........  ..........  ..........  ..........  ..........   [502]
CIN0331M    ..........  ..........  ..........  ..........  ..........   [502]
CIN0318R    ..........  ..........  ..........  ..........  ..........   [502]
CIN0309R    ..........  ..........  ..........  ..........  ..........   [502]

                                        Transmembrane Region
CIN036514V  KPKWKKGV  ERSDSFEMRI  FKPNNMRARV   [530]
CIN0360V    .......  ..........  ..........   [530]
CIN0360R    .......  ..........  ..........   [530]
CIN0327M    .......  ..........  ..........   [530]
CIN0327R    .......  ..........  ..........   [530]
CIN0331M    . .......  ..........  ..........   [530]
CIN0318R    .......  ..........  ..........   [530]
CIN0309R    .......  ..........  ..........   [530]
```

Intracytoplasmic Region

Figure 4. *Continued*

for field use. Pathogenesis, cell-virus interaction, and vaccine development are other areas that require immediate attention.

REFERENCES

1. **Arankalle, V. A., S. P. Shrotri, A. M. Walimbe, Hanumaih, S. D. Pawar, and A. C. Mishra.** 2005. G, N and P gene-based analysis of Chandipura viruses isolated during an encephalitis epidemic in India. *Emerg. Infect. Dis.* **11:**123–126.
2. **Bhatt, P. N., and F. M. Rodrigues.** 1967. Chandipura virus: a new arbovirus isolated in India from patients with febrile illness. *Indian J. Med. Res.* **55:**1295–1305.
3. **Chadha, M. S., V. A. Arankalle, R. S. Jadi, M. V. Joshi, J. P. Thakare, P. V. M. Mahadev, and A. C. Mishra.** 2005. An outbreak of Chandipura virus encephalitis in Eastern district of Gujarat State, India. *Am. J. Trop. Med. Hyg.* **73:**566–570.
4. **Dhanda, V., F. M. Rodrigues, and S. N. Ghosh.** 1970. Isolation of Chandipura virus from sandflies in Aurangabad. *Indian J. Med. Res.* **58:**79–180.
5. **Dragunova, J., and J. Závada.** 1979. Cross-neutralization between vesicular stomatitis virus type Indiana and Chandipura virus. *Acta Virol.* **23:**319–328.
6. **Fontinelle, D., M. Traore-Lamizana, J. Trouillet, A. Leclerc, M. Mondo, Y. Ba, J. P. Digoutte, and H. G. Zeller.** 1994. First isolations of arboviruses from Phlebotomine sand flies in West Africa. *Am. J. Trop. Med. Hyg.* **50:**570–574.
7. **Gadkari, D. A., and C. R. Pringle.** 1980. Temperature-sensitive mutants of Chandipura virus. I. Inter- and intragroup complementation. *J. Virol.* **33:**100–106.
8. **Gadkari, D. A., and C. R. Pringle.** 1980. Temperature-sensitive mutants of Chandipura virus. II. Phenotypic characteristics of the six complementation groups. *J. Virol.* **33:**107–114.
9. **Geevarghese, G., V. A. Arankalle, R. Jadi, P. Kanojia, M. V. Joshi, and A. C. Mishra.** 2005. Detection of Chandipura virus from sandflies of Sergentomyia sp. (Diptera: Phlebotomidae) in Karimnagar district, Andhra Pradesh, India. *J. Med. Entomol.* **42:**495–496.
10. **Ilkal, M. A., M. K. Goverdhan, P. S. Shetty, C. D. Tupe, M. S. Mavale, and V. Dhanda.** 1991. Susceptibility of four species of mosquitoes to Chandipura virus and its detection by immunofluorescence. *Acta Virol.* **35:**27–32.
11. **John, T. J.** 2003. Outbreak of killer brain disease in children: mystery or missed diagnosis? *Indian Pediatr.* **40:**863–869.
12. **Jortner, B. S., P. N. Bhatt, and G. B. Sollitare.** 1973. Experimental Chandipura virus infection in mice. I. Virus assay and light microscopic studies with emphasis on neuropathologic observations. *Acta Neuropathol.* (Berlin) **23:**320–325.
13. **Kelkar, S. D.** 1976. Antibody response to Chandipura virus in experimental animals. *Indian J. Med. Res.* **64:**814–823.
14. **Kemp, G. E.** 1975. Viruses other than arenaviruses from West African wild mammals: factors affecting transmission to man and domestic animals. *Bull. W. H. O.* **52:**615–620.
15. **Khan, N.** 1954. Jamshedpur fever. *Indian J. Med. Sci.* **8:**597–608.
16. **Masters, P. S., and A. K. Banerjee.** 1987. Sequences of Chandipura virus N and NS genes: evidence for high mutability of the NS gene within vesiculovirus. *Virology* **157:**298–306.
17. **Pant, U., A. B. Sudeep, and S. S. Athawale.** 1992. Susceptibility of *Aedes krombeini* cell line to some arboviruses. *Indian J. Med. Res.* **95:**239–244.
18. **Pawar, S. D., A. Singh, S. V. Gangodkar, and B. L. Rao.** 2005. Propagation of Chandipura virus in chick embryos. *Indian J. Exp. Biol.* **43:**930–932.
19. **Peiris, J. S., W. P. Dittus, and C. B. Ratnayake.** 1993. Seroepidemiology of dengue and other arboviruses in a natural population of toque macaques (*Macaca sinica*) at Polonnaruwa, Sri Lanka. *J. Med. Primatol.* **22:**240–245.
20. **Raha, T., E. Samal, A. Majumder, S. Basak, D. Chattopadhyay, and D. J. Chattopadhyay.** 2000. N terminal region of P protein of Chandipura virus is responsible for phosphorylation-mediated homodimerization. *Protein Eng.* **13:**437–444.
21. **Ramchandra Rao, T., K. R. P. Singh, V. Dhanda, and P. N. Bhatt.** 1967. Experimental transmission of Chandipura virus by mosquitoes. *Indian J. Med. Res.* **55:**1306–1310.

22. **Rao, B. L., A. Basu, N. S. Wairagkar, M. M. Gore, V. A. Arankalle, J. P. Thakare, R. S. Jadi, K. A. Rao and A. C. Mishra.** 2004. A large outbreak of acute encephalitis with high fatality rate in children in Andhra Pradesh, India, in 2003, associated with Chandipura virus. *Lancet* **364:**869–874.
23. **Rodrigues, F. M.** 1984. Epidemiology of Japanese encephalitis in India, a brief overview, p. 1–9. *In Proceedings of the National Conference on Japanese Encephalitis.* Indian Council of Medical Research, New Delhi, India.
24. **Rodrigues, F. M., M. R. Patankar, K. Banerjee, P. N. Bhatt, M. K. Goverdhan, K. M. Pavri, and M. Vittal.** 1972. Etiology of the 1965 epidemic of febrile illness in Nagpur city, Maharashtra state, India. *Indian J. Med. Res.* **46:**173–179.
25. **Rodrigues, J. J., P. B. Singh, D. S. Dave, R. Prasan, V. Ayachit, B. H. Shaikh, and K. M. Pavri.** 1983. Isolation of Chandipura virus from the blood in acute encephalopathy syndrome. *Indian J. Med. Res.* **77:**303–307.
26. **Shaikh, N. J., N. S. Wairagkar, S. V. Reddy, J. P. Thakre, and D. A. Gadkari.** 2002. Acute encephalitis without rash in Warangal, Andhra Pradesh and Vadodara, Gujarat associated with measles virus. *J. Assoc. Physicians India* **50:**1198.
27. **Sokhei, C. H., and V. R. Obukhova.** 1984. Susceptibility of laboratory animals to the Chandipura and Isfahan viruses. *Vopr. Virusol.* **29:**290–294.
28. **Tesh, R. B., and G. B. Modi.** 1983. Growth and transovarial transmission of Chandipura virus (Rhabdoviridae: Vesiculovirus) in *Phlebotomus papatasi. Am. J. Trop. Med. Hyg.* **32:**621–623.
29. **Traore-Lamizana, M., D. Fontenille, M. Diallo, Y. Ba, H. G. Zeller, M. Mondo, F. Adam, J. Thonon, and A. Maiga.** 2001. Arbovirus surveillance from 1990 to 1995 in the Barkedji area (Ferlo) of Senegal, a possible natural focus of Rift Valley fever virus. *J. Med. Entomol.* **38:**480–492.
30. **Wairagkar, N. S., N. J. Shaikh, D. Ghosh, R. K. Ratho, S. Singhi, R. C. Mahajan, and D. A. Gadkari.** 2001. Isolation of measles virus from cerebrospinal fluid of children with acute encephalopathy without rash. *Indian Pediatr.* **38:**589–595.
31. **Walker, P. J., and K. Kongsuwan.** 1999. Deduced structural model for animal rhabdovirus glycoproteins. *J. Gen. Virol.* **80:**1211–1220.
32. **Wilks, C. R., and J. A. House.** 1986. Susceptibility of various animals to the Vesiculoviruses Isfahan and Chandipura. *J. Hyg. Lond.* **97:**359–368.

Emerging Infections 7
Edited by W. M. Scheld, D. C. Hooper, and J. M. Hughes
© 2007 ASM Press, Washington, D.C.

Chapter 8

Emergence of Novel Retroviruses

Nathan D. Wolfe, William M. Switzer, and Walid Heneine

Retroviruses are a large and diverse group of enveloped RNA viruses in the family *Retro-viridae* that replicate in a unique way, using a viral reverse transcriptase enzyme to transcribe the RNA genome into linear double-stranded DNA. Retroviruses can either be exogenous in nature, replicating independently of the host genome, or they can exist endogenously as proviral DNA integrated in the germ line of the host. As such, retroviruses can be transmitted either as infectious virions (exogenously) or as endogenous proviral DNA passed from parent to offspring via the germ line.

Taxonomically, retroviruses are divided into two subfamilies: the *Orthoretrovirinae*, composed of six genera (*Alpha-, Beta-, Gamma-, Delta-,* and *Epsilonretrovirus* and *Lentivirus*), and the *Spumaretrovirinae*, composed of only the genus *Spumavirus* (foamy virus) (30). Exogenous retroviruses of simian origin and potential public health significance are found in both retrovirus subfamilies, including the type D simian retrovirus (*Betaretrovirus*), simian (STLV) and human (HTLV) T-lymphotropic viruses (*Deltaretrovirus*), simian (SIV) and human (HIV) immunodeficiency viruses (lentiviruses), and simian foamy virus (SFV) (*Spumavirus*) (30). Retroviruses typically cause lifelong, persistent infections with long periods of clinical latency prior to disease development.

EMERGENCE OF PANDEMIC HUMAN RETROVIRUSES

The emergence of new pandemics can be conceptualized as a series of steps leading from exposure to global spread (Fig. 1). Exposure to the viruses of other animals is a frequent event, with the majority of such exposure events not leading to successful infection. Among viruses capable of causing zoonotic infections, defined for the purposes of this chapter as primary infections resulting from direct animal exposure, only some are capable of secondary spread. Even viruses capable of causing both zoonotic infections and

Nathan D. Wolfe • Departments of Epidemiology, International Health, and Molecular Microbiology and Immunology, Bloomberg School of Public Health, Johns Hopkins University, Baltimore, MD 21205. ***William M. Switzer and Walid Heneine*** • Laboratory Branch, Division of HIV/AIDS Prevention, National Center for HIV, Hepatitis, STD, and TB Prevention, Centers for Disease Control and Prevention, MS G-45, Atlanta, GA 30333.

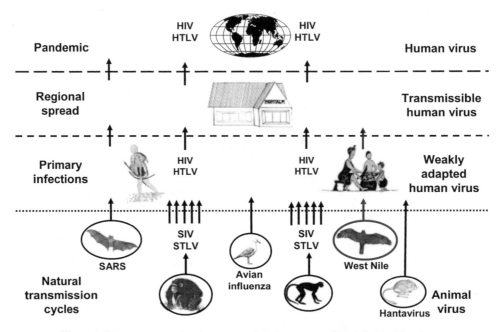

Figure 1. Diagram representing the process of viral emergence. Step 1 (bottom) is primary infection or successful cross-species transmission from the wild-animal reservoir to humans. Step 2 is local secondary transmission between humans, leading to regional spread. Step 3 is pandemic spread from a regional epidemic into the global population. Examples of various zoonotic infections, including simian retroviruses, are shown, with arrows indicating the level of transmission at each step (represented by horizontal dashed lines).

some secondary cases are often of limited public health significance, due to the fact that they are poorly adapted to the new host (3). Emergence can occur only following successful cross-species transmission of a virus, defined here as sustained transmission in the new host. Identifying the frequency of virus transmission at each of these stages, as well as the factors that permit movement from stage to stage, is the ultimate goal of the study of disease emergence and holds the potential to improve our ability to predict disease emergence.

It has been clear for some time that the emergence of the pandemic human retroviruses, HIV and HTLV, resulted from the introduction of multiple independent viruses from nonhuman primates (NHPs) to humans (Fig. 1). Phylogenetic studies of HIV type 1 (HIV-1) and HIV-2, along with their counterpart SIVs, have shown that HIV is the result of as many as eight independent introductions from African monkeys and apes (4, 22). Similarly, HTLV type 1 (HTLV-1) and HTLV-2 originated independently and are related to distinct lineages of STLV type 1 (STLV-1) and STLV-2, respectively, with HTLV-1 having resulted from multiple independent introductions of STLV-1 into human populations (19, 32, 41, 43, 47, 53). Clearly, then, NHP retroviruses have the potential for successful cross-species transmission. Nevertheless, the factors that allow retroviruses that exist in NHP reservoirs to be capable of successful cross-species transmission and emergence in human populations remain largely unknown and unstudied. An important limitation of studies of viruses that are already circulating within host populations is the fact that, while they can provide clear evidence that viruses have been introduced in the past, they do not indicate the frequency or extent of zoonosis. The approach advocated here focuses on the study of individuals who are highly exposed to the blood and body fluids of primates, either through contact in laboratories and primate centers or through the hunting and butchering of wild NHP game, and the detailed follow-up of individuals with zoonotic infections and their contacts for evidence of secondary transmission (49, 58). Such studies have the potential to push the field toward an understanding of the steps of retrovirus emergence. Understanding the factors that allow retrovirus zoonosis, secondary spread, and successful cross-species transmission has the potential to clarify how the existing pandemic retroviruses emerged and, perhaps more importantly, how to prevent the emergence of future retroviruses.

Human Infections with Simian Foamy Viruses

Spumaviruses, also known as foamy viruses, have been isolated from many different species of mammals (37). Foamy viruses from NHPs are referred to as SFVs (37). SFVs tend to be widespread across species and have been identified with high prevalence in many Old and New World monkeys, apes, and prosimians (27, 37). In captivity, more than 70% of adult NHPs are infected with SFV (27, 37). Less is known about the prevalence of SFVs in wild-living primates, but rates as high as 62% have been observed in some species (13, 27, 31). The wide distribution of SFVs among a variety of NHPs has been shown recently to be the result of cospeciation of SFV with the primate host, suggesting an ancient infection (51).

SFV has a broad host range and can infect many types of cells from a variety of animal species in vitro, including humans, resulting in cytopathology and cell death. Persistent infection of cell lines with SFV has also been reported (37). Although SFV infection in one orangutan with encephalopathy was reported, there have been no clinical diseases associated with foamy virus infection in other species of NHPs (33). The pathogenicity of SFV in many species is unclear, and no direct association between infection and disease has been proven (37). The persistent and nonpathogenic nature of SFV infection may be related to the ancient cospeciation of this virus with NHPs (51). Although cross-species transfer of SFV has been reported between NHP species, it is unclear if these infections lead to disease in the new host, as occurs with SIV and STLV (5, 19, 22, 51).

Latent SFV provirus DNA has been found in most cells and tissues of persistently infected animals, with infectious isolates obtained mainly from the oral mucosa and blood (17, 27, 37, 39). Contact with these two body fluids has been implicated in horizontal transmission of SFV, such as occurs with biting and licking, though sexual transmission is also suspected to occur (7, 10, 37). More recently, viral RNA was found in the feces of 75% of wild-living chimpanzees, suggesting that contact with feces, especially mucocutaneously, may also increase the risk of SFV infection (31). Evidence of vertical transmission has been reported in a dam and offspring chimpanzee pair, though additional data are needed to confirm this route of transmission (50). Newborn and infant primates test negative upon losing passive maternal antibodies but acquire infection when they become juveniles, presumably by contact with infected adults (7, 10, 37).

In 1971, a foamy virus was isolated from an African patient with nasopharyngeal carcinoma (1). This viral isolate was given many designations, such as human syncytial

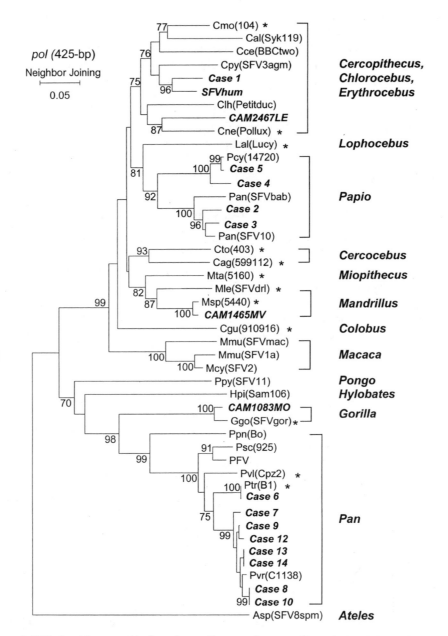

Figure 2. SFVs found in occupationally and naturally exposed persons. Shown is the phylogenetic analysis of SFV polymerase (*pol*) sequences derived from peripheral blood lymphocytes by PCR and sequence analysis described in detail elsewhere (50, 59). Zoonotic human infections with SFVs are shown in bold italics, with CAM indicating those from Cameroon. The numbers shown at branch nodes represent bootstrap percentages from 1,000 replicates; only values greater than 70% are shown. Branch lengths are proportional to the evolutionary distances (scale bar) between the taxa. The primate taxonomic nomenclature used here is defined elsewhere (21). NHPs were coded by using the first letter of the genus and the first two letters of the species names, with their house names or codes within parentheses. Asterisks indicate NHPs native to Cameroon. Cmo, *Cercopithecus mona*

virus, human syncytium-forming virus, human spumaretrovirus, and human foamy virus. Because it precedes the discovery of HIV-1 and HTLV-1, this report may represent the first evidence of a retrovirus detected in a human. However, more recent work has shown that human foamy virus is phylogenetically related to chimpanzee-type SFV, suggesting that it is of chimpanzee origin (25, 50), and thus, it was recently renamed the prototype foamy virus (PFV) (24). To date, it remains uncertain whether PFV represents a genuine foamy virus isolate from a cross-species infection or a laboratory contaminant accidentally introduced during the reportedly prolonged isolation process.

Early studies described a relatively high rate of seroreactivity to PFV among human populations, but these studies lacked definitive evidence of human infection and were not subsequently confirmed (2, 24, 37, 46, 56). Improved diagnostic assays have not documented evidence of foamy virus infection in large numbers of persons in the general population (2, 46). In contrast, screening of primate handlers and researchers exposed to NHPs and retroviruses of NHP origin revealed a substantial prevalence of SFV in this population and pointed out the high risk of cross-species transmission of SFV to humans exposed to primates (24, 50).

Our study at the Centers for Disease Control and Prevention (CDC), which provides voluntary testing for simian retroviruses for persons working at zoos and primate centers, has identified 14 of 418 (3.4%) workers tested as being infected with SFV (50). The infected persons were both men and women working at zoos and research institutions with different occupations, including veterinarians, animal handlers, and scientists (50). Sequence analysis of the SFVs found in the peripheral blood mononuclear cells of these persons showed that the infections originated from African green monkeys ($n = 1$), baboons ($n = 4$), and chimpanzees ($n = 9$) (Fig. 2). In a separate study, 4 of 133 persons (3%) who worked with mammals, including NHPs, were found to be seropositive for SFV in an anonymous serosurvey of 322 zoo workers (44). SFV antigen-specific Western blot assays suggested that the SFV infections of these four persons may have originated from apes (44). Additional studies identified SFV infections in two other workers who were infected with either an African green monkey-like SFV or a chimpanzee-like SFV (24, 37, 45). SFV screening of 46 exposed Canadian workers also identified two seropositive workers (4.3%), including one with a macaque-type SFV infection (9).

The SFV-infected workers generally reported working with the primate species that was the source of their SFV and in many cases recalled receiving injuries from these primate species, such as bites and scratches (9, 24, 50). Some workers, however, did not report any

---

(mona monkey); Cal, *Cercopithecus albogularis* (Sykes monkey); Cce, *Cercopithecus cephus* (red-eared guenon); Cpy, *Chlorocebus pygerythrus* (vervet); Clh, *Cercopithecus lhoesti* (L'Hoest's monkey); Cne, *Cercopithecus neglectus* (De Brazza's guenon); Lal, *Lophocebus albigena* (grey-cheeked mangabey); Pcy, *Papio cynocephalus* (yellow baboon); Pan, *Papio anubis* (olive baboon); Cto, *Cercocebus torquatus* (red-capped mangabey); Cag, *Cercocebus agilis* (agile mangabey); Mta, *Miopithecus talapoin* (talapoin monkey); Mle, *Mandrillus leucophaeus* (drill); Msp, *Mandrillus sphinx* (mandrill); Cgu, *Colobus guereza* (mantled guereza); Mmu, *Macaca mullata* (rhesus macaque); Mcy, *Macaca cyclopsis* (Formosan rock macaque); Ppy, *Pongo pygmaeus* (Bornean orangutan); Hpi, *Hylobates pileatus* (pileated gibbon); Ggo, *Gorilla gorilla* (Western lowland gorilla); Ppn, *Pan paniscus* (bonobo); Psc, *Pan troglodytes schweinfurthii* (East African chimpanzee); Pvl, *Pan troglodytes vellerosus* (Nigerian chimpanzee); Ptr, *Pan troglodytes troglodytes* (Central African chimpanzee); Pvr, *Pan troglodytes verus* (West African chimpanzee); Asp, *Ateles* sp. (spider monkey).

specific injuries, and therefore, it is unclear if transmission of SFV to humans from expo-sure to NHP bodily fluids may occur more casually than previously thought (50).

The high seroprevalence of SFV infection documented in workers exposed occupation-ally to NHPs in zoos and primate centers has raised questions about whether SFV infects human populations in natural settings. Recently, a study of 1,099 bushmeat hunters in Cameroon who reported a history of hunting or butchering primates and/or keeping pri-mates as pets documented a 1% SFV seroprevalence. SFV infections in these studies were determined by phylogenetic analysis to have originated from mandrills, De Brazza's mon-keys, and gorillas, which are all NHP species found in Cameroon and commonly hunted in the region (Fig. 2) (59). Additional evidence of SFV infection in primate hunters was re-ported recently and documented gorilla- and chimpanzee-type SFV infections in two Ban-tus and one Baka pygmy from southern Cameroon (12). The gorilla SFV-infected persons in this study reported having received significant bite wounds from gorillas (12). Another study of 82 workers exposed to Asian macaques around temples in Indonesia reported an SFV infection of cynomolgus macaque origin, consistent with the prevalence of this NHP species in the area (28). Overall, these results show that SFV is actively crossing into hu-mans, document susceptibility to infection by at least seven different SFV clades, and demonstrate the wide geographic distribution of cross-species infection among exposed humans in North America, Europe, Central Africa, and Asia. Although NHPs are also found in South America and SFV infection of these New World primates has been demon-strated (37), there is currently no information available to determine if zoonotic SFV in-fection also occurs in this region.

While several studies have now documented the emergence of SFV among humans (9, 12, 24, 45, 50, 59), less is known about the ability of the virus to be transmitted among humans and to cause disease. Data available from the CDC study of primate workers show that the spouses of six infected men remained uninfected after 9 to 19 years, suggesting that the virus may not be easily transmitted sexually from males to females or following less intimate exposures (50). However, more data are needed to fully assess the transmis-sion of SFV. Specimens were not available from spouses and close contacts of SFV-infected women identified in the CDC study to determine if transmission occurs from female to male or from mother to child (50).

The consistent finding of SFV in the peripheral blood mononuclear cells of persistently infected persons raises questions about the possibility of spread of these viruses following exposure via blood donations from infected persons. It is noteworthy that 11 case patients in the CDC study reported being blood donors, and 6 of these persons were confirmed to be SFV infected at the time of donation by testing of archived sera (50). A retrospective study of recipients of blood products from a blood donor infected with chimpanzee-like SFV failed to identify evidence of SFV infection in two recipients of red cells, one recipi-ent of filtered red cells, and one recipient of platelets (8). However, these blood products were all leukocyte reduced, which may help to explain the absence of transmission seen in this study, since leukocytes are reservoirs for SFV in the blood. Thus, more data are needed to better define the risks for SFV transmission through donated blood.

Although SFV is nonpathogenic in naturally infected NHPs (37), the significance of SFV infection in humans is poorly defined. The introduction of SFV infections into humans is of concern, because changes in the pathogenicities of simian retroviruses following cross-species infection are well documented, since both HIV-1 and HIV-2 emerged from benign SIV infections in the natural primate hosts (4, 22). Published findings from different studies of SFV-infected humans suggest that these are asymptomatic infections, which is consistent with natural SFV infections of NHPs (24, 50). However, the limited number of cases, short duration of follow-up, and, more importantly, selection biases in the enrolling health workers to identify cases all limit the ability to identify potential disease associations (24, 50). The incidence of disease in SFV-infected persons may be low, may follow long latency periods, or may be associated with specific SFV clades that have not yet been identified. Additional studies, such as long-term follow-up of SFV-infected humans, are needed to better assess the clinical outcomes of SFV infection and to define the public health implications of these infections.

Identification of HTLV-3 and HTLV-4

The transmission of SFV to humans exposed to NHPs raises questions about whether other simian retroviruses are also being transmitted to persons with primate exposure. We have recently examined the diversity of HTLVs among primate bushmeat hunters in Cameroon who had documented SFV infections and who thus may be at risk for infection with additional simian retroviruses. We then looked for evidence of HTLVs of possible simian origin in these primate hunters. HTLV-1 and HTLV-2 endemically infect humans (5, 19, 60). HTLVs have been spread globally to at least 22 million persons sexually, from mother to child, and by exposure to contaminated blood through transfusions and injecting drug use (5, 19, 60). HTLV-1 causes adult T-cell leukemia, HTLV-1-associated myelopathy/tropical spastic paraparesis, and other inflammatory diseases in about 2 to 5% of those infected (19, 60). HTLV-2 is less pathogenic than HTLV-1 and has been associated with a neurologic disease similar to HTLV-1-associated myelopathy/tropical spastic paraparesis (5). HTLVs are antigenically and genetically closely related to STLVs, which are composed of three major groups: STLV-1, -2, and -3 (16, 18–20). STLV has been found in more than 33 species of African and Asian Old World primates, both in captivity and in the wild (14, 16, 18, 29, 32, 34–36, 52-54). STLV-1 has been implicated in the development of T-cell lymphomas and leukemia in NHPs (26, 55). Previous studies showing close phylogenetic relationships between HTLV-1 and STLV-1 in the same geographic region have suggested that HTLV-1 originated from multiple cross-species infections with STLV-1 (19, 32, 41–43, 53).

Our recently reported study of HTLV diversity among primate hunters from Cameroon led to the identification of two new HTLVs and thus demonstrated that HTLV diversity is far greater than previously thought (57). In that study, 930 samples were screened for HTLV by serologic testing and PCR amplification. Two new viruses that are distinct from HTLV-1 and HTLV-2 were discovered (57). The first HTLV clustered phylogenetically within the diversity of STLV-3 and represents the first human member of the group. This virus was named HTLV-3 because of its genetic similarity to STLV-3 (Fig. 3) (57). The second unique HTLV discovered in this population was distinct from HTLV-1, -2, and -3 and all STLVs and appears to have evolved independently over a long period (Fig. 3) (57). The virus was designated HTLV-4. While viruses similar to HTLV-4 are likely to be present in NHPs, more work is needed with improved diagnostic assays to identify the simian counterpart of this new virus. Recently, a second HTLV-3 was identified in a Bakola pygmy from southern Cameroon (Fig. 3) (11). This person also reported frequent exposure

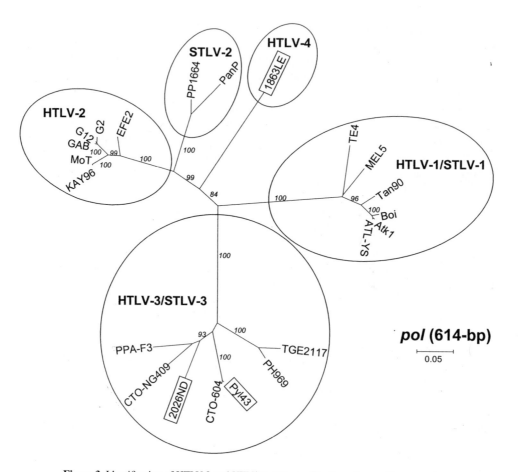

Figure 3. Identification of HTLV-3 and HTLV-4, two novel human viruses. Shown are the phylogenetic relationships of HTLV and STLV polymerase (*pol*) sequences (614 bp) by neighbor-joining analysis as described in detail elsewhere (57). The sequences of the new HTLV-3 and HTLV-4 viruses are shown in boxes. Support for the branching order was determined by 1,000 bootstrap replicates; only values of 60% or more are shown. Branch lengths are proportional to the evolutionary distances (scale bar) between the taxa.

to NHPs and was infected with an HTLV-3 most similar to an STLV-3 found in a red-capped mangabey from Cameroon (11, 35). Combined with a history of STLVs crossing from primates to humans and a wide geographic distribution of STLV-3 across Africa (14, 19, 20, 34–36, 41–43, 47, 52–54), these results suggest that HTLV-3 infection may be more widespread than has been suspected.

Consistent with previous results, many STLV-1-like infections were also identified in our study, confirming the active and frequent transmission and spread of STLV-1 among humans (32, 42, 57). The viruses found in these individuals included strains genetically similar to STLV-1 from mandrills (*Mandrillus sphinx*), gorillas (*Gorilla gorilla gorilla*), chimpanzees (*Pan troglodytes*), and colobus (*Piliocolobus badius*) and crested mona (*Cercopithecus pogonias*) monkeys (29, 32, 42, 57).

Health examinations of participants and collection of information regarding person-to-person contact were not included in either study that identified the new HTLV-3 and HTLV-4 viruses; thus, an assessment of either disease associations or secondary transmission of these novel HTLV infections was not possible (11, 57). Therefore, clinical evaluations and longitudinal epidemiologic studies of persons infected with HTLV-3, HTLV-4, and STLV-1-like viruses are needed to determine if these viruses cause disease and are transmissible among humans, as occurs with the other HTLVs (5, 19, 60). Although STLV-3 has been reported to transform or immortalize human CD4$^+$ lymphocytes in vitro (20), further studies are needed to determine both the cellular tropism of HTLV-3 and HTLV-4 and the abilities of these viruses to transform lymphocytes.

HTLV is screened for in blood banks in the United States and Europe but is not typically screened for in Africa; thus, further spread of these viruses among Central Africans may be facilitated by blood donations from infected persons. The finding that HTLV-3 and HTLV-4 are serologically indistinguishable from HTLV-1 and HTLV-2 by current assays may explain why these viruses were not previously identified and highlights the need for improved diagnostic assays to reliably and accurately detect them (57). Although plasma samples from the HTLV-3- and HTLV-4-infected persons were detected by an enzyme-linked immunosorbent assay containing purified HTLV-1 and HTLV-2 viral lysates (57) or by an HTLV-1 immunofluorescence assay (11), the overall sensitivities of these screening methods for detecting these new viruses are not known. Similarly, the sensitivity of detecting HTLV-3 and HTLV-4 by using screening assays employing recombinant proteins or synthetic peptides is also not known.

FACTORS INFLUENCING RETROVIRUS ZOONOSIS AND EMERGENCE

There are a number of factors that have the potential to influence retrovirus zoonosis, secondary spread, and subsequent emergence. Exposure to the blood and body fluids of nonhuman primates is required for zoonosis. Such exposure can be readily studied in both captive- and wild-animal settings (49, 58). Exposure to the blood and body fluids of nonhuman primates also represents a possible point of intervention in attempting to limit retrovirus zoonosis. Nevertheless, exposure cannot be the sole determinant of retrovirus emergence. Of the individuals who are exposed to the blood and body fluids of nonhuman primates, only a small percentage are infected with zoonotic retroviruses (9, 11, 24, 28, 44, 50, 57, 59). In addition, some individuals who show clear evidence of exposure—for example, through a positive Western blot result—have negative viral PCR results (11, 12, 50, 59). Such discordant results may be due to many factors, including PCR diagnostics that are either too specific or not sufficiently sensitive.

Another possible explanation is that host genetic factors may play a role in determining whether exposed individuals go on to have active zoonotic infections. During the past few years, a number of cellular viral defense mechanisms have been documented, some of which appear to inhibit viral zoonosis. One such gene, the APOBEC host gene, causes lentivirus hypermutation and can thereby limit viral infection (23). The lentivirus Vif protein deactivates APOBEC, allowing infection, but only in a species-specific manner. For example, HIV Vif deactivates human APOBEC (thereby allowing infection in humans), but it does not deactivate the APOBEC genes of other primate species, effectively limiting the potential for successful cross-species infections in novel hosts (23, 48). One possible explanation for the occurrence of low levels of zoonosis in particular retrovirus taxa could be the presence of polymorphisms in APOBEC and other host restriction genes, such as Trim5 alpha, which may make particular individuals in a novel host species more susceptible to cross-species infection (23, 48). Such a pattern might be expected to contribute to sporadic low-prevalence zoonotic infections that may not be likely to cause secondary spread. Recently, SFVs have also been shown to be inhibited by APOBEC cytidine deaminases, which may help explain both the low level of viral replication in persistently infected NHPs and humans and the apparent difficulty of secondary spread from zoonotically infected humans (15, 40).

Virus evolution and adaptation are also likely to play important roles in determining whether primary zoonotic infections have the potential to cause secondary transmission. Mutation rates and a propensity for recombination, for example, are mechanisms which may allow viruses to generate genetic diversity, which provides the fuel for adaptation to novel host species (38) and which may increase the probability that a zoonotic infection will have the potential for secondary spread. In addition to playing a direct role in retrovirus emergence, patterns of host-virus evolution may also provide clues to the potential that viruses have for successful cross-species transmission (38).

The interaction of virus evolution and host behavior may also play an important role in retrovirus emergence, with changes in host behavior providing novel conditions that facilitate retrovirus emergence. Such changes can occur on evolutionary or contemporary time scales. For example, the majority of primates are not carnivorous, but hominoids evolved the ability to hunt (with humans, chimpanzees, and bonobos likely sharing a common ancestor who hunted). The evolution of hunting among hominoids may have played an important role in the emergence of retroviruses. For example, chimpanzee SIV (SIVcpz) resulted from the recombination of SIVs from two monkey species (red-capped mangabeys and greater spot-nosed monkeys) (6). It seems probable that chimpanzees' propensity for hunting monkeys contributed to multiple simultaneous infections, which provided the opportunity for the recombination of SIV required for successful cross-species transmission. In addition, a range of contemporary circumstances, such as blood transfusions and intravenous drug use, provide novel opportunities for secondary transmission. Such "artificial" chains of secondary transmission have the potential to prolong the period in which virus can adapt to novel hosts or recombine with previously existing viruses, potentially increasing the frequency at which zoonotic infections can emerge.

CONCLUSIONS

The work described here among individuals who are highly exposed to the blood and body fluids of NHPs has demonstrated that a much broader range of retroviruses than previously thought are capable of causing primary zoonotic infections among humans and that such zoonotic transmission occurs on a regular basis. Three new retroviruses previously undocumented in humans, including the simian foamy viruses, HTLV-3, and HTLV-4, have all been identified in persons exposed to the blood and body fluids of NHPs. The regular occurrence of primary primate retrovirus infections suggests that zoonosis per se may not be the rate-limiting step in pandemic retrovirus emergence and that other factors, such as viral adaptation and evasion of cellular-level host defense against viruses probably play important roles in successful cross-species transmission and pandemic human retrovirus emergence.

These findings reinforce the need for defining the public health implications of the emergence of the new retroviruses and for ongoing surveillance efforts aimed at documenting and predicting the retrovirus emergence process. More research is needed to define disease outcomes and the level of spread of these newly recognized retroviruses. In order to understand factors associated with retrovirus emergence, and in particular what characteristics distinguish viruses capable of only primary zoonotic infections from those capable of more substantial spread, monitoring of highly exposed individuals and their contacts will be necessary. If done in a more comprehensive way, such "hunter cohorts" also may have the potential to identify novel retroviruses prior to emergence, or early in the process, in order to provide an opportunity for early intervention. Systems for monitoring retrovirus emergence may have the added benefit of helping to determine if SIVs or other pathogens continue to cause new zoonotic infections among humans.

Acknowledgments. The use of trade names is for identification only and does not imply endorsement by the U.S. Department of Health and Human Services, the Public Health Service, or the Centers for Disease Control and Prevention. The findings and conclusions in this report are those of the authors and do not necessarily represent the views of the Centers for Disease Control and Prevention.

REFERENCES

1. **Achong, B. G., P. W. A. Mansell, M. A. Epstein, and P. Clifford.** 1971. An unusual virus in cultures from a human nasopharyngeal carcinoma. *J. Natl. Cancer Inst.* **46:**299–302.
2. **Ali, M., G. P. Taylor, R. J. Pitman, D. Parker, A. Rethwilm, R. Cheingsong-Popov, J. N. Weber, P. D. Bieniasz, J. Bradley, and M. O. McClure.** 1996. No evidence of antibody to human foamy virus in widespread human populations. *AIDS Res. Hum. Retrovir.* **12:**1473–1483.
3. **Antia, R., R. R. Regoes, J. C. Koella, and C. T. Bergstrom.** 2003. The role of evolution in the emergence of infectious diseases. *Nature* **426:**658–661.
4. **Apetrei, C., D. L. Robertson, and P. Marx.** 2004. The history of SIVs and AIDS: epidemiology, phylogeny, and biology of isolates from naturally SIV infected non-human primates (NHP) in Africa. *Front. Biosci.* **9:**225–254.
5. **Araujo, A., and W. W. Hall.** 2004. Human T-lymphotropic virus type II and neurological disease. *Ann. Neurol.* **56:**10–19.
6. **Bailes, E., F. Gao, F. Bibollet-Ruche, V. Courgnaud, M. Peeters, P. A. Marx, B. H. Hahn, and P. M. Sharp.** 2003. Hybrid origin of SIV in chimpanzees. *Science* **300:**1713.
7. **Blewett, E. L., D. H. Black, N.W. Lerche, G. White, and R. Eberle.** 2000. Simian foamy virus infections in a baboon breeding colony. *Virology* **278:**183–193.
8. **Boneva, R. S., A. Grindon, S. Horton, W. M. Switzer, V. Shanmugam, A. Hussain, V. Bhullar, W. Heneine, M. Chamberland, T. M. Folks, and L. E. Chapman.** 2002. Simian foamy virus infection in a blood donor. *Transfusion* **42:**886–891.
9. **Brooks, J. I., E. W. Rudd, R. G. Pilon, J. M. Smith, W. M. Switzer, and P. A. Sandstrom.** 2002. Cross-species retroviral transmission from macaques to human beings. *Lancet* **360:**387–388.
10. **Broussard, S. R., A. G. Comuzzie, K. L. Leighton, M. M. Leland, E. M. Whitehead, and J. S. Allan.** 1997. Characterization of new simian foamy viruses from African nonhuman primates. *Virology* **237:**349–359.
11. **Calattini, S., S. A. Chevalier, R. Duprez, S. Bassot, A. Froment, R. Mahieux, and A. Gessain.** 2005. Discovery of a new human T-cell lymphotropic virus (HTLV-3) in Central Africa. *Retrovirology* **2:**30.
12. **Calattini, S., P. Mauclere, P. Tortevoye, A. Froment, A. Saib, and A. Gessain.** 2004. Interspecies transmission of simian foamy viruses from chimpanzees and gorillas to Bantous and Pygmy hunters in southern Cameroon, p. 7–8. In *Abstracts of the 5th International Foamy Virus Conference.*

13. **Calattini, S., E. Nerrienet, P. Mauclere, M. C. Georges-Courbot, A. Saib, and A. Gessain.** 2004. Natural simian foamy virus infection in wild-caught gorillas, mandrills and drills from Cameroon and Gabon. *J. Gen. Virol.* **85:**3313–3317.

14. **Courgnaud, V., S. Van Dooren, F. Liegeois, X. Pourrut, B. Abela, S. Loul, E. Mpoudi-Ngole, A. Vandamme, E. Delaporte, and M. Peeters.** 2004. Simian T-cell leukemia virus (STLV) infection in wild primate populations in Cameroon: evidence for dual STLV type 1 and type 3 infection in agile monkeys. *J. Virol.* **78:**4700–4709.

15. **Delebecque, F., R. Suspene, S. Calattini, N. Casartelli, A. Saib, A. Froment, S. Wain-Hobson, A. Gessain, J. P. Vartanian, and O. Schwartz.** 2006. Restriction of foamy viruses by APOBEC cytidine deaminases. *J. Virol.* **80:**605–614.

16. **Digilio, L., A. Giri, N. Cho, J. Slattert, P. Markham, and G. Franchini.** 1997. The simian T-lymphotropic/leukemia virus from *Pan paniscus* belongs to the type 2 family and infects Asian macaques. *J. Virol.* **71:** 3684–3692.

17. **Falcone, V., J. Leupold, J. Clotten, E. Urbanyi, O. Herchenroder, W. Spatz, B. Volk, N. Bohm, A. Toniolo, D. Neumann-Haefelin, and M. Schweizer.** 1999. Sites of simian foamy virus persistence in naturally infected African green monkeys: latent provirus is ubiquitous, whereas viral replication is restricted to the oral mucosa. *Virology* **257:**7–14.

18. **Fultz, P. N.** 1994. Simian T-lymphotropic virus type 1, p. 111–131. *In* J. A. Levy (ed.), *The Retroviridae,* vol. 3. Plenum Press, New York, N.Y.

19. **Gessain, A., and R. Mahieux.** 2000. Epidemiology, origin and genetic diversity of HTLV-1 retrovirus and STLV-1 simian affiliated retrovirus. *Bull. Soc. Pathol. Exot.* **93:**163–171.

20. **Goubau, P., M. Van Brussel, A. M. Vandamme, H. F. Liu, and J. Desmyter.** 1994. A primate T-lymphotropic virus, PTLV-L, different from human T-lymphotropic viruses types I and II, in a wild-caught baboon (*Papio hamadryas*). *Proc. Natl. Acad. Sci. USA* **91:**2848–2852.

21. **Groves, C.** 2001. *Primate Taxonomy.* Smithsonian Institution Press, Washington, D.C.

22. **Hahn, B. H., G. M. Shaw, K. M. De Cock, and P. M. Sharp.** 2000. AIDS as a zoonosis: scientific and public health implications. *Science* **287:**607–614.

23. **Harris, R. S., and M. T. Liddament.** 2004. Retroviral restriction by APOBEC proteins. *Nat. Rev. Immunol.* **4:**868–877.

24. **Heneine, W., M. Schweizer, P. Sandstrom, and T. Folks.** 2003. Human infection with foamy viruses. *Curr. Top. Microbiol. Immunol.* **277:**181–196.

25. **Herchenröder, O., R. Renne, D. Loncar, E. K. Cobb, K. K. Murthy, J. Schneider, A. Mergia, and P. A. Luciw.** 1994. Isolation, cloning, and sequencing of simian foamy viruses from chimpanzees (SFVcpz): High homology to human foamy virus (HFV). *Virology* **201:**187–199.

26. **Hubbard, G. B., J. P. Mone, J. S. Allan, K. J. Davis, M. M. Leland, P. M. Banks, and B. Smir.** 1993. Spontaneously generated non-Hodgkin's lymphoma in twenty-seven simian T-cell leukemia virus type 1 antibody-positive baboons. *Lab. Anim. Sci.* **43:**301–309.

27. **Hussain, A. I., V. Shanmugam, V. B. Bhullar, B. E. Beer, D. Vallet, A. Gautier-Hion, N. Wolfe, W. B. Karesh, A. M. Kilbourn, Z. Tooze, W. Heneine, and W. M. Switzer.** 2003. Screening for simian foamy virus infection by using a combined antigen Western blot assay: evidence for a wide distribution among Old World primates and identification of four new divergent viruses. *Virology* **309:**248–257.

28. **Jones-Engel, L., G. A. Engel, M. A. Schillaci, A. Rompis, A. Putra, K. G. Suaryana, A. Fuentes, B. Beer, S. Hicks, R. White, B. Wilson, and J. S. Allan.** 2005. Primate to human retroviral transmission in Asia. *Emerg. Infect. Dis.* **11:**1028–1035.

29. **Leendertz, F. H., S. Junglen, C. Boesch, P. Formenty, E. Couacy-Hymann, V. Courgnaud, G. Pauli, and H. Ellerbrok.** 2004. High variety of different simian T-cell leukemia virus type 1 strains in chimpanzees (*Pan troglodytes verus*) of the Tai National Park, Cote d'Ivoire. *J. Virol.* **78:**4352–4356.

30. **Linial, M. L., H. Fan, B. Hahn, R. Löwer, J. Neil, S. Quackenbush, A. Rethwilm, P. Sonigo, J. Stoye, and M. Tristem.** 2004. *Retroviridae,* p. 421–440. *In* C. M. Fauquet, M. A. Mayo, J. Maniloff, U. Desselberger, and L. A. Ball (ed.), *Virus Taxonomy. Eighth Report of the International Committee on Taxonomy of Viruses.* Elsevier, London, United Kingdom.

31. **Liu, W., M. L. Santiago, B. F. Keele, Y. Li, F. Bibollet-Ruche, Y. Chen, P. A. Goepfert, W. M. Switzer, S. Clifford, E. Mpoudi, C. Sanz, M. L. Wilson, N. Gross-Camp, H. M. McClure, E. Bailes, P. M. Sharp, C. Boesch, V. Smith, M. Worobey, R. Wrangham, M. Peeters, J. F. Y. Brookfield, G. M. Shaw, and B. H. Hahn.** 2005. Simian foamy virus infection in wild chimpanzees, abstr. 259. *HIV Pathogenesis Keystone Symposium.*

32. **Mahieux, R., C. Chappey, M. C. Georges-Courbot, G. Dubreuil, P. Mauclere, A. Georges, and A. Gessain.** 1998. Simian T-cell lymphotropic virus type 1 from *Mandrillus sphinx* as a simian counterpart of human T-cell lymphotropic virus type 1 subtype D. *J. Virol.* **72:**10316–10322.

33. **McClure, M. O., P. D. Bieniaz, T .F. Schulz, I. L. Chrystie, G. Simpson, A. Aguzzi, J. G. Hoad, A. Cunningham, J. Kirkwood, and R. A. Weiss.** 1994. Isolation of a new foamy retrovirus from orangutans. *J. Virol.* **68:**7124–7130.

34. **Meertens, L., and A. Gessain.** 2003. Divergent simian T-cell lymphotropic virus type 3 (STLV-3) in wild-caught *Papio hamadryas papio* from Senegal: widespread distribution of STLV-3 in Africa. *J. Virol.* **77:** 782–789.

35. **Meertens, L., R. Mahieux, P. Mauclere, J. Lewis, and A. Gessain.** 2002. Complete sequence of a novel highly divergent simian T-cell lymphotropic virus from wild caught red-capped mangabeys (*Cercocebus torquatus*) from Cameroon: a new primate T-lymphotropic virus type 3 subtype. *J. Virol.* **76:**259–268.

36. **Meertens, L., V. Shanmugam, A. Gessain, B. E. Beer, Z. Tooze, W. Heneine, and W. M. Switzer.** 2003. A novel, divergent simian T-cell lymphotropic virus type 3 in a wild-caught red-capped mangabey (*Cercocebus torquatus torquatus*) from Nigeria. *J. Gen. Virol.* **84:**2723–2727.

37. **Meiering, C. D., and M. L. Linial.** 2001. Historical perspective of foamy virus epidemiology and infection. *Clin. Microbiol. Rev.* **14:**165–176.

38. **Moya, A., E. C. Holmes, and F. Gonzalez-Candelas.** 2004. The population genetics and evolutionary epidemiology of RNA viruses. *Nat. Rev. Microbiol.* **2:**279–288.

39. **Murray, S. M., L. J. Picker, M. K. Axthelm, and M. L. Linial.** 2006. Expanded tissue targets for foamy virus replication with simian immunodeficiency virus-induced immunosuppression. *J. Virol.* **80:** 663–670.

40. **Russell, R. A., H. L. Wiegand, M. D. Moore, A. Schafer, M. O. McClure, and B. R. Cullen.** 2005. Foamy virus Bet proteins function as novel inhibitors of the APOBEC3 family of innate antiretroviral defense factors. *J. Virol.* **79:**8724–8731.

41. **Salemi, M., J. Desmyter, and A. M. Vandamme.** 2000. Tempo and mode of human and simian T-lymphotropic virus (HTLV/STLV) evolution revealed by analyses of full-genome sequences. *Mol. Biol. Evol.* **17:**374–386.

42. **Salemi, M., S. Van Dooren, E. Audenaert, E. Delaporte, P. Goubau, J. Desmyter, and A. M. Vandamme.** 1998. Two new human T-lymphotropic virus type I phylogenetic subtypes in seroindeterminates, a Mbuti pygmy and a Gabonese, have closest relatives among African STLV-I strains. *Virology* **246:**277–287.

43. **Salemi, M., S. Van Dooren, and A. M. Vandamme.** 1999. Origin and evolution of human and simian T-cell lymphotropic viruses. *AIDS Rev.* **1:**131–139.

44. **Sandstrom, P. A., K. O. Phan, W. M. Switzer, T. Fredeking, L. Chapman, W. Heneine, and T. M. Folks.** 2000. Simian foamy virus infection among zoo keepers. *Lancet* **355:**551–552.

45. **Schweizer M., V. Falcone, J. Gange, R. Turek, and D. Neumann-Haefelin.** 1997. Simian foamy virus isolated from an accidentally infected human individual. *J. Virol.* **71:**4821–4824.

46. **Schweizer, M., R. Turek, H. Hahn, A. Schliephake, K. O. Netzer, G. Eder, M. Reinhardt, A. Rethwilm, and D. Neumann-Haefelin.** 1995. Markers of foamy virus (FV) infections in monkeys, apes, and accidentally infected humans: appropriate testing fails to confirm suspected FV prevalence in man. *AIDS Res. Hum. Retrovir.* **11:**161–170.

47. **Slattery, J. P., G. Franchini, and A. Gessain.** 1999. Genomic evolution, patterns of global dissemination, and interspecies transmission of human and simian T-cell leukemia/lymphotropic viruses. *Genome Res.* **9:** 525–540.

48. **Song, B., H. Javanbakht, M. Perron, D. H. Park, M. Stremlau, and J. Sodroski.** 2005. Retrovirus restriction by TRIM5 alpha variants from Old World and New World primates. *J. Virol.* **79:**3930–3937.

49. **Sotir, M., W. Switzer, C. Schable, J. Schmitt, C. Vitek, and R. F. Khabbaz.** 1997. Risk of occupational exposure to potentially infectious nonhuman primate materials and to simian immunodeficiency virus. *J. Med. Primatol.* **26:**233–240.

50. **Switzer, W. M., V. Bhullar, V. Shanmugam, M. Cong, B. Parekh, N. W. Lerche, J. L. Yee, J. J. Ely, R. Boneva, L. E. Chapman, T. M. Folks, and W. Heneine.** 2004. Frequent simian foamy virus infection in persons occupationally exposed to nonhuman primates. *J. Virol.* **78:**2780–2789.

51. **Switzer, W. M., M. Salemi, V. Shanmugam, V. Bhullar, F. Gao, B. Beer, D. Vallet, A. Gautier-Hion, Z. Tooze, C. Kuilken, F. Villinger, and W. Heneine.** 2005. Ancient co-speciation of simian foamy virus and primates. *Nature* **434:**376–380.

52. **Takemura, T., M. Yamashita, M. K. Shimada, S. Ohkura, T. Shotake, M. Ikeda, T. Miura, and M. Hayami.** 2002. High prevalence of simian T-lymphotropic virus type L in wild Ethiopian baboons. *J. Virol.* **76:**1642–1648.

53. **Vandamme, A. M., M. Salemi, and J. Desmyter.** 1998. The simian origins of the pathogenic human T-cell lymphotropic virus type 1. *Trends Microbiol.* **6:**477–483.

54. **Van Dooren, S., V. Shanmugam, V. Bhullar, B. Parekh, A. M. Vandamme, W. Heneine, and W. M. Switzer.** 2004. Identification in gelada baboons (*Theropithecus gelada*) of a distinct simian T-cell lymphotropic virus 3 with a broad range of Western blot reactivity. *J. Gen. Virol.* **85:**507–551.

55. **Voevodin, A., E. Samilchuk, H. Schatzl, E. Boeri, and G. Frachini.** 1996. Interspecies transmission of macaque simian T-cell leukemia/lymphoma virus type 1 in baboons results in an outbreak of malignant lymphoma. *J. Virol.* **70:**1633–1639.

56. **Weiss, R. A.** 1988. Foamy retroviruses: a virus in search of a disease. *Nature* **333:**497–498.

57. **Wolfe, N. D., W. Heneine, J. K. Carr, A. D. Garcia, V. Shanmugan, U. Tamoufe, J. N. Torimiro, A. T. Prosser, M. LeBreton, E. Mpoudi-Ngole, F. E. McCutchan, D. L. Birx, T. M. Folks, D. S. Burke, and W. M. Switzer.** 2005. Emergence of unique primate T-lymphotropic viruses among central African bushmeat hunters. *Proc. Natl. Acad. Sci. USA* **102:**7994–7999.

58. **Wolfe, N. D., T. A. Prosser, J. K. Carr, U. Tamoufe, E. Mpoudi-Ngole, J. N. Torimiro, M. LeBreton, F. E. McCutchan, D. L. Birx, and D. S. Burke.** 2004. Exposure to nonhuman primates in rural Cameroon. *Emerg. Infect. Dis.* **10:**2094–2099.

59. **Wolfe, N. D., W. M. Switzer, J. K. Carr, V. B. Bhullar, V. Shanmugan, U. Tamoufe, A. T. Prosser, J. N. Torimiro, A. Wright, E. Mpoudi-Ngole, F. E. McCutchan, D. L. Birx, T. M. Folks, D. S. Burke, and W. Heneine.** 2004. Naturally acquired simian retrovirus infections in central African hunters. *Lancet* **363:** 932–937.

60. **Yamashita, M., E. Ido, T. Miura, and M. Hayami.** 1996. Molecular epidemiology of HTLV-I in the world. *J. Acquir. Immune Defic. Syndr. Hum. Retrovirol.* **13**(Suppl. 1):S124–S131.

Emerging Infections 7
Edited by W. M. Scheld, D. C. Hooper, and J. M. Hughes
© 2007 ASM Press, Washington, D.C.

Chapter 9

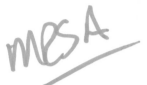

Community-Associated Methicillin-Resistant *Staphylococcus aureus*

Susan E. Crawford, Susan Boyle-Vavra, and Robert S. Daum

Staphylococcus aureus is a pathogen associated with a wide range of community- and hospital-associated diseases, ranging from relatively trivial skin and soft tissue infections to severe sepsis with high mortality (82). The organism may be found in the nasopharyngeal or skin flora of 25 to 40% of otherwise healthy children and adults (129).

Penicillin was the first highly effective antimicrobial compound active against *S. aureus*. However, β-lactamase-producing strains emerged soon after the use of penicillin became widespread (11, 113). The plasmid-borne gene for β-lactamase production conferred resistance to penicillin and could be found in most *S. aureus* isolates by the end of World War II. The trend of increasing resistance to penicillin has continued to this day, with about 95% of clinical isolates resistant to this and related compounds.

Antibiotics relatively resistant to β-lactamase-induced hydrolysis (e.g., methicillin or oxacillin) were introduced in the 1960s. Resistance to them, however, was recognized almost immediately (64), and within a year after their introduction, additional reports of strains resistant to these antibiotics emerged in Europe and Australia (7, 10). These resistant strains were called "methicillin-resistant *Staphylococcus aureus*" (MRSA), a term that implied cross-resistance to all β-lactams, including a wide range of penicillins and cephalosporins. MRSA isolates first appeared in the United States in 1961, and by the late 1970s, MRSA outbreaks were reported in large urban tertiary-care teaching hospitals (8, 12, 107). From the 1970s to the late 1990s, the prevalence of asymptomatic MRSA colonization and symptomatic infection slowly increased, but the causative isolates remained largely confined to health care environments and to the personal ecologies of the patients who frequented them. Risk factors for MRSA colonization or disease other than exposure to a hospital or long-term health care facility included antibiotic use in the past 12 months, contact with a household member who had a risk factor for MRSA acquisition, chronic disease, and nonmedicinal intravenous-drug use (13, 126). Therapeutic options to treat MRSA were few; vancomycin, a glycopeptide antibiotic, was pressed into heavy service in the treatment of MRSA infections and was called the "antibiotic of last resort."

Susan E. Crawford, Susan Boyle-Vavra, and Robert S. Daum • Department of Pediatric Infectious Diseases, University of Chicago, 5841 S. Maryland, MC 6054, Chicago, IL 60637.

EPIDEMIOLOGY

In the past decade, this view of MRSA epidemiology has changed. No longer confined to hospital environments or isolated only from patients with identifiable risk factors, MRSA strains now circulate in the community among previously healthy patients with no risk factors for acquisition of "hospital-associated" MRSA (HA-MRSA). These community isolates differ from HA-MRSA in their epidemiology and spectrum of disease. Their rapidly increasing prevalence has also created a need for reconsideration of basic therapeutic paradigms.

Reports of MRSA infections first identified in the community emerged in several geographic locations in the 1990s (54, 57, 84, 95, 114). The early reports were initially thought to reflect the carriage of MRSA from hospital environments into the community. In support of this interpretation, many community-onset MRSA infections were identified in persons with known risk factors for acquisition of MRSA in the hospital, including recent hospitalization, residence in a long-term care facility, dialysis, recent surgery, indwelling catheters or devices, and intravenous-drug use (33, 77, 118, 119, 120).

A distinct phenomenon, however, was subsequently observed when "community-associated" MRSA (CA-MRSA) cases were reported among patients, predominantly children, without these typical risk factors (27, 53, 57, 59, 60). At the University of Chicago Children's Hospital, the prevalence of CA-MRSA infections among children without predisposing risk for MRSA requiring hospitalization for serious *S. aureus* infections increased from 10 per 100,000 admissions in 1988 to 1990 to 259 per 100,000 admissions in 1993 to 1995 (57) and remained high in a follow-up study performed in 1998 and 1999 (59). In this context, risk was defined as the presence of any of the following: previous hospitalization or antimicrobial therapy within 6 months of the date of MRSA isolation, a history of endotracheal intubation, an underlying chronic disorder, presence of an indwelling venous or urinary catheter, a history of any surgical procedure, or notation in the medical record of a household contact with an identified risk factor.

This same dramatic increase in CA-MRSA disease has now been observed by many others, and outbreaks of disease have occurred among members of sports teams and in prisons and military units (18, 24, 25, 35, 42, 79, 105, 111, 112).

Several clinical and epidemiologic factors initially suggested that the newly recognized CA-MRSA isolates differed from HA-MRSA strains. In addition to MRSA disease being found in persons without the traditional risk factors, the CA-MRSA isolates had antibiotic susceptibility profiles distinct from those of HA-MRSA isolates (57, 114). Whereas the isolation of MRSA in the hospital often dictated the use of vancomycin because of its multiple antibiotic resistance phenotype, community strains were usually susceptible to a variety of non-β-lactam antimicrobials. This finding suggested that therapeutic options for CA-MRSA infections might be expanded to include treatment with clindamycin, trimethoprim-sulfamethoxazole, or doxycycline, options infrequently considered previously in the treatment of hospital-acquired MRSA infections. Later investigations revealed the evolutionary basis for these differences in antibiotic susceptibilities among the community and hospital MRSA strains.

The further observation was made that CA-MRSA disease syndromes resembled those caused by "community-associated" methicillin-susceptible *S. aureus* (CA-MSSA), rather than those seen as a result of HA-MRSA infections (57). Like CA-MSSA, the majority of identified disease caused by CA-MRSA consisted of skin and soft tissue infections, such as boils, furuncles, and abscesses (57, 96, 112, 133). HA-MRSA typically caused infections such as bacteremia associated with an indwelling venous device, postoperative wound infections, or ventilator-associated pneumonia (96). It quickly became apparent that CA-MRSA also caused relatively infrequent but severe invasive diseases, such as necrotizing pneumonia, necrotizing fasciitis, osteomyelitis, and a septic shock syndrome characterized by multiorgan involvement with high mortality among children (2, 22, 52, 91). The similarity in presentation between CA-MSSA and CA-MRSA suggested that the genetic backgrounds of the "CA" *S. aureus* isolates might be similar, as was later confirmed by molecular typing methods.

DISEASE BURDEN

With the recognition of CA-MRSA as a distinct, emerging etiologic agent, reports of outbreaks of CA-MRSA infections across the country and beyond became numerous. A large burden of CA-MRSA disease was reported by prison and jail systems in California, Texas, Mississippi, and Georgia. Outbreaks in these facilities have suggested that conditions in the prison and jail systems might facilitate the spread of CA-MRSA isolates (5, 25, 35, 105). Indeed, hypothesized factors that probably aid in the spread of MRSA include suboptimal personal hygiene, poor access to medical care, infrequent or inadequate laundering of clothing, and limited or restricted access to soap (25). It has been proposed that jails and prisons serve as reservoirs for MRSA in which short inmate stays may provide sufficient time for transmission of CA-MRSA and conditions may facilitate an increase in prevalence with easy spread and return of the isolates into the community. Proposals to diminish the spread of CA-MRSA include skin infection screening and monitoring, culturing of relevant lesions, administration of appropriate antibiotics, improving inmate hygiene, and improving access to medical care. Many issues in the roles of the jail and prison require additional study and definition.

Outbreaks among players on high school, college, and professional sports teams have also occurred. Several individuals have required hospitalization and temporary exclusion from play (24, 71, 79). Contact sports, including wrestling and football, appear to increase the risk of MRSA transmission, and players with the most intense person-to-person contact (e.g., linemen and linebackers in football) have had a higher risk for disease (71, 100). Even members of teams in which skin-to-skin contact was minimal have experienced problems; multiple cases of CA-MRSA infection among members of a fencing club led to the hypothesis that contaminated equipment worn by multiple players might be responsible for transmission (24).

Additional sites where close contact has provided opportunity for the spread of CA-MRSA include military training centers (19, 135) and day care centers (1, 122). The need for improved hygiene, increased monitoring of skin lesions, and improved awareness of the overall problem are issues raised by each of these outbreaks.

Outbreaks have provided incentives to examine the epidemiology of CA-MRSA in closer detail. Additionally, evidence of increasing endemic occurrence of CA-MRSA infections has been provided through MRSA surveillance performed in several communities. Surveillance by the Community Health Network of San Francisco (20) tracked MRSA infections from 1996 to 2002 and found that the number of MRSA isolates increased from

160 in 1996 to 563 in 2002. Eighty-two percent of the total number of MRSA infections from 1998 to 2002 above the baseline rate in 1996 to 1997 could be attributable to CA-MRSA, as defined by an organism isolated in the outpatient setting or within 72 hours of hospitalization. Confirmation that the organisms were indeed "community onset-type" organisms was provided by genotyping to show that the responsible isolates were not "feral" descendents of hospital isolates migrating into the community (see "Bacterial Genetic Investigations" below). The University of California at San Francisco has established a unique clinic specifically for the evaluation and treatment of skin and soft tissue infections (the Integrated Skin and Soft Tissue Clinic) due to the large number of patients requiring physician visits and operating room time for incision and drainage of abscesses caused by CA-MRSA (133).

More evidence to substantiate the idea that CA-MRSA infections and the overall burden of *S. aureus* infections are both dramatically increasing was provided by investigators at Driscoll Children's Hospital in Corpus Christi, Texas. Purcell et al. documented an increase in the number of infections caused by CA-MRSA in their institution from 9 in 1999 to 459 in 2003 (111, 112). The number of MRSA cases almost doubled in 1 year, from 282 infections in 2002 to 467 infections in 2003, with 98% of the infections due to CA-MRSA. Importantly, these increases were directly translated into similar increases in the overall burden of *S. aureus* disease. At Texas Children's Hospital in Houston, similar increases in both the absolute number of community-acquired *S. aureus* infections and the percentage of CA-MRSA compared with all *S. aureus* infections increased in a 3-year period. The percentage of CA-MRSA isolates increased from 71.5% (551 of 771 *S. aureus* isolates) in year 1 to 76.4% (1,193 of 1,562 isolates) in year 3 (69). Other centers have experienced similar increases in the disease burden due to CA-MRSA. This dramatic increase in the *S. aureus* burden and CA-MRSA has not occurred in all geographic locales. Centers already experiencing the increase, however, have continued to do so, and their numbers have relentlessly increased with time.

Certain individuals appear to be at higher risk for CA-MRSA disease. In prospective surveillance performed in Baltimore and Atlanta, children younger than 2 years of age had a higher risk for disease than others (48). In the same study African-Americans had a higher risk than whites in Atlanta, but this difference did not hold true in Baltimore. Other studies have suggested a relatively higher incidence of disease among Pacific Islanders, American Indians, and Alaskan Natives (4, 55). Factors that may contribute to the disease burden in certain populations include increased prevalence of certain underlying diseases or differences in socioeconomic factors (e.g., household/community crowding or decreased access to medical care). Study design may have influenced the results and conclusions from some of these studies. For example, a definition of CA-MRSA that includes only MRSA obtained from persons without risk factors for hospital-acquired MRSA may exclude individuals infected with isolates that are genetically defined CA-MRSA isolates (see "Bacterial Genetic Investigations" below). Members of certain populations also may not be sampled or cultured with the same frequency as others.

BACTERIAL GENETIC INVESTIGATIONS

Important genetic phenomena are believed to be responsible for the phenotypic differences observed in comparisons of CA-MRSA and HA-MRSA isolates. Methicillin resistance is conferred by the *mecA* gene, which encodes penicillin-binding protein 2a (PBP2a), an enzyme catalyzing transpeptidation of *S. aureus* peptidoglycan. PBP2a has low affinity for β-lactam antibiotics. PBP2a, in partnership with native *S. aureus* PBP2, allows the synthesis of peptidoglycan even in the presence of a β-lactam antimicrobial, thus rendering the bacteria resistant to β-lactam antibiotics (26, 109).

mecA is located on a mobile genetic island called the staphylococcal chromosomal cassette *mec* (SCC*mec*) (61), which is present in all MRSA isolates with a single exception (132). The SCC*mec* cassette contains a *mec* complex consisting of *mecA* and its variably present regulatory elements *mecR1* and *mecI*, and *ccr* genes that encode recombinases responsible for the excision of SCC*mec* and its integration into the staphylococcal chromosome. The MecR1 protein binds to β-lactam antibiotics with subsequent proteolytic cleavage of MecI (134). This cleavage of MecI results in derepression of *mecA*, enabling the transcription of *mecA*.

These SCC*mec* elements have been found in multiple *S. aureus* backgrounds, although the mechanism for their movement from strain to strain is not known. Site-specific chromosomal integration of an SCC*mec* element is the genetic event that converts a methicillin-susceptible *S. aureus* strain into a methicillin-resistant strain. Molecular testing of *Staphylococcus epidermidis* isolates dating from 1973 to 1983 also revealed the presence of SCC*mec* elements in that species, suggesting that interspecies transfer of those genetic elements from *S. epidermidis* to *S. aureus* may have occurred (130). SCC elements lacking *mecA* found in *Staphylococcus hominis* (70) and *S. epidermidis* (94) have lent credence to the idea that coagulase-negative species act as a reservoir for the variable DNA sequences found in SCC*mec* elements.

Initial characterization of SCC*mec* elements from MRSA isolates revealed three types in which the DNA sequences of the *ccr* genes (*ccr* complex) and the molecular anatomies of the *mecA* complexes differed (61). SCC*mec* types II and III contained genes that mediated resistance to non-β-lactam antibiotics, consistent with the multidrug resistance phenotype found among HA-MRSA isolates. For example, SCC*mec* type II contains the *ermA* gene, which confers resistance to erythromycin and inducible or constitutive resistance to clindamycin, as well as resistance determinants for cadmium and neomycin (61).

The three SCC*mec* element types initially characterized were 34, 53, and 67 kb in size and were identified in a survey of HA-MRSA isolates (61). Their sizes were believed to limit facile transfer of the elements to different strains on a frequent basis. Thus, prior to the mid-1990s, dissemination of MRSA relied upon transfer of the entire bacterium, implying potential effectiveness for hospital infection control measures.

In contrast, CA-MRSA strains most often contain the novel SCC*mec* type IV, a 21- to 24-kb element, smaller and probably more mobile than the types II and III found in HA-MRSA isolates. Moreover, five of the six sequenced SCC*mec* IV elements (IVa, GenBank accession numbers AB063172 and NC_003923; IVb, accession number AB063173; IVc, accession numbers AY271717 and AB096217; and IVe, accession number AJ810121) lacked antibiotic resistance genes other than the *mecA* gene, consistent with the CA-MRSA phenotype of susceptibility to multiple non-β-lactam antibiotics (36, 83, 93); one had a gentamicin resistance determinant at the left extremity (strain MR108, accession number AB096217). CA-MRSA strains containing the type IV element often remain susceptible to clindamycin, in part because the sequenced type IV elements are not known to contain the *erm* gene (61). Clindamycin-resistant CA-MRSA strains may have acquired the *erm* gene, though the location of the *erm* gene has not yet been elucidated (29). More frequently, erythromycin resistance is detected in CA-MRSA strains, as other genetic elements mediating erythromycin resistance, such as *msrA*, can be found elsewhere on a plasmid or in the *S. aureus* genome (18, 29).

SCC*mec* IV has been found in multiple *S. aureus* genetic backgrounds, supporting the hypothesis that it is readily transferred from strain to strain (36, 103, 115). Although both HA-MRSA and CA-MRSA clones can spread as the entire bacterium is transferred, it is suspected that CA-MRSA clones can increase in number as MSSA backgrounds acquire the SCC*mec* type IV element (93).

Recently, another SCC*mec* type, type V, that appears similar to type IV in size (27 kb) and probably in mobility has been discovered. Type V was first identified in several strains from Australia, where it had already entered three *S. aureus* genetic backgrounds (sequence types 45, 8, and 152) (31). A V-like (type V_T) element was subsequently identified in multiply resistant sequence type 59 CA-MRSA strains in Taipei, Taiwan, and was the predominant background found in CA-MRSA in Taipei (15). Thus, there are now five different SCC*mec* elements that have been described, designated SCC*mec* I to V. Additionally, an SCC*mec* element described by Oliveira et al. in strain HDE288 (104), originally described as SCC*mec* IV, cannot actually be classified among types I through V (Table 1). New SCC*mec* genetic elements are being discovered, as the SCC*mec* elements appear to evolve rapidly; recent characterization of strains from patients in Ireland has revealed seven novel variants of extant SCC*mec* element types (123). The rapid evolution of these elements may make current SCC*mec* nomenclature strategies inadequate for classification.

Different methods have been employed to define the genetic background and characteristics of *S. aureus* strains. Pulsed-field gel electrophoresis (PFGE) has been used to follow rapid evolutionary events in the *S. aureus* genome. It is especially useful for assessing the relatedness of strains in an outbreak and for determining the clonal repertoires of strains in the community. A classification system that categorizes strains by their PFGE restriction fragment patterns into lineages designated USA 100, USA 200, etc., has been described and is in wide use (88). Another isolate-fingerprinting technique, multilocus sequence typing (MLST), provides information on slower-paced evolution of *S. aureus* strains, because polymorphisms in the partial sequences of the seven housekeeping genes examined by this

Table 1. Classification scheme of SCC*mec* elements

SCC *mec* type	*ccr* complex	*ccr* gene	*mec* complex
I	1	AB1	B
II	2	AB2	A
III	3	AB3	A
IV[a]	2	AB2	B
V	5	C_1	C2
V_T	5	C_2	C2
HDE288	4	AB4	B

[a]Type IV elements have been subtyped, e.g., a to g, according to polymorphisms in the left extremity of the element, the so-called L-C region, and the right extremity, the so-called I-R region (62, 73, 82, 93, 122). A unified nomenclature system does not exist, however. Both uppercase and lowercase letters have been used, and they sometimes refer to different things; e.g., SCC*mec* IVa has a different DNA sequence from SCC*mec* IVA.

method are well conserved (41). CA-MRSA and HA-MRSA often have distinct PFGE and MLST patterns, although some overlap exists.

TOXIN GENES AND PATHOPHYSIOLOGY OF DISEASE

The toxin gene repertoire among CA-MRSA isolates has been hypothesized to contribute to the difference in disease spectra between CA-MRSA and HA-MRSA (97). A survey of 16 toxin genes known to be present in genomically sequenced *S. aureus* strains revealed that important differences can be identified when HA-MRSA and CA-MRSA isolates are compared. Six exotoxin genes were found significantly more often among CA-MRSA isolates, and seven were found significantly more often among HA-MRSA strains (97). The exotoxin genes more commonly found in CA-MRSA isolates included *lukS-PV/lukF-PV*, *sea*, *seb*, *sec*, *seh*, and *sek*. It is not clear which of these, if any, confer special virulence characteristics on CA-MRSA isolates.

Two toxin genes present particularly frequently in CA-MRSA isolates, *lukS-PV/lukF-PV*, which encode the Panton-Valentine leukocidin (PVL), have been suspected to play important roles in the virulence of CA-MRSA organisms. PVL is a synergohymenotropic toxin that disrupts the integrity of polymorphonuclear leukocytes, and perhaps other cells. The toxin is hypothesized to cause neutropenia and extensive tissue damage, perhaps mediated by the release of toxic products from neutrophils. The PVL genes are transferred from strain to strain by one of several bacteriophages (98). They insert at a site-specific chromosomal location that is distinct from the SCC*mec* element insertion site.

PVL is not a newly identified toxin, but the epidemiology of *S. aureus* isolates carrying the PVL genes has changed (51, 106). The genes encoding PVL were found in only about 1 to 2% of unselected MSSA isolates (89, 110). However, when disease-causing MSSA isolates were examined, the genes encoding PVL were found in 93% of isolates obtained from patients with furunculosis and 85% of isolates from patients with community-acquired *S. aureus* pneumonia (32, 78). In contrast, *S. aureus* isolates obtained from blood rarely contain the PVL genes (89). PVL genes have also been associated with isolates causing empyema and a distinctive necrotizing pneumonia (44, 52). In a case-control study of MSSA and MRSA isolates causing community-acquired *S. aureus* pneumonia, isolates containing the PVL genes caused more severe disease characterized by hemoptysis, tissue necrosis, and higher morbidity and mortality than isolates that lacked the genes (50).

Data on the prevalence of PVL genes among colonizing CA-MRSA strains obtained by the National Health and Nutrition Survey in 2001 and 2002 suggest that PVL genes are less frequently found among colonizing CA-MRSA strains. This population-based survey detected MRSA carriage in 75 of 9,622 surveyed individuals, with 37 of the 75 MRSA isolates (50%) containing SCC*mec* type IV and 38 containing SCC*mec* type II. Of the 37 people colonized with SCC*mec* type IV-containing strains, only 6 (16%) carried the genes encoding PVL, and none of the SCC*mec* type II-containing strains contained these genes. Additionally, among asymptomatic CA-MRSA isolates colonizing the noses of military personnel, the genes encoding PVL were present in 58% of the strains (40). Nasal swabs collected from 500 healthy children at a Tennessee clinic presenting for a health maintenance visit found that 46, or 9.2%, of the children had nasal colonization with MRSA; only 10, or 22%, of these strains contained the genes for PVL (34). Thus, the presence of PVL in

CA-MRSA strains does not appear to be necessary for colonization and presumably, therefore, spread.

Although the PVL genes are not consistently present in nasal-colonization strains obtained from otherwise healthy individuals, there is a strong correlation between the presence of PVL genes and CA-MRSA disease isolates. Isolates from a case series of patients with necrotizing fasciitis and necrotizing myositis all contained PVL genes, and these, along with *lukD* and *lukE*, were the only toxin genes detected among the 14 MRSA disease isolates (91). CA-MRSA isolates obtained from children and adults with necrotizing pneumonia have also been found to contain *lukS-PV/lukF-PV* (44, 93). Among disease-causing CA-MRSA isolates, 77 to 100% contain the PVL genes (92, 97, 103, 127).

The CA-MRSA epidemic has been fueled by multiple *S. aureus* genetic backgrounds containing the PVL genes. Analysis of CA-MRSA strains containing SCC*mec* IV from the United States and Australia found PVL in five different CA-MRSA backgrounds defined by MLST (103). Analysis of 117 CA-MRSA disease-causing strains from the United States, France, Switzerland, Australia, New Zealand, and Western Samoa found that the CA-MRSA strains uniformly contained both SCC*mec* type IV and the PVL loci (127). These CA-MRSA isolates belonged to six different clonal groups, as defined by PFGE and MLST. These data support the notion that the dramatic increase in CA-MRSA disease largely represents the spread of multiple and diverse *S. aureus* genetic backgrounds rather than the spread of a single clone. Moreover, SCC*mec* IV and PVL together seem to confer a selective advantage for pathogenicity. It is not at present understood why the prevalence of PVL among CA-MRSA strains is so high, as the genes encoding PVL are not believed to be transferred with the SCC*mec* IV complex. Recently, PVL genes were also found in SCC*mec* type V_T strains from patients and healthy children in Taiwan (15). It is also not understood why the spread of CA-MRSA strains containing PVL has occurred so rapidly, whereas disease-causing MSSA strains containing PVL are not known to have increased rapidly. Further research is needed to understand these phenomena.

CLINICAL PRESENTATION

Asymptomatic colonization is the most frequent outcome of host interaction with *S. aureus*. Among symptomatic patients, skin and soft tissue infections represent the majority of the disease burden due to CA-MRSA (48, 69). The Centers for Disease Control and Prevention (CDC) conducted population-based prospective surveillance and determined that 77% of 1,647 CA-MRSA infections in Baltimore and Atlanta were skin and soft tissue infections (48). Furuncles, carbuncles, and deep skin abscesses are most common. These skin infections are characterized by local warmth, induration, tenderness, and erythema with or without fluctuance. Dermonecrotic lesions are often initially thought to be brown recluse spider bites or other insect bites, causing delay in diagnosis and treatment. This history is often given by patients even in areas of the country outside the habitat of spiders whose bites can produce similar dermonecrosis. CA-MRSA skin lesions can rapidly progress in size and severity; fever and signs of systemic illness are variably present. In one prospective series of patients presenting to an urban medical center emergency department, half of all skin infections and 75% of all *S. aureus* skin infections were due to MRSA, nearly all of which carried SCC*mec* IV and the PVL genes (46).

The mainstay of treatment for skin abscesses is incision and drainage of the lesion (80). Before the epidemic CA-MRSA era, studies had supported the notion that adjunctive antibiotic therapy was unnecessary in uncomplicated cases of *S. aureus* abscesses, particularly small ones, but data regarding the precise rates of successful treatment, prevention of complications, and recurrence rates of CA-MRSA lesions have been inconclusive. One retrospective study suggested that incision and drainage alone of abscess-equivalent lesions <5 cm in diameter is adequate therapy, but this conclusion assumes the ineffectiveness of "inappropriate" antibiotics, with which many of the patients were also treated (75). Surrounding cellulitis, large lesions, fever, systemic illness, and comorbid conditions suggest the need for adjunctive antimicrobial therapy.

CA-MRSA can also cause more severe disease and has been implicated in several invasive-disease syndromes, including pneumonia with empyema, necrotizing pneumonia, necrotizing fasciitis, septic thrombophlebitis with pulmonary embolization, and severe sepsis syndrome (44, 91, 93). Although some of these invasive-disease syndromes had been previously described with MSSA (50, 78), they appear to be more frequently associated with CA-MRSA. In the CDC prospective surveillance mentioned previously, 6% of CA-MRSA cases were considered "invasive," including bacteremia, septic arthritis, osteomyelitis, and pneumonia (48).

CA-MRSA pneumonia characterized by rapidly progressing respiratory distress, hemoptysis, necrotizing features best viewed by computerized axial tomography (CT), and empyema requiring decortication has been described among children and adults with increased frequency. Patients with CA-MRSA necrotizing pneumonia/empyema present with a syndrome characterized by an influenza or influenza-like prodrome, high fever, leukopenia, respiratory failure, and shock (44). Infection with influenza virus or other viruses may predispose to invasion and infection by colonizing CA-MRSA strains. Chest radiography may reveal lobar or patchy consolidation with or without pneumatoceles. The pneumonia may be classified as "necrotizing" if the chest CT shows a consolidative infiltrate, destruction of normal lung architecture, and loss of tissue enhancement. Necrotizing pneumonia due to CA-MRSA (or CA-MSSA) carrying the genetic determinants for PVL is associated with increased morbidity and mortality compared with community-acquired pneumonia (CAP) due to *S. aureus* strains lacking PVL (50). Suspicion of CA-MRSA pneumonia should be raised when patients present with rapidly progressing respiratory distress, severe systemic illness, or the presence of pleural effusion by radiography or ultrasound. Early signs or predictors of CA-MRSA pneumonia as the etiology would be of clinical use but have yet to be identified (Fig. 1 and 2).

Empiric treatment of suspected CAP has been complicated by the emergence of CA-MRSA as an etiology. Guidelines for empirical therapy for CAP often do not include antimicrobials that successfully treat CA-MRSA, and determination of the etiologic agent of pneumonia is often unsuccessful or impractical. Addition of vancomycin is suggested for the empirical treatment regimen of ill patients with CAP. The presence of a pleural effusion necessitates thoracentesis and drainage, as well as evaluation of the pleural fluid in an effort to diagnose empyema.

Severe sepsis due to CA-MRSA has been increasingly recognized (2, 22, 73, 93). Our definition of severe sepsis includes isolation of *S. aureus* from a clinically important site, hypotension (systolic blood pressure below the fifth percentile for age for children or less than 90 mm Hg for adults), and respiratory distress syndrome or respiratory failure, plus

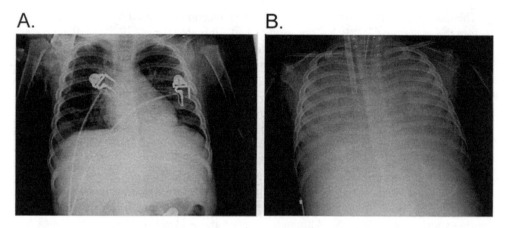

Figure 1. (A) A 2-year-old child with a history of asthma presented to the hospital with tachypnea and fever. The chest X-ray shown here showed patchy airspace disease in the left base, interpreted to be patchy atelectasis associated with asthma. (B) Less than 24 h later, the child's condition had rapidly deteriorated. This chest X-ray shows bilateral airspace opacification of both lungs. MRSA was isolated from the airway of this child and from the lungs at postmortem examination.

clinical or laboratory evidence of abnormal function of the central nervous system, liver, kidneys, muscles, or skin or hemostasis (or a combination thereof), usually in the presence of leukopenia or thrombocytopenia (2). Shock in the presence of pneumonia and purpura fulminans have also been documented. Severe sepsis may be rapidly progressive and result in death. Necrotizing pneumonia is always or nearly always present (Fig. 1). Initial treatment with antibiotics later found to be ineffective against the infecting MRSA strains may have contributed to the deaths of some patients, but death has resulted even when appropriate antibiotics were administered at presentation. The syndrome is often initially suspected to be meningococcemia or toxic shock syndrome. Autopsy results have revealed bilateral adrenal hemorrhage consistent with the Waterhouse-Friderichsen syndrome (2), most commonly associated with meningococcemia. *S. aureus* sepsis is a newly identified cause. Antibiotic therapy directed against MRSA should now be included in the empirical regimen for any patient presenting with sepsis and/or purpura fulminans.

Osteomyelitis, pyomyositis, septic arthritis, necrotizing fasciitis, septic thrombophlebitis, and orbital infections are other syndromes ascribed to CA-MRSA. Most reports have described disease in children, but adults have also been affected (44, 91). Empiric antibiotic coverage for any suspected *S. aureus* syndrome should now include agents active against CA-MRSA.

ASYMPTOMATIC COLONIZATION

When MRSA disease began to be recognized among previously healthy patients without risk for MRSA, it was presumed that asymptomatic MRSA colonization must also be occurring in the general population. Indeed, among healthy children visiting an outpatient health care center for routine care and children visiting a pediatric emergency room

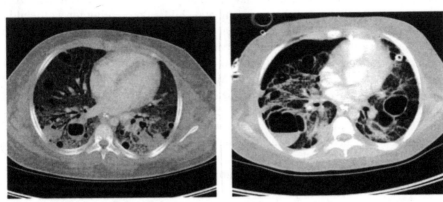

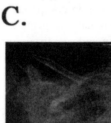

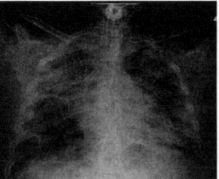

Figure 2. (A) Chest CT of an 8-year-old boy, 1 week after he presented to the hospital with MRSA necrotizing pneumonia. This CT shows extensive opacification and ground-glass appearance of both lungs and multiple pneumatoceles, all due to severe necrotizing pneumonia. (B) Chest CT of the same patient 6 weeks later, showing extensive destruction of normal lung architecture and an anterior pneumothorax. (C) Chest radiograph of the same patient 2 months after presentation, when the patient had recovered from his acute illness. This radiograph shows patchy airspace opacities and numerous pneumatoceles bilaterally.

for an urgent issue, the carrier rates of MRSA were about 1% (60, 125). The National Health and Nutrition Survey surveyed a cross-section of the general population in 2001 and 2002 and also found that about 1% of children and adults carried MRSA among their nasal flora (http://www.cdc.gov/nchs/nhanes.htm). About half of these strains contained SCC*mec* IV, and about half contained SCC*mec* II. Both studies were performed relatively early in the CA-MRSA epidemic, and colonization rates may have subsequently increased. Cultures taken from asymptomatic subjects without risk factors for MRSA colonization in Taiwan from 1997 to 2002 found a colonization rate of 5% (15). Interestingly, a majority of those colonizing strains contained SCC*mec* IV and lacked the PVL loci, whereas a small subset contained SCC*mec* V_T carrying the PVL determinants. A 2004 Tennessee study of nasal colonization among 500 children presenting for well-child care found a startlingly high MRSA colonization rate of 9.2%, dramatically increased from the 0.8% found in 2001 (34).

Persons asymptomatically colonized with CA-MRSA seem to be at higher risk for *S. aureus* disease than those colonized with MSSA. Ellis et al. found that, among military recruits, those with CA-MRSA nasal colonization had a relative risk of 10.7 for developing clinical infection compared with those colonized with CA-MSSA ($P < 0.001$) (40). Of nine CA-MRSA-colonized participants who developed subsequent infection, eight were colonized with a PVL-positive strain and presented with abscesses, whereas the participant colonized with a PVL-negative strain presented with cellulitis. The MSSA isolates in this study were not characterized further to determine if they contained the PVL determinants.

The presence of the PVL genetic determinants among CA-MRSA isolates may be responsible for the differences in the risk of infection compared with PVL-negative HA-MRSA or PVL-negative MSSA. MSSA strains harboring the genes for PVL have also caused necrotizing pneumonia, sepsis, and skin and soft tissue infections. Further definition of the risk of infection among those colonized with PVL-positive CA-MRSA may have important prognostic and therapeutic implications.

THERAPY FOR CA-MRSA INFECTIONS

The CA-MRSA epidemic has complicated the selection of empirical antibiotic therapy for presumed *S. aureus* infections. The impossibility of clinically distinguishing between infections caused by CA-MSSA and CA-MRSA dictates that clinicians become familiar with the frequencies of CA-MRSA in their respective communities. In areas where the burden of CA-MRSA disease is significant (some have suggested that CA-MRSA strains are >10% of *S. aureus* strains [6]), empirical β-lactam therapy is no longer appropriate. Local resistance rates can be tracked by monitoring hospital clinical microbiology reports and outbreaks investigated by local public health departments. The recommended increased frequency of obtaining diagnostic cultures will also be of value in determining antibiotic susceptibilities.

Whereas treatment of often multiply resistant hospital-associated MRSA called vancomycin into heavy use, options for treatment of CA-MRSA are currently broader. Any antibiotic use has the potential to select for resistant strains, and CA-MRSA may not always remain susceptible to drugs currently available, as suggested by the presence of multidrug-resistant SCC*mec* type IV- and type V-containing CA-MRSA strains in Taiwan (15). The selection of empirical antibiotic therapy should reflect the local rate of methicillin resistance, the disease syndrome, the severity of illness, and the clinical implications of transiently choosing suboptimal therapy before culture and susceptibility results are known. Figure 2 illustrates an approach to the management of skin and soft tissue infections when CA-MRSA is among the likely etiologies. Empirical therapy for possible CA-MRSA invasive disease, including necrotizing pneumonia, septic arthritis, osteomyelitis, necrotizing fasciitis, and severe sepsis, can follow the Fig. 3 paradigms for moderate and severe illness.

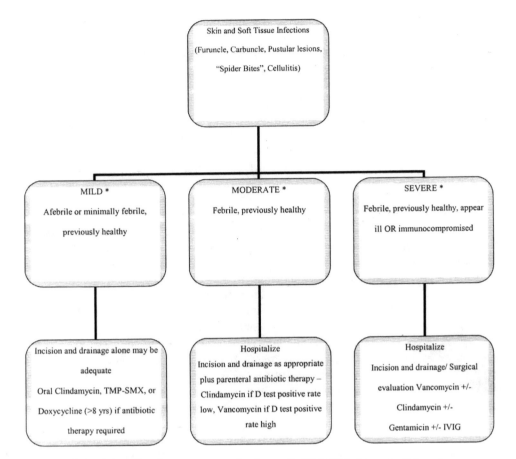

Figure 3. Paradigm for management of patients with CA-MRSA skin and soft tissue infections. The designations mild, moderate, and severe refer to the levels of clinical acuity.

The therapy for possible CA-MRSA disease involves the use of agents, many of which have not been in wide use for *S. aureus* infections prior to the CA-MRSA epidemic. Some relevant clinical properties of these agents are reviewed below.

Clindamycin

Clindamycin is a lincosamide antimicrobial that inhibits protein synthesis at the chain elongation step by interfering with transpeptidation by the 50S ribosomal subunit. It has activity against gram-positive organisms, including *S. aureus*, *Streptococcus pneumoniae*, *Streptococcus pyogenes*, and anaerobic organisms. While most HA-MRSA isolates are resistant to clindamycin, most CA-MRSA isolates are susceptible. A retrospective chart evaluation of patients treated for MRSA infection suggested that clindamycin was effective in treating invasive infections. Outcomes were comparable to those in patients with MSSA infections who were treated with β-lactams (87). Clindamycin is known for its poor taste as an oral suspension and its potential for precipitating *Clostridium difficile* colitis, and some have remained reluctant to use it. Its advantages, however, include its availability in both oral and intravenous formulations; good tissue penetration, especially into skin and bone; and a lower cost than some alternative therapies.

Characterization of CA-MRSA strains obtained early in the epidemic found that many were resistant only to β-lactams, making clindamycin a reliable choice for therapy. However, reports of increasing erythromycin and clindamycin resistance among community strains have emerged (68).

Clindamycin-susceptible, erythromycin-resistant *S. aureus* (clindamycin-erythromycin-discordant) isolates may reflect several molecular scenarios. Resistance to these antibiotics is commonly mediated by the *erm* gene, giving rise to the so-called macrolide, lincosamide, streptogramin B phenotype (3). These three structurally distinct compounds all interfere with protein synthesis by binding to a common target on the 23S rRNA. The *erm* gene product modifies the common binding target by methylating a critical adenine residue on ribosomal RNA. Expression of *erm* is normally repressed unless it is induced by a 14- or 15-member macrolide, e.g., erythromycin, via a translational attenuation mechanism. Because lincosamides (clindamycin) and streptogramin B do not induce the *erm* gene, isolates that express *erm* only after erythromycin induction are phenotypically resistant to macrolides but test susceptible to lincosamide (clindamycin) and streptogramin B antibiotics. In the presence of a mutation upstream of *erm*, the production of the methylase gene product proceeds without an inducer, and these mutants express a constitutive macrolide, lincosamide, streptogramin B phenotype. Even when inducible *erm* expression is present and clindamycin susceptibility is reported, clindamycin can select for constitutive *erm* expression. Clindamycin treatment failures have been reported under these circumstances (45, 76, 87). Although the frequency is not known, failure is likely to be infrequent.

The potential for clindamycin treatment failure can be assessed by performance of a tandem erythromycin-clindamycin disk diffusion test on all erythromycin-resistant, clindamycin-susceptible *S. aureus* isolates. Guidelines for performance of this "D test" have been published by the Clinical and Laboratory Standards Institute (formerly NCCLS) (99). The D test is performed by placing clindamycin and erythromycin disks at an edge-to-edge distance of 15 to 20 mm. The appearance of a D-shaped zone of clearing around the clindamycin disk indicates the presence of the *erm* gene and erythromycin-induced clindamycin resistance. If the D test is positive, clinicians should be aware that treatment with clindamycin may result in clinical treatment failure (Fig. 4). Clindamycin-susceptible, erythromycin-resistant isolates with a negative D test may contain an efflux pump specific to erythromycin, encoded by another gene called *msrA*. Clindamycin treatment is appropriate for these strains. The proportion of D-test-positive CA-MRSA isolates varies geographically (16, 45), although few data are available that directly address this issue.

Clindamycin has another potential advantage in the treatment of suspected toxin-mediated disease, such as necrotizing fasciitis, necrotizing pneumonia, toxic shock syndrome, and severe sepsis, due to its potent suppression of bacterial protein synthesis. Many experts have argued, therefore, for its hypothetical superiority in toxin-mediated syndromes, although explicit data are lacking. Advocates for clindamycin in this setting often combine it with oxacillin (in areas with low prevalence of MRSA) or vancomycin.

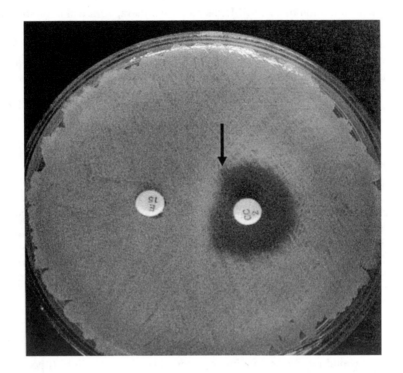

Figure 4. A "D test" is performed on isolates that are resistant to erythromycin but susceptible to clindamycin in order to evaluate the potential for treatment failure when using clindamycin. Blunting of the clindamycin zone of inhibition (marked by a vertical arrow) indicates the presence of an *erm* gene in the test isolate that is inducible by erythromycin.

Clindamycin is bacteriostatic and therefore probably should not be used in the treatment of endocarditis or other intravascular *S. aureus* infections.

Trimethoprim-Sulfamethoxazole

Trimethoprim-sulfamethoxazole (TMP-SMX) interferes with the biosynthesis of tetrahydrofolic acid, essential for microbial synthesis of proteins and nucleotides. Many experts believe that mild to moderate skin infections caused by CA-MRSA can be effectively managed by this fixed antibiotic combination. Lack of clinical experience in using TMP-SMX for *S. aureus* infections and lack of controlled trials supporting its use limit the confidence of some clinicians in this treatment regimen. A study conducted among intravenous-drug users suggested that TMP-SMX might be as effective as vancomycin for *S. aureus* infection, although vancomycin was superior for the treatment of endocarditis (86). A retrospective chart review of patients with cutaneous CA-MRSA infections concluded that a combination of TMP-SMX and rifampin was an effective treatment for cutaneous CA-MRSA infection (63), whereas use of TMP-SMX alone resulted in only a 50% clinical cure rate.

An important limitation of TMP-SMX as empirical therapy for a skin or soft tissue infection is its lack of activity against some strains of group A streptococci. Thus, if group A streptococcal infection is a consideration, e.g., in a patient with cellulitis, TMP-SMX may not be a good choice. Common side effects of TMP-SMX include rash and urticaria. More rarely, clinicians should be alert for the more serious Stevens-Johnson syndrome, hematologic abnormalities, and hepatotoxicity.

Tetracyclines

The long-acting tetracycline derivatives doxycycline, minocycline, and tigecycline have also been considered for the treatment of MRSA. Tigecycline is a novel tetracycline analogue approved by the U.S. Food and Drug Administration in 2005. Comparison of tigecycline with aztreonam plus vancomycin for the treatment of skin and skin structure infections showed equivalence between the two treatments (17). Case series report an 85% success rate in treatment of CA-MRSA infections with minocycline or doxycycline, but randomized trials have not been performed (116). These agents are generally not indicated for use in children younger than 8 years of age due to concern about discoloration of bones and teeth. Oral and intravenous formulations of tetracycline derivatives are available, but tigecycline is available only as an intravenous formulation.

Vancomycin and Related Glycopeptides

Vancomycin is a glycopeptide antimicrobial agent that inhibits the synthesis and assembly of cell wall peptidoglycan by binding to terminal D-Ala–D-Ala lipid II peptide precursors. Vancomycin underwent a marked increase in use when the spread of nosocomial MRSA occurred worldwide and for many years was called the "antibiotic of last resort." It is available only in an intravenous preparation. Adverse effects, including nephrotoxicity, require serum drug level monitoring, especially when other nephrotoxic agents are given concurrently. A histamine-like reaction, known as "red-man syndrome," associated with vancomycin infusion can be avoided by pretreatment with an antihistamine and slowed infusion. Vancomycin should be considered for children with serious suspected MRSA infections, including severe sepsis; toxic shock syndrome; necrotizing pneumonia; intravascular infections, such as septic thrombophlebitis or endocarditis; and necrotizing fasciitis.

Concern about vancomycin resistance is rising, since *S. aureus* isolates with so-called intermediate susceptibility to vancomycin (VISA) have been recovered (21, 124) in association with treatment failure. VISA isolates are believed to occur more frequently than is currently documented, because clinical microbiology laboratories often do not perform the necessary tests to detect intermediate susceptibility (47). Moreover, in 2002, the Centers for Disease Control and Prevention reported the first documented infection caused by high-level vancomycin-resistant *S. aureus* (VRSA) that contained the *vanA* vancomycin resistance genes from enterococci (23, 28, 128). Four additional VRSA isolates have been found subsequently. VRSA isolates are also unreliably detected by routine clinical microbiology laboratory methods.

Another glycopeptide antimicrobial, teicoplanin, is not licensed in the United States but appears to offer no advantage over vancomycin for treatment of staphylococcal infections.

Dalbavancin is a glycopeptide antibiotic with a long half-life currently under investigation for use in the treatment of infections with gram-positive aerobic and anaerobic bacteria. Phase 3 trials in the treatment of skin and soft tissue infections in adults have been completed, but the results are not yet available.

BEYOND VANCOMYCIN

Linezolid

Linezolid is the first agent in a new class of antimicrobials called the oxazolidinones that act to inhibit the initiation step of protein synthesis. Linezolid has broad in vitro activity against β-lactam- and glycopeptide-susceptible and -resistant gram-positive bacteria, including MRSA, VISA, VRSA, and vancomycin-resistant enterococci. Treatment with linezolid has resulted in outcomes similar to those of treatment with vancomycin in patients with skin and soft tissue infections and pneumonia caused by resistant gram-positive organisms, including MRSA. Acquired resistance to linezolid in *S. aureus* has thus far been exceedingly rare. Linezolid is well tolerated in the pediatric population (37, 67, 131). It is available in intravenous and oral forms, and oral bioavailability is approximately 100%, allowing transition from intravenous to oral therapy. Unfortunately, linezolid is very expensive compared with alternative antibiotics. Because it is bacteriostatic against *S. aureus*, it is also not the preferred treatment option in endocarditis and meningitis, for which a bactericidal agent is preferred (30, 117).

Use of linezolid has been associated with reversible neutropenia, anemia, and thrombocytopenia. Monitoring of neutrophils, hemoglobin, and platelets should occur weekly in patients receiving linezolid, particularly if therapy extends beyond 2 weeks; in those with preexisting myelosuppression; or in those receiving other drugs that produce bone marrow suppression. Prolonged use of linezolid has also been associated with optic and peripheral neuropathies.

Quinupristin-Dalfopristin (Synercid)

Quinupristin-dalfopristin is a fixed combination of group B and group A streptogramins. Both of these antibiotics bind to the 50S subunit of the bacterial ribosome and have a bactericidal effect resulting from inhibition of protein synthesis. Synercid has in vitro activity against staphylococci, streptococci, and enterococci, excluding *Enterococcus faecalis*. In two randomized open-label trials, the bacteriologic success rate for treatment of gram-positive skin and skin structure infections with quinupristin-dalfopristin was lower than with the standard therapy group (cefazolin, oxacillin, or vancomycin) (101).

ADJUNCTIVE THERAPIES

Intravenous immunoglobulin has been suggested for use in supportive treatment of toxin-mediated diseases, such as toxic shock syndrome (9, 121). The severe, rapidly progressive course in children and adults with necrotizing pneumonia, severe sepsis, and shock due to CA-MRSA may be due in part to toxin-mediated effects. One brand of commercially available intravenous immunoglobulin (IVIG) was found to contain antibody directed against recombinant PVL (49), and thus, IVIG may have a role in limiting toxin-mediated effects. IVIG neutralizes pore formation and the cytolytic effect of PVL in vitro (49). Clinical trials evaluating the effectiveness of IVIG in CA-MRSA necrotizing pneumonia and severe sepsis are warranted.

PREVENTIVE MEASURES

S. aureus has its primary ecologic niche in the anterior nares. It has been assumed, but not proven, that the same is true for CA-MRSA. Skin-to-skin contact is likely the primary mechanism for transfer of a colonizing or skin and soft tissue infection isolate from one host to another, as evidenced by outbreaks among sports teams and those in close-contact quarters. Preventive measures have focused on decreasing transmission through improved hygiene, including strict wound care, proper disposal of contaminated items, covering unhealed wounds, and hand washing. Some sports teams have increased efforts to schedule equipment washing, discouraged towel sharing, restricted infected members from play until lesions are healed, and encouraged good hygiene among team members (24, 100). No single measure has proven successful, although outbreaks have been curtailed after the institution of multiple measures such as these. Several correctional facilities are also instituting increased access to soap and water and improved attention to skin lesions to prevent the spread of CA-MRSA, as recommended by the Federal Bureau of Prisons (25).

Eradication of colonization by MRSA has also been suggested as a strategy to prevent recurrent disease and possibly to control outbreaks. Many have attempted decolonization in outbreak situations, but few randomized controlled trials have evaluated the efficacies of various medications and washes in the eradication of *S. aureus* carriage (14, 81). Most eradication strategies proposed to eliminate MRSA carriage have been extrapolated from studies evaluating decolonization of MSSA. Some washes considered effective in decreasing MSSA colonization, such as chlorhexidine, may not have the same effectiveness against MRSA (65, 66).

Intranasal mupirocin ointment appears to have the most success in decreasing *S. aureus* nasal colonization, with a subsequent decrease in carriage at other body sites. A 5-day application of intranasal mupirocin showed good results in short-term eradication. However, recolonization occurred in at least half of subjects within months (38, 39, 43). Recolonization and concern about the development of resistance limit its widespread use at present (90).

Selective treatment of high-risk populations, including dialysis patients, surgical patients, and those with recurrent *S. aureus* infections, in order to prevent disease has also been attempted. Preoperative treatment of patients with intranasal mupirocin did not significantly reduce the overall rate of postoperative *S. aureus* surgical site infections compared with placebo (108). However, treatment did significantly decrease the rate of all nosocomial *S. aureus* infections among the patients who were *S. aureus* carriers. Implementation of this prophylaxis would necessitate screening patients for *S. aureus* nasal carriage prior to treatment.

Washing in dilute bleach (1 teaspoon per gallon of water) twice a week in conjunction with nasal mupirocin has also been suggested as a potentially effective means for decreasing colonization (68), but it has not yet been critically evaluated.

Simultaneous use of any proposed intervention to decrease colonization by all close contacts is likely to be necessary, as it is has been hypothesized that close contacts within a household have high transmission rates (58). Randomized trials evaluating the efficacy, safety, and long-term results of various agents will be necessary before decolonization strategies can be routinely recommended.

DEFINING CA-MRSA

Definitions of CA-MRSA have varied and have been inconsistently used (118). Distinguishing HA-MRSA from CA-MRSA is useful in defining the changing epidemiology, identifying those at risk, and choosing empirical antibiotic therapy when required. The most commonly used definition has been based on time, with the designation of CA-MRSA assigned to an MRSA isolate obtained in the outpatient setting or in the first 48 to 72 hours of hospitalization. Because a substantial number of MRSA isolates actually have an epidemiologic link to the hospital setting, such a temporal definition may have limited use in predicting the clinical or microbiological characteristics of the organism. PFGE and MLST data suggest that some MRSA strains isolated in the community are of hospital origin, and furthermore, as the CA-MRSA epidemic has continued, movement of community strains into the hospital has likely occurred. For example, an outbreak in a neonatal intensive-care unit was promulgated by so-called CA-MRSA isolates containing SCC*mec* IV and resulted in severe illness characterized by pneumonia and sepsis (56). Additionally, in Western Australia, CA-MRSA isolates containing SCC*mec* IV were responsible for an outbreak of nosocomial infections (102), and at Harbor-UCLA Medical Center, CA-MRSA isolates have become the major clone accounting for nosocomial *S. aureus* infections (85). A decrease in multidrug resistance among hospital MRSA isolates has also been documented in the National Nosocomial Infections Surveillance System, consistent with the appearance of community MRSA strains in the hospital (72).

The presence or absence of traditional MRSA risk factors, including previous admission to a hospital, residence in a long-term care facility, recent surgery, history of MRSA colonization or infection, or presence of an indwelling device, has also been used to distinguish HA-MRSA from CA-MRSA. For example, some have defined a CA-MRSA isolate as one identified in the outpatient setting or within 72 h of hospitalization in the absence of traditional risk factors. This definition of CA-MRSA is the one currently used by the CDC (http://www.cdc.gov). Even using a combined temporal and risk factor definition, however, may not predict the molecular characteristics of the MRSA isolate. In MRSA surveillance at our institution, we have found that most patients with MRSA have some identifiable risk, whether the organism is obtained from a hospital or community origin (S. Crawford et al., unpublished data).

FUTURE DIRECTIONS

Many questions remain as CA-MRSA colonization and disease become more prevalent. Insight into the mechanism of transfer of resistance elements and toxin genomic islands may provide clues as to why the burden of CA-MRSA disease has increased so rapidly. Available preventive measures currently rely upon good hygiene and wound care and, although important, are unlikely to succeed in the community. Further investigation of decolonization methods is needed. *S. aureus* vaccine candidates are under investigation. New target candidates for vaccines and therapy, perhaps directed against important toxins, may provide hope for preventing and treating disease.

CONCLUSIONS

CA-MRSA disease is an emerging infectious disease responsible for a large disease burden. CA-MRSA isolates have different genetic elements and toxin genes than HA-MRSA, and these differences are considered to be responsible for the variations in epidemiology and disease. It is not understood what factors have led to the emergence of PVL-positive MRSA, nor why it appears that the disease burden has appeared so rapidly, as PVL is not a newly recognized virulence factor. Attention to hygiene and strict adherence to contact precautions in institutional settings are the current guidelines in place to prevent spread. Awareness of the increasing prevalence of CA-MRSA in relation to *S. aureus* disease is crucial. Culturing suspected *S. aureus* infections is now necessary to guide antibiotic therapy, and local prevalence rates and resistance patterns should guide clinicians in choosing empirical therapy. Early recognition of CA-MRSA disease is important but difficult; CA-MRSA must now be recognized as a possible cause of necrotizing pneumonia, sepsis, and other invasive life-threatening diseases.

REFERENCES

1. **Adcock, P. M., P. Pastor, F. Medley, J. E. Patterson, and T. V. Murphy.** 1998. Methicillin-resistant *Staphylococcus aureus* in two child care centers. *J. Infect. Dis.* **78:**577–580.
2. **Adem, P. V., C. P. Montgomery, A. N. Husain, T. K. Koogler, V. Arangelovich, M. Humilier, S. Boyle-Vavra, and R. S. Daum.** 2005. *Staphylococcus aureus* sepsis and the Waterhouse-Friderichsen syndrome in children. *N. Engl. J. Med.* **353:**1245–1251.
3. **Arthur, M., A. Brisson-Noel, and P. Courvalin.** 1987. Origin and evolution of genes specifying resistance to macrolide, lincosamide and streptogramin antibiotics: data and hypotheses. *J. Antimicrob. Chemother.* **20:**783–802.
4. **Baggett, H. C., T. W. Hennessy, K. Rudolph, D. Bruden, A. Reasonover, A. Parkinson, R. Sparks, R. M. Donian, P. Martinez, K. Mongkolrattanothai, and J. C. Butler.** 2004. Community-onset methicillin-resistant *Staphylococcus aureus* associated with antibiotic use and the cytotoxin Panton-Valentine leukocidin during a furunculosis outbreak in rural Alaska. *J. Infect. Dis.* **189:**1565–1573.
5. **Baillargeon, J., M. F. Kelley, C. T. Leach, G. Baillargeon, and B. H. Pollock.** 2004. Methicillin-resistant *Staphylococcus aureus* infection in the Texas prison system. *Clin. Infect. Dis.* **38:**e92–e95.
6. **Baker, C. J., and R. W. Frenck.** 2004. Change in management of skin/soft tissue infections needed. *AAP News* **25:**105.
7. **Barber, M.** 1961. Methicillin-resistant staphylococci. *J. Clin. Pathol.* **14:**385.
8. **Barrett, F. F., R. F. McGehee, and M. Finland.** 1968. Methicillin-resistant *Staphylococcus aureus* at Boston City Hospital. *N. Engl. J. Med.* **279:**441–448.
9. **Barry, W., L. Hudgins, S. T. Donta, and E. L. Pesanti.** 1992. Intravenous immunoglobulin therapy for toxic shock syndrome. *JAMA* **267:**3315–3316.
10. **Benner, E. J., and F. H. Kayser.** 1968. Growing clinical significance of methicillin-resistant *Staphylococcus aureus*. *Lancet* **ii:**741–744.
11. **Bondi, A., Jr., and C. C. Dietz.** 1945. Penicillin resistant staphylococci. *Proc. Soc. Exp. Biol. Med.* **60:**55.
12. **Boyce, J. M., and W. A. Causey.** 1982. Increasing occurrence of methicillin-resistant *Staphylococcus aureus* in the United States. *Infect. Control* **3:**377–383.
13. **Boyce, J. M.** 1989. Methicillin-resistant *Staphylococcus aureus*: detection, epidemiology, and control measures. *Infect. Dis. Clin. N. Am.* **3:**901–913.
14. **Boyce, J. M.** 2001. MRSA patients: proven methods to treat colonization and infection. *J. Hosp. Infect.* **48**(Suppl. A):S9–S14.
15. **Boyle-Vavra, S., B. Ereshefsky, C. C. Wang, and R. S. Daum.** 2005. Successful multiresistant community-associated methicillin-resistant *Staphylococcus aureus* lineage from Taipei, Taiwan, that carries either the novel staphylococcal chromosome cassette *mec* (SCC*mec*) type VT or SCC*mec* type IV. *J. Clin. Microbiol.* **43:**4719–4730.

16. **Braun, L., D. Craft, R. Williams, F. Tuamokumo, and M. Ottolini.** 2005. Increasing clindamycin resistance among methicillin-resistant *Staphylococcus aureus* in 57 northeast United States military treatment facilities. *Pediatr. Infect. Dis. J.* **24**:622–626.

17. **Breedt, J., J. Teras, J. Gardovskis, F. J. Maritz, T. Vaasna, D. P. Ross, M. Gioud-Paquet, N. Dartois, E. J. Ellis-Grosse, E. Loh and the Tigecycline 305 cSSSI Study Group.** 2005. Safety and efficacy of tigecycline in treatment of skin and skin structure infections: results of a double-blind phase 3 comparison study with vancomycin-aztreonam. *Antimicrob. Agents Chemother.* **49**:4658–4666.

18. **Buckingham, S. C., L. K. McDougal, L. D. Cathey, K. Comeaux, A. S. Craig, S. K. Fridkin, and F. C. Tenover.** 2004. Emergence of community-associated methicillin-resistant *Staphylococcus aureus* at a Memphis, Tennessee children's hospital. *Pediatr. Infect. Dis. J.* **23**:619–624.

19. **Campbell, K. M., A. F. Vaughn, K. L. Russell, B. Smith, D. L. Jimenez, C. P. Barrozo, J. R. Minarcik, N. F. Crum, and M. A. Ryan.** 2004. Risk factors for community-associated methicillin-resistant *Staphylococcus aureus* infections in an outbreak of disease among military trainees in San Diego, California, in 2002. *J. Clin. Microbiol.* **42**:4050–4053.

20. **Carleton, H. A., B. A. Diep, E. D. Charlebois, G. F. Sensabaugh, and F. Perdreau-Remington.** 2004. Community-adapted methicillin-resistant *Staphylococcus aureus* (MRSA): population dynamics of an expanding community reservoir of MRSA. *J. Infect. Dis.* **190**:1730–1738.

21. **Centers for Disease Control and Prevention.** 1997. *Staphylococcus aureus* with reduced susceptibility to vancomycin—United States, 1997. *Morb. Mortal. Wkly. Rep.* **46**:765–766.

22. **Centers for Disease Control and Prevention.** 1999. Four pediatric deaths from community-acquired methicillin-resistant *Staphylococcus aureus*: Minnesota and North Dakota, 1997–1999. *Morb. Mortal. Wkly. Rep.* **48**:707–710.

23. **Centers for Disease Control and Prevention.** 2002. Vancomycin-resistant *Staphylococcus aureus*—Pennsylvania, 2002. *Morb. Mortal. Wkly. Rep.* **51**:902.

24. **Centers for Disease Control and Prevention.** 2003. Methicillin-resistant *Staphylococcus aureus* infections among competitive sports participants—Colorado, Indiana, Pennsylvania, and Los Angeles County, 2000–2003. *Morb. Mortal. Wkly. Rep.* **52**:793–795.

25. **Centers for Disease Control and Prevention.** 2003. Methicillin-resistant *Staphylococcus aureus* infections in correctional facilities—Georgia, California, and Texas, 2001–2003. *Morb. Mortal. Wkly. Rep.* **52**:992–996.

26. **Chambers, H. F.** 1988. Methicillin-resistant staphylococci. *Clin. Microbiol. Rev.* **1**:173–186.

27. **Chambers, H. F.** 2001. The changing epidemiology of *Staphylococcus aureus*? *Emerg. Infect. Dis.* **7**:178–182.

28. **Chang, S., D. M. Sievert, J. C. Hageman, et al.** 2003. Infection with vancomycin-resistant *Staphylococcus aureus* containing the *vanA* resistance gene. *N. Engl. J. Med.* **348**:1342–1347.

29. **Chavez-Bueno, S., B. Bozdogan, K. Katz, K. L. Bowlware, N. Cushion, D. Cavuoti, N. Ahmad, G. H. McCracken, Jr., and P. C. Appelbaum.** 2005. Inducible clindamycin resistance and molecular epidemiologic trends of pediatric community-acquired methicillin-resistant *Staphylococcus aureus* in Dallas, Texas. *Antimicrob. Agents Chemother.* **49**:2283–2288.

30. **Chiang, F. Y., and M. Climo.** 2003. Efficacy of linezolid alone or in combination with vancomycin for treatment of experimental endocarditis due to methicillin-resistant *Staphylococcus aureus*. *Antimicrob. Agents Chemother.* **47**:3002–3004.

31. **Coombs, G. W., G. R. Nimmo, J. M. Bell, F. Huygens, F. G. O'Brien, M. J. Malkowski, J. C. Pearson, A. J. Stephens, P. M. Giffard, and the Australian Group for Antimicrobial Resistance.** 2004. Genetic diversity among community methicillin-resistant *Staphylococcus aureus* strains causing outpatient infections in Australia. *J. Clin. Microbiol.* **42**:4735–4743.

32. **Couppie, P., B. Cribier, G. Prevost, E. Grosshans, and Y. Peimont.** 1994. Leukocidin from *Staphylococcus aureus* and cutaneous infections: an epidemiologic study. *Arch. Dermatol.* **130**:1208–1209.

33. **Craven, D. E., A. I. Rixinger, T. A. Goularte, and W. R. McCabe.** 1986. Methicillin-resistant *Staphylococcus aureus* bacteremia linked to intravenous drug abusers using a "shooting gallery." *Am. J. Med.* **80**:770–775.

34. **Creech, C. B., D. S. Kernodle, A. Alsentzer, C. Wilson, and K. M. Edwards.** 2005. Increasing rates of nasal carriage of methicillin-resistant *Staphylococcus aureus* in healthy children. *Pediatr. Infect. Dis. J.* **24**:617–621.

35. **Culpepper, R., R. Nolan, S. Chapman, A. Kennedy, and M. Currier.** 2001. Methicillin-resistant *Staphylococcus aureus* skin or soft tissue infections in a state prison—Mississippi, 2000. *Morb. Mortal. Wkly. Rep.* **50**:919–922.

36. **Daum, R. S., T. Ito, K. Hiramatsu, F. Hussain, K. Mongkolrattanothai, M. Jamklang, and S. Boyle-Vavra.** 2002. A novel methicillin-resistance cassette in community-acquired methicillin-resistant *Staphylococcus aureus* isolates of diverse genetic backgrounds. *J. Infect. Dis.* **186:**1344–1347.

37. **Deville, J. G., S. Adler, P. H. Azimi, B. A. Jantausch, M. R. Morfin, S. Beltran, B. Edge-Padbury, S. Naberhuis-Stehouwer, and J. B. Bruss.** 2003. Linezolid versus vancomycin in the treatment of known or suspected resistant gram-positive infections in neonates. *Pediatr. Infect. Dis. J.* **22**(Suppl. 9)**:**S158–S163.

38. **Doebbeling, B. N., D. L. Breneman, H. C. Neu, R. Aly, B. G. Yangco, H. P. Holley, Jr., R. J. Marsh, M. A. Pfaller, J. E. McGowan, Jr., B. E. Scully, et al.** 1993. Elimination of *Staphylococcus aureus* nasal carriage in health care workers: analysis of six clinical trials with calcium mupirocin ointment. *Clin. Infect. Dis.* **17:**466–474.

39. **Doebbeling, B. N., D. R. Reagan, M. A. Pfaller, A. K. Houston, R. J. Hollis, and R. P. Wenzel.** 1994. Long-term efficacy of intranasal mupirocin ointment. A prospective cohort study of *Staphylococcus aureus* carriage. *Arch. Intern. Med.* **154:**1505–1508.

40. **Ellis, M. W., D. R. Hospenthal, D. P. Dooley, P. J. Gray, and C. K. Murray.** 2004. Natural history of community-acquired methicillin-resistant *Staphylococcus aureus* colonization and infection in soldiers. *Clin. Infect. Dis.* **39:**971–979.

41. **Enright, M. C., N. P. Day, C. E. Davies, S. J. Peacock, and B. G. Spratt.** 2000. Multilocus sequence typing for characterization of methicillin-resistant and methicillin-susceptible clones of *Staphylococcus aureus*. *J. Clin. Microbiol.* **38:**1008–1015.

42. **Fergie, J. E., and K. Purcell.** 2001. Community-acquired methicillin-resistant *Staphylococcus aureus* infections in South Texas children. *Pediatr. Infect. Dis. J.* **20:**860–863.

43. **Fernandez, C., C. Gaspar, A. Torrellas, A. Vindel, J. A. Saez-Nieto, F. Cruzet, and L. Aguilar.** 1995. A double-blind, randomized, placebo-controlled clinical trial to evaluate the safety and efficacy of mupirocin calcium ointment for eliminating nasal carriage of *Staphylococcus aureus* among hospital personnel. *J. Antimicrob. Chemother.* **35:**399–408.

44. **Francis, J. S., M. C. Doherty, U. Lopatin, C. P. Johnston, G. Sinha, T. Ross, M. Cai, N. N. Hansel, T. Perl, J. R. Ticehurst, K. Carroll, D. L. Thomas, E. Nuermberger, and J. G. Bartlett.** 2005. Severe community-onset pneumonia in healthy adults caused by methicillin-resistant *Staphylococcus aureus* carrying the Panton-Valentine leukocidin genes. *Clin. Infect. Dis.* **40:**100–107.

45. **Frank, A. L., J. F. Marcinak, P. D. Mangat, J. T. Tjhio, S. Kelkar, P. C. Schreckenberger, and J. P. Quinn.** 2002. Clindamycin treatment of methicillin-resistant *Staphylococcus aureus* infections in children. *Pediatr. Infect. Dis. J.* **21:**530–534.

46. **Frazee, B. W., J. Lynn, E. D. Charlebois, L. Lambert, D. Lowery, and F. Perdreau-Remington.** 2005. High prevalence of methicillin-resistant *Staphylococcus aureus* in emergency department skin and soft tissue infections. *Ann. Emerg. Med.* **45:**311–320.

47. **Fridkin, S. K., J. Hageman, L. K. McDougal, J. Mohammed, W. R. Jarvis, T. M. Perl, F. C. Tenover, and the Vancomycin-Intermediate *Staphylococcus aureus* Epidemiology Study Group.** 2003. Epidemiological and microbiological characterization of infections caused by *Staphylococcus aureus* with reduced susceptibility to vancomycin, United States, 1997–2001. *Clin. Infect. Dis.* **36:**429–439.

48. **Fridkin, S. K., J. C. Hageman, M. Morrison, L. T. Sanza, K. Como-Sabetti, J. A. Jernigan, K. Harriman, L. H. Harrison, R. Lynfield, M. M. Farley, and the Active Bacterial Core Surveillance Program of the Emerging Infections Program Network.** 2005. Methicillin-resistant *Staphylococcus aureus* disease in three communities. *N. Engl. J. Med.* **352:**1436–1444.

49. **Gauduchon, V., G. Cozon, F. Vandenesch, A. L. Genestier, N. Eyssade, S. Peyrol, J. Etienne, and G. Lina.** 2004. Neutralization of *Staphylococcus aureus* Panton Valentine leukocidin by intravenous immunoglobulin in vitro. *J. Infect. Dis.* **189:**346–353.

50. **Gillet, Y., B. Issartel, P. Vanhems, J. C. Fournet, G. Lina, M. Bes, F. Vandenesch, Y. Piemont, N. Brousse, D. Floret, and J. Etienne.** 2002. Association between *Staphylococcus aureus* strains carrying the gene for Panton-Valentine leukocidin and highly lethal necrotising pneumonia in young immunocompetent patients. *Lancet* **359:**753–759.

51. **Gladstone, G. P., and W. E. Van Heyningen.** 1957. Staphylococcal leucocidins. *Br. J. Exp. Pathol.* **38:**123–137.

52. **Gonzalez, B. E., K. G. Hulten, M. K. Dishop, L. B. Lamberth, W. A. Hammerman, E. O. Mason, Jr., and S. L. Kaplan.** 2005. Pulmonary manifestations in children with invasive community-acquired *Staphylococcus aureus* infection. *Clin. Infect. Dis.* **41:**583–590.

53. **Gorak, E. J., S. M. Yamada, and J. D. Brown.** 1999. Community-acquired methicillin-resistant *Staphylococcus aureus* in hospitalized adults and children without known risk factors. *Clin. Infect. Dis.* **29:**797–800.

54. **Gottlieb, R. D., M. K. Shah, D. C. Perlman, and C. P. Kimmelman.** 1992. Community-acquired methicillin-resistant *Staphylococcus aureus* infections in otolaryngology. *Otolaryngol. Head Neck Surg.* **107:**434–437.

55. **Groom, A. V., D. H. Wolsey, T. S. Naimi, K. Smith, S. Johnson, D. Boxrud, K. A. Moore, and J. E. Cheek.** 2001. Community-acquired methicillin-resistant *Staphylococcus aureus* in a rural American Indian community. *JAMA* **286:**1201–1205.

56. **Healy, C. M., K. G. Hulten, D. L. Palazzi, J. R. Campbell, and C. J. Baker.** 2004. Emergence of new strains of methicillin-resistant *Staphylococcus aureus* in a neonatal intensive care unit. *Clin. Infect. Dis.* **39:**1460–1466.

57. **Herold, B. C., L. C. Immergluck, M. C. Maranan, D. S. Lauderdale, R. E. Gaskin, S., Boyle-Vavra, C. D. Leitch, and R. S. Daum.** 1998. Community-acquired methicillin-resistant *Staphylococcus aureus* in children with no identified predisposing risk. *JAMA* **279:**593–598.

58. **Hollis, R. J., J. L. Barr, B. N. Doebbeling, M. A. Pfaller, and R. P. Wenzel.** 1995. Familial carriage of methicillin-resistant *Staphylococcus aureus* and subsequent infection in a premature neonate. *Clin. Infect. Dis.* **21:**328–332.

59. **Hussain, F. M., S. Boyle-Vavra, C. D. Bethel, and R. S. Daum.** 2000. Current trends in community-acquired methicillin-resistant *Staphylococcus aureus* at a tertiary care pediatric facility. *Pediatr. Infect. Dis. J.* **19:**1163–1166.

60. **Hussain, F. M., S. Boyle-Vavra, and R. S. Daum.** 2001. Community-acquired methicillin-resistant *Staphylococcus aureus* colonization in healthy children attending an outpatient pediatric clinic. *Pediatr. Infect. Dis. J.* **20:**763–767.

61. **Ito, T., Y. Katayama, K. Asada, N. Mori, K. Tsutsumimoto, C. Tiensasitorn, and K. Hiramatsu.** 2001. Structural comparison of three types of staphylococcal cassette chromosome *mec* integrated in the chromosome in methicillin-resistant *Staphylococcus aureus*. *Antimicrob. Agents Chemother.* **45:**1323–1336.

62. **Ito, T., K. Okuma, X. X. Ma, H. Yuzawa, and K. Hiramatsu.** 2003. Insights on antibiotic resistance of *Staphylococcus aureus* from its whole genome: genomic island SCC. *Drug Resist. Updates* **6:**41–52.

63. **Iyer, S., and D. H. Jones.** 2004. Community-acquired methicillin-resistant *Staphylococcus aureus* skin infection: a retrospective analysis of clinical presentation and treatment of a local outbreak. *J. Am. Acad. Dermatol.* **50:**854–858.

64. **Jevons, M. P.** 1961. "Celbenin"-resistant staphylococci. *Br. Med. J.* **i:**124.

65. **Kampf, G., R. Jarosch, and H. Ruden.** 1998. Limited effectiveness of chlorhexidine based hand disinfectants against methicillin-resistant *Staphylococcus aureus* (MRSA). *J. Hosp. Infect.* **38:**297–303.

66. **Kampf, G.** 2004. The value of using chlorhexidine soap in a controlled trial to eradicate MRSA in colonized patients. *J. Hosp. Infect.* **58:**86–87.

67. **Kaplan, S. L., S. L. Deville Kaplan, J. G. Deville, R. Yogev, M. R. Morfin, E. Wu, S. Adler, B. Edge-Padbury, S. Naberhuis-Stehouwer, J. B. Bruss, and the Linezolid Pediatric Study Group.** 2003. Linezolid versus vancomycin for treatment of resistant Gram-positive infections in children. *Pediatr. Infect. Dis. J.* **22:**677–686.

68. **Kaplan, S. L.** 2005. Personal communication.

69. **Kaplan, S. L., K. G. Hulten, B. E. Gonzalez, W. A. Hammerman, L. Lamberth, J. Versalovic, and E. O. Mason, Jr.** 2005. Three-year surveillance of community-acquired *Staphylococcus aureus* infections in children. *Clin. Infect. Dis.***40:**1785–1791.

70. **Katayama, Y., F. Takeuchi, T. Ito, X. X. Ma, Y. Ui-Mizutani, I. Kobayashi, and K. Hiramatsu.** 2003. Identification in methicillin-susceptible *Staphylococcus hominis* of an active primordial mobile genetic element for the staphylococcal cassette chromosome *mec* of methicillin-resistant *Staphylococcus aureus*. *J. Bacteriol.* **185:**2711–2722.

71. **Kazakova, S. V., J. C. Hageman, M. Matava, A. Srinivasan, L. Phelan, B. Garfinkel, T. Boo, S. McAllister, J. Anderson, B. Jensen, D. Dodson, D. Lonsway, L. K. McDougal, M. Arduino, V. J. Fraser, G. Killgore, F. C. Tenover, S. Cody, and D. B. Jernigan.** 2005. A clone of methicillin-resistant *Staphylococcus aureus* among professional football players. *N. Engl. J. Med.* **352:**468–475.

72. **Klevens, R. M., J. R. Edwards, F. C. Tenover, L. C. McDonald, T. Horan, R. Gaynes, and the National Nosocomial Infections Surveillance System.** 2006. Changes in the epidemiology of methicillin-resistant *Staphylococcus aureus* in intensive care units in US hospitals, 1992–2003. *Clin. Infect. Dis.* **42:**389–391.

73. **Kravitz, G. R., D. J. Dries, M. L. Peterson, and P. M. Schlievert.** 2005. Purpura fulminans due to *Staphylococcus aureus*. *Clin. Infect. Dis.* **40:**941–947.

74. **Kwon, N. H., D. T. Park, J. S. Moon, W. K. Jung, S. H. Kim, J. M. Kim, S. K. Hong, H. C. Koo, Y. S. Joo, and Y. H. Park.** 2005. Staphylococcal cassette chromosome *mec* (SCC*mec*) characterization and molecular analysis for methicillin-resistant *Staphylococcus aureus* and novel SCC*mec* subtype IVg isolated from bovine milk in Korea. *J. Antimicrob. Chemother.* **56:**624–632.

75. **Lee, M. C., A. M. Rios, M. F. Aten, A. Mejias, D. Cavuoti, G. H, McCracken, Jr., and R. D. Hardy.** 2004. Management and outcome of children with skin and soft tissue abscesses caused by community-acquired methicillin-resistant *Staphylococcus aureus*. *Pediatr. Infect. Dis. J.* **23:**123–127.

76. **Levin, T. P., B. Suh, P. Axelrod, A. L. Truant, and T. Fekete.** 2005. Potential clindamycin resistance in clindamycin-susceptible, erythromycin-resistant *Staphylococcus aureus*: report of a clinical failure. *Antimicrob. Agents Chemother.* **49:**1222–1224.

77. **Levine, D. P., R. D. Cushing, J. Jui, and W. J. Brown.** 1982. Community-acquired MRSA endocarditis in the Detroit Medical Center. *Ann. Intern. Med.* **97:**330–338.

78. **Lina, G., Y. Peimont, F. Godail-Gamot, M. Bes, M. O. Peter, V. Gauduchon, F. Vandenesch, and J. Etienne.** 1999. Involvement of Panton-Valentine leukocidin-producing *Staphylococcus aureus* in primary skin infection and pneumonia. *Clin. Infect. Dis.* **29:**1128–1132.

79. **Lindenmayer, J. M., S. Schoenfeld, R. O'Grady, and J. K. Carney.** 1998. Methicillin-resistant *Staphylococcus aureus* in a high school wrestling team and the surrounding community. *Arch. Intern. Med.* **158:**895–899.

80. **Llera, J. L., and R. C. Levy.** 1985. Treatment of cutaneous abscess: a double-blind clinical study. *Ann. Emerg. Med.* **14:**15–19.

81. **Loeb, M., C. Main, C. Walker-Dilks, and A. Eady.** 2003. Antimicrobial drugs for treating methicillin-resistant *Staphylococcus aureus* colonization. *Cochrane Database Syst. Rev.* **2003**(4):CD003340.

82. **Lowy, F. D.** 1998. *Staphylococcus aureus* infections. *N. Engl. J. Med.* **339:**520–532.

83. **Ma, X. X., T. Ito, C. Tiensasitorn, M. Jamklang, P. Chongtrakool, S. Boyle-Vavra, R. S. Daum, and K. Hiramatsu.** 2002. Novel type of staphylococcal cassette chromosome *mec* identified in community-acquired methicillin-resistant *Staphylococcus aureus* strains. *Antimicrob. Agents Chemother.* **46:**1147–1152.

84. **Maguire, G. P., A. D. Arthur, P. J. Boustead, B. Dwyer, and B. J. Currie.** 1996. Emerging epidemic of community-acquired methicillin-resistant *Staphylococcus aureus* infection in the Northern Territory. *Med. J. Aust.* **164:**721–723.

85. **Maree, C. M., R. S. Daum, S. Boyle-Vavra, K. Matayoshi, and L. G. Miller.** 2005. Rapid temporal increase in community-acquired methicillin-resistant *S. aureus* strains causing nosocomial infections. Presented at the Interscience Conference on Antimicrobial Agents and Chemotherapy, Washington, D.C., December 2005.

86. **Markowitz, N., E. L. Quinn, and L. D. Saravolatz.** 1992. Trimethoprim-sulfamethoxazole compared with vancomycin for the treatment of *Staphylococcus aureus* infection. *Ann. Intern. Med.* **117:**390–398.

87. **Martinez-Aguilar, G., W. A. Hammerman, E. O. Mason, Jr., and S. L. Kaplan.** 2003. Clindamycin treatment of invasive infections caused by community-acquired, methicillin-resistant, and methicillin-susceptible *Staphylococcus aureus* in children. *Pediatr. Infect. Dis. J.* **22:**593–598.

88. **McDougal, L. K., C. D. Steward, G. E. Killgore, J. M. Chaitram, S. K. McAllister, and F. C. Tenover.** 2003. Pulsed-field gel electrophoresis typing of oxacillin-resistant *Staphylococcus aureus* isolates from the United States: establishing a national database. *J. Clin. Microbiol.* **41:**5113–5120.

89. **Melles, D. C., R. F. Gorkink, H. A. Boelens, S. D. Snijders, J. K. Peeters, M. J. Moorhouse, P. J. van der Spek, W. B. van Leeuwen, G. Simons, H. A. Verbrugh, and A. van Belkum.** 2004. Natural population dynamics and expansion of pathogenic clones of *Staphylococcus aureus*. *J. Clin. Investig.* **114:**1732–1740.

90. **Miller, M. A., A. Dascal, J. Portnoy, and J. Mendelson.** 1996. Development of mupirocin resistance among methicillin-resistant *Staphylococcus aureus* after widespread use of nasal mupirocin ointment. *Infect. Control Hosp. Epidemiol.* **17:**811–813.

91. **Miller, L. G., F. Perdreau-Remington, G. Rieg, S. Mehdi, J. Perlroth, A. S. Bayer, A. W. Tang, T. O. Phung, and B. Spellberg.** 2005. Necrotizing fasciitis caused by community-associated methicillin-resistant *Staphylococcus aureus* in Los Angeles. *N. Engl. J. Med.* **352:**1445–1453.

92. **Mishaan, A. M., E. O. Mason, Jr., G. Martinez-Aguilar, W. Hammerman, J. J. Propst, J. R. Lupski, P. Stankiewicz, S. L. Kaplan, and K. Hulten.** 2005. Emergence of a predominant clone of community-acquired *Staphylococcus aureus* among children in Houston, Texas. *Pediatr. Infect. Dis. J.* **24:**201–206.

93. **Mongkolrattanothai, K., S. Boyle, M. D. Kahana, and R. S. Daum.** 2003. Severe *Staphylococcus aureus* infections caused by clonally related community-acquired methicillin-susceptible and methicillin-resistant isolates. *Clin. Infect. Dis.* **37:**1050–1058.

94. **Mongkolrattanothai, K., S. Boyle, T. V. Murphy, and R. S. Daum.** 2004. Novel non-*mecA*-containing staphylococcal chromosomal cassette composite island containing *pbp4* and *tagF* genes in a commensal staphylococcal species: a possible reservoir for antibiotic resistance islands in *Staphylococcus aureus*. *Antimicrob. Agents Chemother.* **48:**1823–1836.

95. **Moreno, F., C. Crisp, J. H. Jorgensen, and J. E. Patterson.** 1995. Methicillin-resistant *Staphylococcus aureus* as a community organism. *Clin. Infect. Dis.* **21:**1308–1312.

96. **Naimi, T. S., K. H. LeDell, D. J. Boxrud, A. V. Groom, C. D. Steward, S. K. Johnson, J. M. Besse, C. O'Boyle, R. N. Danila, J. E. Cheek, M. T. Osterholm, K. A. Moore, and K. E. Smith.** 2001. Epidemiology and clonality of community-acquired methicillin-resistant *Staphylococcus aureus* in Minnesota, 1996–1998. *Clin. Infect. Dis.* **33:**990–996.

97. **Naimi, T. S., K. H. LeDell, K. Como-Sabetti, S. M. Borchardt, D. J. Boxrud, J. Etienne, S. K. Johnson, F. Vandenesch, S. Fridkin, C. O'Boyle, R. N. Danila, and R. Lynfield.** 2003. Comparison of community- and health care-associated methicillin-resistant *Staphylococcus aureus* infection. *JAMA* **290:**2976–2984.

98. **Narita, S., J. Kaneko, J. Chiba, Y. Piemont, S. Jarraud, J. Etienne, and Y. Kamio.** 2001. Phage conversion of Panton-Valentine leukocidin in *Staphylococcus aureus*: molecular analysis of a PVL-converting phage, phiSLT. *Gene* **268:**195–206.

99. **NCCLS.** 2004. *Performance Standards for Antimicrobial Susceptibility Testing: 12th Informational Supplement.* NCCLS document M100-S14. NCCLS, Wayne, Pa.

100. **Nguyen, D. M., L. Mascola, and E. Brancoft.** 2005. Recurring methicillin-resistant *Staphylococcus aureus* infections in a football team. *Emerg. Infect. Dis.* **11:**526–532.

101. **Nichols, R. L., D. R. Graham, S. L. Barriere, A. Rodgers, S. E. Wilson, M. Zervos, D. L. Dunn, B. Kreter, et al.** 1999. Treatment of hospitalized patients with complicated gram-positive skin and skin structure infections: two randomized, multicentre studies of quinupristin/dalfopristin versus cefazolin, oxacillin or vancomycin. *J. Antimicrob. Chemother.* **44:**263–273.

102. **O'Brien, F. G., J. W. Pearman, M. Gracey, T. V. Riley, and W. B. Grubb.** 1999. Community strain of methicillin-resistant *Staphylococcus aureus* involved in a hospital outbreak. *J. Clin. Microbiol.* **37:** 2858–2862.

103. **Okuma, K., K. Iwakawa, J. D. Turnidge, W. B. Grubb, J. M. Bell, F. G. O'Brien, G. W. Coombs, J. W. Pearman, F. C. Tenover, M. Kapi, C. Tiensasitorn, T. Ito, and K. Hiramatsu.** 2002. Dissemination of new methicillin-resistant *Staphylococcus aureus* clones in the community. *J. Clin. Microbiol.* **40:** 4289–4294.

104. **Oliveira, D. C., A. Tomasz, and H. de Lencastre.** 2001. The evolution of pandemic clones of methicillin-resistant *Staphylococcus aureus*: identification of two ancestral genetic backgrounds and the associated *mec* elements. *Microb. Drug Resist.* **7:**349–361.

105. **Pan, E. S., B. A. Diep, H. A. Carleton, E. D. Charlebois, G. F. Sensabaugh, B. L. Haller, and F. Perdreau-Remington.** 2003. Increasing prevalence of methicillin-resistant *Staphylococcus aureus* infection in California jails. *Clin. Infect. Dis.* **37:**1384–1388.

106. **Panton, P. N., and F. C. O. Valentine.** 1932. Staphylococcal toxin. *Lancet* **i:**506–508.

107. **Peacock, J. E., Jr., F. J. Marsik, and R. P. Wenzel.** 1980. Methicillin-resistant *Staphylococcus aureus*: introduction and spread within a hospital. *Ann. Intern. Med.* **93:**526–532.

108. **Perl, T. M., J. J. Cullen, R. P. Wenzel, M. B. Zimmerman, M. A. Pfaller, D. Sheppard, J. Twombley, P. P. French, L. A. Herwaldt, and the Mupirocin and the Risk of *Staphylococcus aureus* Study Team.** 2002. Intranasal mupirocin to prevent postoperative *Staphylococcus aureus* infections. *N. Engl. J. Med.* **346:**1871–1877.

109. **Pinho, M. G., H. de Lencastre, and A. Tomasz.** 2001. An acquired and a native penicillin-binding protein cooperate in building the cell wall of drug-resistant staphylococci. *Proc. Natl. Acad. Sci. USA* **98:** 10886–10891.

110. **Prevost, G., P. Couppie, P. Prevost, S. Gayet, P. Petiau, B. Cribier, H. Monteil, and Y. Piemont.** 1995. Epidemiological data on *Staphylococcus aureus* strains producing synergohymenotropic toxins. *J. Med. Microbiol.* **42:**237–245.

111. **Purcell, K., and J. E. Fergie.** 2002. Exponential increase in community-acquired methicillin-resistant *Staphylococcus aureus* infections in South Texas children. *Pediatr. Infect. Dis. J.* **21:**988–999.

112. **Purcell, K., and J. Fergie.** Epidemic of community-acquired MRSA infections: a 13-year study at Driscoll Children's Hospital, abstr. 484. Presented at the annual meeting of the Infectious Diseases Society of America, 2004.

113. **Rammelkamp, C. H., and T. Maxon.** 1942. Resistance of *Staphylococcus aureus* to the action of penicillin. *Proc. Soc. Exp. Biol. Med.* **51:**386.

114. **Riley, T. V., and I. L. Rouse.** 1995. Methicillin-resistant *Staphylococcus aureus* in Western Australia, 1983–1992. *J. Hosp. Infect.* **29:**177–188.

115. **Robinson, D. A., and M. C. Enright.** 2003. Evolutionary models of the emergence of methicillin-resistant *Staphylococccus aureus*. *Antimicrob. Agents Chemother.* **47:**3926–3934.

116. **Ruhe, J. J., T. Monson, R. W. Bradsher, and A. Menon.** 2005. Use of long-acting tetracyclines for methicillin-resistant *Staphylococcus aureus* infections: case series and review of the literature. *Clin. Infect. Dis.* **40:**1429–1434.

117. **Ruiz, M. E., I. C. Guerrero, and C. U. Tuazon.** 2002. Endocarditis caused by methicillin-resistant *Staphylococcus aureus*: treatment failure with linezolid. *Clin. Infect. Dis.* **35:**1018–1020.

118. **Salgado, C. D., B. M. Farr, and D. P. Calfee.** 2003. Community-acquired methicillin-resistant *Staphylococcus aureus*: a meta-analysis of prevalence and risk factors. *Clin. Infect. Dis.* **36:**131–139.

119. **Saravolatz, L. D., N. Markowitz, L. Arking, D. Pohlod, and E. Fisher.** 1982. MRSA: epidemiologic observations during a community-acquired outbreak. *Ann. Intern. Med.* **96:**11–16.

120. **Saravolatz, L. D., D. J. Pohlod, and L. M. Arking.** 1982. Community-acquired methicillin-resistant *Staphylococcus aureus* infections: a new source for nosocomial outbreaks. *Ann. Intern. Med.* **97:**325–329.

121. **Schlievert, P. M.** 2001. Use of intravenous immunoglobulin in the treatment of staphylococcal and streptococcal toxic shock syndromes and related illnesses. *J. Allergy Clin. Immunol.* **108:**S107–S110.

122. **Shahin, R., I. L. Johnson, F. Jamieson, A. McGeer, J. Tolkin, E. L. Ford-Jones, et al.** 1999. Methicillin-resistant *Staphylococcus aureus* carriage in a child care center following a case of disease. *Arch. Pediatr. Adolesc. Med.* **153:**864–868.

123. **Shore, A., A. S. Rossney, C. T. Keane, M. C. Enright, and D. C. Coleman.** 2005. Seven novel variants of the staphylococcal chromosomal cassette *mec* in methicillin-resistant *Staphylococcus aureus* isolates from Ireland. *Antimicrob. Agents Chemother.* **49:**2070–2083.

124. **Smith, T. L., M. L. Pearson, K. R. Wilcox, C. Cruz, M. V. Lancaster, B. Robinson-Dunn, F. C. Tenover, M. J. Zervos, J. D. Band, E. White, W. R. Jarvis, et al.** 1999. Emergence of vancomycin resistance in *Staphylococcus aureus*. *N. Engl. J. Med.* **340:**493–501.

125. **Suggs, A. H., M. C. Maranan, S. Boyle-Vavra, and R. S. Daum.** 1999. Methicillin-resistant and borderline methicillin-resistant asymptomatic *Staphylococcus aureus* colonization in children without identifiable risk factors. *Pediatr. Infect. Dis. J.* **18:**410–414.

126. **Thompson, R. L., I. Cabezudo, and R. P. Wenzel.** 1982. Epidemiology of nosocomial infections caused by methicillin-resistant *Staphylococcus aureus*. *Ann. Intern. Med.* **97:**309–317.

127. **Vandenesch, F., T. Naimi, M. C. Enright, G. Lina, G. R. Nimmo, H. Heffernan, N. Liassine, M. Bes, T. Greenland, M. E. Reverdy, and J. Etienne.** 2003. Community-acquired methicillin-resistant *Staphylococcus aureus* carrying Panton-Valentine leukocidin genes: worldwide emergence. *Emerg. Infect. Dis.* **9:**978–984.

128. **Whitener, C. J., S. Y. Park, F. A. Browne, L. J. Parent, K. Julian, B. Bozdogan, P. C. Appelbaum, J. Chaitram, L. M. Weigel, J. Jernigan, L. K. McDougal, F. C. Tenover, and S. K. Fridkin.** 2004. Vancomycin-resistant *Staphylococcus aureus* in the absence of vancomycin exposure. *Clin. Infect. Dis.* **38:**1049–1055.

129. **Williams, R. E. O.** 1963. Healthy carriage of *Staphylococcus aureus*: its prevalence and importance. *Bacteriol. Rev.* **27:**56–71.

130. **Wisplinghoff, H., A. E. Rosato, M. C. Enright, M. Noto, W. Craig, and G. L. Archer.** 2003. Related clones containing SCC*mec* type IV predominate among clinically significant *Staphylococcus epidermidis* isolates. *Antimicrob. Agents Chemother.* **47:**3574–3579.

131. **Yogev, R., L. E. Patterson, S. L. Kaplan, M. R. Morfin, A. Martin, B. Edge-Padbury, S. Naberhuis-Stehouwer, and J. B. Bruss.** 2003. Linezolid for the treatment of complicated skin and skin structure infections in children. *Pediatr. Infect. Dis. J.* **22**(Suppl. 9):S172–S177.

132. **Yoshida, R., K. Kuwahara-Arai, T. Baba, L. C. Cui, J. F. Richardson, and K. Hiramatsu.** 2003. Physiological and molecular analysis of a *mecA*-negative *Staphylococcus aureus* clinical strain that expresses heterogeneous methicillin resistance. *J. Antimicrob. Chemother.* **51:**247–255.

133. **Young, D. M., H. W. Harris, E. D. Charlebois, H. Chambers, A. Campbell, F. Pedreau-Remington, C. Lee, M. Mankani, R. Mackersie, and W. P. Schecter.** 2004. An epidemic of methicillin-resistant *Staphylococcus aureus* soft tissue infections among medically underserved patients. *Arch. Surg.* **139:**947–953.

134. **Zhang, H. Z., C. J. Hackbarth, K. M. Chansky, and H. F. Chambers.** 2001. A proteolytic transmembrane signaling pathway and resistance to beta-lactams in staphylococci. *Science* **291:**1962–1965.

135. **Zinderman, C. E., B. Conner, M. A. Malakooti, J. E. LaMar, A. Armstrong, and B. K. Bohnker.** 2004. Community-acquired methicillin-resistant *Staphylococcus aureus* among military recruits. *Emerg. Infect. Dis.* **10:**941–944.

Emerging Infections 7
Edited by W. M. Scheld, D. C. Hooper, and J. M. Hughes
© 2007 ASM Press, Washington, D.C.

Chapter 10

Carbapenem Resistance in *Klebsiella pneumoniae* and Other Members of the Family *Enterobacteriaceae*

Simona Bratu and John Quale

Bacteria belonging to the family *Enterobacteriaceae* are important nosocomial pathogens. In intensive-care areas, *Klebsiella pneumoniae* and *Enterobacter* spp. are frequent causes of respiratory tract, urinary tract, and bloodstream infections (57, 64). Over the past 2 decades, *K. pneumoniae* possessing extended-spectrum β-lactamases (ESBLs), which confer resistance to cephalosporins and aztreonam, have emerged (10). In several large series, cephalosporin resistance in *K. pneumoniae* ranged from approximately 11 to 34% (20, 27, 53, 58). Data from the National Nosocomial Infections Surveillance indicate that ~20% of *K. pneumoniae* isolates collected in 2004 were resistant to third-generation cephalosporins, a 47% increase from the preceding 5-year period (12). Many of the ESBL-possessing *K. pneumoniae* isolates are also resistant to fluoroquinolones and aminoglycosides (20, 27, 53), limiting therapeutic options. In large surveillance studies, carbapenem-resistant *K. pneumoniae* isolates were exceedingly unusual (20, 27, 53, 58), and carbapenems have been considered the recommended agents for therapy of severe infections due to these pathogens.

Enterobacteriaceae with reduced susceptibility to carbapenems are an emerging, worldwide problem. In most cases, the reduced carbapenem susceptibility is attributable to acquisition of one of a variety of β-lactamases with carbapenem-hydrolyzing properties.

β-LACTAMASES ASSOCIATED WITH RESISTANCE TO CARBAPENEMS IN *ENTEROBACTERIACEAE*

Class C β-Lactamases

Resistance to carbapenems in enteric gram-negative bacilli can arise from a variety of mechanisms. Several reports have documented carbapenem resistance in *Enterobacter* spp. due to production of the chromosomal class C β-lactamase coupled with diminished permeability (9, 13, 16, 31, 55, 69). Since the chromosomal β-lactamase in *Enterobacter*

Simona Bratu and John Quale • Division of Infectious Diseases, SUNY Downstate Medical Center, Brooklyn, NY 11203.

spp. can hydrolyze imipenem only slowly, decreasing the entry of carbapenems into the periplasmic space is essential for the development of high-level resistance (9). In several studies, carbapenem susceptibility was restored once the selective pressure of imipenem was removed (2, 31, 69). Rare isolates of *Proteus mirabilis* (38, 61), *Providencia rettgeri* (55), and *Citrobacter freundii* (36) have been noted to be carbapenem resistant. Resistance in these isolates was attributed to a combination of increased β-lactamase production and reduced porin expression, although altered penicillin-binding proteins may also have been contributory (61).

The combination of β-lactamases and porin changes has also been documented as an important factor in carbapenem-resistant *K. pneumoniae* (4, 11, 15, 37). Isolates of *K. pneumoniae* that acquired a class C β-lactamase and lost a 40- to 42-kDa outer membrane protein have been noted to have reduced imipenem susceptibility (4, 11, 37). Two major porins have been described in *K. pneumoniae*, OmpK35 and OmpK36 (21). Loss of OmpK35 has been noted in ESBL-possessing *K. pneumoniae* (21). The expression of the β-lactamase SHV-2, along with diminished OmpK36 production, was demonstrated to adversely affect the MIC of imipenem (15, 37); restoration of OmpK36 was associated with a reduction in the MICs of imipenem and meropenem (37). This porin was also important in restoring cefepime and cefoxitin susceptibilities in ESBL producers but had no effect on ceftazidime (37). A third porin, OmpK37, may be important for the entry of carbapenem antibiotics, but it is not typically expressed in most clinical isolates (17).

Class B Metallo-β-Lactamases

Carbapenem resistance can be mediated by the acquisition of carbapenem-hydrolyzing β-lactamases. The class B metallo-β-lactamases are capable of hydrolyzing virtually all β-lactams (with the exception of aztreonam) and require the presence of zinc cations at their active site. Two major classes of metallo-β-lactamases have been identified: the IMP and the VIM families. Metallo-β-lactamases have been especially problematic in areas of eastern Asia and southern Europe and have been most frequently encountered in isolates of *Pseudomonas aeruginosa* and *Acinetobacter baumannii* (25, 32, 59, 60). For example, in Korea, VIM-type enzymes in *P. aeruginosa* and IMP and VIM enzymes in *A. baumannii* have been recovered (32). While clonal spread of *P. aeruginosa* and *A. baumannii* strains carrying VIM β-lactamases has been documented, multiple strains of *A. baumannii* with IMP metallo-β-lactamases were found (32). The experience involving the spread of metallo-β-lactamases in southern Europe parallels that in eastern Asia. In Italy, 6.5% of all *P. aeruginosa* isolates were found to be carrying either VIM or IMP metallo-β-lactamases (60). Different *P. aeruginosa* strains possessed multiple integrons, indicating increased mobility of these β-lactamases (60). Several reports have documented the spread of metallo-β-lactamases to other gram-negative bacilli, including *Enterobacteriaceae*.

In Japan, IMP enzymes have been recovered from isolates of *Serratia marcescens* and *Enterobacter* spp. and conferred resistance to ceftazidime and imipenem (Table 1) (25, 29, 59). Occasional isolates of *K. pneumoniae* carrying IMP metallo-β-lactamases have also been recovered in Japan (29, 59). In another investigation, 1.2% of over 3,000 isolates of *K. pneumoniae* in Taiwan possessed bla_{IMP-8} (68). One report from Australia documented the presence of bla_{IMP-4} in *K. pneumoniae* and *Escherichia coli* isolates with reduced

Table 1. Class B metallo-β-lactamases found in *Enterobacteriaceae*

Bacterium	β-Lactamase	No. of isolates	Location	Reference
S. marcescens	IMP	9	Japan	59
	IMP-1, IMP-11	4	Japan	25
	IMP-1	144	Japan	29
Enterobacter spp.	IMP-1	NS^a	Japan	29
	IMP-8	20	Taiwan	67
	VIM-4	1	Italy	35
K. pneumoniae	IMP	1	Japan	59
	IMP-1	1	Singapore	28
	IMP-4	1	Australia	50
	IMP-8	17	Taiwan	68
	VIM-4	1	Italy	35
E. coli	IMP-1	NS	Japan	29
	IMP-4	1	Australia	50
	VIM-1	1	Greece	39
C. freundii	IMP-1	NS	Japan	29
	VIM-2	1	Taiwan	67

^{a}NS, not stated.

susceptibility to carbapenems (50). Finally, a single isolate of *K. pneumoniae* with $bla_{\text{IMP-1}}$ was reported from Singapore (28).

Metallo-β-lactamases belonging to the VIM group have also been found in *Enterobacteriaceae* (Table 1). In Taiwan, approximately 3% of *Enterobacter cloacae* isolates had $bla_{\text{IMP-8}}$ and 0.3% of *C. freundii* isolates had $bla_{\text{VIM-2}}$ (67). Identification of $bla_{\text{VIM-4}}$ in isolates of *K. pneumoniae* and *E. cloacae* from a patient in Italy has been reported (35). Finally, an isolate of *E. coli* from Greece was found to possess VIM-1; this isolate also possessed a class C β-lactamase (39).

The presence of metallo-β-lactamases in *Enterobacteriaceae* has not always been associated with overt carbapenem resistance (unlike many *P. aeruginosa* or *A. baumannii* isolates with metallo-β-lactamases). For example, all of the isolates of *E. cloacae* with $bla_{\text{IMP-8}}$ from Taiwan were susceptible to imipenem and meropenem (67). In addition, of 17 $bla_{\text{IMP-8}}$-positive *K. pneumoniae* isolates collected in Taiwan (68), only 2 were resistant to carbapenems. The *E. coli* transconjugants with $bla_{\text{IMP-8}}$ also remained susceptible to carbapenems (68). Similarly, an *E. coli* transformant with $bla_{\text{IMP-4}}$ had an increase in the MIC of imipenem from 0.38 to only 1.5 μg/ml (14), and an *E. coli* transformant with $bla_{\text{IMP-1}}$ had an MIC of imipenem of 2 μg/ml (28). One isolate of *K. pneumoniae* with $bla_{\text{IMP-1}}$ was found to show confluent growth below an imipenem concentration of 3 μg/ml and scattered colonies up to 32 μg/ml (28). Both variants possessed similar imipenem-hydrolyzing activities; however, the highly resistant variant lacked a 39-kDa outer membrane protein (28).

Similar observations have been noted for *Enterobacteriaceae* with VIM β-lactamases. The *E. coli* clinical isolate from Greece with $bla_{\text{VIM-1}}$ had imipenem and meropenem MICs of 8 and 2 μg/ml, respectively (39); this isolate carried an AmpC-type β-lactamase ($bla_{\text{CMY-2}}$) as well. The isolates of *K. pneumoniae* and *E. cloacae* with $bla_{\text{VIM-4}}$ had imipenem MICs in the susceptible range, although the MIC increased when a higher in-oculum was employed (35).

The spread of metallo-β-lactamases to *Enterobacteriaceae* clearly poses a challenge for detection, since carbapenem resistance may not be evident. How the presence of these enzymes in *Enterobacteriaceae* with carbapenem MICs in the susceptible range affects the utility of carbapenem therapy remains unknown.

Class A and D β-Lactamases

As with the class C β-lactamases, the class A and D β-lactamases belong to the serine group of enzymes because they possess a serine moiety at the active site. Several groups of the class D OXA-type β-lactamases have been found to possess carbapenem-hydrolyzing properties (49). The first group consists of the closely related OXA-23 and OXA-27; the second cluster includes OXA-24, -25, -26, and -40. Most isolates carrying these enzymes have been *A. baumannii* from patients in Europe and Brazil (49). A unique carbapenem-hydrolyzing enzyme, OXA-48, has been recovered in a carbapenem-resistant strain of *K. pneumoniae* from Turkey (47). This isolate also carried other β-lactamases and lacked a 36-kDa outer membrane protein, all contributing to high-level β-lactam resistance.

A few class A β-lactamases have been found to possess hydrolytic activity against carbapenems (Table 2). Sme-1 was first identified from an isolate of *S. marcescens* in London

Table 2. Class A carbapenem-hydrolyzing β-lactamases found in *Enterobacteriaceae*

Bacterium	β-Lactamase(s)	No. of isolates	Location(s)	Reference(s)
S. marcescens	Sme-1	1	England	44
	Sme-1, Sme-2	25	Minnesota, California, Massachusetts	54
Enterobacter spp.	IMI-1	2	California	56
	NmcA	1	France	45
	NmcA	1	Washington State	52
	KPC-2	4	Massachusetts	24
	KPC-2, KPC-3	3	New York	5
K. pneumoniae	GES-4	1	Greece	62
	KPC-1	1	North Carolina	70
	KPC-2	4	Maryland	41, 42
	KPC-2	18	New York	3
	KPC-2	29	New York	6
	KPC-2, KPC-3	62	New York	8
	KPC-3	24	New York	65
K. oxytoca	KPC-2	1	New York	71
	KPC-2	1	New York	3
E. coli	KPC-3	7	New Jersey	23
S. enterica	KPC-2	1	Maryland	40

in 1985, before clinical use of carbapenems became widespread (44). Sme-1 and Sme-2 were subsequently recovered from carbapenem-resistant isolates of *S. marcescens* from several cities in the United States (54), but to date, there have been no further reports of these enzymes. These isolates were resistant to imipenem but not to ceftazidime (44, 54). A second β-lactamase, IMI-1, was detected in two clinical isolates of *E. cloacae* from patients hospitalized in California in 1984 (56). These isolates were resistant to imipenem but not to meropenem or ceftazidime (56). A third enzyme, NmcA, has been recovered from isolates of *E. cloacae* from Europe (43, 45) and North America (52). The β-lactamases NmcA and IMI-1 and their regulatory genes were closely related, and both preferentially hydrolyzed imipenem (45, 56). Another enzyme, GES-2, was found in a single isolate of *P. aeruginosa* from South Africa (51). One clinical isolate of *K. pneumoniae* harboring the GES-4 β-lactamase has been identified from Greece (62). This isolate exhibited high-level resistance to most β-lactam antibiotics, including extended-spectrum cephalosporins, carbapenems, and aztreonam. In addition, it was resistant to other non-β-lactam antibiotics, including aminoglycosides, trimethoprim, sulfonamides, and tetracyclines (62).

Enterobacteriaceae carrying KPC β-lactamases are emerging and pose serious challenges to therapy. To date, only members of the family *Enterobacteriaceae* have been found to possess KPC-type β-lactamases. The first of these enzymes to be recognized, KPC-1, was recovered from an isolate of *K. pneumoniae* in North Carolina (70). The imipenem and meropenem MICs for this isolate were 16 µg/ml, and susceptibility to imipenem was restored with the addition of clavulanic acid, a property characteristic of class A β-lactamases (70). In addition to carbapenems, this isolate was resistant to cephalosporins, aztreonam, and penicillins.

Soon after the initial description of KPC-1, reports documenting isolates with KPC-2 surfaced. KPC-2 differs from KPC-1 by a single amino acid change. Four unrelated strains of *K. pneumoniae* from Baltimore, Maryland, collected from 1998 to 1999 were found to possess KPC-2 (41, 42). An imipenem-resistant isolate of *Salmonella enterica*, also from Maryland in 1998, was found to carry KPC-2 (40). A strain of *Klebsiella oxytoca*, isolated from a patient in New York in 1998, possessed KPC-2 and was resistant to carbapenems and cephalosporins (71). From 1997 to 2002, sporadic isolates of *K. pneumoniae* and *K. oxytoca* with KPC-2 were identified in various hospitals in New York City (3); the imipenem MICs for these isolates ranged from 4 to >64 µg/ml. By 2003 to 2004, hospital-wide outbreaks involving KPC-2-possessing *K. pneumoniae* isolates were reported in New York City (6). In one survey conducted in 2004, 24% of *K. pneumoniae* isolates from four New York City hospitals were found to carry KPC enzymes (8).

Isolates of *Enterobacter* spp. carrying KPC-2 have been recovered in Boston (24) and New York City (5). Recently, strains of *E. cloacae* and *E. coli* from a patient in France have also been found to have KPC-2 (S. Petrella, M. Renard, R. Bismuth, L. Bodin, V. Jarlier, and W. Sougakoff, *Abstr. 13th Eur. Congr. Clin. Microbiol. Infect. Dis.*, abstr. O288, 2003). Both of these isolates had reduced susceptibility to imipenem, and neither possessed a plasmid encoding the KPC β-lactamase.

A third related enzyme, KPC-3, differs from KPC-2 by a single amino acid change. An outbreak of *K. pneumoniae* with KPC-3 occurred from 2000 to 2001 in one New York City hospital (65). The imipenem MICs for these isolates ranged from 2 to 16 µg/ml, and all were resistant to cephalosporins (65). KPC-3 was also identified in isolates of *K. pneumoniae* in other hospitals in New York City (8). KPC-3 has been identified in a small number of isolates of *E. cloacae* (5) and *E. coli* (23).

As with *Enterobacteriaceae* possessing metallo-β-lactamases, the presence of a KPC-type enzyme does not always result in carbapenem resistance. None of the four isolates of *K. pneumoniae* with bla_{KPC-2} collected in Baltimore (42) were frankly resistant to carbapenems, but they did have uncharacteristically elevated MICs to these antibiotics (~1 to 8 μg/ml). Other isolates of *K. pneumoniae* (3, 6, 8) and some *Enterobacter* spp. (5, 24) with bla_{KPC-2} have been reported with carbapenem MICs below the breakpoint for resistance. Also, *E. coli* transformants often have MICs of imipenem that remain in the susceptible range (24, 40, 65).

KPC-possessing bacteria that do have high-level carbapenem resistance frequently have additional factors contributing to their resistance. *Klebsiella* spp. with bla_{KPC-2} also had other β-lactamases (3), including TEM-1, SHV-1, SHV-7, SHV-12, and inhibitor-resistant TEM-30. The imipenem-resistant isolate of *K. pneumoniae* with bla_{KPC-1} underexpressed the outer membrane porin OmpK35 (70), a characteristic of some ESBL-possessing *K. pneumoniae* isolates (21). This isolate (70) also possessed other β-lactamases (TEM-1 and SHV-29). The *K. pneumoniae* isolates with bla_{KPC-3} were also found to lack the OmpK35 porin (65). However, not all *Klebsiella* spp. with bla_{KPC} have obvious porin defects (6, 71), although other β-lactamases (e.g., TEM-1, SHV-11, and SHV-46) have been present.

BIOCHEMICAL AND KINETIC PROPERTIES OF THE CARBAPENEM-HYDROLYZING ENZYMES

The class B metallo-β-lactamases hydrolyze carbapenems, cephalosporins, and penicillins but do not hydrolyze monobactams. They are not inhibited by clavulanic acid, sulbactam, or tazobactam but are inhibited by EDTA and thiol compounds. Kinetic data for several important carbapenem-hydrolyzing β-lactamases are listed in Table 3. Carbapenems have been noted to be good substrates for IMP (14, 30) and VIM (19, 48) β-lactamases, with hydrolytic efficiencies (k_{cat}/K_m) typically greater for imipenem than for meropenem. Kinetic data for OXA-48, found in a clinical isolate of *K. pneumoniae* from Turkey, demonstrated greater hydrolytic activity against carbapenems than other class D carbapenem-hydrolyzing enzymes (47). The activity of OXA-48 was inhibited by NaCl and only weakly inhibited by clavulanic acid, tazobactam, and sulbactam (47).

Characterization studies of KPC-1 (70) and KPC-2 (71) have demonstrated the highest k_{cat} values for cephaloridine. Hydrolysis of imipenem is 25 to 35 times slower than for cephaloridine, and hydrolysis of meropenem is slower than that of imipenem (70, 71). Both KPC enzymes had the greatest affinity for meropenem, and the hydrolytic efficiencies of imipenem and meropenem were approximately 30% of that for cephaloridine. Cefoxitin and ceftazidime had the lowest rates of hydrolysis (70, 71). Compared to another class A carbapenem-hydrolyzing β-lactamase, Sme-1, KPC-1 possess a serine-to-threonine amino acid change at position 237 (70). This amino acid substitution may explain the lower imipenem hydrolysis rate but greater activity against cephalosporins observed with KPC-1 (70). Clavulanic acid and tazobactam both inhibited KPC-1 and KPC-2, with tazobactam a better inhibitor (70, 71).

Table 3. Kinetic parameters of various carbapenem-hydrolyzing β-lactamases

β-Lactamase	K_m (μM)				k_{cat}/K_m (μM^{-1} s^{-1})				Reference
	Penicillin	Ceftazidime	Imipenem	Meropenem	Penicillin	Ceftazidime	Imipenem	Meropenem	
IMP-1	520	44	39	10	0.62	0.18	1.2	0.12	30
IMP-4	365	28	42	12	NR	NR	NR	NR	14
VIM-1	841	794	1.5	48	0.034	0.076	1.3	0.27	19
VIM-2	49	98	10	5	1.14	0.9	0.99	0.28	48
OXA-48	40	5,100	14	200	6.1	0.001	0.145	0.0005	47
Sme-1	16.7	NR^a	202	13.4	1.16	NR	0.52	0.66	54
Sme-2	17.7	NR	313	9.6	1.2	NR	0.44	0.76	54
IMI-1	64	270	170	26	0.56	0.000024	0.52	0.38	56
KPC-1	23	94	81	12	1.4	0.001	0.15	0.25	70
KPC-2	27	NR	51	15	1.9	NR	0.29	0.27	71

^{a}NR, not reported.

GENETIC ARRANGEMENTS ASSOCIATED WITH
CARBAPENEM-HYDROLYZING β-LACTAMASES

Most of the metallo-β-lactamases have been located on integrons and plasmids, which facilitates their transmission among gram-negative bacteria (49). When other resistance genes are incorporated into the integron, an efficient package encoding multidrug resistance develops.

For example, in geographically distinct locations in Italy, *P. aeruginosa* isolates carrying integron-associated bla_{VIM-1} and bla_{IMP-13} have been recovered (60). Other resistance gene cassettes (*aacA4* and *aadA1*) were found within the integrons in some of the isolates (60). Isolates of *E. coli* and *K. pneumoniae* had a 150-kb plasmid harboring a class 1 integron with bla_{IMP-4}; bla_{TEM-1} and bla_{SHV-12} were on separate plasmids in the *E. coli* and the *K. pneumoniae* isolates (50). Similarly, bla_{IMP} genes from different genera of bacteria in Japan were found associated with an integrase gene and with an aminoglycoside-modifying gene (59).

The metallo-β-lactamases belonging to the VIM family have also resided on integrons, frequently with other resistance gene cassettes (48, 49). A bla_{VIM-2} gene from *P. aeruginosa* resided within a class 1 integron on a 45-kb plasmid that also conferred resistance to sulfonamides (48). An isolate of *E. coli* possessed a bla_{VIM-1} gene that was part of a class 1 integron on a 50-kb plasmid (39). Included in the integron were the gene cassettes *aacA7*, *aadA*, and *dhfrI*, encoding resistance to aminoglycosides and trimethoprim (39).

Most OXA-type enzymes that possess carbapenem-hydrolyzing properties are also within class 1 integrons (49). The bla_{OXA-48} enzyme found in *K. pneumoniae* (47) was on a 70-kb plasmid but was not integron associated; however, it did possess an insertion sequence that included a promoter for gene expression.

In an isolate of *K. pneumoniae*, the genetic sequence for bla_{GES-4} was carried within a class 1 integron on an 80-kb conjugative plasmid (62). Also located in this integron was the aminoglycoside resistance gene *aacA4* (62).

Genes encoding KPC β-lactamases are also frequently identified on transmissible elements, occasionally with other resistance genes. The bla_{KPC-1} gene resided on a 50-kb plasmid (70). Unlike the other class A carbapenem-hydrolyzing genes bla_{Sme-1} (44), bla_{IMI-1} (56), and bla_{Nmc-A} (43), bla_{KPC-1} did not appear to have a positive LysR regulatory gene in its vicinity (70). No other resistance genes were identified on the plasmid with bla_{KPC-1}. Upstream from bla_{KPC-1} were alterations in the proposed promoter region, suggesting involvement of alternative transcription factors (70).

An isolate of *S. enterica* (40) harbored bla_{KPC-2} on a plasmid that also conferred resistance to streptomycin, trimethoprim, and sulfonamides. The flanking regions encoded proteins associated with putative transposases (40). Similarly, *K. oxytoca* carried bla_{KPC-2} that resided on a 70-kb conjugative plasmid (71). This plasmid also had genes that encoded four other β-lactamases and resistance to gentamicin and tobramycin (71). Located upstream from this bla_{KPC-2} was an insertion sequence that could stimulate transposase- and cointegrase-associated reactions (71). The similar flanking genetic sequences in *S. enterica* and *K. oxytoca* suggest that bla_{KPC-2} resides on a transmissible element. *Enterobacter* spp. with bla_{KPC-2} on a 65-kb plasmid (24) and *K. pneumoniae* with bla_{KPC-3} on a 75-kb plasmid that also transferred resistance to amikacin and gentamicin (65) have been reported.

The association of many of these genes with mobile genetic structures facilitates their spread and will undoubtedly provide a challenge to control efforts.

CLINICAL AND MOLECULAR EPIDEMIOLOGY

The largest collection of *K. pneumoniae* isolates with metallo-β-lactamases has been reported from Taiwan (68). Approximately 1% of all isolates were found to carry an IMP β-lactamase; pulsed-field gel electrophoresis was performed on these isolates and documented largely clonal spread of the pathogens. Most of the patients with these resistant *K. pneumoniae* isolates were located in intensive-care areas, and several patients had received β-lactams prior to the culture (68).

Virtually all patients with KPC-possessing pathogens have been described as debilitated and severely ill and have often resided in an intensive-care area (6, 65). These resistant bacteria are often acquired after a prolonged period of hospitalization, and patients have often received multiple courses of antimicrobials (6). In one review of 60 patients, most had received fluoroquinolones or β-lactam antibiotics (6), although only 20% had previously received a carbapenem.

The nosocomial outbreaks involving KPC-possessing *K. pneumoniae* isolates have occurred in New York City. Of 18 isolates of *K. pneumoniae* with bla_{KPC-2} collected from seven hospitals in two New York City boroughs, 12 belonged to a single ribotype, suggesting carriage between health care facilities (3). An outbreak occurring from 2000 to 2001 involving 24 patients infected with *K. pneumoniae* with KPC-3 was centered in intensive-care units at one hospital (65). Most of these isolates were identified by pulsed-field gel electrophoresis as belonging to one predominant strain (65); aggressive infection control measures were successful in controlling this outbreak. However, by 2003 to 2004, KPC-possessing *K. pneumoniae* isolates were located in 10 different New York hospitals (7), documenting the ease of interhospital spread of these pathogens. Two outbreaks of KPC-2-possessing *K. pneumoniae* that occurred in 2003 and 2004 involved strains that belonged to similar ribotypes (6). These outbreaks were hospital-wide, without an obvious epidemiological link (6). By 2004, KPC-possessing *K. pneumoniae* was endemic at four New York City hospitals, and 88% of the isolates belonged to the same ribotype (8).

DETECTION OF *K. PNEUMONIAE* WITH CARBAPENEM-HYDROLYZING β-LACTAMASES

Successfully controlling the spread of *K. pneumoniae* (and other *Enterobacteriaceae*) possessing carbapenem-hydrolyzing β-lactamases requires accurate identification of these isolates. Significant difficulty has been noted in identifying *Enterobacteriaceae* with metallo-β-lactamases. Carbapenem susceptibility testing is not a reliable method, since many isolates have MICs below the breakpoint for resistance (66, 67, 68). To screen for metallo-β-lactamases, simplified methods that employ thiol compounds (e.g., 2-mercaptopropionic acid [MPA] and sodium mercaptoacetic acid) or EDTA have been developed. These compounds inhibit metallo-β-lactamases and augment the zone of inhibition around a β-lactam disk or Etest strip. Unfortunately, no single screening test appears to be applicable to all isolates potentially carrying metallo-β-lactamases (33, 63,

66). For double-disk diffusion tests, using EDTA as the β-lactamase inhibitor appeared to improve detection of metalloenzymes in *P. aeruginosa*, whereas MPA and sodium mercaptoacetic acid were superior inhibitors for detection in *A. baumannii* (33). However, methods that employ a double disk with ceftazidime and either MPA or EDTA did not accurately detect metallo-β-lactamases in *Enterobacteriaceae* (1, 66). For *P. aeruginosa* isolates with a variety of β-lactamases, an Etest strip containing imipenem and imipenem plus EDTA detected 94% of isolates with metallo-β-lactamases, with a specificity of 95% (63). A positive result using the Etest method is defined as a decrease of ≥3 twofold dilutions in the MIC of imipenem when combined with EDTA (63). However, isolates that are not frankly resistant to imipenem (as is the case for most *Enterobacteriaceae*) may not be detected by this method (66).

Similarly, detection of KPC-possessing *K. pneumoniae* may be difficult. As previously noted, occasional KPC-possessing isolates were reported to remain susceptible to carbapenems (3, 42, 65). In a surveillance study in New York City, nine isolates, or 3.3% of all ESBL-producing *K. pneumoniae* isolates, were identified with the KPC-2 β-lactamases (6). For several isolates, the MICs of imipenem were lower when tested by the broth microdilution method than by the Etest, and a significant inoculum effect on the MIC of imipenem was observed (6). In a surveillance study involving four hospitals (8), also in New York City, 42% of 257 single-patient isolates possessed ESBLs, and 24% possessed KPC β-lactamases (the vast majority were KPC-2). A pronounced inoculum effect was observed on the broth microdilution MIC for imipenem (8). The inoculum effect was less pronounced for meropenem, and no such effect was seen for ertapenem (8). Importantly, the clinical microbiology laboratories identified 15% of these KPC-possessing *K. pneumoniae* isolates as susceptible to imipenem; the isolates were highly resistant when tested by Etest or disk diffusion assays (8). It was suggested that, due to the extremely mucoid nature of some *K. pneumoniae* isolates, inoculum preparation using a wand technique for broth microdilution susceptibility testing may not deliver an adequate concentration of bacteria. Therefore, imipenem susceptibility results may be misleadingly low. It was recommended that (i) the wand technique not be used for inoculum preparation of mucoid colonies and (ii) ertapenem or meropenem be reported as the class agent for carbapenem susceptibility testing in areas where KPC-possessing *K. pneumoniae* isolates are present (8). In addition, disk diffusion or Etest assays could be used to confirm carbapenem susceptibility. Finally, an inoculum effect on the MIC of imipenem has also been observed with two isolates of *Enterobacter* spp. possessing KPC-2 (5). Whether similar recommendations need to be made for this genus remains unknown. To date, KPC-possessing *Enterobacter* spp. remain unusual, even where *K. pneumoniae* strains with KPC β-lactamases are endemic (8).

THERAPY OF INFECTIONS DUE TO
CARBAPENEM-RESISTANT *K. PNEUMONIAE*

Given the multidrug resistance of most of these pathogens, therapy of carbapenem-resistant *K. pneumoniae* remains difficult. Although *K. pneumoniae* with VIM and IMP β-lactamases may remain susceptible to carbapenems, and a small number of patients have apparently been successfully treated with a carbapenem (68), it is unproven that this class of antibiotic retains clinical usefulness. The MICs of imipenem for isolates with metallo-β-lactamases may be elevated when tested with a higher inoculum (35), and these isolates can easily acquire additional mechanisms of resistance (porin deficits and other β-lactamases). Therefore, treatment of serious infections due to VIM- or IMP-possessing *K. pneumoniae* with carbapenems should be undertaken with caution. Although aztreonam is not affected by metallo-β-lactamases, isolates of *K. pneumoniae* often possess other β-lactamases, causing resistance to this antibiotic (68). Occasional isolates may remain susceptible to fluoroquinolones or aminoglycosides (28, 39, 59, 68). Although most reports do not include data for the polymyxins (28, 39, 59, 68), it is anticipated that many *Enterobacteriaceae* with metallo-β-lactamases would be susceptible to colistin or polymyxin B. However, these agents would not be active against isolates of *S. marcescens*.

Therapy of infections due to KPC-possessing pathogens is equally difficult. Isolates reported as susceptible to imipenem may have had an inadequate inoculum for microbroth testing; these isolates are highly resistant when tested by the disk diffusion or Etest method. As with isolates with metallo-β-lactamases, carbapenem therapy of infections due to KPC-possessing bacteria cannot be recommended, even if the MICs are below the breakpoint for resistance by conventional testing methods. Although KPC enzymes are class A β-lactamases that are inhibited by clavulanic acid and tazobactam, virtually all isolates are highly resistant to the β-lactam–β-lactamase inhibitor combinations (3, 6, 7, 8, 65). The combination of imipenem and clavulanic acid generally lowers the imipenem MIC by several twofold dilutions, but probably not enough to be clinically relevant (7, 65). The vast majority of KPC-possessing isolates are also resistant to fluoroquinolones and trimethoprim-sulfamethoxazole (3, 6, 7, 8, 23, 65, 71), and only about half remain susceptible to amikacin (Table 4). Approximately 60% of KPC-possessing *K. pneumoniae* isolates from New York City are susceptible to gentamicin, and this agent provides bactericidal activity in time-kill experiments (7). Although many isolates are reported to be susceptible to tetracycline or doxycycline (6, 7, 65), the MICs hover around the breakpoint for susceptibility and time-kill experiments do not suggest that this is an effective regimen (7). However, the glycylcycline antibiotic tigecycline is active against many *Enterobacteriaceae* (46), including KPC-possessing *K. pneumoniae* (6, 7). The clinical usefulness of this antibiotic against these resistant pathogens remains to be determined.

Table 4. Susceptibility results for 62 KPC-possessing *K. pneumoniae* isolates[a]

Antibiotic	MIC$_{50}$ (µg/ml)	MIC$_{90}$ (µg/ml)	Range (µg/ml)	% Susceptible	% Intermediate	% Resistant
Piperacillin-tazobactam	>256	>256	>256	0	0	100
Cefotetan	64	>256	16->256	15	34	51
Ceftazidime	>256	>256	32->256	0	2	98
Cefepime	>256	>256	16->256	0	5	95
Gentamicin	4	64	1->256	65	3	32
Amikacin	64	128	2->256	6	6	88
Ciprofloxacin	>32	>32	8->32	0	0	100
Doxycycline	8	16	4->256	32	50	18
Polymyxin B	2	8	0.5->16	73	0	27

[a]Reproduced with permission from reference 8.

The increasing drug resistance among nosocomial gram-negative pathogens has renewed interest in the polymyxins (18). The revival of polymyxin B and colistin (polymyxin E) has been prompted by the emergence of multidrug-resistant *P. aeruginosa* and *A. baumannii* (18, 34). Approximately 90% of KPC-possessing *K. pneumoniae* isolates are susceptible to polymyxin B, and the antibiotic exhibits a concentration-dependent killing effect (6, 7). The addition of rifampin to polymyxin B provided bactericidal activity in 15/16 tested isolates in one report and resulted in a lower inhibitory concentration of polymyxin B (7).

Although there are no comparative studies examining the outcomes of infections with KPC-possessing *K. pneumoniae*, adverse outcomes have been noted in some studies, possibly due to the lack of an established effective regimen. In one outbreak, 8 of 14 patients with infections with KPC-3-positive *K. pneumoniae* died, at least in part due to the infection (65). In one uncontrolled series involving patients with bacteremia due to KPC-2-carrying *K. pneumoniae*, eight of nine patients receiving ineffective therapy experienced an adverse clinical or microbiological outcome. In contrast, two of eight patients treated with an effective regimen (generally an aminoglycoside or polymyxin B) experienced a poor outcome (6). A single case report has also documented a successful outcome with colistin therapy for multidrug-resistant *K. pneumoniae* septicemia (26).

CONTROL STRATEGIES

Outbreaks involving *K. pneumoniae* with carbapenem-hydrolyzing β-lactamases have involved a relatively small number of strains (6, 7, 8, 65, 68). Infection control measures should be the mainstay for controlling these outbreaks. Aggressive infection control measures were reported to be successful in controlling an outbreak of KPC-possessing *K. pneumoniae* in an intensive-care unit (65). However, hospital-wide outbreaks may be more difficult to control and may persist despite infection control measures (6). This failure may be due in part to the difficulty clinical laboratories have had in identifying KPC-positive isolates based on carbapenem resistance, as noted above. Also, in outbreak settings, asymptomatic gastrointestinal colonization with KPC-positive *K. pneumoniae* may be common, as occurs with ESBL-possessing pathogens and vancomycin-resistant enterococci. Relying on clinical cultures to identify all patients harboring these pathogens may be misleading and will likely reveal only the tip of the iceberg. Routine surveillance studies may be necessary to identify all patients with carbapenem-resistant *K. pneumoniae*. In one small surveillance study involving an outbreak of KPC-2 *K. pneumoniae* in three intensive-care areas, 39% of patients were found to have gastrointestinal colonization (6). Of these patients, only 14% had preceding clinical cultures with a carbapenem-resistant *K. pneumoniae* isolate. Unfortunately, no commercially available medium is appropriate for screening of stool cultures for carbapenem-resistant *K. pneumoniae*.

Antibiotic control strategies are often an important component of methods to reduce antibiotic resistance. Given the multidrug resistance of many of these isolates (6, 68), it is difficult to pinpoint one class of antibiotics that may be encouraging the emergence of these strains. In addition to carbapenems, the VIM, IMP, and KPC β-lactamases can hydrolyze a wide variety of β-lactams. Pressure from overall β-lactam use (22), and not solely carbapenems, is suggested by the absence of carbapenem receipt in many patients harboring these pathogens (3, 6, 40). The fact that other carbapenem-hydrolyzing enzymes emerged prior to the commercial release of carbapenems also suggests that other properties of these enzymes may justify their existence (44, 56) or that other antibiotics in nature could be substrates and exert selection pressures. Also complicating potential antibiotic control strategies is the fact that other resistance genes often accompany the carbapenemase gene, including those for other β-lactamases (71), amikacin (65), gentamicin (65, 71), streptomycin (40), tobramycin (71), and trimethoprim-sulfamethoxazole (40). Because of these associations, it has been suggested that selective pressure from non-β-lactam antibiotics (e.g., aminoglycosides) may encourage concomitant carbapenem resistance (24). It is likely that broad antibiotic control programs that include multiple classes of antibiotics will be needed to help control the spread of these multidrug-resistant pathogens.

CONCLUSIONS

There has been a global emergence of *K. pneumoniae* and other *Enterobacteriaceae* possessing carbapenem-hydrolyzing β-lactamases. *Enterobacteriaceae* with metallo-β-lactamases have emerged in eastern Asia and southern Europe, and isolates with KPC-type β-lactamases have emerged in the northeastern United States. Nosocomial outbreaks with these pathogens have been documented, confirming their ability to spread rapidly in the hospital setting. Because many of the outbreaks have involved a small number of strains of *K. pneumoniae*, infection control strategies are of paramount importance. Unfortunately, there have been significant obstacles to the detection of *K. pneumoniae* with metallo-β-lactamases and KPC β-lactamases. Many of these pathogens are not overtly resistant to carbapenem antibiotics; therefore, reliance on carbapenem susceptibility testing for detection may be misleading. Also, no commercially available medium has been considered appropriate for screening for gastrointestinal colonization. Given the multidrug-resistant nature of these bacteria, defining an effective therapeutic regimen has been difficult. Often, the polymyxins are resorted to for therapy of serious infections; however, resistance to polymyxins has also been documented. Future studies will need to address more effective methods of detection and the development of novel therapeutic modalities.

REFERENCES

1. **Arakawa, Y., N. Shibata, K. Shibayama, H. Kurokawa, T. Yagi, H. Fujiwara, and M. Goto.** 2000. Convenient test for screening metallo-β-lactamase-producing gram-negative bacteria by using thiol compounds. *J. Clin. Microbiol.* **38:**40–43.

2. **Bornet, C., A. Davin-Regli, C. Bosi, J.-M. Pages, and C. Bollet.** 2000. Imipenem resistance of *Enterobacter aerogenes* mediated by outer membrane permeability. *J. Clin. Microbiol.* **38:**1048–1052.

3. **Bradford, P. A., S. Bratu, C. Urban, M. Visalli, N. Mariano, D. Landman, J. J. Rahal, S. Brooks, S. Cebular, and J. Quale.** 2004. Emergence of carbapenem-resistant *Klebsiella* species possessing the class A carbapenem-hydrolyzing KPC-2 and inhibitor-resistant TEM-30 β-lactamases in New York City. *Clin. Infect. Dis.* **39:**55–60.

4. **Bradford, P. A., C. Urban, N. Mariano, S. J. Projan, J. J. Rahal, and K. Bush.** 1997. Imipenem resistance in *Klebsiella pneumoniae* is associated with the combination of ACT-1, a plasmid-mediated AmpC β-lactamase, and the loss of an outer membrane protein. *Antimicrob. Agents Chemother.* **41:**563–569.

5. **Bratu, S., D. Landman, M. Alam, E. Tolentino, and J. Quale.** 2005. Detection of KPC carbapenem-hydrolyzing enzymes in *Enterobacter* spp. from Brooklyn, New York. *Antimicrob. Agents Chemother.* **49:**776–778.

6. **Bratu, S., D. Landman, R. Haag, R. Recco, A. Eramo, M. Alam, and J. Quale.** 2005. Rapid spread of carbapenem-resistant *Klebsiella pneumoniae* in New York City: A new threat to our antibiotic armamentarium. *Arch. Intern. Med.* **165:**1430–1435.

7. **Bratu, S., P. Tolaney, U. Karamudi, J. Quale, M. Mooty, S. Nichani, and D. Landman.** 2005. Carbapenemase-producing *Klebsiella pneumoniae* in Brooklyn, NY: molecular epidemiology and in-vitro activity of polymyxin B and other agents. *J. Antimicrob. Chemother.* **56:**128–132.

8. **Bratu, S., M. Mooty, S. Nichani, D. Landman, C. Gullans, B. Pettinato, U. Karumudi, P. Tolaney, and J. Quale.** 2005. Emergence of KPC-possessing *Klebsiella pneumoniae* in Brooklyn, New York: epidemiology and recommendations for detection. *Antimicrob. Agents Chemother.* **49:**3018–3020.

9. **Bush, K., S. K. Tanaka, D. P. Bonner, and R. B. Sykes.** 1985. Resistance caused by decreased penetration of β-lactam antibiotics into *Enterobacter cloacae*. *Antimicrob. Agents Chemother.* **27:**555–560.

10. **Canton, R., T. M. Coque, and F. Baquero.** 2003. Multi-resistant Gram-negative bacilli: from epidemics to endemics. *Curr. Opin. Infect. Dis.* **16:**315–325.

11. **Cao, V. T. B., G. Arlet, B. M. Ericsson, A. Tammelin, P. Courvalin, and T. Lambert.** 2000. Emergence of imipenem resistance in *Klebsiella pneumoniae* owing to combination of plasmid-mediated CMY-4 and permeability alteration. *J. Antimicrob. Chemother.* **46:**895–900.

12. **Centers for Disease Control and Prevention.** 2004. National Nosocomial Infections Surveillance (NNIS) System Report, data summary from January 1992 through June 2004. *Am. J. Infect. Control* **32:**470–485.

13. **Chow, J. W., and D. M. Shlaes.** 1991. Imipenem resistance associated with the loss of a 40 kDa outer membrane protein in *Enterobacter aerogenes*. *J. Antimicrob Chemother.* **28:**499–504.

14. **Chu, Y.-W., M. Afzal-Shah, E. T. S. Houang, M.-F. I. Palepou, D. J. Lyon, N. Woodford, and D. M. Livermore.** 2001. IMP-4, a novel metallo-β-lactamase from nosocomial *Acinetobacter* spp. collected in Hong Kong between 1994 and 1998. *Antimicrob. Agents Chemother.* **45:**710–714.

15. **Crowley, B., V. J. Benedi, and A. Domenech-Sanchez.** 2002. Expression of SHV-2 β-lactamase and of reduced amounts of OmpK36 porin in *Klebsiella pneumoniae* results in increased resistance to cephalosporins and carbapenems. *Antimicrob. Agents Chemother.* **46:**3679–3682.

16. **de Champs, C., C. Henquell, D. Guelon, D. Sirot, N. Gazuy, and J. Sirot.** 1993. Clinical and bacteriological study of nosocomial infections due to *Enterobacter aerogenes* resistant to imipenem. *J. Clin. Microbiol.* **31:**123–127.

17. **Domenech-Sanchez, A. S. Hernandez-Alles, L. Martinez-Martinez, V. J. Benedi, and S. Alberti.** 1999. Identification and characterization of a new porin gene of *Klebsiella pneumoniae*: its role in β-lactam antibiotic resistance. *J. Bacteriol.* **181:**2726–2732.

18. **Falagas, M. E. and S. K. Kasiakou.** 2005. Colistin: the revival of polymyxins for the management of multidrug-resistant Gram-negative bacterial infections. *Clin. Infect. Dis.* **40:**1333–1341.

19. **Franceschini, N., B. Caravelli, J. D. Docquier, M. Galleni, J. M. Frere, G. Amicosante, and G. M. Rossolini.** 2000. Purification and biochemical characterization of the VIM-1 metallo-beta-lactamase. *Antimicrob. Agents Chemother.* **44:**3003–3007.

20. **Hanberger, H., J.-A. Garcia-Rodriguez, M. Gobernado, H. Goossens, L. E. Nilsson, M. J. Struelens, and the French and Portuguese ICU Study Groups.** 1999. Antibiotic susceptibility among aerobic Gram-negative bacilli in intensive care units in 5 European countries. *JAMA* **281:**67–71.

21. **Hernandez-Alles, S., S. Alberti, D. Alvarez, A. Domenech-Sanchez, L. Martinez-Martinez, J. Gil, J. M. Tomas, and V. J. Benedi.** 1999. Porin expression in clinical isolates of *Klebsiella pneumoniae*. *Microbiology* **145:**673–679.

22. **Hirakata, Y., K. Izumikawa, T. Yamaguchi, H. Takemura, H. Tanaka, R. Yoshida, J. Matsuda, M. Nakano, K. Tomono, S. Maesaki, M. Kaku, Y. Yamada, S. Kamihira, and S. Kohno.** 1998. Rapid detection and evaluation of clinical characteristics of emerging multiple-drug-resistant gram-negative rods carrying the metallo-β-lactamase gene *bla*$_{IMP}$. *Antimicrob. Agents Chemother.* **42:**2006–2011.

23. **Hong, T., E. S. Moland, B. Abdalhamid, N. D. Hanson, J. Wang, C. Sloan, D. Fabian, A. Farajallah, J. Levine, and K. S. Thomson.** 2005. *Escherichia coli*: development of carbapenem resistance during therapy. *Clin. Infect. Dis.* **40:**e84–e86.

24. **Hossain, A., M. J. Ferraro, R. M. Pino, R. B. Dew III, E. S. Moland, T. J. Lockhart, K. S. Thomson, R. V. Goering, and N. D. Hanson.** 2004. Plasmid-mediated carbapenem hydrolyzing enzyme KPC-2 in *Enterobacter* sp. *Antimicrob. Agents Chemother.* **48:**4438–4440.

25. **Jones, R. N., L. M. Desphande, J. M. Bell, J. D. Turnidge, S. Kohno, Y. Hirakata, Y. Ono, Y. Miyazawa, S. Kawakama, M. Inoue, Y. Hirata, and M. A. Toleman.** 2004. Evaluation of the contemporary occurrence

rates of metallo-β-lactamases in multidrug-resistant gram-negative bacilli in Japan: report from the SENTRY Antimicrobial Surveillance Program (1998–2002). *Diagn. Microbiol. Infect. Dis.* **49:**289–294.

26. **Karabinis, A., E. Paramythiotou, D. Mylona-Petropoulou, A. Kalogeromitros, N. Katsarelis, F. Kontopidou, I. Poularas, and H. Malamou-Lada.** 2005. Colistin for *Klebsiella pneumoniae*-associated sepsis. *Clin. Infect. Dis.* **38:**e7–e9.

27. **Karlowsky, J. A. , M. E. Jones, C. Thornsberry, I. R. Friedland, and D. F. Sahm.** 2003. Trends in antimicrobial susceptibilities among *Enterobacteriaceae* isolated from hospitalized patients in the United States from 1998 to 2001. *Antimicrob. Agents Chemother.* **47:**1672–1680.

28. **Koh, T. H., L. H. Sng, G. S. Babini, N. Woodford, D. M. Livermore, and L. M. C. Hall.** 2001. Carbapenem-resistant *Klebsiella pneumoniae* in Singapore producing IMP-1 β-lactamase and lacking an outer membrane protein. *Antimicrob. Agents Chemother.* **45:**1939–1940.

29. **Kurokawa, H., T. Yagi, N. Shibata, K. Shibayama, and Y. Arakawa.** 1999. Worldwide proliferation of carbapenem-resistant gram-negative bacteria. *Lancet* **354:**955.

30. **Laraki, N., N. Franceschini, G. M. Rossolini, P. Santucci, C. Meunier, E. de Pauw, G. G. Amicosante, J. M. Frere, and M. Galeni.** 1999. Biochemical characterization of the *Pseudomonas aeruginosa* 101/1477 metallo-β-lactamase IMP-1 produced by *Escherichia coli*. *Antimicrob. Agents Chemother.* **43:**902–906.

31. **Lee, E. H., M. H. Nicolas, M. D. Kitzis, G. Pialoux, E. Collatz, and L. Gutmann.** 1991. Association of two resistance mechanisms in a clinical isolate of *Enterobacter cloacae* with high-level resistance to imipenem. *Antimicrob. Agents Chemother.* **35:**1093–1098.

32. **Lee, K., G. Y. Ha, B. M. Shin, J. J. Kim, J. O. Kang, S. J. Jang, D. Y. Yong, Y. Chong, and the Korean Nationwide Surveillance of Antimicrobial Resistance (KONSAR) Group.** 2004. Metallo-β-lactamase-producing gram-negative bacilli in Korean Nationwide Surveillance of Antimicrobial Resistance Group hospitals in 2003: continued prevalence of VIM-producing *Pseudomonas* spp. and increase in IMP-producing *Acinetobacter* spp. *Diagn. Microbiol. Infect. Dis.* **50:**51–58.

33. **Lee, K., Y. S. Lim, D. Yong, J. H. Yum, and Y. Chung.** 2003. Evaluation of the Hodge test and the imipenem-EDTA double-disk synergy test for differentiating metallo-β-lactamase-producing isolates of *Pseudomonas* spp. and *Acinetobacter* spp. *J. Clin. Microbiol.* **41:**4623–4629.

34. **Levin, A. S., A. A. Barone, J. Penco, M. V. Santos, I. S. Marinho, E. A. G. Arruda, E. I. Manrique, and S. F Costa.** 1999. Intravenous colistin as therapy for nosocomial infections caused by multidrug-resistant *Pseudomonas aeruginosa* and *Acinetobacter baumannii*. *Clin. Infect. Dis.* **28:**1008–1011.

35. **Luzzaro, F., J.-D. Docquier, C. Colinon, A. Endimiani, G. Lombardi, G. Amicosante, G. M. Rossolini, and A. Toniolo.** 2004. Emergence in *Klebsiella pneumoniae* and *Enterobacter cloacae* clinical isolates of the VIM-4 metallo-β-lactamase encoded by a conjugative plasmid. *Antimicrob. Agents Chemother.* **48:**648–650.

36. **Mainardi, J.-L., P. Mugnier, A. Coutrot, A. Buu-Hoi, E. Collatz, and L. Gutmann.** 1997. Carbapenem resistance in a clinical isolate of *Citrobacter freundii*. *Antimicrob. Agents Chemother.* **41:**2352–2354.

37. **Martinez-Martinez, L., A. Pascual, S. Hernandez-Alles, D. Alvarez-Diaz, A. I. Suarez, J. Tran, V. J. Benedi, and G. A. Jacoby.** 1999. Roles of β-lactamases and porins in activities of carbapenems and cephalosporins against *Klebsiella pneumoniae*. *Antimicrob. Agents Chemother.* **43:**1669–1673.

38. **Mehtar, S., A. Tsakris, and T. L. Pitt.** 1991. Imipenem resistance in *Proteus mirabilis*. *J. Antimicrob. Chemother.* **28:**612–615.

39. **Miriagou, V., E. Tzelepi, D. Gianneli, and L. S. Tzouvelekis.** 2003. *Escherichia coli* with a self-transferable, multiresistant plasmid coding for metallo-β-lactamase VIM-1. *Antimicrob. Agents Chemother.* **47:**395–397.

40. **Miriagou, V., L. S. Tzouvelekis, S. Rossiter, E. Tzelepi, F. J. Angulo, and J. M. Whichard.** 2003. Imipenem resistance in a *Salmonella* clinical strain due to plasmid-mediated class A carbapenemase KPC-2. *Antimicrob. Agents Chemother.* **47:**1297–1300.

41. **Moland, E. S., J. A. Black, J. Ourada, M. D. Reisbig, N. D. Hanson, and K. S. Thomson.** 2002. Occurrence of newer β-lactamases in *Klebsiella pneumoniae* isolates from 24 U.S. hospitals. *Antimicrob. Agents Chemother.* **46:**3837–3842.

42. **Moland, E. S., N. D. Hanson, V. L. Herrera, J. A. Black, T. J. Lockhart, A. Hossain, J. J. Johnson, R. V. Goering, and K. S. Thomson.** 2003. Plasmid-mediated, carbapenem-hydrolysing β-lactamase, KPC-2, in *Klebsiella pneumoniae* isolates. *J. Antimicrob. Chemother.* **51:**711–714.

43. **Naas, T., and P. Nordmann.** 1994. Analysis of a carbapenem-hydrolyzing class A β-lactamase from *Enterobacter cloacae* and of its LysR-type regulatory protein. *Proc. Natl. Acad. Sci.* **91:**7693–7697.

44. **Naas, T., L. Vandel, W. Sougakoff, D. M. Livermore, and P. Nordmann.** 1994. Cloning and sequence analysis of the gene for a carbapenem-hydrolyzing class A β-lactamase, Sme-1, from *Serratia marcescens* S6. *Antimicrob. Agents Chemother.* **38:**1262–1270.

45. **Nordmann, P., S. Mariotte, T. Naas, R. Labia, and M. H. Nicolas.** 1993. Biochemical properties of a carbapenem-hydrolyzing β-lactamase from *Enterobacter cloacae* and cloning of the gene into *Escherichia coli. Antimicrob. Agents Chemother.* **37:**939–946.

46. **Peterson, P. J., N. V. Jacobus, W. J. Weiss, P. E. Sum, and R. T. Testa.** 1999. In vitro and in vivo antibacterial activities of a novel glycylcycline, the 9-*t*-butylglycylamido derivative of minocycline (GAR-936). *Antimicrob. Agents Chemother.* **43:**738–744.

47. **Poirel, L., C. Heritier, V. Tolun and P. Nordmann.** 2004. Emergence of oxacillinase-mediated resistance to imipenem in *Klebsiella pneumoniae. Antimicrob. Agents Chemother.* **48:**15–22.

48. **Poirel, L., T. Naas, D. Nicolas, L. Collet, S. Bellais, J. D. Cavallo, and P. Nordmann.** 2000. Characterization of VIM-2, a carbapenem-hydrolyzing metallo-beta-lactamase, and its plasmid- and integron-borne gene from a *Pseudomonas aeruginosa* clinical isolate in France. *Antimicrob. Agents Chemother.* **44:**891–897.

49. **Poirel, L., and P. Nordmann.** 2002. Acquired carbapenem-hydrolyzing beta-lactamases and their genetic support. *Curr. Pharmaceut. Biotechnol.* **3:**117–121.

50. **Poirel, L., J. N. Pham, L. Cabanne, B. J. Gatus, S. M. Bell, and P. Nordmann.** 2004. Carbapenem-hydrolysing metallo-β-lactamases from *Klebsiella pneumoniae* and *Escherichia coli* isolated in Australia. *Pathology* **36:**366–367.

51. **Poirel, L., G. F. Weldhagen, T. Naas, C. De Champs, M. G. Dove, and P. Nordmann.** 2001. GES-2, a class A β-lactamase from *Pseudomonas aeruginosa* with increased hydrolysis of imipenem. *Antimicrob. Agents Chemother.* **45:**2598–2603.

52. **Pottumarthy, S., E. Smith Moland, S. Juretschko, S. R. Swanzy, K. S. Thomson, and T. R. Fritsche.** 2003. NmcA carbapenem-hydrolyzing enzyme in *Enterobacter cloacae* in North America. *Emerg. Infect. Dis.* **9:**999–1002.

53. **Quale, J., D. Landman, P. A. Bradford, M. Visalli, J. Ravishankar, C. Flores, D. Mayorga, K. Vangala, and A. Adedeji.** 2002. Molecular epidemiology of a citywide outbreak of extended-spectrum β-lactamase-producing *Klebsiella pneumoniae* infection. *Clin. Infect. Dis.* **35:**834–841.

54. **Queenan, A. M., C. Torres-Viera, H. S. Gold, Y. Carmeli, G. M. Eliopoulos, R. C. Moellering, Jr., J. P. Quinn, J. Hindler, A. A. Medeiros, and K. Bush.** 2000. SME-type carbapenem-hydrolyzing class A beta-lactamases from geographically diverse *Serratia marcescens* strains. *Antimicrob. Agents Chemother.* **44:**3035–3039.

55. **Raimondi, A., A. Traverso, and H. Nikaido.** 1991. Imipenem- and meropenem-resistant mutants of *Enterobacter cloacae* and *Proteus rettgeri* lack porins. *Antimicrob. Agents Chemother.* **35:**1174–1180.

56. **Rasmussen, B. A., K. Bush, D. Keeney, Y. Yang, R. Hare, C. O'Gara, and A. A. Medeiros.** 1996. Characterization of IMI-1 beta-lactamase, a class A carbapenem-hydrolyzing enzyme from *Enterobacter cloacae. Antimicrob. Agents Chemother.* **40:**2080–2086.

57. **Richards, M. J., J. R. Edwards, D. H. Culver, R. P. Gaynes, and the National Nosocomial Infections Surveillance System.** 1999. Nosocomial infections in medical intensive care units in the United States. *Crit. Care Med.* **27:**887–892.

58. **Sader, H. S., D. J. Biedenbach, and R. N. Jones.** 2003. Global patterns of susceptibility for 21 commonly utilized antimicrobial agents tested against 48,440 *Enterobacteriaceae* in the SENTRY Antimicrobial Surveillance Program (1997–2001). *Diagn. Microbiol. Infect. Dis.* **47:**361–364.

59. **Senda, K., Y. Arakawa, S. Ichiyama, K. Nakashima, H. Ito, S. Ohsuka, K. Shimokata, N. Kato, and M. Ohta.** 1996. PCR detection of metallo-β-lactamase gene (bla_{IMP}) in gram-negative rods resistant to broad-spectrum β-lactams. *J. Clin. Microbiol.* **34:**2909–2913.

60. **Toleman, M. A., D. Biedenbach, D. M. C. Bennett, R. N. Jones, and T. R. Walsh.** 2005. Italian metallo-β-lactamases: a national problem? Report from the SENTRY Antimicrobial Surveillance Programme. *J. Antimicrob. Chemother.* **55:**61–70.

61. **Villar, H. E., F. Danel, and D. M. Livermore.** 1997. Permeability to carbapenems of *Proteus mirabilis* mutants selected for resistance to imipenem or other β-lactams. *J. Antimicrob. Chemother.* **40:**365–370.

62. **Vourli, S., P. Giakkoupi, V. Miriagou, E. Tzelepi, A. C. Vatopoulos, and L. S. Tzouvelekis.** 2004. Novel GES/IBC extended-spectrum beta-lactamase variants with carbapenemase activity in clinical enterobacteria. *FEMS Microbiol. Lett.* **234:**209–213.

63. **Walsh, T. R., A. Bolmström, A. Qwärnström, and A. Gales.** 2002. Evaluation of a new Etest for detecting metallo-β-lactamases in routine clinical testing. *J. Clin. Microbiol.* **40:**2755–2759.

64. **Weber, D. J., R. Raasch, and W. A. Rutala.** 1999. Nosocomial infections in the ICU. *Chest* **115**(Suppl.)**:** 34S–41S.

65. **Woodford, N., P. M. Tierno, Jr., K. Young, L. Tysall, M.-F. I. Palepou, E. Ward, R. E. Painter, D. F. Suber, D. Shungu, L. L. Silver, K. Inglima, J. Kornblum, and D. M. Livermore.** 2004. Outbreak of *Klebsiella pneumoniae* producing a new carbapenem-hydrolyzing class A β-lactamase, KPC-3, in a New York medical center. *Antimicrob. Agents Chemother.* **48:**4793–4799.

66. **Yan, J.-J., J.-J. Wu, S.-H. Tsai, and C.-L. Chuang.** 2004. Comparison of the double-disk, combined disk, and E-test methods for detecting metallo-β-lactamases in gram-negative bacilli. *Diagn. Microbiol. Infect. Dis.* **49:**5–11.

67. **Yan, J.-J., W.-C. Ko, C.-L. Chuang, and J.-J. Wu.** 2002. Metallo-β-lactamase-producing *Enterobacteriaceae* isolates in a university in Taiwan: prevalence of IMP-8 in *Enterobacter cloacae* and first identification of VIM-2 in *Citrobacter freundii*. *J. Antimicrob. Chemother.* **50:**503–511.

68. **Yan, J.-.J., W.-C. Ko, S.-H. Tsai, H. M. Wu, and J.-J. Wu.** 2001. Outbreak of infection with multidrug-resistant *Klebsiella pneumoniae* carrying bla_{IMP-8} in a university medical center in Taiwan. *J. Clin. Microbiol.* **39:**4433–4439.

69. **Yigit, H., G. J. Anderson, J. W. Biddle, C. D. Steward, J. K. Rasheed, L. L. Valera, J. E. McGowen, Jr., and F. C. Tenover.** 2002. Carbapenem resistance in a clinical isolate of *Enterobacter aerogenes* is associated with decreased expression of OmpF and OmpC porin analogs. *Antimicrob. Agents Chemother.* **46:** 3817–3822.

70. **Yigit, H., A. M. Queenan, G. J. Anderson, A. Domenech-Sanchez, J. W. Biddle, C. D. Steward, S. Alberti, K. Bush, and F. C. Tenover.** 2001. Novel carbapenem-hydrolyzing beta-lactamase, KPC-1, from a carbapenem-resistant strain of *Klebsiella pneumoniae*. *Antimicrob. Agents Chemother.* **45:**1151–1161.

71. **Yigit, H., A. M. Queenan, J. K. Rasheed, J. W. Biddle, A. Domenech-Sanchez, S. Alberti, K. Bush, and F. C. Tenover.** 2003. Carbapenem-resistant strain of *Klebsiella oxytoca* harboring carbapenem-hydrolyzing β-lactamase KPC-2. *Antimicrob. Agents Chemother.* **47:**3881–3889.

Emerging Infections 7
Edited by W. M. Scheld, D. C. Hooper, and J. M. Hughes
© 2007 ASM Press, Washington, D.C.

Chapter 11

The Emerging Role of Klebsiellae in Liver Abscess

Joseph Rahimian and Jin-Town Wang

EPIDEMIOLOGY OF PLA

Pyogenic liver abscess (PLA) was described as early as the writings of Hippocrates (400 B.C.E.). He based prognosis on the type of fluid recovered from the draining of the abscess, noting that ". . . if the pus which is discharged be pure and white, the patients recover . . . but if it resemble the lees of oil as it flows, they die" (2). In 1938, Ochsner et al. (63) described the treatment and mortality of patients with PLA and recommended surgical treatment as the primary treatment modality. In their review of 575 collected cases, PLA was most commonly a complication of acute appendicitis, which accounted for 34% of cases. The disease predominantly affected young men and was associated with high mortality. Surgery remained the therapy of choice until the mid-1980s, when percutaneous drainage was shown to be a safe and less invasive alternative (4, 6, 30, 39, 40, 67, 70).

There has been no clear temporal trend in the incidence of PLA, which has remained fairly constant, ranging in most studies from 0.008 to 0.03% of hospital admissions (63, 65, 68). The mean age of patients with PLA has increased, with most recent reports showing a mean age of 55 to 60 years (4, 9, 10, 41, 44, 70, 74, 75). Most studies have also been consistent in finding either a slight predominance of male patients or an equal male-to-female ratio (4, 11, 41, 44, 62, 75), in contrast to the large male predominance in the Ochsner et al. study (63). These findings are likely related to changes in the cause of PLA. While most cases were related to appendicitis in the past, underlying biliary disease has now been found to be the most common cause in many recent studies (4, 9, 10, 11, 67, 70, 72). Other causes of PLA include neoplastic disease, hematogenous spread during bacteremia, and abdominal trauma. Many cases are labeled as cryptogenic, with no cause identified, despite an appropriate workup.

The majority of organisms involved in PLA originate from the gastrointestinal tract. Table 1 lists the most common organisms recovered from several PLA studies. In the majority of cases, *Escherichia coli* was the predominant pathogen recovered from abscess culture. Prior to 2004, only four studies found *Klebsiella pneumoniae* to be the single

Joseph Rahimian • Department of Infectious Diseases, St. Vincent's Hospital, New York, NY 10011.
Jin-Town Wang • Department of Microbiology, National Taiwan University Hospital, Taipei 10016, Taiwan.

Table 1. Characteristics of PLA studies

Study (reference)	Period of study	No. of patients	Age (yr)	% Solitary	% Right sided	% Positive blood cultures	% with diabetes	Predominant organism
Ochsner et al. (63)	1928–1937	47	30–39[a]	54	68	55–60		E. coli
Huang et al. (44)	1952–1972	80	60	40	38			E. coli
de la Maza et al. (32)	1959–1968	55	60–80[a]					E. coli
Rubin et al. (68)	1961–1973	53	70+					E. coli
Lazarchick et al. (50)	1960–1970	75	51–60[a]	52	74	43	16	E. coli
Greenstein et al. (41)	1967–1982	38	56	50	68			K. pneumoniae
McDonald et al. (58)	1968–1982	55	53[a]	60		50	16	E. coli
Moore-Gillon et al. (60)	1970–1980	16				64		Streptococcus
Land et al. (48)	1973–1980	31	60–69[a]	92	76	56		Streptococcus
Branum et al. (11)	1970–1986	73	50–60[a]	59	70		11	E. coli, K. pneumoniae
Bertel et al. (9)	1977–1984	39	56–60[a]	56	69			Streptococcus
Barnes et al. (7)	1979–1985	48	40–49[a]	73	58	48	27	E. coli
Huang et al. (44)	1973–1993	153	56	52	63			K. pneumoniae
Giorgio et al. (40)	1979–1992	147	45	65	63			E. coli
Yinnon et al. (75)	1979–1992	30	55	26	64			K. pneumoniae
Seeto and Rockey (70)	1979–1994	142	51–60[a]	61	58		15	E. coli
Bissada and Bateman (10)	1982–1989	27	56	59	56	44		
Koneru et al. (47)	1987–1990	15		40	67	55		E. coli
Yang et al. (74)	1988–1992	97	56	84	61		43	K. pneumoniae
Alvarez et al. (4)	1985–1997	133	60	73	71	57	13	E. coli
Rahimian et al. (67)	1993–2003	79	56	77	71	37	15	K. pneumoniae

[a]Number or range represents median age rather than mean.

predominant pathogen recovered. Of these studies, one was from Taiwan (74) and one was from Israel (75). Only two studies from the United States published prior to 2004 found *Klebsiella* to be the predominant pathogen. The study by Greenstein et al. (41) recovered *Klebsiella* from 27% of cases. Of the 14 cases in which *Klebsiella* was recovered, 7 (50%) were monomicrobial and 7 (50%) were polymicrobial. The study by Huang et al. (44) showed that during the initial study period (1952 to 1972), *E. coli* was the predominant organism recovered, but in the second half of the study (1973 to 1993), *Klebsiella* was the predominant organism (though by only a small margin, followed by streptococci). The study suggested that *Klebsiella* was becoming a more common pathogen in cases of PLA. This pattern was further demonstrated in a 2004 study in which Rahimian et al. (67) recovered *Klebsiella* in 29% of the cases, making it the predominant organism recovered. Among cases in which a pathogen was recovered from the abscess culture, the pathogen was *Klebsiella* in 43% of cases. Also of interest was the fact that in the majority of cases in which *Klebsiella* was recovered, it was the only pathogen (78% of cases). Therefore, the percentage of PLA cases caused by *Klebsiella* alone was substantially greater in this study than in any prior study from the United States. In 2005, Lederman and Crum (51) again found that *Klebsiella* was the most common pathogen recovered, accounting for 30% of the total cases and 40% of cases where an organism was recovered. Together, these two studies demonstrate that *Klebsiella* has become the most common pathogen involved in PLA cases in the United States in recent years.

The highest rates of *Klebsiella* recovery were from Taiwan, where 82% of cases were caused by *Klebsiella* (74). The reason for this dramatic finding is unclear. However, the above-mentioned studies suggest that the epidemiological changes may not be limited to one geographic area. The higher rate of *K. pneumoniae* monomicrobial PLA may reflect an evolution in the United States in the etiology of liver abscesses, with changes noted over the past 15 years in reports from Taiwan. It is also possible that the higher rate of *Klebsiella* involvement in the study by Rahimian et al. (67) may simply be a reflection of the recent increase in the Asian population in New York City, where the study was conducted. Indeed, Asian patients were overrepresented among cases of PLA at both institutions where the study was conducted, and this overrepresentation was statistically significant in one of the two institutions. It is unclear whether genetic differences in susceptibility, socioeconomic factors, or yet-unidentified differences account for the overrepresentation of PLA, including those caused by *K. pneumoniae*, among the Asian population.

The study by Yang et al. (74) also showed a high rate of diabetes (43%) among patients with PLA. Another study from Taiwan also found a high rate of diabetes (45%) among patients with PLA (28). Table 1 lists the prevalences of diabetes among patients with PLA from various studies. The higher rate of diabetes seen in Taiwan have not been noted among studies in the United States, where rates of diabetes range from 10% to 27%.

THE EXPERIENCE IN TAIWAN

Since 1980, *K. pneumoniae* has emerged as the predominant pathogen causing PLA in Taiwan (15, 21, 25, 49, 52, 53, 74). Before 1970, PLA caused by *K. pneumoniae* was extremely rare in Taiwan. An early study of 141 cases from 1957 to 1969 reported that amebic liver abscesses were much more common than pyogenic liver abscesses (80% and 20%, respectively) and that the causative organisms of 17 culture-positive PLA cases were *E. coli*

(41%), staphylococci (23%), streptococci (18%), *Proteus* (12%), and *Pseudomonas* (6%) (19). There were no cases of *Klebsiella* causing liver abscess in that study. From 1970 to 1980, *K. pneumoniae* emerged as a more common pathogen in PLA, both in the United States (41, 58, 68) and in Taiwan (25). The increased rates of *Klebsiella* in reports from the United States during this period are shown above. After 1980, however, the percentage of *K. pneumoniae* among PLA cases in Taiwan further increased and far surpassed that seen in reports from the United States. Recovery rates of *K. pneumoniae* rose from 50.8% in one study from 1979 to 1987 ($n = 179$) (21) to 69.8% in another study from 1981 to 1986 ($n = 43$) (15). While these numbers were notably higher than those seen in the United States, the frequency of *K. pneumoniae* as a causative organism continued to rise in Taiwan. One study of 320 cases from 1986 to 1992 found *K. pneumoniae* in 80.6% of the cases (52), while another study of 42 cases from 1992 to 1993 found *K. pneumoniae* in 80.9% (53). The highest recovery rate was seen in a study of 97 patients from 1988 to 1992, in which *K. pneumoniae* was recovered from 82.1% of the patients (74) (Fig. 1). In contrast, there has been no comparable increase in *K. pneumoniae* cases in the United States during the same period. However, there is some evidence that this may be changing, as demonstrated by the study by Rahimian et al. (67). In that report, *K. pneumoniae* was identified in 50% of Asian patients with PLA but in only 27% of non-Asian patients in New York. In a recent study, Lederman and Crum (51) reviewed *K. pneumoniae* PLA cases reported in the United States since 1966 and also noted an increasing number of cases. They reviewed 20 cases from 1999 to 2003 in San Diego and found *K. pneumoniae* to be the most commonly recovered organism, accounting for 6 (30%) cases. Their study provides further evidence of an increasing role of *K. pneumoniae* in cases of PLA in the United States. Furthermore, they noted a trend toward increased recovery of *K. pneumoniae* among Filipinos compared to Caucasians. Of seven cases involving Filipino patients, an organism was recovered in six. In four of the six cases (67%), the organism was

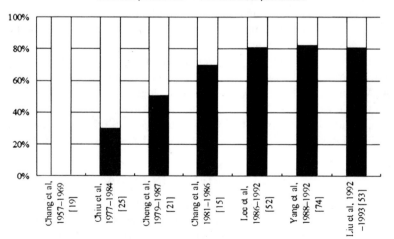

Figure 1. Changing epidemiology of pyogenic liver abscess in Taiwan. The graph shows the percentage of *K. pneumoniae* among pyogenic liver abscesses in Taiwan.

K. pneumoniae. While this is a small sample size, it suggests that the higher rates of *Klebsiella* recovery are influenced in part by membership in certain subpopulations in the United States. There are no studies from the Philippines addressing rates of *K. pneumoniae* recovery from PLA, but it may be that rates in that country parallel the increasing rates seen in countries such as Taiwan and that the higher rates of *Klebsiella* recovery in the United States are in part due to the Asian population.

The reasons why *K. pneumoniae* has emerged as the predominant pathogen causing PLA in Taiwan remains unclear. One possible contributing factor is the documented systemic overuse of amoxicillin and ampicillin in both agriculture and medical practice in Taiwan since the 1970s (16, 18, 43). In the early 1970s, nearly all gram-negative bacterial isolates from agricultural animals in Taiwan were susceptible to the aminopenicillins. Chang (18) reported that among 320 *E. coli* strains isolated from 285 raw milk samples in four major agricultural counties from September 1972 through May 1973, only 5 strains (1.6%) were resistant to aminopenicillins. However, after the use of these antimicrobial agents in animal farming became widespread in the late 1970s and early 1980s, there was a change in the susceptibility profiles. Hsu et al. (43) reported that among 98 nontyphoid *Salmonella* strains isolated from 724 randomly selected pigs from 11 pig farms distributed throughout Taiwan from September 1979 through May 1980, as many as 45 strains (45.9%) were resistant to ampicillin. Because *K. pneumoniae* is constitutively resistant to these aminopenicillins (1), their systemic overuse might eliminate susceptible microorganisms and encourage the colonization of *K. pneumoniae* in both humans and animals. In keeping with this hypothesis, community-acquired thoracic empyema and lung abscess in Taiwan have also shown similar changes in bacteriologic profiles, with an increasing proportion of cases being caused by *K. pneumoniae* (20, 73). While previous studies implicated anaerobes in the predominant etiology of lung abscesses, in the study by Wang et al. (73), *K. pneumoniae* was the most common cause and was recovered in 33% of cases. Among bacterial isolates recovered from transthoracic aspirates, recovery of *K. pneumoniae* increased from 4.6% from 1985 to 1990 to 21% from 1996 to 2003. Diabetes mellitus was again found to be associated with recovery of *Klebsiella*, as seen in the PLA cases from Taiwan. Meningitis is another disease process that has shown a similar change in epidemiology. While *Streptococcus pneumoniae* was previously the most common bacterial cause, after 1995, *Klebsiella pneumoniae* replaced *S. pneumoniae* as the leading pathogen causing community-acquired meningitis in Taiwanese adults (34, 71) (Fig. 2).

MICROBIOLOGY AND THE ROLES OF THE *magA* GENE AND CAPSULAR SEROTYPE IN PATHOGENESIS

K. pneumoniae is one of the most common gram-negative bacteria isolated in the clinical microbiology laboratory. It is a frequent cause of nosocomial infections, such as urinary tract infections, nosocomial pneumonia, and abdominal infections. It is also a cause of community-acquired pneumonia and has frequently been described among particular populations, such as alcoholics, diabetics, and those with chronic obstructive pulmonary disease. The organism has a high propensity for abscess formation. It is naturally resistant to ampicillin and carbenicillin, and many hospital strains now demonstrate resistance to multiple classes of antibiotics. It does not appear that the more resistant strains of

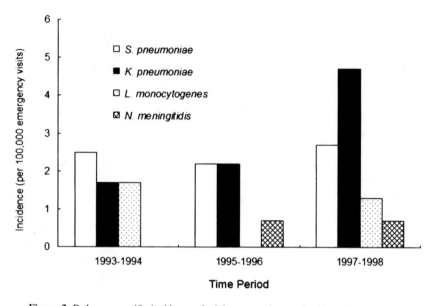

Figure 2. Pathogen-specific incidence of adult community-acquired bacterial meningitis diagnosed at National Taiwan University Hospital during the periods from 1993 to 1994, 1995 to 1996, and 1997 to 1998.

K. pneumoniae are involved in the majority of PLA cases. Rahimian et al. (67) found only one isolate that was an extended-spectrum beta-lactamase (ESBL) producer. A study from Taiwan found that of 160 *K. pneumoniae* isolates from PLA patients, none was an ESBL-producing organism (72). Another study from Taiwan also found no ESBL-producing isolates among 51 cases of PLA caused by *K. pneumoniae* (17).

Early studies on the emerging role of *K. pneumoniae* in PLA focused on host factors, such as diabetes mellitus and glucose intolerance (14, 23, 54, 72). Diabetes mellitus and/or glucose intolerance could be detected in up to 75% of the cases (72). This association has led to speculation that the diabetic patient is at increased risk for this specific organism and disease process. However, in recent years, bacterial virulence has been found to play an important role in the pathogenesis of the disease (29, 33, 37, 38, 46). A multinational prospective study revealed a global difference in clinical patterns of community-acquired *K. pneumoniae* bacteremia, with a distinctive form of *K. pneumoniae* infection causing liver abscess, endophthalmitis, and meningitis almost exclusively in Taiwan (46). Fung et al. (38) found that the prevalence of serotype K1 among bacteremic *K. pneumoniae* isolates (30.8%) in Taiwan was much higher than those reported by other investigators worldwide. They also found that *K. pneumoniae* strains with serotypes K1 and K2 were associated with PLA (63.4% and 14.2% of PLA cases, respectively). Interestingly, nearly all (12 of 14) strains causing liver abscess with metastatic endophthalmitis were serotype K1 (37).

Because these data suggested that there could be some *K. pneumoniae* strains carrying specific virulence factors involved in PLA, researchers began to study bacterial genetics. Fang et al. (33) observed a higher mucoviscosity in strains that caused primary PLA than in those that did not (52 of 53 and 9 of 52, respectively; $P < 0.0001$). They also developed a string test for rapid and objective screening of mucoviscosity. A virulence gene in a reference clinical isolate, NTUH-K2044 (which caused primary PLA and metastatic meningitis in an otherwise healthy 40-year-old man), was identified by using transposon mutagenesis to create a mutant library and to screen mutants with decreased mucoviscosity. This gene was called *magA* (mucoviscosity-associated gene A). The prevalence of *magA* was significantly higher in PLA strains than in noninvasive strains (52 of 53 and 14 of 52, respectively; $P < 0.0001$). The wild-type NTUH-K2044 strain produced a mucoviscous exopolysaccharide web, actively proliferated in nonimmune human serum, resisted phagocytosis, and caused liver microabscess and meningitis in mice (Fig. 3). However, *magA* mutants lost the exopolysaccharide web and became extremely serum sensitive, phagocytosis susceptible, and avirulent to mice (Fig. 3). Virulence was restored by complementation using a *magA*-containing plasmid. Therefore, *magA* fits Koch's postulates as a virulence gene (33). A *magA*-negative control strain, MGH-78578 (which was the cause of fatal pneumonia in a hospitalized patient and was selected for a complete genome-sequencing project at Washington University, St. Louis, Mo. [http://genome.wustl.edu/projects/bacterial/ ?kpneumoniae1]) could not proliferate in nonimmune human serum and was avirulent to mice (33).

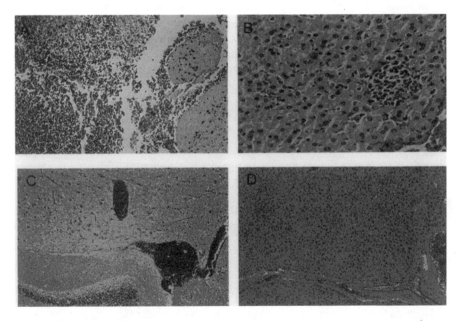

Figure 3. (A and B) Histopathology in the liver and brain of a mouse inoculated with 10^5 CFU of *K. pneumoniae* NTUH-K2044, examined on day 9 after inoculation (hematoxylin and eosin stain; magnification, ×100 [A] versus ×200 [B]). (C and D) Histopathology in the liver and brain of a mouse inoculated with 10^5 CFU of *K. pneumoniae magA* mutant, examined on day 9 after inoculation (hematoxylin and eosin stain; magnification, ×100). Panels A and B show severe meningitis and liver microabscess; panels C and D show normal histology.

Sequences of the *magA* flanking region revealed a 33-kb fragment that was absent in MGH78578 (Fig. 4). Further studies revealed that *magA* is located within a *cps* gene cluster, and that these *cps* loci are specific genetic determinants of serotype K1 in *K. pneumoniae* (29). Therefore, studies based on the capsular serotype seem to be in agreement with the genetic studies.

The presence of *magA* and its flanking 33-kb region suggested the existence of genomic heterogeneity between PLA-associated and noninvasive *K. pneumoniae* strains. The same research group constructed a microarray using a phagemid library of NTUH-K2044 (26, 56). Comparisons of DNA and RNA hybridization signals between four PLA strains and three noninvasive strains revealed two chromosomal regions that were present in PLA strains but not in noninvasive strains or in MGH 78578. The first region was found to be associated with allantoin metabolism and was therefore called the *allS* region. The second region was associated with iron acquisition and was therefore called the *kfu* (*Klebsiella* ferric uptake) region. Knockout of these two regions did not affect the 50% lethal dose in mice by intraperitoneal inoculation. However, the virulence of Δ*allS* and Δ*kfu* mutants decreased by 100 times when intragastric inoculations were performed. Histological examinations of mice that died after intragastric inoculation showed larger abscesses in the liver than in mice that died after intraperitoneal inoculation (Fig. 5). The mode of entry of *K. pneumoniae* into the blood and liver was not documented. However, bacterial cells enter the bloodstream through M cells (26) or due to minor mucosal injuries of the gastrointestinal tract. The fact that larger abscesses were found after intragastric than after intraperitoneal inoculation supported the hypothesis that *K. pneumoniae* gained entry into the bloodstream via the gastrointestinal tract (55). Because all of the venous return in the gastrointestinal tract is collected by the portal vein into the liver, many bacteria are likely to be trapped in the liver by Kupffer cells. However, the invasive strains were resistant to phagocytosis and serum killing. This property may have resulted in the subsequent formation of liver abscesses (56).

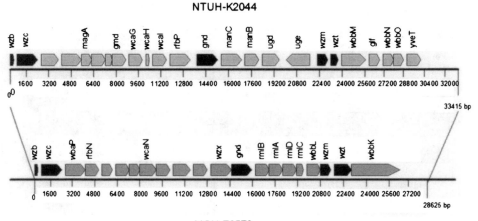

Figure 4. Sequences of the *magA* flanking region revealed a 33-kb fragment, which was replaced with a 28-kb fragment in MGH78578.

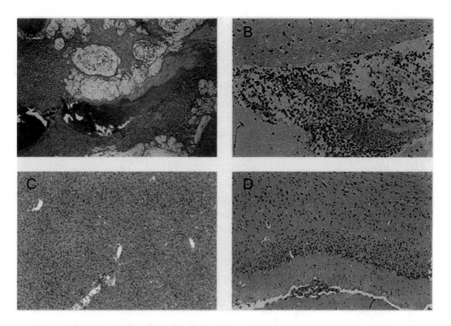

Figure 5. Histological examination of the livers and brains of mice. *K. pneumoniae* was given to mice by intragastric inoculation at a dose of 10^4 CFU. (A and B) Mice inoculated with NTUH-K2044. (C and D) Mice inoculated with MGH 78578. (A) Severe liver abscess (hematoxylin and eosin stain; magnification, ×40). (B) Meningitis and brain abscess (hematoxylin and eosin stain; magnification, ×100). (C and D) Normal histology (hematoxylin and eosin stain; magnification, ×100).

Interestingly, all three regions, *magA*, *allS*, and *kfu*/PTS, were found to be present in each of the strains causing PLA with metastatic endophthalmitis or meningitis (56). Therefore, *magA* is strongly associated with metastatic endophthalmitis or meningitis, and PLA with metastatic complications seems to be caused by *K. pneumoniae* strains of the same genotype. However, in patients with *K. pneumoniae* meningitis without PLA, more than 50% of the strains were *magA* negative. The pathogenesis of non-PLA *K. pneumoniae* meningitis might therefore be different.

After the isolation of *magA*, two recent *K. pneumoniae* strains isolated from PLA cases occurring in Western countries were proven to be *magA* positive: one was in the United States (36), and the other was in Belgium (45). The Belgian case also involved endophthalmitis and bacteremia. These preliminary results suggest that the PLA strain might be genetically the same worldwide. It also suggests that the same strain accounting for the increase in *K. pneumoniae* PLA cases seen in Taiwan will likely influence the microbiology of PLA in other parts of the world, including the United States. Future cases from these areas will likely involve the associated septic complications. However, more studies are required to confirm the role of *magA* in PLA cases from Western countries. To date, there has been one report of endophthalmitis and meningitis associated with *K. pneumoniae* PLA in the United States (69); however, the strain was not available for genetic study.

CLINICAL FEATURES

The most common signs and symptoms of PLA are fever, right upper quadrant pain, and chills (4, 9, 10, 11, 41, 44, 48, 57, 67, 74, 75). The most common laboratory abnormalities are a low albumin level, elevated alkaline phosphatase, and an elevated white blood cell count (10, 11, 17, 44, 48, 67, 70). The majority of patients have lesions in the right lobe of the liver (Table 1). Although many cases of PLA involve multiple abscesses, single abscesses predominate in 50% to 70% of cases (Table 1). Cases involving multiple abscesses appear to be associated with a higher mortality rate. Chou et al. (28) reviewed 483 cases and found a mortality rate of 22.1% in cases with multiple abscesses compared to 12.8% in cases with solitary abscesses. Several other studies have also noted a higher mortality rate with multiple abscesses (42, 50, 66). Another study demonstrated higher mortality among polymicrobial abscesses than in cases where only one organism was recovered (31% and 21%, respectively) (41). Positive blood cultures have been associated with increased mortality in several studies (4, 41, 44, 70). The rates of recovery of bacteria from blood cultures range from 37% to 64% of cases (Table 1). Recovery of organisms from blood has increased since the report by Ochsner et al., in which most blood cultures were sterile (63). At times, organisms recovered from blood may be the only isolate available to guide therapy. However, in many cases, abscess culture grows organisms different from or in addition to those recovered from blood. The percentage of cases in which blood and abscess cultures are concordant is only 47% to 70% (7, 48, 67). Therefore, attempts should be made to obtain abscess cavity culture when possible.

In a clinical study, Chang and Chou (14) reported that, compared with PLA caused by other bacteria, PLA caused by *K. pneumoniae* was significantly more likely to be monomicrobial (95% and 50%, respectively), and patients were more likely to have diabetes mellitus as an underlying disease (66% and 19%, respectively). Cases caused by *K. pneumoniae*, however, were significantly less likely to have biliary tract disease as the predisposing factor (21% versus 75%). A study in Denmark showed that liver cirrhosis was a risk factor for PLA (59). However, the majority of *K. pneumoniae* PLAs in Taiwan were not complications of biliary tract disease or cirrhosis. Yang et al. (74) reported that the percentage of cases with preexisting biliary tract disease as the predisposing factor was up to 36%, but the remaining 64% of cases were "cryptogenic" (i.e., without identifiable hepatobiliary or intra-abdominal pathology). Thus, PLA cases caused by *K. pneumoniae* in Taiwan appear to be a clinically heterogeneous group; in 21 to 36% of the cases, preexisting biliary tract diseases predisposed patients to the development of PLA, while the remaining 64 to 79% of cases were cryptogenic or primary. The pathogeneses of these cases might involve other yet-unspecified bacterial and/or host factors.

Primary *K. pneumoniae* PLA is not merely a disease of the liver. There appears to be a tendency to develop systemic fulminant septic metastatic complications in approximately 10% of the cases (3, 12, 13, 23, 31, 54, 61, 64, 69, 72). Cheng et al. (23) reported that among 187 patients with PLA, 23 patients (12%) developed septic metastatic lesions, including 14 cases (60.8%) of endophthalmitis or uveitis, 10 cases (43.4%) of pulmonary abscess and/or emboli, 6 cases (26.0%) of purulent meningitis and/or brain abscess, 5 cases (21.7%) of bacteriuria and/or prostate abscess, 2 cases (8.6%) of osteomyelitis and/or pyogenic arthritis, and 1 case (4.3%) of psoas abscess. Metastatic endophthalmitis and meningitis are often associated with devastating consequences (3, 12, 13, 23, 27, 31, 54, 61, 64, 69). Metastatic endophthalmitis almost always leads to blindness, with some cases requiring evisceration unless promptly (generally within 24 hours) treated with appropriate systemic and intravitreal antibiotics (27). In cases of community-acquired *K. pneumoniae* meningitis, 80% of patients died or entered a vegetative state. The major determinant of the prognosis was whether the first dose of an appropriate antibiotic was administered before consciousness deteriorated to a Glasgow coma score of 7 points or less (35).

TREATMENT AND OUTCOMES

Mortality rates have decreased substantially over the past several decades. While Ochsner et al. described a mortality rate of 72.3%, one of the most recent studies described a mortality rate of only 2.5% (67). The decreasing mortality rate is likely due in part to improved imaging techniques, as well as improved microbiologic identification and increased use of percutaneous drainage.

While several studies have shown that percutaneous drainage is safe and effective, few studies have compared this intervention to surgical therapy. The cure rates and mortality rates using these interventions have been highly variable. Bergamini et al. (8) found surgical intervention to be associated with a lower mortality rate than with percutaneous drainage (29% and 50%, respectively), with the highest mortality rate seen in patients treated with antibiotics alone (67%). Huang et al. (44) also found surgical intervention to be associated with a lower mortality rate than percutaneous drainage (14 and 26%, respectively). However, both of these studies were initiated in 1973. More recent studies have shown percutaneous drainage to have a lower mortality rate than surgical intervention. Seeto and Rockey (70) found that percutaneous drainage was successful in 76% of cases, with a 6% mortality rate, while surgical intervention had an overall success rate of 61%, with a 13% mortality rate. In the last 5 years of the study, the cure rate in the percutaneous-drainage group increased to 90%, with only a 5% mortality rate. This study also reported that cases treated with antibiotics alone had the highest mortality. Alvarez Perez et al. (4) found a 13% mortality rate with both surgical and percutaneous drainage, with the highest mortality rate again being found in patients treated with antibiotics alone. However, despite the similar mortality rates in the percutaneous and surgical groups, the former had a higher rate of treatment failure (27 and 19%, respectively). Unfortunately, it is extremely difficult to compare these treatment modalities. Surgery was more often done in the earlier years of each study, and the higher mortality rates may therefore be confounded by other factors. On the other hand, patients who were not sent for surgery may have been too ill to tolerate the procedure; therefore, the groups receiving percutaneous drainage or antibiotics alone may reflect a more severely ill patient population. Furthermore, many studies have included patients treated with needle aspiration in the same group as those treated with catheter drainage. A randomized trial comparing the surgical and percutaneous interventions is necessary, though it is unlikely to occur, given the impressive cure rates seen with percutaneous drainage in recent years. At this time, all primary PLA cases caused by *K. pneumoniae* in Taiwan appear to be community acquired, and the causative *K. pneumoniae* strains are nearly universally susceptible to all cephalosporins and aminoglycosides by routine disk susceptibility testing (17, 72, 74). Nevertheless, cumulative evidence has shown that the first- and second-generation cephalosporins are suboptimal choices for treatment. The MICs of cefazolin, cefuroxime, and cefmetazole inhibiting 90% of *K. pneumoniae* strains causing primary PLA were reported to be 2, 4, and 1 µg/ml, respectively.

These values are much higher than the MICs of cefotaxime, cefepime, cefpirome, and aztreonam (0.06 µg/ml) (17). The insufficient penetration of cefazolin, cefuroxime, and cefmetazole into cerebrospinal and vitreous fluids (5) is also a serious disadvantage in the face of a systemic infection caused by invasive *K. pneumoniae* strains capable of invading the central nervous system. A retrospective study showed that patients receiving extended-spectrum cephalosporins for the treatment of *K. pneumoniae* PLA had a significantly lower incidence (6.3%) of metastatic infections, respiratory failure, or death 72 h after admission than patients receiving cefazolin with or without gentamicin (37.3%) ($P < 0.001$) (24). The same study also identified other independent factors preventing the development of metastatic infections, respiratory failure, or death. These included a normal platelet count, alkaline phosphatase less than 300 U/liter, no gas formation in the abscess, and early drainage of the liver abscesses (22, 24). Thus, appropriate and timely drainage of PLA, in addition to an extended-spectrum cephalosporin, appears to be important in order to obtain the best possible outcome.

The emerging role of *Klebsiella* in PLA also suggests that some regimens previously used for PLA, such as ampicillin with gentamicin, may not be optimal choices of therapy. Given the intrinsic resistance of *Klebsiella* to ampicillin and the poor uptake of gentamicin into bacterial cells in low-pH environments, extended-spectrum penicillins and cephalosporins may be more suitable treatment options. For ESBL-containing strains, carbapenems may be considered. Ophthalmologic and neurological evaluations should be part of the initial evaluation of patients with documented *K. pneumoniae* PLA, especially for strains that are found to be *magA* positive. Failure to recognize metastatic endophthalmitis and/or meningitis within 24 hours of onset may delay the appropriate management and lead to devastating consequences.

The optimal duration of treatment for PLA remains unclear. Most studies have used at least 2 weeks of intravenous antibiotics, followed by oral therapy. Some have developed a standardized approach to PLA, using 3 weeks of intravenous therapy followed by 1 to 2 months of oral therapy (72).

CONCLUSIONS

While cases of pyogenic liver abscesses have been reported in the literature for many years, there have been many changes in the epidemiology of the disease. Over the past several decades, patient age has increased, there is no longer as significant a male predominance as there used to be, and there has been a change in the underlying diseases seen in PLA cases. Mortality has decreased dramatically in cases of PLA, perhaps because of changing underlying causes, improved diagnostic capabilities, and more optimal therapies.

Recently, a new change in the epidemiology of the disease has occurred. *K. pneumoniae* has become by far the most common pathogen recovered from these infections in areas such as Taiwan and has been recovered with increasing frequency in other areas, as well. The most recent studies suggest that it is currently the most common cause of PLA in the United States. Diabetes mellitus has emerged as a possible risk factor, though the extent and significance of this association remains unclear. In Taiwan, serotype K1 has been associated with endophthalmitis and meningitis, creating a unique syndrome that has only recently been noted. Recently, virulence factors, such as that encoded by the *magA* gene, have been identified. Strains with *magA* are also strongly associated with metastatic complications, such as endophthalmitis and meningitis. It will be interesting to see if this syndrome is noted with increasing frequency in other areas of the world, as well. The increasing role of *Klebsiella* does not appear to be limited to cases of PLA, as *Klebsiella* is also being recovered with increasing frequency from cases of lung abscesses. These changes have important implications for management and treatment.

Acknowledgments. We thank Chi-Tai Fang and Chester Lerner for assistance with the content and preparation of the manuscript.

REFERENCES

1. **Abbott, S.** 1999. *Klebsiella, Enterobacter, Citrobacter*, and *Serratia*, p. 475–482. *In* P. R. Murray, E. J. Baron, M. A. Pfaller, F. C. Tenover, and R. H. Yolken (ed.), *Manual of Clinical Microbiology*, 7th ed. ASM Press, Washington, D.C.
2. **Adams, F.** 1886. *The Genuine Works of Hippocrates*. W. Wood and Company, New York, N.Y.
3. **Aguilar, J., A. Cruz, and C. Ortega.** 1994. Multiple hepatic and pulmonary abscesses caused by *Klebsiella pneumoniae*. *Enferm. Infecc. Microbiol. Clin.* **12:**270–271.
4. **Alvarez Perez, J. A., J. J. Gonzalez, R. F. Baldonedo, L. Sanz, G. Carreno, A. Junco, J. I. Rodriguez, M. D. Martinez, and J. I. Jorge.** 2001. Clinical course, treatment, and multivariate analysis of risk factors for pyogenic liver abscess. *Am. J. Surg.* **181:**177–186.
5. **Andes, D. R., and W. A. Craig.** 2005. Cephalosporins, p. 294–310. *In* G. L. Mandell, J. E. Bennett, and R. Dolin (ed.), *Principles and Practice of Infectious Diseases*, 6th ed. Elsevier, Philadelphia, Pa.
6. **Attar, B., H. Levendoglu, and H. S. Cuasay.** 1986. CT-guided percutaneous aspiration and catheter drainage of pyogenic liver abscesses. *Am. J. Gastroenterol.* **81:**550–555.
7. **Barnes, P. F., K. M. De Cock, T. N. Reynolds, and P. W. Ralls.** 1987. A comparison of amebic and pyogenic abscess of the liver. *Medicine* (Baltimore) **66:**472–483.
8. **Bergamini, T. M., G. M. Larson, M. A. Malangoni, and J. D. Richardson.** 1987. Liver abscess: review of 12-year experience. *Am. Surg.* **52:**596–599.
9. **Bertel, C. K., J. A. van Heerden, and P. F. Sheedy II.** 1986. Treatment of pyogenic hepatic abscesses. Surgical vs percutaneous drainage. *Arch. Surg.* **121:**554–558.
10. **Bissada, A. A., and J. Bateman.** 1991. Pyogenic liver abscess: a 7-year experience in a large community hospital. *Hepatogastroenterology* **38:**317–320.
11. **Branum, G. D., G. S. Tyson, M. A. Branum, and W. C. Meyers.** 1990. Hepatic abscess. Changes in etiology, diagnosis, and management. *Ann. Surg.* **212:**655–662.
12. **Cahill, M., B. Chang, and A. Murray.** 2000. Bilateral endogenous bacterial endophthalmitis associated with pyogenic hepatic abscess. *Br. J. Ophthalmol.* **84:**1436.
13. **Casanova, C., J. A. Lorente, F. Carrillo, E. P. Rodriguez, and N. Nunez.** 1989. *Klebsiella pneumoniae* liver abscess associated with septic endophthalmitis. *Arch. Intern. Med.* **149:**1467.
14. **Chang, F. Y., and M. Y. Chou.** 1995. Comparison of pyogenic liver abscesses caused by *Klebsiella pneumoniae* and non-*K. pneumoniae* pathogens. *J. Formos. Med. Assoc.* **94:**232–237.
15. **Chang, F. Y., M. Y. Chou, R. L. Fan, and M. F. Shaio.** 1988. A clinical study of *Klebsiella* liver abscesses. *J. Formos. Med. Assoc.* **87:**282–287.
16. **Chang, S. C., H. J. Chang, and M. S. Lai.** 1999. Antibiotic usage in primary care units in Taiwan. *Int. J. Antimicrob. Agents* **11:**23–30.
17. **Chang, S. C., C. T. Fang, P. R. Hsueh, Y. C. Chen, and K. T. Luh.** 2000. *Klebsiella pneumoniae* isolates causing liver abscess in Taiwan. *Diagn. Microbiol. Infect. Dis.* **37:**279–284.
18. **Chang, S. H.** 1975. *Escherichia coli* isolation from raw milk in central and southern Taiwan and their susceptibility to drugs. *Chin. J. Microbiol.* **8:**142–145.
19. **Chang, W. Y., and C. Y. Chen.** 1970. Clinical observation of liver abscess. *J. Formos. Med. Assoc.* **69:**670–708.
20. **Chen, K. Y., P. R. Hsueh, Y. S. Liaw, P. C. Yang, and K. T. Luh.** 2000. A 10-year experience with bacteriology of acute thoracic empyema with emphasis on *Klebsiella pneumoniae* in patients with diabetes mellitus. *Chest* **117:**1685–1689.

21. **Cheng, D. L., Y. C. Liu, M. Y. Yen, C. Y. Liu, F. W. Shi, and L. S. Wang.** 1989. Causal bacteria of pyogenic liver abscess. *J. Formos. Med. Assoc.* **88:**1008–1011.

22. **Cheng, D. L., Y. C. Liu, M. Y. Yen, C. Y. Liu, F. W. Shi, and L. S. Wang.** 1990. Pyogenic liver abscess: clinical manifestations and value of percutaneous catheter drainage treatment. *J. Formos. Med. Assoc.* **89:**571–576.

23. **Cheng, D. L., Y. C. Liu, M. Y. Yen, C. Y. Liu, and R. S. Wang.** 1991. Septic metastatic lesions of pyogenic liver abscess: association with *Klebsiella pneumoniae* bacteremia in diabetic patients. *Arch. Intern. Med.* **151:**1557–1559.

24. **Cheng, H. P., L. K. Siu, and F. Y. Chang.** 2003. Extended-spectrum cephalosporin compared to cefazolin for treatment of *Klebsiella pneumoniae*-caused liver abscess. *Antimicrob. Agents Chemother.* **47:**2088–2092.

25. **Chiu, C. T., D. Y. Lin, C. S. Wu, et al.** 1987. A clinical study on pyogenic liver abscess. *J. Formos. Med. Assoc.* **86:**405–412.

26. **Chou, C. H., C. H. Lee, L. C. Ma, C. T. Fang, S. C. Chang, and J. T. Wang.** 2004. Isolation of a chromosomal region of *Klebsiella pneumoniae* associated with allantoin metabolism and liver infection. *Infect. Immun.* **72:**3783–3792.

27. **Chou, F. F., and H. K. Kou.** 1996. Endogenous endophthalmitis associated with pyogenic hepatic abscess. *J. Am. Coll. Surg.* **182:**33–36.

28. **Chou, F. F., S. M. Sheen-Chen, Y. S. Chen, and M. C. Chen.** 1997. Single and multiple pyogenic liver abscesses: clinical course, etiology, and result of treatment. *World J. Surg.* **21:**384–389.

29. **Chuang, Y. P., C. T. Fang, S. Y. Lai, S. C. Chang, and J. T. Wang.** 2006. Genetic determinants of capsular serotype K1 of *Klebsiella pneumoniae* causing primary liver abscess. *J. Infect. Dis.* **193:**645-654.

30. **Civardi, G., C. Filice, M. Caremani, and A. Giorgio.** 1992. Hepatic abscesses in immunocompromised patients: ultrasonically guided percutaneous drainage. *Gastrointest. Radiol.* **17:**175–178.

31. **Couez, D., E. Libon, M. Wasteels, G. Derue, and J. P. Gilbeau.** 1991. *Klebsiella pneumoniae* liver abscess with septic endophthalmitis: the role of computed tomography. *J. Belge Radiol.* **74:**41–44.

32. **de la Maza, L., F. Naeim, and L. Berman.** 1974. The changing etiology of liver abscess. *JAMA* **227:**161–163.

33. **Fang, C. T., Y. P. Chuang, C. T. Shun, S. C. Chang, and J. T. Wang.** 2004. A novel virulence gene in *Klebsiella pneumoniae* strains causing primary liver abscess and septic metastatic complications. *J. Exp. Med.* **199:**697–705.

34. **Fang, C. T., S. C. Chang, P. R. Hsueh, Y. C. Chen, W. Y. Shau, and K. T. Luh.** 2000. Microbiologic features of adult community-acquired bacterial meningitis in Taiwan. *J. Med. Assoc.* **99:**300–304.

35. **Fang, C. T., Y. C. Chen, S. C. Chang, W. Y. Shau, and K. T. Luh.** 2000. *Klebsiella pneumoniae* meningitis: timing of antimicrobial therapy and prognosis. *Q. J. Med.* **93:**45–53.

36. **Fang, F. C., N. Sandler, and S. J. Libby.** 2005, Liver abscess caused by *magA*⁺ *Klebsiella pneumoniae* in North America. *J. Clin. Microbiol.* **43:**991–992.

37. **Fung, C. P., F. Y. Chang, S. C. Lee, B. S. Hu, B. I. T. Kuo, C. Y. Liu, M. Ho, and L. K. Siu.** 2002. A global emerging disease of *Klebsiella pneumoniae* liver abscess: is serotype K1 an important factor for complicated endophthalmitis? *Gut* **50:**420–424.

38. **Fung, C. P., B. S. Hu, F. Y. Chang, et al.** 2000. A 5-year study of the seroepidemiology of *Klebsiella pneumoniae*: high prevalence of capsular serotype K1 in Taiwan and implication for vaccine efficacy. *J. Infect. Dis.* **181:**2075–2079.

39. **Gerzof, S. G., W. C. Johnson, A. H. Robbins, and D. C. Nabseth.** 1985. Intrahepatic pyogenic abscess: treatment by percutaneous drainage. *Am. J. Surg.* **149:**487–494.

40. **Giorgio, A., L. Tarantino, N. Mariniello, G. Francica, E. Scala, P. Amoroso, A. Nuzzo, and G. Rizzatto.** 1995. Pyogenic liver abscesses: 13 years of experience in percutaneous needle aspiration with US guidance. *Radiology* **195:**122–124.

41. **Greenstein, A. J., D. Lowenthal, G. S. Hammer, F. Schaffner, and A. H. Aufses, Jr.** 1984. Continuing changing patterns of disease in pyogenic liver abscess: a study of 38 patients. *Am. J. Gastroenterol.* **79:**217–226.

42. **Heymann, A. D.** 1979. Clinical aspects of grave pyogenic abscesses of the liver. *Surg. Gynecol. Obstet.* **149:**209–213.

43. **Hsu, F. S., L. L. Chuech, and Y. M. Shen.** 1983. Isolation, serotyping and drug resistance of *Salmonella* in scouring pigs in Taiwan. *Chinese J. Microbiol. Immunol.* **16:**283–290.

44. **Huang, C. J., H. A. Pitt, P. A. Lipsett, F. A. Osterman, K. D. Lillemoe, J. L. Cameron, and G. D. Zuidemo.** 1996. Pyogenic hepatic abscess. Changing trends over 42 years. *Ann. Surg.* **223:**600–609.

45. **Karama, E. M., F. Willermain, X. Janssen, J. T. Wang, and S. van den Wijngaert.** Endogenous endophthalmitis complicating *K. pneumoniae* liver abscess in Europe. Submitted for publication.

46. **Ko, W. C., D. L. Paterson, A. J. Sagnimeni, D. Hansen, D. Von Gottberg, S. Mohapatra, J. M. Caseelas, H. Goossens, L. Mulazimoglu, T. Gordon, K. Klugman, J. G. McCormack, and V. L. Yu.** 2002. Community-acquired *Klebsiella pneumoniae* bacteremia: global differences in clinical patterns. *Emerg. Infect. Dis.* **8:**160–166.

47. **Koneru, S., G. Peskin, and V. Sreenivas.** 1994. Pyogenic hepatic abscess in a community hospital. *Am. Surg.* **60:**278–281.

48. **Land, M. A., M. Moinuddin, and A. L. Bisno.** 1985. Pyogenic liver abscess: changing epidemiology and prognosis. *South. Med. J.* **78:**1426–1430.

49. **Lau, Y. J., B. S. Hu, W. L. Wu, Y. H. Lin, H. Y. Chang, and Z. Y. Shi.** 2000. Identification of a major cluster of *Klebsiella pneumoniae* isolates from patients with liver abscess in Taiwan. *J. Clin. Microbiol.* **38:**412–414.

50. **Lazarchick, J., N. De Souza, D. Nichols, and J. Washington.** 1973. Pyogenic liver abscess. *Mayo Clin. Proc.* **45:**349–355.

51. **Lederman, E. R., and N. F. Crum.** 2005. Pyogenic liver abscess with a focus on *Klebsiella pneumoniae* as a primary pathogen: an emerging disease with unique clinical characteristics. *Am. J. Gastroenterol.* **100:**322–331.

52. **Lee, T. Y., Y. L. Wan, and C. C. Tsai.** 1994. Gas-forming liver abscess: radiological findings and clinical significance. *Abdom. Imaging* **19:**47–52.

53. **Liu, Y. C., D. L. Cheng, and Y. S. Chen.** 1996. A pilot study of oral fleroxacin once daily compared with conventional therapy in patients with bacterial liver abscess, p. 296. *In Proceedings of the 7th International Congress for Infectious Diseases.* BMJ Publishing Group, London, United Kingdom.

54. **Liu, Y. C., D. L. Cheng, and C. L. Lin.** 1986. *Klebsiella pneumoniae* liver abscess associated with septic endophthalmitis. *Arch. Intern. Med.* **146:**1913–1916.

55. **Lu, L., and W. A. Walker.** 2001. Pathologic and physiologic interactions of bacteria with the gastrointestinal epithelium. *Am. J. Clin. Nutr.* **73:**1124S–1130S.

56. **Ma, L. C., C. T. Fang, C. Z. Lee, C. T. Shun, and J. T. Wang.** 2005. Genomic heterogeneity in *Klebsiella pneumoniae* strains associated with primary pyogenic liver abscess and metastatic infections. *J. Infect. Dis.* **192:**117–128.

57. **McDonald, A. P., and R. J. Howard.** 1980. Pyogenic liver abscess. *World J. Surg.* **4:**369–380.

58. **McDonald, M. I., G. R. Corey, H. A. Gallis, and D. T. Durack.** 1984. Single and multiple pyogenic liver abscesses. *Medicine* **63:**291–302.

59. **Molle, I., A. M. Thulstrup, H. Vilstrup, and H. T. Sorensen.** 2001. Increased risk and case fatality rate of pyogenic liver abscess in patients with liver cirrhosis: a nationwide study in Denmark. *Gut* **48:**260–263.

60. **Moore-Gillon, J. C., S. J. Eykyn, and I. Phillips.** 1981. Microbiology of pyogenic liver abscess. *Br. Med. J.* **283:**819–821.

61. **Naito, T., T. Kawakami, M. Tsuda, T. Ebe, S. Sekiya, H. Isonuma, T. Matsumoto, and K. Watanabe.** 1999. A case of endophthalmitis and abscesses in the liver and the lung caused by *Klebsiella pneumoniae*. *Kansenshogaku Zasshi* **73:**935–938.

62. **Neoptolemos, J. P., D. S. Macpherson, J. Holm, and D. P. Fossard.** 1982. Pyogenic liver abscess: a study of forty-four cases in two centres. *Acta Chir. Scand.* **148:**415–421.

63. **Ochsner, A., M. DeBakey, and S. Murray.** 1938. Pyogenic abscess of the liver. *Am. J. Surg.* **40:**292–314.

64. **Ohmori, S., K. Shiraki, K. Ito, H. Inoue, T. Ito, T. Sakai, K. Takase, and T. Nakano.** 2002. Septic endophthalmitis and meningitis associated with *Klebsiella pneumoniae* liver abscess. *Hepatol. Res.* **22:**307–312.

65. **Perera, M. R., A. Kirk, and P. Noone.** 1980. Presentation, diagnosis, and management of liver abscess. *Lancet* **i:**629–632.

66. **Pitt, H. A., and G. D. Zuidema.** 1975. Factors influencing mortality in the treatment of pyogenic hepatic abscesses. *Surg. Gynecol. Obstet.* **140:**228.

67. **Rahimian, J., T. Wilson, V. Oram, and R. Holzman.** 2004. Pyogenic liver abscess: recent trends in etiology and mortality. *Clin. Infect. Dis.* **39:**1654–1659.

68. **Rubin, R., M. Swartz, and R. Malt.** 1974. Hepatic abscess: changes in clinical, bacteriologic and therapeutic aspects. *Am. J. Med.* **57:**601–610.

69. **Saccente, M.** 1999. *Klebsiella pneumoniae* liver abscess, endophthalmitis, and meningitis in a man with newly recognized diabetes mellitus. *Clin. Infect. Dis.* **29:**1570–1571.

70. **Seeto, R. K., and D. C. Rockey.** 1996. Pyogenic liver abscess. Changes in etiology, management, and outcome. *Medicine* (Baltimore) **75:**99-113.

71. **Tang, L. M., S. T. Chen, W. C. Hsu, and R. K. Lyu.** 1999. Acute bacterial meningitis in adults: a hospital-based epidemiological study. *Q. J. Med.* **92:**719–725.

72. **Wang, J. H., Y. C. Liu, S. S. Lee, et al.** 1998. Primary liver abscess due to *Klebsiella pneumoniae* in Taiwan. *Clin. Infect. Dis.* **26:**1434–1438.

73. **Wang, J. L., K. Y. Chen, C. T. Fang, P. R. Hsueh, P. C. Yang, and S. C. Chang.** 2005. Changing bacteriology of adult community-acquired lung abscess in Taiwan: *Klebsiella pneumoniae* versus anaerobes. *Clin. Infect. Dis.* **40:**915–922.

74. **Yang, C. C., C. Y. Chen, X. Z. Lin, T. T. Chang, J. S. Shin, and C. Y. Lin.** 1993. Pyogenic liver abscess in Taiwan: emphasis on gas-forming liver abscess in diabetics. *Am. J. Gastroenterol.* **88:**1911–1915.

75. **Yinnon, A. M., I. Hadas-Halpern, M. Shapiro, and C. Hershko.** 1994. The changing clinical spectrum of liver abscess: the Jerusalem experience. *Postgrad. Med. J.* **70:**436–439.

Emerging Infections 7
Edited by W. M. Scheld, D. C. Hooper, and J. M. Hughes
© 2007 ASM Press, Washington, D.C.

Chapter 12

Conjugate Vaccines as Probes To Define the Burden of Pneumococcal and *Haemophilus influenzae* Type b Pneumonia as Well as the Role of Viruses in the Pathogenesis of Pneumonia

Keith P. Klugman and Shabir A. Madhi

The diagnosis of the etiology of pneumonia is challenging, particularly in children, from whom infected sputa are rarely available and for whom a urinary antigen test is not a useful diagnostic tool (1). Invasive approaches, such as lung taps, may increase the yield of pathogens (31), but they are limited to specific cases in which obvious consolidation on X rays is peripheral, allowing access to aspiration by a needle. Recent advances in vaccines against the major bacterial pathogens causing pneumonia allow us to use these vaccines as probes within the context of randomized trials or case control studies to determine the vaccine-preventable burden of pneumonia. These approaches also allow us to define the roles of these pathogens in a variety of clinical endpoints and to explore in a novel way the interaction of bacteria with viruses in the pathogenesis of pneumonia.

Hib CONJUGATE VACCINE

Studies on the role of conjugate vaccine as a probe to define the burden of pathogen-specific pneumonia were pioneered in The Gambia by Kim Mulholland and colleagues, who showed that *Haemophilus influenzae* type b (Hib) conjugate could reduce the burden of radiologically proven pneumonia by 21% (95% confidence interval [CI], 5 to 35%) in vaccine recipients compared to controls in a randomized clinical trial (26). A retrospective analysis of a Hib conjugate vaccine trial in Chile produced similar results 22% (95% CI, −7 to 43%) (19), and point estimates of efficacy in Brazilian (9) and Colombian (10) case control trials pointed to similar reductions (31% [95% CI, −9 to 57%] and 55% [95% CI, 7 to 78%], respectively) (Table 1). The higher estimates of efficacy in the case-control studies

Keith P. Klugman • Hubert Department of Global Health, Rollins School of Public Health, and Division of Infectious Diseases, School of Medicine, Emory University, 1518 Clifton Rd., Rm. 720, Atlanta, GA 30322.
Shabir A. Madhi • Respiratory and Meningeal Pathogens Research Unit, Chris Hani-Baragwanath Hospital, Old Nurses Home, 1st Floor, West Wing, Bertsham, Gauteng 2013, South Africa.

Table 1. Conjugate vaccine studies as probes of X-ray confirmed bacterial pneumonia etiology

Vaccine[a]	Site (reference)	Type of study	Vaccine efficacy (%)	95% CI (%)[b]
Hib conjugate PRP-T (ITT)	The Gambia (26)	Individually randomized	21	5 to 35
PRP-T (ITT)	Indonesia (12)	Cluster randomized	−5	NS
PRP-T (PP)	Chile (19)	Cluster randomized	22	−7 to 43
PRP-CRM$_{197}$	Brazil (9)	Case control	31	−9 to 57
PRP-T	Colombia (10)	Case control	55	7 to 78
Pneumococcal conjugate 7-valent CRM$_{197}$ (ITT)	California (5)	Individually randomized	18	5 to 29
	Navajo (27)	Cluster randomized	<0	NS
Non-HIV-infected; 9-valent CRM$_{197}$ (ITT)	South Africa (16)	Individually randomized	20	2 to 35
HIV-infected; 9-valent CRM$_{197}$ (ITT)	South Africa (16)	Individually randomized	13	−7 to 29
9-valent CRM$_{197}$ (ITT)	The Gambia (8)	Individually randomized	35	26 to 43

[a]ITT, intent to treat; PP, per protocol.
[b]NS, not significant.

may reflect a bias toward less access to immunization in the cases, although in the Colombian study (10), access to measles-mumps-rubella vaccine was not significantly greater among controls, and the increased efficacy may have been due to stringent criteria for defining bacterial pneumonia among hospitalized cases. In some parts of the world, such as Southeast Asia, the Hib contribution to the pneumonia burden may be modest relative to those of other pathogens. A Hib vaccine probe study in Lombok, Indonesia, failed to find a significant fraction of X-ray-confirmed pneumonia that could be prevented by the Hib conjugate vaccine (12). The study, however, suggested the possibility that Hib might cause a small fraction of the very large burden of pneumonia in that rural community. The vaccine prevented 4% (95% CI, 0.7 to 7.1%) of largely community-diagnosed clinical pneumonia, thus preventing 1,561 (95% CI, 270 to 2,853) cases per 10^5 child-years from an incidence in controls of 39,516 per 10^5 child-years (12). In contrast, in The Gambia, where surveillance was primarily health facility based and the community was more periurban, there was a reduction of only 110 cases per 10^5 child-years in the vaccinated arm compared to an incidence of 2,500 in the placebo arm (26). Studies based in more urban areas thus underestimate the fraction of disease preventable by Hib vaccine.

PNEUMOCOCCAL CONJUGATE VACCINE

Two conjugate pneumococcal vaccine formulations have been tested in randomized trials against pneumonia endpoints: a seven-valent vaccine consisting of serotypes 4, 6B, 9V, 14, 18C, 19F, and 23F and a nine-valent formulation with the addition of serotypes 1 and 5. Both vaccines have the carbohydrate capsular material conjugated to the diphtheria toxoid mutant CRM$_{197}$. The seven- and nine-valent pneumococcal conjugate vaccines have been shown to be highly efficacious in the prevention of pneumococcal bacteremia. Rates of protection in excess of 90% were found in children (mostly with bacteremia alone) in northern California (4), while efficacies against bacteremic pneumonia and meningitis were >80% in Navajo (28), South African (16), and Gambian (8) children.

Pneumonia remains the leading cause of death for children globally (3). As the pneumococcus is likely the major preventable cause of pneumonia, all four trials of pneumococcal conjugate vaccine with an invasive-disease endpoint have addressed the vaccine impact against pneumonia (Table 1). A retrospective analysis of pneumonia cases in the northern California trial revealed a vaccine efficacy of 20% against pneumonia reported as consolidation on X ray (5). In an attempt to standardize the X-ray endpoint of pneumonia in conjugate vaccine trials, the WHO convened a working group that has produced guidelines for this diagnosis (6).

Using this approach, the three subsequent pneumococcal conjugate vaccine clinical trials have reported efficacies ranging from no efficacy in the Navajo (27) to 25% efficacy in per-protocol analyses in South Africa (16) and 37% in The Gambia (8). There was remarkable concordance in the point estimates of vaccine efficacy from the periurban environments of Soweto (16) in Africa and San Francisco in northern California (5). There was less concordance in the rural studies. The lack of impact on pneumonia in the Navajo trial (27) may reflect poor coverage of the seven-valent vaccine in a community in which many "adult" strains circulate to children. Both the Soweto and northern California studies included children at the point of primary care, while the Navajo study concentrated recruitment on hospitalized children. It is possible that in an environment in which community access to antibiotics is good, hospitalized children may reflect nonresponsive (mainly viral) pneumonias. This cluster-randomized trial also lacked power to find a level of protection on the order of 20%. The high impact of the nine-valent conjugate in rural Gambia (8) may reflect an increased fraction of bacterial pathogens causing pneumonia in children without early access to antibiotics and with delayed exposure to the health care system.

The effect of living in a rural versus urban area in terms of childhood mortality and potential for vaccine impact is well illustrated by the two large trials of conjugate vaccines in The Gambia. The Hib vaccine trial (26) was conducted in the western part of the country, which is periurban around the capital, while the pneumococcal trial (8) was conducted in the eastern, more remote, rural part of the country. Mortality in the more urban Hib trial conducted from 1993 to 1996 was 2/1,000 enrolled children, compared to 28/1,000 children in the per-protocol analysis of all-cause mortality in the rural area. Although the mortality surveillance was more complete in the rural study, the 14-fold-increased mortality detected there suggests a huge difference between urban and rural mortalities in a single small country. A 16% drop in all-cause mortality was found among recipients of the pneumococcal conjugate vaccine (8). The vaccine could thus be used as a probe to measure impact on mortality in that study.

The specificity of the endpoint of clinical trials is important to avoid misclassification bias (13), which reduces the apparent efficacy of the intervention. In an attempt to increase the specificity of the X-ray consolidation WHO endpoint, the data from the South African trial were reanalyzed in a blinded analysis using acute serum measures of procalcitonin and C-reactive protein (CRP) (20) (Table 2). These data show that vaccine efficacy increases as the specificity of the endpoint increases, thus increasing the power of vaccine studies to document an impact against pneumonia. These data also suggest that the true efficacy of pneumococcal conjugate vaccine against vaccine serotype pneumococcal pneumonia may be in excess of 64% (20) (as pneumonia caused by other bacterial pathogens

Table 2. Data from a South African trial analyzed using procalcitonin and CRP[a]

Outcome measure[b]	Children not infected with HIV					Children infected with HIV				
	No. receiving PnCV[e] (n = 18,633)	No. receiving placebo (n = 18,626)	Vaccine efficacy (%)	95% CI (%)	P value	No. receiving PnCV (n = 1,289)	No. receiving placebo (n = 1,288)	Vaccine efficacy (%)	95% CI (%)	P value
CXR-AC	132	167	21	1, 37	0.04	139	153	9	-13, 27	0.38
CXR-AC + PCT ≥ 2 ng/ml	40	52	23	-16, 49	0.21	61	83	27	-1, 47	0.06
CXR-AC + PCT ≥ 4 ng/ml	23	37	38	-5, 63	0.07	43	65	34	3, 55	0.03
CXR-AC + PCT ≥ 5 ng/ml	19	35	46	5, 69	0.03	41	61	33	1, 54	0.04
CXR-AC + CRP < 40 mg/liter	68	82	17	-14, 40	0.25	74	69	-7	-32, 28	0.67
CXR-AC + CRP ≥ 40 mg/liter	64	85	25	-4, 46	0.08	65	84	23	-6, 44	0.10
CXR-AC + CRP ≥ 80 mg/liter	42	61	31	-2, 54	0.06	51	71	28	-2, 50	0.06
CXR-AC + CRP ≥ 120 mg/liter	28	45	38	0, 61	0.05	40	61	35	3, 56	0.03
CXR-AC + CRP ≥ 120 mg/liter + PCT ≥ 5 ng/ml	9	25	64	23, 83	0.006	21	44	52	20, 71	0.004
Bacteremic pneumococcal pneumonia[c]	5	8	38	-91, 80	0.42	17	31	45	1, 70	0.04
Vaccine serotype pneumococcal pneumonia[d]	2	6	67	-65, 93	0.18	7	17	59	1, 83	0.04

[a]Reprinted from reference 20 with permission. CXR-confirmed alveolar consolidation is based on World Health Organization guidelines for interpretation. Point estimates differ from those previously published because only children with chest X-ray (CXR)-confirmed pneumonia for whom sera for CRP and procalcitonin measurements were available are included.
[b]CXR-AC, CXR-confirmed alveolar consolidation; PCT, procalcitonin.
[c]Pneumonia associated with growth from blood of S. pneumoniae of any serotype.
[d]Pneumonia associated with growth from blood of S. pneumoniae of vaccine serotype.
[e]PnCV, pneumococcal conjugate vaccine.

and by nonvaccine serotypes would be expected to also cause consolidation on X ray and high levels of procalcitonin and CRP, thus confounding and lowering the point estimate of true vaccine efficacy against vaccine serotypes).

The burden of pneumonia prevented by conjugate pneumococcal vaccine may be underestimated by consideration only of the vaccine impact against X-ray-confirmed pneumonia. Once again, analyses of the South African data suggest that the burden of disease prevented, or vaccine-attributable reduction (VAR) in disease burden, is higher against clinically confirmed pneumonia than against X-ray-confirmed disease (23). Even though the point estimates of efficacy are similar, the greater VAR observed for clinical pneumonia means that this outcome was more sensitive than radiologically confirmed pneumonia in detecting the burden of pneumonia prevented by vaccination (23) (Table 3). Using the outcome of VAR in all lower respiratory tract infection (LRTI) episodes as a benchmark, chest radiography detected 46.1% (95% CI, 40.7 to 51.6%) of pneumococcal lower respiratory tract infections prevented by vaccination. In The Gambia, the sensitivity of chest X-ray-confirmed pneumonia to detect the burden of pneumococcal LRTI prevented by vaccination was 76.5% (95% CI, 50.1 to 93.2%) (8). Clinical pneumonia endpoints should attempt to exclude cases of bronchiolitis against which no vaccine efficacy can be shown (23). A CRP level of ≥40 mg/dl may be a more useful measure than an X ray to define the vaccine-preventable fraction of pneumonia in children (22).

CONJUGATE VACCINE EFFICACY AGAINST PNEUMONIA ASSOCIATED WITH HIV

Vaccine efficacy against invasive disease in human immunodeficiency virus (HIV)-infected children is approximately 60%, and although the point estimate of efficacy against pneumonia in this group of children is lower (13%) than it is in non-HIV-infected children (20%) (16), once all clinically diagnosed cases are included, the vaccine efficacy in that group (15%) has the greatest public health impact in terms of burden of disease prevented (2,573 cases per 10^5 child-years versus 267 per 10^5 child-years in non-HIV-infected children) (23). The impact of Hib conjugate vaccine on pneumonia in HIV-infected children has not been established, although the vaccine has activity against invasive Hib disease in these children similar to that of pneumococcal conjugate (24).

HERD IMMUNITY

There is abundant evidence that conjugate pneumococcal vaccines reduce the carriage of vaccine serotypes (15) and in that way reduce the burden of invasive disease in the elderly (32). By inference, therefore, the vaccine should prevent both bacteremic and non-bacteremic pneumococcal pneumonia by herd immunity. However, its efficacy against nonbacteremic pneumonia, while clear in immunized children, has yet to be confirmed in adult populations or nonvaccinated siblings living with immunized children. As the burden of pneumonia in the elderly and in very young infants is significant, with pneumonia the leading infectious cause of death in adults and very young infants (3), such analyses may reveal the largest potential disease reduction impact of this vaccine and greatly increase the cost-effectiveness of immunizing children with the vaccine. A significant herd immunity

Table 3. Estimated efficacies of a nine-valent pneumococcal conjugate vaccine in preventing pneumococcal pneumonia in hospitalized HIV-infected and non-HIV-infected children, by analysis[a]

Outcome measure	Intent-to-treat analysis							Per-protocol analysis		
	No. of vaccine recipients (n = 19,922)	No. of placebo recipients (n = 19,914)	Vaccine efficacy[b] (%) (95% CI)	P[c]	Incidence in placebo group[d]	VAR[e]	Power[f] (%)	No. of vaccine recipients (n = 18,245)	No. of placebo recipients (n = 19,914)	Vaccine efficacy (%) (95% CI)
Clinical LRTI	1,493	1,646	9 (3–15)	0.004	3,565	336	81	858	970	11 (3–19)
Clinical pneumonia	975	1,162	16 (9–23)	0.00003	2,517	410	99	544	679	20 (10–28)
Bronchiolitis	650	643	−1 (−11 to 10)	0.85	1,392	−13	<5	431	419	−3 (−15 to 11)
WHO-defined AC[g]	356	428	17 (4–28)	0.01	927	155	72	251	303	17 (2–30)
WHO-defined mild pneumonia	232	192	−17 (−32 to 0)	0.05	416	−86	48	155	117	−23 (−41 to −4)
WHO-defined mild pneumonia without wheezing	100	105	5 (−25 to 28)	0.72	227	11	5	56	64	13 (−25 to 39)
WHO-defined severe pneumonia	916	1,043	12 (4–20)	0.003	2,259	279	83	511	618	17 (7–26)
WHO-defined severe pneumonia without wheezing	598	697	14 (5–23)	0.02	1,509	215	80	310	383	19 (6–30)
Bacteremic pneumococcal pneumonia										
All	22	39	44 (5–67)	0.03	85	37	58	16	29	45 (−2 to 70)
Associated with a vaccine serotype	9	23	61 (16–82)	0.01	50	30	60	8	16	50 (−17 to 79)
IPPV[h] for LRTI	18	28	36 (−16 to 64)	0.14	61	22	26	8	9	11 (131 to 66)
Death due to LRTI	161	160	−1 (−20 to 24)	0.96	346	−2	<5	67	68	1 (−38 to 30)

[a]Reprinted from reference 23 with permission. For definitions of outcome measures, see "Methods" in reference 23.
[b]For a definition of vaccine efficacy, see "Methods" in reference 23.
[c]P value is for number of vaccine recipients versus number of placebo recipients.
[d]Incidence rate in the placebo group, expressed as number of cases per 10^5 child-years of observation.
[e]Expressed as number of cases per 10^5 child-years of observation.
[f]Power to detect a difference with 95% confidence.
[g]AC, alveolar consolidation, confirmed by chest radiograph findings.
[h]IPPV, intermittent positive-pressure mechanical ventilation.

effect of routine immunization with Hib conjugate vaccine on invasive Hib disease has recently been shown in The Gambia (2), which also suggests that the burden of vaccine-preventable pneumonia may be greater than that predicted by randomized trials.

INTERACTION BETWEEN BACTERIA AND VIRUSES IN THE PATHOGENESIS OF PNEUMONIA

A consistent finding in studies of pediatric viral pneumonia has been evidence of bacterial coinfection (14, 17, 18). More recently, the same observation has been made for episodes of community-acquired pneumococcal pneumonia diagnosed by culture and PCR, 31% of which have involved coinfection with a virus (25).

Influenza-like illness within the previous 7 to 28 days has been shown to be a significant risk (odds ratio, 12.4; 95% CI, 1.7 to 306) for subsequent admission for pneumococcal pneumonia (29). The mechanism of the interaction may be as varied as the synergy between the pneumococcus and the influenza virus on apoptosis of neutrophils (11); virus-induced interleukin-1 and tumor necrosis factor upregulation of the platelet-activating factor receptor, which mediates bacterial invasion (7); or the influenza virus strain neuraminidase activity, which degrades mucin and enhances secondary pneumococcal pneumonia in mice (30).

The vaccine probe approach allows direct investigation of the concurrence of bacterial and viral pathogens in children with pneumonia. The first such vaccine probe approach to this interaction demonstrated that a remarkable 31% of virus-associated pneumonia in hospitalized children is prevented by pneumococcal conjugate vaccine (21). As shown in Table 4, clinically diagnosed hospital-acquired pneumonia cases associated with influenza virus, parainfluenza virus, and respiratory syncytial virus infections were all reduced in children who had received pneumococcal conjugate vaccine (21). These estimates of the concurrence of bacterial and viral infections are clearly underestimates, as they do not reflect interactions with bacteria other than the pneumococcus, they do not take into account nonvaccine serotypes or replacement disease with those serotypes, and they presume 100% vaccine efficacy against vaccine serotypes.

The mechanism of protection is thought to be the prevention of pneumococcal superinfection in children for whom exposure to these viruses increases susceptibility to pneumococcal infection. Pneumococcal conjugate vaccine has no impact on World Health Organization-defined mild pneumonia (23), suggesting that most of these infections are viral without bacterial superinfection. A number of inferences can be drawn from these data (21). Children (and possibly adults) hospitalized with presumed viral pneumonia require antibiotics, even if the bacterial superinfection cannot be confirmed by culture. The approach to a global pandemic of influenza should include a stockpile of antibiotics with which to treat hospitalized patients. In addition, preparedness for an influenza pandemic should include widespread vaccination with effective bacterial vaccines that would confer protection against pneumonia and that are not reliant on pandemic influenza vaccine availability. Conjugate vaccines are also an important adjunct to vaccination of children against influenza to prevent endemic disease, and they have the advantage that long-term protection can be achieved without annual vaccinations. Finally, these data suggest that community-acquired viral bronchiolitis does not require antibiotics, as the vaccine does not prevent a significant fraction of these episodes.

Table 4. Percentage efficacies of pneumococcal conjugate vaccine by per-protocol analysis in fully immunized infants[a]

Clinical diagnosis	All children[b]				Non-HIV-infected children[c]				HIV-infected children[c]			
	No. receiving vaccine (n = 18,245)	No. receiving placebo (n = 18,268)	Efficacy (%) (95% CI)	P value	No. receiving vaccine (n = 17,065)	No. receiving placebo (n = 17,086)	Efficacy (%) (95% CI)	P value	No. receiving vaccine (n = 1,180)	No. receiving placebo (n = 1,182)	Efficacy (%) (95% CI)	P value
Total no. of pneumonia cases[d]	544	679	20 (10, 28)	0.00009	348	452	23 (11, 33)	0.0002	181	210	14 (−4, 28)	0.1
Pneumonia with alveolar consolidation	251	303	17 (2, 30)	0.03	119	158	25 (4, 40)	0.02	128	140	8 (−15, 27)	0.5
Pneumonia without identified virus[e]	419	486	14 (2, 24)	0.03	252	299	16 (0, 29)	0.05	167	187	11 (−8, 26)	0.3
Any identified virus-associated pneumonia[f]	160	231	31 (15, 43)	0.0004	111	167	33 (15, 48)	0.0008	44	57	23 (−14, 47)	0.2
Influenza A	31	56	45 (14, 64)	0.01	21	32	34 (−14, 62)	0.1	9	21	57 (7, 80)	0.03
RSV	90	115	22 (−3, 41)	0.08	64	94	32 (6, 50)	0.02	22	17	−30 (−143, 31)	0.4
PIV types 1–3	24	43	44 (8, 66)	0.02	16	27	41 (−10, 68)	0.09	8	16	50 (−17, 78)	0.1
Adenovirus	14	15	7 (−94, 55)	0.9	9	13	31 (−62, 70)	0.4	5	2	−150 (−1,188, 51)	0.3

[a] Reprinted from reference 21 with permission.
[b] Includes children whose HIV status was unknown.
[c] Although the number of children receiving vaccine or placebo is known, the denominators of HIV-infected and non-HIV-infected children are estimated as 6.47% and 93.53%, respectively (see the Supplementary Methods of reference 21 online for the basis of this estimate).
[d] First episodes are shown; thus, a child with episodes of pneumonia both associated with and not associated with a virus is counted in that category for each first episode, but only once in the total number of pneumonia cases.
[e] Includes episodes of pneumonia that tested negative for all of the respiratory viruses examined.
[f] Includes the first episode of any identified virus-associated pneumonia, including influenza B virus.

CONCLUSIONS

Although the diagnosis of bacterial pneumonia in individual patients remains difficult, the efficacy of conjugate vaccines in the prevention of pneumonia in children provides a novel tool to establish the fraction of respiratory illness that is preventable by the vaccine and, by inference, provides for the first time evidence of the true role of bacteria in the pathogenesis of pneumonia.

REFERENCES

1. **Adegbola, R., S. Obaro, E. Biney, and B. Greenwood.** 2001. Evaluation of Binax now *Streptococcus pneumoniae* urinary antigen test in children in a community with a high carriage rate of pneumococcus. *Pediatr. Infect. Dis. J.* **20:**718–719.
2. **Adegbola, R. A., O. Secka, G. Lahai, N. Lloyd-Evans, A. Njie, S. Usen, C. Oluwalana, S. Obaro, M. Weber, T. Corrah, K. Mulholland, K. McAdam, B. Greenwood, and P. J. Milligan.** 2005. Elimination of *Haemophilus influenzae* type b (Hib) disease from The Gambia after the introduction of routine immunisation with a Hib conjugate vaccine: a prospective study. *Lancet* **366:**144–150.
3. **Anonymous.** 2005. *World Health Report.* World Health Organization, Geneva, Switzerland.
4. **Black, S., H. Shinefield, B. Fireman, E. Lewis, P. Ray, J. R. Hansen, L. Elvin, K. M. Ensor, J. Hackell, G. Siber, F. Malinoski, D. Madore, I. Chang, R. Kohberger, W. Watson, R. Austrian, K. Edwards, et al.** 2000. Efficacy, safety and immunogenicity of heptavalent pneumococcal conjugate vaccine in children. *Pediatr. Infect. Dis. J.* **19:**187–195.
5. **Black, S. B., H. R. Shinefield, S. Ling, J. Hansen, B. Fireman, D. Spring, J. Noyes, E. Lewis, P. Ray, J. Lee, and J. Hackell.** 2002. Effectiveness of heptavalent pneumococcal conjugate vaccine in children younger than five years of age for prevention of pneumonia. *Pediatr. Infect. Dis. J.* **21:**810–815.
6. **Cherian, T., E. K. Mulholland, J. B. Carlin, H. Ostensen, R. Amin, M. de Campo, D. Greenberg, R. Lagos, M. Lucero, S. A. Madhi, K. L. O'Brien, S. Obaro, and M. C. Steinhoff.** 2005. Standardized interpretation of paediatric chest radiographs for the diagnosis of pneumonia in epidemiological studies. *Bull. W. H. O.* **83:**353–359.
7. **Cundell, D. R., N. P. Gerard, C. Gerard, I. Idanpaan-Heikkila, and E. I. Tuomanen.** 1995. *Streptococcus pneumoniae* anchor to activated human cells by the receptor for platelet-activating factor. *Nature* **377:**435–438.
8. **Cutts, F. T., S. M. Zaman, G. Enwere, S. Jaffar, O. S. Levine, J. B. Okoko, C. Oluwalana, A. Vaughan, S. K. Obaro, A. Leach, K. P. McAdam, E. Biney, M. Saaka, U. Onwuchekwa, F. Yallop, N. F. Pierce, B. M. Greenwood, and R. A. Adegbola.** 2005. Efficacy of nine-valent pneumococcal conjugate vaccine against pneumonia and invasive pneumococcal disease in The Gambia: randomised, double-blind, placebo-controlled trial. *Lancet* **365:**1139–1146.
9. **de Andrade, A. L., J. G. de Andrade, C. M. Martelli, S. A. de Silva, R. M. de Oliveira, M. S. Costa, C. B. Laval, L. H. Ribeiro, and J. L. Di Fabio.** 2004. Effectiveness of *Haemophilus influenzae* b conjugate vaccine on childhood pneumonia: a case-control study in Brazil. *Int. J. Epidemiol.* **33:**173–181.
10. **de la Hoz, F., A. B. Higuera, J. L. Di Fabio, M. Luna, A. G. Naranjo, M. de la Luz Valencia, D. Pastor, and A. J. Hall.** 2004. Effectiveness of *Haemophilus influenzae* type b vaccination against bacterial pneumonia in Colombia. *Vaccine* **23:**36–42.
11. **Engelich, G., M. White, and K. L. Hartshorn.** 2001. Neutrophil survival is markedly reduced by incubation with influenza virus and *Streptococcus pneumoniae*: role of respiratory burst. *J. Leukoc. Biol.* **69:**50–56.
12. **Gessner, B. D., A. Sutanto, M. Linehan, I. G. Djelantik, T. Fletcher, I. K. Gerudug, Ingerani, D. Mercer, V. Moniaga, L. H. Moulton, K. Mulholland, C. Nelson, S. Soemohardjo, M. Steinhoff, A. Widjaya, P. Stoeckel, J. Maynard, and S. Arjoso.** 2005. Incidences of vaccine-preventable *Haemophilus influenzae* type b pneumonia and meningitis in Indonesian children: hamlet-randomised vaccine-probe trial. *Lancet* **365:**43–52.
13. **Jaffar, S., A. Leach, P. G. Smith, F. Cutts, and B. Greenwood.** 2003. Effects of misclassification of causes of death on the power of a trial to assess the efficacy of a pneumococcal conjugate vaccine in The Gambia. *Int. J. Epidemiol.* **32:**430–436.
14. **Juven, T., J. Mertsola, M. Waris, M. Leinonen, O. Meurman, M. Roivainen, J. Eskola, P. Saikku, and O. Ruuskanen.** 2000. Etiology of community-acquired pneumonia in 254 hospitalized children. *Pediatr. Infect. Dis. J.* **19:**293–298.

15. **Klugman, K. P.** 2001. Efficacy of pneumococcal conjugate vaccines and their effect on carriage and antimicrobial resistance. *Lancet Infect. Dis.* **1**:85–91.

16. **Klugman, K. P., S. A. Madhi, R. E. Huebner, R. Kohberger, N. Mbelle, and N. Pierce.** 2003. A trial of a 9-valent pneumococcal conjugate vaccine in children with and those without HIV infection. *N. Engl. J. Med.* **349**:1341–1348.

17. **Korppi, M., M. Leinonen, M. Koskela, P. H. Makela, and K. Launiala.** 1989. Bacterial coinfection in children hospitalized with respiratory syncytial virus infections. *Pediatr. Infect. Dis. J.* **8**:687–692.

18. **Korppi, M., M. Leinonen, P. H. Makela, and K. Launiala.** 1990. Bacterial involvement in parainfluenza virus infection in children. *Scand. J. Infect. Dis.* **22**:307–312.

19. **Levine, O. S., R. Lagos, A. Munoz, J. Villaroel, A. M. Alvarez, P. Abrego, and M. M. Levine.** 1999. Defining the burden of pneumonia in children preventable by vaccination against *Haemophilus influenzae* type b. *Pediatr. Infect. Dis. J.* **18**:1060–1064.

20. **Madhi, S. A., J. R. Heera, L. Kuwanda, and K. P. Klugman.** 2005. Use of procalcitonin and C-reactive protein to evaluate vaccine efficacy against pneumonia. *PLoS Med.* **2**:e38.

21. **Madhi, S. A., and K. P. Klugman.** 2004. A role for *Streptococcus pneumoniae* in virus-associated pneumonia. *Nat. Med.* **10**:811–813.

22. **Madhi, S. A., M. Kohler, L. Kuwanda, C. Cutland, and K. P. Klugman.** 2006. Usefulness of C-reactive protein to define pneumococcal conjugate vaccine efficacy in the prevention of pneumonia. *Pediatr. Infect. Dis. J.* **25**:30–36.

23. **Madhi, S. A., L. Kuwanda, C. Cutland, and K. P. Klugman.** 2005. The impact of a 9-valent pneumococcal conjugate vaccine on the public health burden of pneumonia in HIV-infected and -uninfected children. *Clin. Infect. Dis.* **40**:1511–1518.

24. **Madhi, S. A., K. Petersen, M. Khoosal, R. E. Huebner, N. Mbelle, R. Mothupi, H. Saloojee, H. Crewe-Brown, and K. P. Klugman.** 2002. Reduced effectiveness of *Haemophilus influenzae* type b conjugate vaccine in children with a high prevalence of human immunodeficiency virus type 1 infection. *Pediatr. Infect. Dis. J.* **21**:315–321.

25. **Michelow, I. C., K. Olsen, J. Lozano, N. K. Rollins, L. B. Duffy, T. Ziegler, J. Kauppila, M. Leinonen, and G. H. McCracken, Jr.** 2004. Epidemiology and clinical characteristics of community-acquired pneumonia in hospitalized children. *Pediatrics* **113**:701–707.

26. **Mulholland, K., S. Hilton, R. Adegbola, S. Usen, A. Oparaugo, C. Omosigho, M. Weber, A. Palmer, G. Schneider, K. Jobe, G. Lahai, S. Jaffar, O. Secka, K. Lin, C. Ethevenaux, and B. Greenwood.** 1997. Randomised trial of *Haemophilus influenzae* type-b tetanus protein conjugate vaccine for prevention of pneumonia and meningitis in Gambian infants. *Lancet* **349**:1191–1197.

27. **O'Brien, K. L., A. David, J. Benson, K. Moenne, R. Reid, L. Moulton, S. Katz, A. Parkinson, R. Weatherholtz, C. Donaldson, J. Hackell, R. Kohberger, G. Siber, and M. Santosham.** 2002. Presented at the 3rd International Symposium on Pneumococci and Pneumococcal Diseases, Anchorage, Alaska.

28. **O'Brien, K. L., L. H. Moulton, R. Reid, R. Weatherholtz, J. Oski, L. Brown, G. Kumar, A. Parkinson, D. Hu, J. Hackell, I. Chang, R. Kohberger, G. Siber, and M. Santosham.** 2003. Efficacy and safety of seven-valent conjugate pneumococcal vaccine in American Indian children: group randomised trial. *Lancet* **362**:355–361.

29. **O'Brien, K. L., M. I. Walters, J. Sellman, P. Quinlisk, H. Regnery, B. Schwartz, and S. F. Dowell.** 2000. Severe pneumococcal pneumonia in previously healthy children: the role of preceding influenza infection. *Clin. Infect. Dis.* **30**:784–789.

30. **Peltola, V. T., K. G. Murti, and J. A. McCullers.** 2005. Influenza virus neuraminidase contributes to secondary bacterial pneumonia. *J. Infect. Dis.* **192**:249–257.

31. **Vuori-Holopainen, E., and H. Peltola.** 2001. Reappraisal of lung tap: review of an old method for better etiologic diagnosis of childhood pneumonia. *Clin. Infect. Dis.* **32**:715–726.

32. **Whitney, C. G., M. M. Farley, J. Hadler, L. H. Harrison, N. M. Bennett, R. Lynfield, A. Reingold, P. R. Cieslak, T. Pilishvili, D. Jackson, R. R. Facklam, J. H. Jorgensen, and A. Schuchat.** 2003. Decline in invasive pneumococcal disease after the introduction of protein-polysaccharide conjugate vaccine. *N. Engl. J. Med.* **348**:1737–1746.

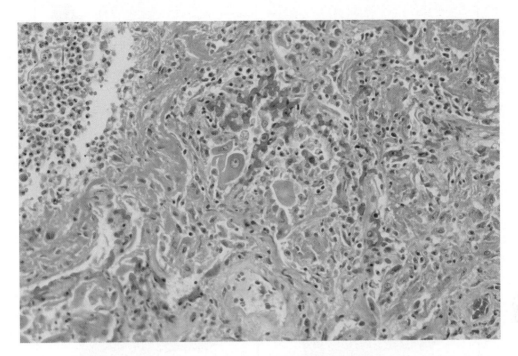

Color Plate 1 (chapter 2). Organizing phase of SARS in the lung. The alveolar lumens are filled with chronic inflammatory cells, reactive pneumocytes, and giant cells. Hematoxylin and eosin stain was used. Original magnification, ×400.

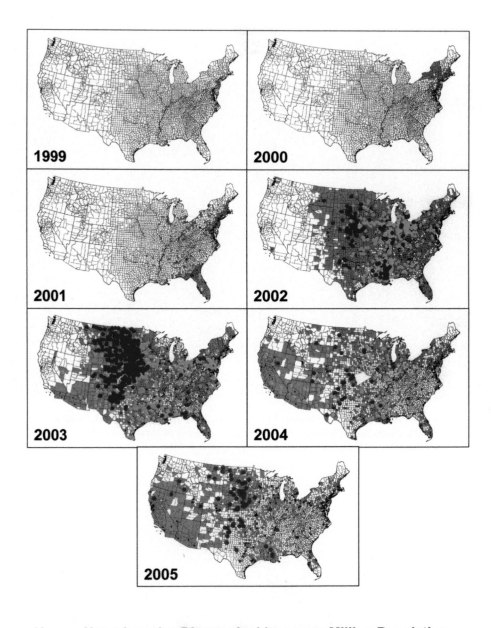

Human Neuroinvasive Disease Incidence per Million Population

• .01-9.99   ● 10-99.99   ● >=100

■ Any WNV Activity (birds, mosquitoes, horses, humans)

Color Plate 2 (chapter 6). WNV in the United States, 1999 to 2005. The incidence of human neuroinvasive disease is indicated by county. Shaded counties have had WNV activity recorded in humans, birds, other vertebrates, or mosquitoes.

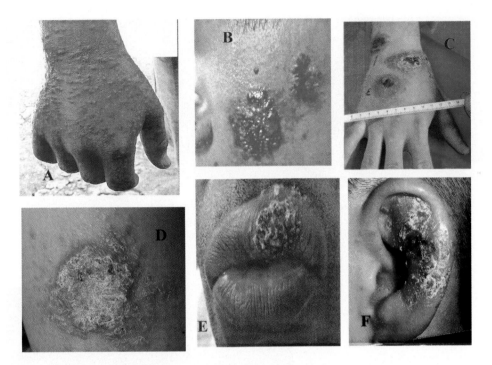

Color Plate 3 (chapter 17). (A) Multiple sand fly bites on a hand (photograph courtesy of R. Coleman, Walter Reed Army Institute of Research); (B) impetiginous facial lesions due to *L. major;* (C) multiple ulceronodular leishmaniasis lesions; (D) scaling plaque leishmanial lesion demonstrating multiple satellite lesions; (E) ulcerative leishmaniasis on the upper lip, showing direct inoculation, not mucosal leishmaniasis; (F) ulcerative lesion due to *L. major* on the helix of the ear.

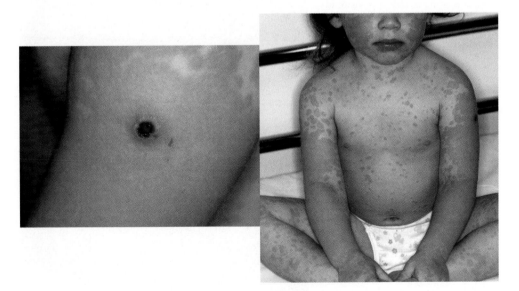

Color Plate 4 (chapter 18). Examples of erythema multiforme. Copyright © Logical Images, Inc.

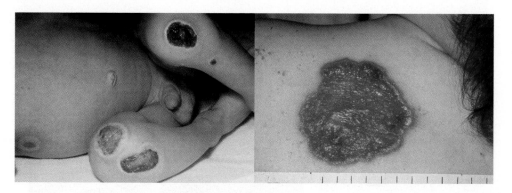

Color Plate 5 (chapter 18). Progressive vaccinia in children with severe combined immunodeficiency. Note the total lack of inflammatory response and the progressive, centripetal nature of spread of the lesion. Copyright © Logical Images, Inc.

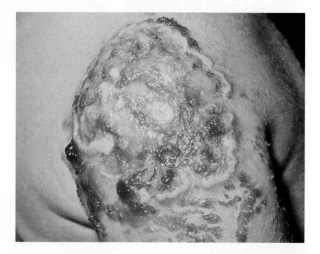

Color Plate 6 (chapter 18). Progressive vaccinia showing another appearance of a progressive lesion in a child with intact antibody synthesis but lacking T-cell function. Copyright © Logical Images, Inc.

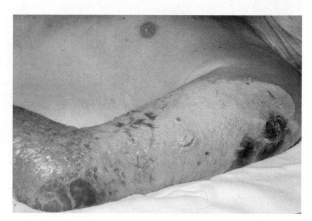

Color Plate 7 (chapter 18). Progressive vaccinia in an adult with lymphosarcoma. Copyright © Logical Images, Inc.

Emerging Infections 7
Edited by W. M. Scheld, D. C. Hooper, and J. M. Hughes
© 2007 ASM Press, Washington, D.C.

Chapter 13

Mycobacterium avium subsp. paratuberculosis and Crohn's Disease

Saleh A. Naser and Najih A. Naser

HISTORY OF CROHN'S DISEASE

Medical historians suggest that Crohn's disease may have first been reported as early as the 1600s, but whether that truly was the first record of the disease will never be known (56). In 1913, T. K. Dalziel described several patients with chronic intestinal disorders that were similar to intestinal tuberculosis, though they were, he believed, suffering from a new disorder. He felt that the disease he had observed had marked similarities to a newly described disease in cattle known at that time as pseudotuberculosis (21). The similarities between the two disorders included phenotypic and pathologic characteristics (13, 20, 21, 43). The signs and symptoms and the conditions of the sufferers, animal and human, were identical. They included abdominal pain, diarrhea, bloody stool, and loss of weight. The anatomical distributions of the diseases and their manifestations and histological characteristics were also similar. At that time, Dalziel was successful in isolating a bacterium from the intestinal tissue of a diseased bovine diagnosed with pseudotuberculosis, confirming the work of H. A. Johne and L. Frothingham in 1895 (53). The bacterium was originally named *Mycobacterium enteritidis chronicae pseudotuberculosae bovis johne* or *Mycobacterium paratuberculosis*, and the most recent nomenclature is *Mycobacterium avium* subsp. *paratuberculosis* (94). Attempts by Dalziel and his associates to culture this bacterium from the intestinal tissue of humans with pseudotuberculosis were unsuccessful (21). It was not until 1932, in a landmark article published by Crohn, Ginzberg, and Oppenheimer, that the disease was recognized as unique and separate from intestinal tuberculosis, and it was reclassified as "Crohn's disease" (20). Unfortunately, B. B. Crohn could not fulfill Koch's postulates in reference to the disease, and the inability to do so caused him and others to believe that Crohn's disease was not caused by an infectious process, similar to intestinal tuberculosis, but was strictly an autoimmune disease. Thus, to this day, the scientific community continues to grapple with the origins of the disease, with

Saleh A. Naser • Department of Molecular Biology and Microbiology, Burnett College for Biomedical Sciences, University of Central Florida, Orlando, FL 32816. *Najih A. Naser* • TransTech Pharma, 4170 Mendenhall Oaks Parkway, High Point, NC 27265.

new technologies sparking renewed interest in the old theory that Crohn's disease will some day be demonstrated to have a mycobacterial etiology.

CLINICAL ASPECTS OF CROHN'S DISEASE

Crohn's disease is an idiopathic chronic granulomatous ileocolitis. Although this inflammatory bowel disease (IBD) was initially described as a segmental disease of the small intestine, it has more recently been found to be associated with the mouth, larynx, esophagus, stomach, colon, skin, muscle, synovial tissue, and bone (13, 42, 43, 47). The characteristic lesions of Crohn's disease are strikingly segmental and patchy. A characteristic symptom of this chronic disease is progressive thickening of the bowel wall caused by fibrosis and narrowing of the lumen, in addition to proliferative changes in the mucosal membranes of the lower gastrointestinal (GI) tract. These proliferative changes lead to the cobblestone appearance of the mucosa frequently observed in Crohn's disease patients and cause various degrees of ulceration (42, 43). A chronic enteritis, Crohn's disease differs from other colitis diseases, including ulcerative colitis (UC), another form of IBD, in that it causes transmural inflammation of the gut characterized by noncaseating granulomas, microfistula formation, and ulcerative fissures (65, 83). Histologically, noncaseating tuberculoid granulomas and extensive lymphocytic infiltrations in the submucosa are important features of the disease, and microfistula formation is a common occurrence (77). Microfistula formation causes severe pain for the patient and provides an internal environment suitable for bacterial colonization and propagation, which can lead to stricture formation. Other common features include pain and tenderness in the lower right quadrant mimicking acute appendicitis. Intestinal stenosis also occurs, causing obstruction of the lumen, abdominal distention, constipation, and occasionally vomiting. Intestinal bleeding due to granulomatous and ulcerative lesions can induce diarrhea, which eventually leads to malabsorption and weight loss (65, 77). Crohn's disease is a lifelong disorder, leaving patients to endure unpredictable periods of relapse and remission. Because there is currently no cure, their quality of life can be severely compromised as a result of these recurring episodes (42).

Crohn's disease has been shown to manifest itself in two distinct forms: perforating and nonperforating (13, 42). This dual clinical presentation of Crohn's disease is analogous to those of two other mycobacterial diseases, leprosy and tuberculosis, which both manifest in two distinct clinical forms: contained and aggressive (13, 20, 42, 43, 47). Interestingly, the symptoms of Crohn's disease appear to be caused in part by immune interference, or immunomodulation reactions, common in *Mycobacterium tuberculosis* infections (57).

CROHN'S DISEASE EPIDEMIOLOGY: INCIDENCE AND PREVALENCE

Crohn's disease emerged perceptibly in Western Europe and North America in the late 1940s and early 1950s, and incidences on both continents have progressively increased since that time. In some areas, such as northeast Scotland, the incidence (11.6 per 100,000 per year) is now approaching an epidemic (58). Because of the slow progression of the disease, there is a wide spectrum of disease activity in patients, ranging from minimal symptoms to severe complications. In addition, physicians differ on the criteria used to determine diagnosis of Crohn's disease as opposed to UC, and frequently the disease is misdiagnosed. Therefore, the actual incidence of Crohn's disease in the United States is difficult to determine, and studies on incidence and prevalence vary greatly. The Crohn's and Colitis Foundation of America has estimated that approximately 1 million Americans have IBD, the category of diseases that includes Crohn's disease and UC, with half of those being Crohn's disease patients (http://www.ccfa.org). The disease is diagnosed equally among men and women and is encountered in American Jews of European descent four to five times more commonly than in the general population (35). Although IBD has long been considered a disease predominantly affecting persons of European descent, the prevalence rate among African Americans has been steadily increasing, approaching that of white sufferers. According to the Crohn's and Colitis Foundation of America, prevalence rates among Hispanics and Asians are lower than those for whites and African Americans.

The only true population-based data concerning the incidence and prevalence of Crohn's disease come from Olmsted County, Minnesota. Loftus et al. estimated that the prevalence of Crohn's disease in Olmsted County was 133 cases per 100,000 persons, and the incidence was 5.8 per 100,000 per year in January 1991 (61). The most disturbing evidence to come out of Olmsted County concerned the increasing incidence of Crohn's disease among young children. Loftus et al. reported no cases of Crohn's disease among people less than 20 years of age in the 1940s and 1950s; however, by 1991, 17% of all Crohn's disease cases were in people under 20 years of age. Welsh researchers found that the number of new cases of Crohn's disease in children increased by 9.1% per year from 1989 to 1993 (19). Other studies have reported that Crohn's disease may afflict around 13 people per 100,000 in the United Kingdom, similar to incidence rates in other countries in Europe (40). The disease is most devastating in children due to their greater nutritional requirements, which are difficult to meet when they are afflicted with a disease that includes nutrient malabsorption among its manifestations. In addition, children with Crohn's disease often experience growth retardation and/or delays in sexual maturity, due to the hormonal imbalance that exists during the course of the disease (76).

CROHN'S DISEASE DIAGNOSIS

Crohn's disease can be diagnosed through a series of physical examinations and tests. Blood tests may be performed to check for anemia, which could indicate bleeding in the GI tract, or to uncover high white blood cell counts indicative of an active inflammatory response. Also, stool samples can be analyzed for the presence of blood, indicating bleeding or infection in the intestines. In addition to blood tests, either or both of the following procedures may be used in diagnosing the disease. An upper GI series may be performed to indicate whether inflammation or other abnormalities of the small intestine are present. An endoscopy or colonoscopy can also be performed to visualize the state of the GI tract in terms of inflammation and fistulization (42, 46, 65). Also, biopsy specimens can be taken during colonoscopy for microscopic analysis. Unfortunately, the tools used in definitively diagnosing Crohn's disease are expensive and invasive. Therefore, it is of utmost importance to determine the etiological agent of the disease, if only to aid in the development of diagnostic techniques that are less invasive for the patient.

TREATMENT OF CROHN'S DISEASE

Treatment of Crohn's disease depends on the location and severity of disease, complications, and response to previous treatment. The most common complication is stricture of the intestine, and surgery to remove the obstructed intestinal area is often performed. However, surgery is not a curative measure, and patients often relapse. It has been accepted for a long time that the goal of treatment of Crohn's disease patients is to control inflammation, correct nutritional deficiencies, and relieve symptoms; therefore, a multifactorial approach is often used. Treatment may include use of anti-inflammatory drugs, such as sulfasalazine and corticosteroids, or immunosuppressive drugs, such as 6-mercaptopurine and azathioprine (48). For patients who do not respond to standard therapies, infliximab, the first drug to be approved specifically for Crohn's disease, is prescribed for the treatment of moderate to severe cases and for the treatment of open, draining fistulas (48). Infliximab is a monoclonal antibody directed against tumor necrosis factor (TNF). TNF is thought to play a role in the inflammation associated with Crohn's disease. Recently, safety concerns have been raised about the ability of infliximab to activate dormant tuberculosis (98). Trials of antibiotics for the treatment of Crohn's disease have also been performed, but with controversial outcomes. Early studies using standard tuberculosis drugs (ethambutol, isoniazid, and pyrazinamide) yielded mixed results. However, use of antibiotics, such as macrolides and rifabutin, has been shown to be effective in the treatment of patients with Crohn's disease (see below). Most recently, successful therapeutic response has been reported following the treatment of Crohn's disease patients with granulocyte-macrophage colony-stimulating factor (24). The efficacies of these therapies are evaluated by monitoring disease signs, symptoms, and quality-of-life indicators, also known as the Crohn's disease activity index.

CROHN'S DISEASE ETIOLOGY: THEORIES AND REALITY

There has been much debate concerning the etiology of Crohn's disease in the scientific literature since Crohn reestablished it as a separate disorder in 1932. Everything from diet and environmental pathogens to autoimmunity and genetic aberrations has been implicated as playing a possible role in the pathology of Crohn's disease. Innovative research using new technologies is beginning to shed light on the true origins of the disease, which may actually involve several etiological factors. Following the review of the main proposed theories below, it will be clear that this chronic enteritis is the result of a genetic predisposition that is exploited by an environmental trigger, namely, a bacterial pathogen, causing an abnormal immune response.

The Genetic Susceptibility Factor

In order to more clearly understand whether Crohn's disease is an inherited or an acquired disorder, many investigators have explored the familial occurrence of the disease. A greater-than-expected incidence for site and clinical type of Crohn's disease within individual families and a pattern of early age of onset and disease complications were correlated when familial cases were compared to isolated cases. These studies support the role of genetic factors in the susceptibility to and pathology of Crohn's disease (3). Statistical rates of disease in siblings and monozygotic twins further implicate a genetic contribution to acquisition of the disease that is equivalent to those in other immune-mediated disorders, such as multiple sclerosis and insulin-dependent diabetes (86). Mixed results were reported when linkage analysis and population-based studies were used in attempts to identify susceptibility genes in inflammatory bowel disease. HLA association studies, as well as molecular genotyping, have produced confusing and inconsistent results. Particular controversies have arisen concerning the putative association of Crohn's disease with the DR5DQ1 haplotype (9). Putative susceptibility loci for Crohn's disease have been identified by genome screening in chromosomes 12q, 1p, 3p, 3q, 5p, 6p, 7q, 14q, 19p, and, recently, 16q (9). The relevant gene on chromosome 16 has been named *NOD2* (nucleotide oligomerization domain) and contains a region encoding 10 leucine-rich repeats at the carboxy terminus of caspase recruitment domains (CARDs). A disease-related mutation truncates the 10th leucine-rich repeat. *NOD2/CARD15* may prove to be a catalyst for genetic and therapeutic advances. Located in the *IBD1* locus on chromosome 16q12, it is thought to encode a disease resistance protein on monocytes, similar to antimicrobial proteins expressed in plants, and it causes susceptibility to intracellular pathogens in patients with Crohn's disease (73). NOD2/CARD15 belongs to a family of intracellular protein receptors called NBS-LRR (for nucleotide-binding site—leucine-rich repeat) that have been demonstrated to recognize the peptidoglycan motif of bacterial pathogens by binding the muramyl dipeptide component. Once activated by the bacterial cell wall, NOD2/CARD15 is capable of inducing NF-κB, a key proinflammatory pathway responsible for the production of cytokines and chemokines. Further experimental data have shown that *NOD2/CARD15* is upregulated by a specific cytokine, namely, TNF-α, thereby amplifying the immune response and facilitating a continuous cycle of inflammation; the overexpression of *NOD2/CARD15* seen in Crohn's disease patients serves to further explain this exaggerated immune response associated with the disease (73). A frameshift mutation in *NOD2/CARD15*, caused by a cytosine insertion, as well as several single-nucleotide polymorphisms, has been shown to decrease the immune system's innate ability to recognize certain pathogens, particularly in cases of ileal Crohn's disease versus colonic disease (73). This selective association is supported by the finding that the *NOD2/CARD15* gene occurs most abundantly in Paneth cells, which are located primarily in the terminal ileum, where they serve as a major host defense against gut microbes (59). Inherited defects in *NOD2/CARD15* have been observed in 30 to 50% of Crohn's disease patients compared to 7 to 20% of healthy controls (51). The positive correlation of *NOD2/CARD15* gene mutations with the occurrence of Crohn's disease provides one of the first physical links between an infectious agent and irregular immune response at the molecular level (73). This has been confirmed in our laboratory, most recently following the culture of *M. avium* subsp. *paratuberculosis* in modified mycobacterial growth indicator tube (MGIT) culture media confirmed by PCR based on the IS*900* gene unique to *M. avium* subsp. *paratuberculosis* from two Crohn's disease patients who exhibited polymorphism in their *CARD15* genes.

Ongoing study in our laboratory using a microarray of approximately 30,000 genes representing the entire human genome and following hybridization with RNA from six Crohn's disease patients, two patients with UC, and eight healthy controls revealed a possible downregulation of the gamma interferon receptor gene *(INFGR1)* exclusively in Crohn's disease patients. Interestingly, the *INFGR1* gene was downregulated in only five (83%) Crohn's disease patients (data presented at the 105th General Meeting of the American Society for Microbiology, 2005). Polymorphisms in the gamma interferon

R1 receptors have also been suggested to predispose to infection with tuberculous and nontuberculous bacteria.

Alterations in Normal Luminal Bacteria

R. B. Sartor (84) has contended that "a normal host could develop a chronic inflammatory response by harboring stable populations of normal fecal bacteria which have subtle pathogenic alterations that may be extremely difficult to detect by standard microbiological techniques." Microbial agents have been suggested to be environmental "triggers," which may initiate the complex inflammatory cascade observed, reactivate quiescent disease, or be responsible for the frequent septic complications of Crohn's disease. Demonstrations have been made using animal models that implicate normal luminal bacteria as triggers of immune-mediated chronic intestinal inflammation, such as that seen in Crohn's disease patients. It has been shown that sporadic cases could be altered by luminal decontamination and subsequent repopulation with "normal" enteric bacteria. However, this evidence could point to possible elimination of the actual etiological agent during broad-spectrum antibiotic decontamination of the lumen, and the theory remains unsubstantiated.

Altered Mucosal-Barrier Function

Researchers speculate that increased intestinal permeability could allow passage of bacterial products, such as lipopolysaccharide, peptidoglycan-polysaccharide, and N-formyl-methionyl-leucyl-phenylalanine, into surrounding tissue, initiating an immune response with intestinal damage and systemic manifestations. Lipopolysaccharide and peptidoglycan-polysaccharide stimulate cytokine synthesis and activate complement, while N-formyl-methionyl-leucyl-phenylalanine acts as a potent chemotactic factor (49). Genetic factors could also be involved in intestinal-permeability defects, based on the observation that patients with quiescent Crohn's disease and two-thirds of their healthy relatives have increased permeability to inert markers (49). However, others have failed to show a significant increase in mucosal permeability to a number of markers in first-degree relatives of Crohn's disease patients (84). Increased mucosal permeability has been shown to be enhanced in Crohn's disease; however, controversy exists in determining whether this is a primary or secondary effect of the disease agent (84).

Disorder in the Host Immune Response

Most Crohn's disease patients demonstrate a different and unexpected immune reaction compared to patients with other infectious diseases. The anergic immune reactions demonstrated in Crohn's disease patients are driven by an elevated Th1 cytokine profile, including interleukin-12 and gamma interferon, which induce a damaging type of chronic inflammation, in contrast to Th2 cytokines, which promote a healing immune response. However, several pathogenic microorganisms have been identified, including *Mycobacterium tuberculosis* and *Mycobacterium leprae*, that have evolved sophisticated measures to circumvent the human immune system, producing similar dysregulated immune responses (13, 43). Some mycobacterial species, like *M. leprae*, actually impede the actions of the cell-mediated immune response by suppressing the production of cytokines in the host (13, 43). Still, some bacterial species possess antigenic epitopes strikingly similar to those of host molecules. These shared components can elicit a perpetual molecular-mimicry state, analogous to the mechanisms of autoimmunity, where bacterial antigens appear as self-antigens, thus escaping detection by the immune system. This phenomenon has been investigated in the case of mycobacterial heat shock proteins and outer envelope polysaccharides, due to their homology to human epitopes. However, concrete evidence of molecular mimicry in these cases has yet to be established. Moreover, antigen-antibody investigations into the Crohn's disease immune response may be hampered by sero-cross-reactivity caused by the many shared antigens among species of mycobacteria. Some pathogenic mycobacteria have up to a 65% cross-reactivity rate as a result of such close homology between their antigens (28). Consequently, statistical results concerning control groups versus test subjects can be skewed by patients unknowingly exposed to different mycobacterial organisms. Therefore, it is imperative to discover immunogenic antigens that are specific to *M. avium* subsp. *paratuberculosis* in order to more thoroughly study the potential of a mycobacterial etiology associated with Crohn's disease. It is bacterial survival strategies such as these, coupled with other determinants, such as the genetic makeup of the host and organism and environmental factors, that serve to cloud a definitive understanding of the immunomodulatory responses that are initiated by mycobacterial infection.

Persistent Infection by Pathogens

Although evidence may indicate a role for resident normal flora in providing a constant antigenic drive for chronic intestinal inflammation in the genetically susceptible host, either through loss of immunological tolerance or because of an intrinsic defect in mucosal-barrier function, it is possible that these host responses are due in large part to persistent pathogen exposure (84). Microorganisms that have been reported to be involved in Crohn's disease pathogenesis include adherent invasive *Escherichia coli, Bacteroides, Clostridium*, members of the *Enterobacteriaceae, Yersinia enterocolitica*, and *Listeria monocytogenes* (50, 54). Each of these microorganisms has been reported in the literature to have a role in Crohn's disease pathogenesis. In addition, a viral etiology of Crohn's disease has been suggested; however, no virus except measles virus has been specifically detected in diseased tissues. A higher prevalence of measles virus in Crohn's disease patients than in control patients has been reported in some studies, but not others (10). However, the possible role of mycobacteria in Crohn's disease pathogenesis has reemerged and is again a topic of debate in the scientific literature, the lay press, and gastroenterology clinics.

M. AVIUM SUBSP. *PARATUBERCULOSIS* AND JOHNE'S DISEASE

The remarkable similarities between Crohn's disease and other well-documented mycobacterioses in humans and animals have kept researchers returning to the theory that the etiology of Crohn's disease is rooted in mycobacterial infection (13, 17, 21, 43, 47). The parallels between Crohn's disease and bovine paratuberculosis infection, or Johne's disease, remain one of the best arguments for this hypothesis. The pathology and signs of Johne's disease were first described as early as 1806, but it was Johne and Frothingham who are said to have first documented these signs as a disease by demonstrating a link between mycobacteria and paratuberculosis in ruminants in 1895 (53). Upon receiving from a local German farmer the tissues of a cow thought to have succumbed to intestinal tuber-culosis, Johne and Frothingham performed a histological examination in which they found an abundance of immune cells in the abnormally thick intestinal mucosa and wall, includ-ing leukocytes and epithelioid cells. Acid-fast staining and microscopic evaluation of the ruminant intestine revealed colonies of acid-fast microorganisms similar to *Mycobac-terium bovis*, the cause of tuberculosis in cattle. Today, scientists have further typed that organism more specifically as *M. avium* subsp. *paratuberculosis*, as mentioned above. *M. avium* subsp. *paratuberculosis* infection in animals has been found among primates, wild rabbits, sheep, goats, bison, and deer (9, 18, 40, 43). Ziehl-Neelsen staining of bacil-lary *M. avium* subsp. *paratuberculosis* has been detected in tissue, peripheral blood, milk, and fecal samples from infected animals (9, 40, 43). *M. avium* subsp. *paratuberculosis* was also detected in the environment, including surface water and chlorinated drinking water (64, 75). The impact of *M. avium* subsp. *paratuberculosis* infection on the global agricultural industry is enormous and is estimated at $1.5 billion per year in the United States alone (9, 40, 43). *M. avium* subsp. *paratuberculosis* infection in animals may spread rapidly through fecal contamination of feed and ingestion of contaminated colostrum. The efficacy of current pasteurization procedures and the thermal tolerance of *M. avium* subsp. *paratuberculosis* have been debated vigorously in the past 3 years. Although the data have been conflicting, the majority of recent studies reported thermal tolerance of *M. avium* subsp. *paratuberculosis* following standard pasteurization (9, 26, 40, 41, 43, 63). Regard-less of the number of *M. avium* subsp. *paratuberculosis* cells surviving in pasteurized milk, beef, and treated drinking water, the zoonotic potential of *M. avium* subsp. *paratuberculo-sis* and its impact on humans are globally critical.

WHY IS *MYCOBACTERIUM AVIUM* SUBSP. *PARATUBERCULOSIS* A LEADING CANDIDATE IN CROHN'S DISEASE ETIOLOGY?

M. avium subsp. *paratuberculosis* is a member of the *Mycobacterium avium* complex, which also includes *Mycobacterium avium* subsp. *avium, Mycobacterium intracellulare*, and *Mycobacterium avium* subsp. *silvaticum. M. avium* subsp. *avium* and *M. intracellulare* have been associated with infections in immunocompromised patients, mainly in those with AIDS. *M. avium* subspecies *silvaticum* has rarely been associated with human infec-tion, and few cases of *M. avium* subsp. *paratuberculosis* infection have been reported in AIDS patients (78). The clinical significance of *M. avium* subsp. *paratuberculosis* lies in its potential association with Crohn's disease.

Mycobacteria and cell wall-deficient (CWD), or spheroplast, organisms were first iso-lated from tissues from patients with Crohn's disease in the 1970s (7). However, Chiodini et al. were the first to report the isolation of CWD *M. avium* subsp. *paratuberculosis* from tissue lesions of Crohn's disease patients (14, 15). The CWD organisms were confirmed as *M. avium* subsp. *paratuberculosis* using the recently discovered IS*900*, a 1.451-kb in-sertion sequence that occurs in approximately 17 copies in the *M. avium* subsp. *paratu-berculosis* genome (62). Different techniques have been used to detect *M. avium* subsp. *paratuberculosis* organisms in patients with Crohn's disease, including culture, culture followed by PCR, and PCR applied directly on bowel tissue. Using culture, *M. avium* subsp. *paratuberculosis* and several other species of mycobacteria, such as members of the *Mycobacterium avium* complex, *Mycobacterium kansasii*, *Mycobacterium chelonae*, and

Mycobacterium fortuitum, have been isolated by several researchers, but only in up to 5% of patients with Crohn's disease and often after incubation for many months or years (14, 15, 39, 45, 62). In many of these studies, spheroplastic forms were obtained, some of which appeared from subsequent studies to be mycobacteria. Inoculation of *M. avium* subsp. *paratuberculosis* isolated from a patient with Crohn's disease caused granulomas of the distal small intestine in goats following oral administration and hepatic and splenic granulomas in mice following intraperitoneal and intravenous injection (96). The application of IS*900* PCR to long-term cultures raised the detection rate of *M. avium* subsp. *paratuberculosis* in the Crohn's disease gut to 30% (66, 97). IS*900* PCR applied directly to DNA extracts of surgically resected gut samples indicated the presence of *M. avium* subsp. *paratuberculosis* in about two-thirds of people with Crohn's disease in 1992 (82). This study was followed by a large number of studies that reported controversial outcomes. At least nine studies concluded that there was an association between Crohn's disease and *M. avium* subsp. *paratuberculosis* (22, 23, 32, 33, 37, 60, 64, 68, 93), and eight studies did not (1, 8, 12, 16, 25, 34, 55, 80).

During late 1990s, our team at the University of Central Florida in Orlando has focused on the development of a microbiologic system that supports culture of a cell wall-deficient form of *M. avium* subsp. *paratuberculosis* from clinical samples from patients with active Crohn's disease. With a modification of a recently developed liquid culture medium known as MGIT (Becton Dickinson), with the addition of sucrose and mycobactin, and incubation at 37°C with 5% CO_2, suspected mycobacterial growth was observed following only 10 to 12 weeks of incubation. IS*900*-based PCR confirmed the isolation of *M. avium* subsp. *paratuberculosis* in the MGIT culture from decontaminated tissue extracts (87). The MGIT system has shown superiority over other mycobacterial cultures, including the popular Bactec system, for primary isolation of *M. avium* subsp. *paratuberculosis* from clinical samples. This study renewed interest in investigating the association of *M. avium* subsp. *paratuberculosis* with Crohn's disease. In addition to the development of a modified MGIT culture system, the advent of nested PCR, reverse transcriptase (RT) PCR, and real-time PCR has provided tools for more sensitive detection of *M. avium* subsp. *paratuberculosis* from Crohn's disease patients. The use of physical disruption in addition to catalytic lysis of *M. avium* subsp. *paratuberculosis* provided a better yield of *M. avium* subsp. *paratuberculosis* nucleic acid, providing additional sensitivity of the IS*900*-based PCR detection systems.

EVIDENCE OF *M. AVIUM* SUBSP. *PARATUBERCULOSIS* IN CROHN'S DISEASE PATIENTS SINCE 2000

Although the results of earlier studies linking *M. avium* subsp. *paratuberculosis* to Crohn's disease varied, most studies published since 2000 have indicated higher detection rates of *M. avium* subsp. *paratuberculosis* in Crohn's disease patients than in controls. Supporting evidence for the involvement of *M. avium* subsp. *paratuberculosis* in Crohn's disease is grouped into several categories: PCR detection of *M. avium* subsp. *paratuberculosis* DNA, PCR detection of *M. avium* subsp. *paratuberculosis* RNA and serum anti-*M. avium* subsp. *paratuberculosis* immunoglobulin G (IgG) antibodies, and detection of *M. avium* subsp. *paratuberculosis* DNA by in situ hybridization and culture of *M. avium* subsp. *paratuberculosis* from tissue, breast milk, and peripheral blood.

PCR Detection of *M. avium* subsp. *paratuberculosis* DNA

As mentioned above, detection of *M. avium* subsp. *paratuberculosis* DNA by PCR directly from clinical samples or from suspect culture requires an optimized cell lysis procedure that maximizes the yield of nucleic acid. Additionally, optimized PCR conditions are necessary, because they lead to better sensitivity and specificity of the assay. Cell lysis may be improved with mechanical disruption of the *M. avium* subsp. *paratuberculosis* cells using the FastPrep ribolyzer system. Optimized PCR requires (i) oligonucleotide primers that target regions of the *M. avium* subsp. *paratuberculosis* genome with minimum secondary-structure formation, (ii) appropriate concentrations of the PCR mixture ingredients, and (iii) an optimal annealing temperature. The inclusion of betaine or dimethyl sulfoxide in the PCR mixture is necessary to diminish formation of secondary structures by either the oligonucleotide primers or the template, considering the rich content of 69% G + C of the *M. avium* subsp. *paratuberculosis* genome. The use of nested PCR adds significantly to the sensitivity of *M. avium* subsp. *paratuberculosis* detection. In fact, the literature confirms that success in detection of *M. avium* subsp. *paratuberculosis* DNA in clinical samples from Crohn's disease patients is due to the use of nested PCR. Studies that reported lack of detection of *M. avium* subsp. *paratuberculosis* DNA in Crohn's disease tissue were based on standard PCR assays and/or conventional culture media. Moreover, the quality of the tissue sample also plays a role in the outcome of the study. Using formaldehyde-preserved tissue samples or paraffin-embedded block tissue is not appropriate for PCR analysis. Inhibitors must be removed, and DNA ultrapurification is needed before PCR analysis is performed on such DNA extracts.

Since 2000, five studies (Table 1) have reported the detection of *M. avium* subsp. *paratuberculosis* DNA by PCR in more patients with Crohn's disease (range, 40% to 92%) than controls (range, 0% to 28%) (6, 18, 79, 70, 79, 81). In the same period, three studies failed to detect *M. avium* subsp. *paratuberculosis* DNA in Crohn's disease patients by PCR (2, 4, 36).

PCR Detection of *M. avium* subsp. *paratuberculosis* RNA

Detection of microbial RNA indicates viability. Mishina et al. (64) reported the detection of *M. avium* subsp. *paratuberculosis* RNA by RT-PCR in eight out of eight tissue samples from Crohn's disease patients compared to two out of four controls. Interestingly,

Table 1. Detection of *M. avium* subsp. *paratuberculosis* DNA in Crohn's disease patients by PCR (2000 to 2005)

Specimen	% *M. avium* subsp. *paratuberculosis* DNA by PCR[a]	Country	Reference
Surgical tissue	83 (CD), 17 (NIBD)	United States	79
Intestinal biopsy specimens	45.2 (CD), 6.3 (NIBD)	United States	18
	40 (CD), 0 (NIBD)	Ireland	81
	92 (CD), 26 (NIBD)	United Kingdom	6
Blood	46 (CD), 45 (UC), 22 (NIBD)	United States	70

[a]NIBD, noninflammatory bowel disease; CD, Crohn's disease.

M. avium subsp. *paratuberculosis* RNA was detected in two control samples from patients with UC. The authors suggested that Crohn's disease and UC may be two forms of one IBD, similar to those reported in leprosy and tuberculosis. In our laboratory, we developed real-time RT-PCR based on oligonucleotide primers derived from the IS*900* unique to *M. avium* subsp. *paratuberculosis*. Our real-time RT-PCR detected *M. avium* subsp. *paratuberculosis* RNA in blood from 3 out of 7 (43%) Crohn's disease subjects, 2 out of 2 (100%) UC subjects, and 1 out of 15 (7%) non-IBD subjects (data not published). Interestingly, the real-time RT-PCR results (done within 12 hours) were similar to results from 12-week culture incubation with nested-PCR confirmation.

Detection of *M. avium* subsp. *paratuberculosis* DNA by In Situ Hybridization

Because *M. avium* subsp. *paratuberculosis* cells in Crohn's disease lack cell walls, acid-fast stains are negative. Alternative methods that are not cell wall based have been sought by our group and others. Since 2000, five studies (Table 2) have reported the detection of *M. avium* subsp. *paratuberculosis* in Crohn's disease tissue by in situ hybridization. *M. avium* subsp. *paratuberculosis* was detected in intestinal tissue in 40% to 100% of these tissues, compared to none in controls (52, 71, 79, 89, 90). Interestingly, *M. avium* subsp. *paratuberculosis* was detected in inflamed tissue, as well as in neighboring healthy tissue, from the same Crohn's disease patient (Fig. 1). In a study in 2000 (87), we were able to visualize an *M. avium* subsp. *paratuberculosis* spheroplast partially reverted into a bacillary form using Ziehl-Neelsen staining. The finding was confirmed recently by Naser et al. (70), following the immunostaining of a 4- to 6-week-old culture inoculated with buffy coat from the blood of Crohn's disease patients using rabbit anti-*M. avium* subsp. *paratuberculosis* IgG antibodies and fluorescence-labeled anti-rabbit secondary antibodies and confocal laser scanning microscopy.

Immunological Response to *M. avium* subsp. *paratuberculosis*

If *M. avium* subsp. *paratuberculosis* is involved in Crohn's disease pathogenesis, an immunological response by patients is naturally expected. Whether it is a cell-mediated response, as expected in a mycobacterial infection, or a humoral immune response, or both, which is most likely, an anti-*M. avium* subsp. *paratuberculosis* host immune response

Table 2. Detection of *M. avium* subsp. *paratuberculosis* in Crohn's disease patients' tissue by fluorescence in situ hybridization (2000 to 2005)

% *M. avium* subsp. *paratuberculosis* DNA[a]	Country	Reference
100 (CD), 0 (NIBD)	United States	71
73 (CD), 0 (NIBD)	Italy	90
40 (CD), 0 (NIBD)	United States	52
67 (CD), 69 (CD), 0 (NIBD)	Italy	89
67 (CD), 0 NIBD	United States	79

[a]NIBD, noninflammatory bowel disease; CD, Crohn's disease.

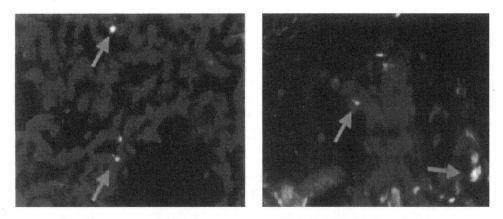

Figure 1. In situ identification of *Mycobacterium avium* subsp. *paratuberculosis* systemic infection in Crohn's disease tissue. *M. avium* subsp. *paratuberculosis* DNA was detected in inflamed tissue (right) and in neighboring healthy tissue (left) from the same patient with active Crohn's disease using an IS*900*-derived DNA probe. The probe was labeled with fluorescein, and hybridization with *M. avium* subsp. *paratuberculosis* DNA was visualized using confocal laser scanning microscopy. The arrows indicate the presence of *M. avium* subsp. *tuberculosis* DNA in tissue.

should be detectable. In the past few years, there has been emphasis on investigating anti-*M. avium* subsp. *paratuberculosis* IgG antibodies in sera from Crohn's disease patients by immunoblotting or enzyme-linked immunosorbent assay. The outcomes have been conflicting, largely due to the choice of the *M. avium* subsp. *paratuberculosis* antigen(s) employed. Our group has identified p35 and p36 recombinant clones expressing 35- and 36-kDa proteins, respectively, from an expression genomic library of *M. avium* subsp. *paratuberculosis* constructed in *E. coli* (11, 27–31, 72, 91, 92). Both antigens have been reported heavily in the literature to be specific to sera from Crohn's disease patients with poor reactivity to control sera. Olsen et al. (74) also reported elevated anti-*M. avium* subsp. *paratuberculosis* antibody response in sera from Crohn's disease patients compared to controls when a 14-kDa protein of *M. avium* subsp. *paratuberculosis* was evaluated. The use of p35, p36, and the 14-kDa antigens clearly produced evidence that supports the association of *M. avium* subsp. *paratuberculosis* with Crohn's disease. There has been speculation about possible partial failure in the cellular immune response in Crohn's disease patients and about the ability to effectively clear *M. avium* subsp. *paratuberculosis* by phagocytosis (85). In our laboratory, we evaluated the presence of *M. avium* subsp. *paratuberculosis* in tissues from 17 Crohn's disease patients and 10 controls. We also evaluated the immunogenicity of polymorphonuclear cells (PMNCs) and mononuclear cells (MNCs) in peripheral blood from 19 Crohn's disease patients and 11 controls. Nested PCR detected the IS*900* gene unique to *M. avium* subsp. *paratuberculosis* in tissues from 15 of 17 (88%) Crohn's disease patients and 4 of 10 (40%) controls ($P < 0.001$). PMNC phagocytosis of fluorescein-labeled viable *M. avium* subsp. *paratuberculosis* was suppressed in 13 of 19 (68%) Crohn's disease patients compared to 0 of 11 controls; the suppression ranged between 6 and 97%. MNC phagocytosis was suppressed in some Crohn's disease patients (5 of 19 [26%]), with no suppression in controls. Plasma inhibitors specific to PMNCs were detected in 9 of 19 (47%) Crohn's disease patients and in 0 of 11 controls. Plasma inhibitors specific to MNCs were detected in 3 of 19 (16%) Crohn's disease patients. In addition to the defect in the ability of PMNCs to phagocytose the bacterium, *M. avium* subsp. *paratuberculosis* was localized peripherally in the cytoplasm of in vitro-infected Crohn's disease PMNCs (Fig. 2). Lymphocyte anergy due to failure to respond normally to phytohematoagglutinin (PHA) was detected in 8 of 19 (42%) Crohn's disease patients. Possible prior exposure to *M. avium* subsp. *paratuberculosis* due to strong reactivity to purified protein derivative was detected in 7 of 11 (64%) Crohn's disease patients with normal PHA responses. Detection of *M. avium* subsp. *paratuberculosis* in tissue and alteration in the abilities of neutrophils and MNCs to respond efficiently to

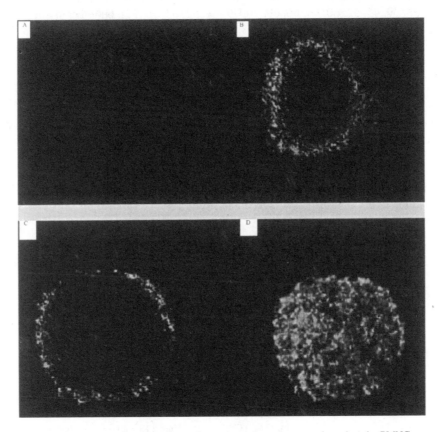

Figure 2. Phagocytosis of *Mycobacterium avium* subspecies *paratuberculosis* by PMNCs from a Crohn's disease patient. In vitro exposure of PMNCs from a Crohn's disease patient and a healthy control to fluorescein isothiocyanate-labeled *M. avium* subsp. *paratuberculosis* illustrates a clear decrease in the numbers of *M. avium* subsp. *paratuberculosis* cells phagocytosed by PMNCs from a Crohn's disease patient (A) compared to cells from a healthy control (C) following a 20-min incubation. Similar results were observed when the exposure was extended to 2 h (B and D). *M. avium* subsp. *paratuberculosis* colocalization in PMNCs from Crohn's disease patients was concentrated in phagosomes close to the cytoplasmic membrane in contrast to PMNCs from healthy subjects, in which *M. avium* subsp. *paratuberculosis* cells were scattered throughout the cytoplasm. The images were taken using confocal laser scanning microscopy.

M. avium subsp. *paratuberculosis* and PHA may be related to the fact that mycobacterial pathogens infect phagocytic cells and consequently activate signals that dysregulate the immune system. The data suggest a possible role for an environmental pathogen in Crohn's disease pathogenesis (unpublished data).

Culture Evidence

Intestinal Tissue

M. avium subsp. *paratuberculosis* has been isolated from surgical tissue and intestinal biopsy specimens from Crohn's disease patients in various parts of the world (1, 6, 22, 23, 33, 37, 38, 39, 45, 52, 60, 64, 66, 69, 70, 79, 81, 82, 87–90, 97), but other studies failed to isolate *M. avium* subsp. *paratuberculosis* from Crohn's disease tissue (2, 8, 12, 18, 25, 34, 55, 80). Since 2000, with the use of the modified MGIT culture medium technique, *M. avium* subsp. *paratuberculosis* has been identified in cultures by IS*900*-based PCR in six of seven (87%) Crohn's disease patients compared to zero of three (0%) controls (87). *M. avium* subsp. *paratuberculosis* was also cultured in MGIT media following 40 weeks of incubation from biopsy specimens from 4 of 20 (20%) Crohn's disease patients compared to 2 of 33 (6%) controls (87). Studies by other groups using similar techniques have also found *M. avium* subsp. *paratuberculosis* to be associated with Crohn's disease samples. Bull and associates identified *M. avium* subsp. *paratuberculosis* in 14 of 33 (42%) biopsy specimens from Crohn's disease patients compared to 3 of 33 (9%) biopsy specimens from controls (6). In addition, *M. avium* subsp. *paratuberculosis* was reported in MGIT cultures of 83% of biopsy specimens from Crohn's disease patients compared to 10% of controls (88) (Table 3).

Table 3. Culture of *M. avium* subsp. *paratuberculosis* from Crohn's disease patients using MGIT culture media (2000 to 2005)

Specimen	No. (%) *M. avium* subsp. *paratuberculosis* in MGIT confirmed by IS*900*[a]	Country	Reference
Surgical tissue	6/7 (86) CD 0/3 (0) NIBD	United States	87
Intestinal biopsy, specimens	4/20 (20) CD 2/33 (6) NIBD	United States	87
	14/33 (42) CD 3/33 (9) NIBD	United Kingdom	6
	25/30 (83) CD 3/29 (10) NIBD	Italy	88
Breast milk	2/2 (100) CD 0/5 (0) Normal	United States	69
Blood	14/28 (50) CD 2/9 (22) UC 0/11 (0) NIBD	United States	70

[a]NIBD, noninflammatory bowel disease; CD, Crohn's disease.

Breast Milk

Due to the similarity between Johne's disease and Crohn's disease and the fact that *M. avium* subsp. *paratuberculosis* in infected animals is excreted into milk, we sought human milk samples from lactating women with active Crohn's disease. To date, *M. avium* subsp. *paratuberculosis* has been cultured from the milk of three women with active Crohn's disease and zero of seven healthy women (69). The impact of this finding on breast-feeding and possible transmission of *M. avium* subsp. *paratuberculosis* from mothers to infants has yet to be determined (Table 3).

Peripheral Blood

The culture of *M. avium* subsp. *paratuberculosis* from breast milk, gall bladder tissue, inflamed and neighboring noninflamed tissue, and lymph node tissue suggested that *M. avium* subsp. *paratuberculosis* infection in Crohn's disease patients is systemic. Consequently, we analyzed buffy coat preparations of blood from 52 subjects. Modified MGIT culture media were incubated for 10 to 12 weeks, followed by microscopic staining and nested-PCR identification. Naser et al. (70) found positive cultures of *M. avium* subsp. *paratuberculosis* from the blood of 14 of 28 (50%) Crohn's disease patients, 2 of 9 (22%) UC patients, and 0 of 11 individuals without inflammatory bowel disease (Table 3). The use of immunosuppressive medication did not correlate with positive blood cultures. A multicenter blind study aimed at analysis of blood samples from Crohn's disease patients and controls is under way.

THERAPEUTIC RESPONSE USING *M. AVIUM* SUBSP. *PARATUBERCULOSIS* ANTIBIOTICS

If *M. avium* subsp. *paratuberculosis* causes Crohn's disease, the inclination is to treat patients with antibiotics and to monitor them for clinical improvement. The problem is that mycobacteria are very difficult to treat, and *M. avium* is harder to treat than most due to the development of multiply drug-resistant strains. Moreover, the CWD form of *M. avium* subsp. *paratuberculosis* in Crohn's disease patients limits the choice of antibiotics, excluding those drugs that target the cell wall. In our laboratory, we evaluated 15 antimycobacterial drugs in vitro against an *M. avium* subsp. *paratuberculosis* clinical isolate. Clarithromycin, a macrolide, was effective in vitro against *M. avium* subsp. *paratuberculosis* growth. However, when regimens of two or three antibiotics were evaluated, a combination of clarithromycin at a lower concentration and rifabutin exhibited excellent synergistic activity against *M. avium* subsp. *paratuberculosis*. In an open clinical trial (92), a total of 36 Crohn's disease patients whose sera tested positive against p35 and p36 recombinant antigens were treated with rifabutin and clarithromycin and followed up for 4 to 17 months. Of the 29 Crohn's disease patients who tolerated the treatment, 21 (72%) sustained clinical improvement and were considered responders. Similar outcomes were reported for other open clinical trials in the United Kingdom and Australia (5, 44). Blinded comparison studies have not yet been performed.

CONCLUSIONS

The mycobacterial theory states that *M. avium* subsp. *paratuberculosis* is a specific pathogen that is a major etiologic agent in Crohn's disease—perhaps not the only infectious agent, but certainly the most prevalent. The *M. avium* subsp. *paratuberculosis* theory embraces all that has been reported about immune dysregulation, predisposing genetic factors, immune deficiency, the role of gut flora, and a compromised mucosal epithelial barrier. *M. avium* subsp. *paratuberculosis* infection in humans with Crohn's disease is known to be systemic (similar to animal paratuberculosis), following the culture of *M. avium* subsp. *paratuberculosis* from tissue, milk, and blood from Crohn's disease patients. Interestingly, *M. avium* subsp. *paratuberculosis* isolates cultured in our laboratory exhibited genetic sharing with *M. avium* subsp. *paratuberculosis* isolates derived from animals with Johne's disease (38, 67). *M. avium* subsp. *paratuberculosis* is believed to behave similarly to *M. tuberculosis* and *M. leprae* and is able to dysregulate immune signaling as one of its evolved survival strategies. Ultimately, optimal treatment of patients with active Crohn's disease will likely require multiple approaches, including immunomodulation.

The mycobacterial theory and its association with Crohn's disease, and perhaps IBD in general, have been considered among the most controversial and vigorously debated subjects in the literature for the past century. The interest in the *M. avium* subsp. *paratuberculosis*-Crohn's disease theory is tremendous, including many who are considered to be outside the gastroenterology community. Perhaps lessons from the *Helicobacter* story have been learned, or perhaps even the skeptics hesitate to exclude a possible *M. avium* subsp. *paratuberculosis* role in IBD etiology. The recent achievement of Marshall and Warren, who received the 2005 Nobel Prize in physiology or medicine for their work on *Helicobacter pylori* and gastric ulcers, may add to the fuel that continues to renew interest in the *M. avium* subsp. *paratuberculosis*-Crohn's disease debate.

Acknowledgments. This work was supported by grant RO1-AI51251-01 from NIH-NIAID.
Special thanks are due to M. Ghonaim for his valuable assistance during the preparation of this chapter.

REFERENCES

1. **Al-Shamali, M., I. Khan, B. Al-Nakib, F. Al-Hassan, and A. S. Mustafa.** 1997. A multiplex polymerase chain reaction assay for the detection of *Mycobacterium paratuberculosis* DNA in Crohn's disease tissue. *Scand. J. Gastroenterol.* **32:**819–823.
2. **Baksh, F. K., S. D. Finkelstein, S. M. Ariyananyagam-Baksh, P. A. Swalsky, E. C. Klein, and J. C. Dunn.** 2004. Absence of *Mycobacterium avium* subsp. *paratuberculosis* in the microdissected granulomas of Crohn's disease. *Mod. Pathol.* **17:**1289–1294.
3. **Bayless, T. M., A. Z. Tokayer, J. M. Polito II, S. A. Quaskey, E. D. Mellits, and M. L. Harris.** 1996. Crohn's disease: concordance for site and clinical type in affected family. *Gastroenterology* **111:** 573–579.
4. **Bernstein, C. N., J. F. Blanchard, P. Rawsthorne, and M. T. Collins.** 2004. Population-based case control study of seroprevalence of *Mycobacterium paratuberculosis* in patients with Crohn's disease and ulcerative colitis. *J. Clin. Microbiol.* **42:**1129–1135.
5. **Borody, T. J., S. Leis, E. F. Warren, and R. Surace.** 2002. Treatment of severe Crohn's disease using antimycobacterial triple therapy—approaching a cure? *Dig. Liver Dis.* **34:**29–38.
6. **Bull, T. J., E. J. McMinn, K. Sidi-Boumedine, A. Skull, D. Durkin, P. Neild, G. Rhodes, R. Pickup, and J. Hermon-Taylor.** 2003. Detection and verification of *Mycobacterium avium* subsp *paratuberculosis* in fresh ileocolonic mucosal biopsy specimens from individuals with and without Crohn's disease. *J. Clin. Microbiol.* **41:**2915–2923.
7. **Burnham, W. R., J. E. Lennard-Jones, J. L. Stanford, and R. G. Bird.** 1978. Mycobacteria as a possible cause of inflammatory bowel disease. *Lancet* **ii:**693–696.

8. **Cellier, C., H. De Beenhouwer, A. Berger, C. Penna, F. Carbonnel, R. Parc, P. H. Cugnenc, Y. Le Quintrec, J. P. Gendre, J. P. Barbier, and F. Portaels.** 1998. *Mycobacterium paratuberculosis* and *Mycobacterium avium* subsp. *silvaticum* DNA cannot be detected by PCR in Crohn's disease tissue. *Gastroenterol. Clin. Biol.* **22:**675–678.

9. **Chacon, O., L. B. Bermudez, and R. G. Barletta.** 2004. Johne's disease, inflammatory bowel disease, and *Mycobactrium paratuberculosis. Annu. Rev. Microbiol.* **58:**329–363.

10. **Chadwick, N., I. J. Bruce, S. Schepelmann, R. E. Pounder, and A. J. Wakefield.** 1998. Measles virus RNA is not detected in inflammatory bowel disease using hybrid capture and reverse transcriptase followed by polymerase chain reaction. *J. Med. Virol.* **55:**305–311.

11. **Chamberlin, W., D. Y. Graham, K. Hulten, H. M. T. El-Zimaity, M. R. Schwartz, S. A. Naser, I. Shafran, and F. A. K. El-Zaatari.** 2001. *Mycobacterium avium* subsp. *paratuberculosis* as one cause of Crohn's disease. *Aliment. Pharmacol. Ther.* **15:**337–346.

12. **Chiba, M., T. Fukushima, Y. Horie, M. Iizuka, and O. Masamune.** 1998. No *Mycobacterium paratuberculosis* detected in intestinal tissue, including Peyer's patches and lymph follicles, of Crohn's disease. *J. Gastroenterol.* **33:**482–487.

13. **Chiodini, R. J.** 1989. Crohn's disease and the mycobacterioses: a review and comparison of two disease entities. *Clin. Microbiol. Rev.* **2:**90–117.

14. **Chiodini, R. J., H. J. Van Kruiningen, R. S. Merkal, W. R. Thayer, Jr., and J. A. Coutu.** 1984. Characteristics of an unclassified *Mycobacterium* species isolated from patients with Crohn's disease. *J. Clin. Microbiol.* **20:**966–971.

15. **Chiodini, R. J., H. J. Van Kruiningen, W. R. Thayer, R. S. Merkal, and J. A. Coutu.** 1984. Possible role of mycobacteria in inflammatory bowel disease. I. An unclassified *Mycobacterium* species isolated from patients with Crohn's disease. *Dig. Dis. Sci.* **29:**1073–1079.

16. **Clarkson, W. K., M. E. Presti, P. F. Petersen, P. E. Zachary, W. X. Fan, C. L. Leonardi, A. M. Vernava, W. E. Longo, and J. M. Kreeger.** 1998. Role of *Mycobacterium paratuberculosis* in Crohn's disease. *Dis. Colon Rectum* **41:**195–199.

17. **Collins, M. T.** 1996. Diagnosis of *paratuberculosis. Vet. Clin. N. Am. Food Anim. Pract.* **12:**357–371.

18. **Collins, M. T., G. Lisby, C. Moser, D. Chicks, S. Christensen, M. Reichelderfer, N. Hoiby, B. A. Harms, O. O. Thomsen, U. Skibsted, and V. Binder.** 2000. Results of multiple diagnostic tests for *Mycobacterium avium paratuberculosis* in patients with inflammatory bowel disease and in controls. *J. Clin. Microbiol.* **38:**4373–4381.

19. **Cosgrove, M.** 1996. The epidemiology of pediatric inflammatory bowel disease. *Arch. Dis. Child.* **74:**460–461.

20. **Crohn, B. B., K. Ginzburg, and G. D. Oppenheimer.** 1932. Regional ileitis: a pathological and clinical entity. *JAMA* **9:**1323–1329.

21. **Dalziel, T. K.** 1913. Chronic interstitial enteritis. *Br. Med. J.* **2:**1068–1070.

22. **Dell'Isola, B., C. Poyart, O. Goulet, J. F. Mougenot, E. Sadoun-Journo, N. Brousse, J. Schmitz, C. Ricour, and P. Berche.** 1994. Detection of *Mycobacterium paratuberculosis* by polymerase chain reaction in children with Crohn's disease. *J. Infect. Dis.* **169:**449–451.

23. **Del Prete, R., M. Quaranta, A. Lippolis, V. Giannuzzi, A. Mosca, E. Jirillo, and G. Miragliotta.** 1998. Detection of *Mycobacterium paratuberculosis* in stool samples of patients with inflammatory bowel disease by IS*900*-based PCR and colorimetric detection of amplified DNA. *J. Microbiol. Methods* **33:**105–114.

24. **Dieckgraefe, B. K., and J. R. Korzenik.** 2002. Treatment of active Crohn's disease with recombinant human-granulocyte-macrophage colony-stimulating factor. *Lancet* **360:**1478–1480.

25. **Dumonceau, J. M., A. Van Gossum, M. Adler, P. A. Fonteyne, J. P. Van Vooren, J. Deviere, and F. Portaels.** 1996. No *Mycobacterium paratuberculosis* found in Crohn's disease using the polymerase chain reaction. *Dig. Dis. Sci.* **41:**421–426.

26. **Ellingson, J. L., J. L. Anderson, J. J. Koziczkowski, R. P. Radcliff, S. J. Sloan, S. E. Allen, and N. M. Sullivan.** 2005. Detection of viable *Mycobacterium avium* subsp. *paratuberculosis* in retail pasteurized whole milk by two culture methods and PCR. *J. Food Prot.* **68:**966–972.

27. **El-Zaatari, F. A., S. A. Naser, L. Engstrand, C. Y. Hachem, and D. Y. Graham.** 1994. Identification and characterization of *Mycobacterium paratuberculosis* recombinant proteins expressed in *E. coli. Curr. Microbiol.* **29:**177–184.

28. **El-Zaatari, F. A. K., S. A. Naser, L. Engstrand, P. E. Burch, C. Y. Hachem, D. L. Whipple, and D. Y. Graham.** 1995. Nucleotide sequence analysis and seroreactivities of the 65K heat shock protein from *Mycobacterium paratuberculosis. Clin. Diagn. Lab. Immunol.* **2:**657–664.

29. **El-Zaatari, F. A. K., S. A. Naser, and D. Y. Graham.** 1997. Characterization of a specific *Mycobacterium paratuberculosis* recombinant clone expressing 35,000-molecular-weight antigen and reactivity with sera from animals with clinical and subclinical Johne's disease. *J. Clin. Microbiol.* **35:**1794–1799.

30. **El-Zaatari, F. A. K., S. A. Naser, D. C. Markesich, D. C. Kalter, L. Engstand, and D. Y. Graham.** 1996. Identification of *Mycobacterium avium* complex in sarcoidosis. *J. Clin. Microbiol.* **34:**2240–2245.

31. **El-Zaatari, F. A., S. A. Naser, K. Hulten, P. Burch, and D. Y. Graham.** 1999. Characterization of *Mycobacterium paratuberculosis* p36 antigen and its seroreactivities in Crohn's disease. *Curr. Microbiol.* **39:**115–119.

32. **Erasmus, D. L., T. C. Victor, P. J. Van Eeden, V. Falck, and P. Van Helden.** 1995. *Mycobacterium paratuberculosis* and Crohn's disease. *Gut* **36:**942.

33. **Fidler, H. M., W. Thurrell, N. M. J. Johnson, G. A. W. Rook, and J. J. McFadden.** 1994. Specific detection of *Mycobacterium paratuberculosis* DNA associated with granulomatous tissue in Crohn's disease. *Gut* **35:**506–510.

34. **Frank, T. S., and S. M. Cook.** 1996. Analysis of paraffin sections of Crohn's disease for *Mycobacterium paratuberculosis* using polymerase chain reaction. *Mod. Pathol.* **9:**32–35.

35. **Friedman, S., and R. S. Blumberg.** 1999. Inflammatory bowel disease, p. 1679–1691. *In* E. Braunwald, S. A. Fauci, D. L. Kasper, S. L. Hauser, and D. L. Longo (ed.), *Harrison's Principles of Internal Medicine*, 15th ed. McGraw-Hill, New York, N.Y.

36. **Fujita, H., Y. Eishi, and I. Ishige.** 2002. Quantitative analysis of bacterial DNA from *Mycobacterium* spp., *Bacteroides vulgatus* and *Escherichia coli* in tissue samples from patients with inflammatory bowel diseases. *J. Gastroenterol.* **37:**509–516.

37. **Gan, H., Q. Ouyang, and H. Bu.** 1997. *Mycobacterium paratuberculosis* in the intestine of patients with Crohn's disease. *Chung Hua Nei Ko Tsa Chih* **36:**228–230.

38. **Ghadiali, A. H., M. Strother, S. A. Naser, E. J. Manning, and S. Sreevatsan.** 2004. *Mycobacterium avium* subsp. *paratuberculosis* strains isolated from Crohn's disease patients and animal species exhibit similar polymorphic locus patterns. *J. Clin. Microbiol.* **42:**5345–5348.

39. **Gitnick, G., J. Collins, B. Beaman, D. Brooks, M. Arthur, T. Imaeda, and M. Palieschesky.** 1989. Preliminary report on isolation of mycobacteria from patients with Crohn's disease. *Dig. Dis. Sci.* **34:**925–932.

40. **Grant, I.** 2005. Zoonotic potential of *Mycobacterium avium* ssp. *paratuberculosis*: the current position. *J. Appl. Microbiol.* **98:**1282–1293.

41. **Grant, I. R., H. J. Ball, and M. T. Rowe.** 2002. Incidence of *Mycobacterium paratuberculosis* in bulk raw and commercially pasteurized cows' milk from approved dairy processing establishments in the United Kingdom. *Appl. Environ. Microbiol.* **68:**2428–2435.

42. **Greenstein, A. J., P. Lachman, D. B. Sachar, J. Springhorn, T. Heimann, H. D. Janowitz, and A. H. Aufses.** 1988. Perforating and non-perforating indications for repeated operations in Crohn's disease: evidence for two clinical forms. *Gut* **29:**588–592.

43. **Greenstein, R. J., and A. J. Greenstein.** 1995. Is there clinical, epidemiological, and molecular evidence for two forms of Crohn's disease? *Mol. Med. Today* **1:**343–348.

44. **Gui, G. P., P. R. Thomas, M. L. Tizard, J. Lake, J. D. Sanderson, and J. Hermon-Taylor.** 1997. Two-year-outcomes analysis of Crohn's disease treated with rifabutin and macrolide antibiotics. *J. Antimicrob. Chemother.* **39:**393–400.

45. **Haagsma, J., C. J. J. Mulder, A. Eger, and G. N. J. Tytgat.** 1991. *Mycobacterium paratuberculosis* isole chez des patients atteints de maladie de Crohn. Resultats preliminaires. *Acta Endosc.* **21:**255–260.

46. **Harvey, R. F., and J. M. Bradshaw.** 1980. A simple index of Crohn's-disease activity. *Lancet* **i:**514.

47. **Hermon-Taylor, J., N. Barnes, C. Clarke, and C. Finlayson.** 1998. *Mycobacterium paratuberculosis* cervical lymphadenitis followed five years later by terminal ileitis similar to Crohn's disease. *Br. Med. J.* **316:**449–453.

48. **Holland, S. M.** 2000. Cytokine therapy of mycobacterial infections. *Adv. Intern. Med.* **45:**431–452.

49. **Hollander, D., C. M. Vadheim, E. Brettholz, G. M. Petersen, T. Delahunty, and J. I. Rotter.** 1986. Increased intestinal permeability in patients with Crohn's disease and their relatives. *Ann. Intern. Med.* **105:**883–885.

50. **Hugot, J. P., C. Alberti, D. Berrebi, E. Bingen, and J. P. Cezard.** 2003. Crohn's disease: the cold chain hypothesis. *Lancet* **362:**2012–2015.

51. **Hugot, J. P., H. Zoulai, and S. Lesage.** 2003. Lessons to be learned from the NOD2 gene in Crohn's disease. *Eur. J. Gastroenterol. Hepatol.* **15:**593–597.

52. **Hulten, K., H. M. El-Zimaity, T. J. Karttunen, A. Almashhrawi, M. R. Schwartz, D. Y. Graham, and F. A. K. El-Zaatari.** 2001. Detection of *M. avium* subsp. *paratuberculosis* in Crohn's disease tissues by *in situ* hybridization. *Am. J. Gastroenterol.* **96:**3222–3224.

53. **Johne, H. A., and L. Frothingham.** 1895. Ein eigenthumlicher fallvon tuberculose beim rind. *Dtsch. Zeitschr. Tiermed. Vergl. Pathol.* **21:**438–454.

54. **Kallinowski, F., A. Wassmer, M. A. Hofmann, D. Harmsen, J. Heesemann, H. Karch, C. H. Herfarth, and H. J. Buhr.** 1998. Prevalence of enteropathogenic bacteria in surgically treated chronic inflammatory bowel disease. *Hepatol. Gastroenterol.* **45:**1552–1558.

55. **Kanazawa, K., Y. Haga, O. Funakoshi, H. Nakajima, A. Munakata, and Y. Yoshida.** 1999. Absence of *Mycobacterium paratuberculosis* DNA in intestinal tissues from Crohn's disease by nested polymerase chain reaction. *J. Gastroenterol.* **34:**200–206.

56. **Kirsner, J.** 1984. Crohn's disease. *JAMA* **251:**80–81.

57. **Kucharzik, T., N. Lugering, H. Weigelt, M. Adolf, W. Domschke, and R. Stoll.** 1996. Immunoregulatory properties of IL-13 in patients with inflammatory bowel disease: comparison with IL-4 and IL-10. *Clin. Exp. Immunol.* **104:**483–490.

58. **Kyle, J.** 1992. Crohn's disease in the Northeastern and Northern Isles of Scotland: an epidemiological review. *Gastroenterology* **103:**392–399.

59. **Lala, S., Y. Ogura, C. Osborne, S. Y. Hor, A. Bromfield, S. Davies, O. Ogunbiyi, G. Nunez, and S. Keshav.** 2003. Crohn's disease and the NOD2 gene: a role for Paneth cells. *Gastroenterology* **125:**47–57.

60. **Lisby, C. M. G., J. Andersen, K. Engbaek, and V. Binder.** 1994. *Mycobacterium paratuberculosis* in intestinal tissue from patients with Crohn's disease demonstrated by a nested primer polymerase chain reaction. *Scand. J. Gastroenterol.* **29:**923–929.

61. **Loftus, E. V., Jr., M. D. Silverstein, W. J. Sandborn, W. J. Tremaine, W. S. Harmsen, and A. R. Zinsmeister.** 1998. Crohn's disease in Olmsted County, Minnesota, 1940–1993: incidence, prevalence, and survival. *Gastroenterology* **114:**1161–1168.

62. **McFadden, J., J. Collins, B. Beaman, M. Arthur, and G. Gitnick.** 1992. Mycobacteria in Crohn's disease: DNA probes identify the wood pigeon strain of *Mycobacterium avium* and *Mycobacterium paratuberculosis* from human tissue. *J. Clin. Microbiol.* **30:**3070–3073.

63. **Millar, D., J. Ford, J. D. Sanderson, S. Withey, M. Tizard, T. Doran, and J. Hermon-Taylor.** 1996. IS*900* PCR to detect *Mycobacterium paratuberculosis* in retail milk supplies of whole pasteurized cows' milk in England and Wales. *Appl. Environ. Microbiol.* **62:**3446–3452.

64. **Mishina, D., P. Katsel, S. T. Brown, E. C. A. M. Gilberts, and R. J. Greenstein.** 1996. On the etiology of Crohn's disease. *Proc. Natl. Acad. Sci. USA* **93:**9816–9820.

65. **Modigliani, R. J., Y. Mary, J. F. Simon, A. Cortot, J. C. Soule, and J. P. Gendre.** 1990. Clinical, biological and endoscopic picture of attacks of Crohn's disease. *Gastroenterology* **98:**811–818.

66. **Moss, M. T., J. D. Sanderson, M. L. V. Tizard, J. Hermon-Taylor, F. A. K. El-Zaatari, D. C. Markesich, and D. Y. Graham.** 1992. Polymerase chain reaction of *Mycobacterium paratuberculosis* and *Mycobacterium avium* subsp. *silvaticum* in long term cultures from Crohn's disease and control tissues. *Gut* **33:**1209–1213.

67. **Motiwala, A. S., M. Strother, A. Amonsin, B. Byrum, S. A. Naser, J. R. Stabel, W. P. Shulaw, J. B. Bannantine, V. Kapur, and S. Sreevatsan.** 2003. Molecular epidemiology of *Mycobacterium avium* subspecies *paratuberculosis*: evidence for limited strain diversity, strain sharing, and identification of unique targets for diagnosis. *J. Clin. Microbiol.* **41:**2015–2026.

68. **Murray, A., J. Oliaro, M. M. T. Schlup, and V. S. Chadwick.** 1995. *Mycobacterium paratuberculosis* and inflammatory bowel disease: frequency distribution in serial colonoscopic biopsies using the polymerase chain reaction. *Microbios* **83:**217–228.

69. **Naser, S. A., D. Schwartz, and I. Shafran.** 2000. Isolation of *Mycobacterium avium* subsp. *paratuberculosis* from breast milk of Crohn's disease patients. *Am. J. Gastroenterol.* **95:**1094–1095.

70. **Naser, S. A., G. Ghobrial, C. Romero, and J. F. Valentine.** 2004. Culture of *Mycobacterium avium* subspecies *paratuberculosis* from the blood of patients with Crohn's disease. *Lancet* **364:**1039–1044.

71. **Naser, S. A., I. Shafran, D. Schwartz, F. El-Zaatari, and J. Biggerstaff.** 2002. In situ identification of mycobacteria in Crohn's disease patient tissue using confocal laser scanning microscopy. *Mol. Cell. Probes* **16:**41–48.

72. **Naser, S. A., K. Hulten, I. Shafran, D. Y. Graham, and F. A. El-Zaatari.** 2000. Specific seroreactivity of Crohn's disease patients against p35 and p36 antigens of *M. avium* subsp. *paratuberculosis*. *Vet. Microbiol.* **77:**497–504.

73. Ogura, Y., D. K. Bonen, N. Inohara, D. L. Nicolae, F. F. Chen, R. Ramos, H. Britton, T. Moran, R. Karaliuskas, R. H. Duerr, J. P. Achkar, S. R. Brant, T. M. Bayless, B. S. Kirschner, S. B. Hanauer, G. Nunez, and J. H. Cho. 2001. A frame shift mutation in NOD2 associated with susceptibility to Crohn's disease. *Nature* **411:**603–606.

74. Olsen, I., H. G. Wiker, E. Johnson, H. Langeggan, and L. J. Reitan. 2001. Elevated antibody responses in patients with Crohn's disease against a 14-kDa secreted protein purified from *Mycobacterium avium* subsp. *paratuberculosis. Scand. J. Infect. Dis.* **53:**198–203.

75. Pickup, R. W., G. Rhodes, S. Arnott, K. Sidi-Boumedine, T. Bull, A. Weightman, M. Hurley, and J. Hermon-Taylor. 2005. *Mycobacterium avium* subsp. *paratuberculosis* in the catchment area and water of the River Taff in South Wales, United Kingdom, and its potential relationship to clustering of Crohn's disease cases in the city of Cardiff. *Appl. Environ. Microbiol.* **71:**2130–2139.

76. Postuma, R., and S. P. Moroz. 1985. Pediatric Crohn's disease. *J. Pediatr. Surg.* **20:**478–482.

77. Present, D. H., P. Rutgeerts, and S. Targan. 1999. Infliximab for the treatment of fistulas in patients with Crohn's disease. *N. Engl. J. Med.* **340:**1398–1405.

78. Richter, E., J. Wessling, N. Lugering, W. Domschke, and S. Rusch-Gerdes. 2002. *Mycobacterium avium* subsp. *paratuberculosis* infection in a patient with HIV, Germany. *Emerg. Infect. Dis.* **8:**729–731.

79. Romero, C., A. Hamdi, J. F. Valentine, and S. A. Naser. 2005. Evaluation of surgical tissue from patients with Crohn's disease for the presence of *Mycobacterium avium* subspecies *paratuberculosis* DNA by *in situ* hybridization and nested polymerase chain reaction. *Inflamm. Bowel Dis.* **11:**116–125.

80. Rowbotham, D. S., N. P. Mapstone, L. K. Trejdosiewicz, P. D. Howdle, and P. Quirke. 1995. *Mycobacterium paratuberculosis* DNA not detected in Crohn's disease tissue by fluorescent polymerase chain reaction. *Gut* **37:**660–667.

81. Ryan, P., M. W. Bennett, S. Aarons, G. Lee, J. Race K. Collins, G. C. O'Sullivan, J. O'Connell, and F. Shanahan. 2002. PCR detection of *Mycobacterium paratuberculosis* in Crohn's disease granulomas isolated by laser capture microdissection. *Gut* **51:**665–670.

82. Sanderson, J. D., M. T. Moss, M. L. Tizard, and J. Hermon-Taylor. 1992. *Mycobacterium paratuberculosis* DNA in Crohn's disease tissue. *Gut* **33:**890–896.

83. Sands, B. E. 2004. From symptoms to diagnosis: clinical distinctions among various forms of intestinal inflammation. *Gastroenterology* **126:**1518–1532.

84. Sartor, R. B. 2005. Role of commensal enteric bacteria in the pathogenesis of immune-mediated intestinal inflammation: lessons from animal models and implications for translational research. *J. Pediatr. Gastroenterol. Nutr.* **1:**30–31.

85. Sartor, R. B. 2005. Does *Mycobacterium avium* subspecies *paratuberculosis* cause Crohn's disease? *Gut* **54:**896–898.

86. Satsangi, J., D. P. Jeweel, W. M. C. Rosenberg, and J. I. Bell. 1994. Genetics of inflammatory bowel disease: a progress report. *Gut* **35:**696–700.

87. Schwartz, D., I. Shafran, C. Romero, C. Piromalli, J. Biggerstaff, N. Naser, W. Chamberlin, and S. A. Naser. 2000. Use of short-term culture for identification of *Mycobacterium avium* subsp. *paratuberculosis* in tissue from Crohn's disease patients. *Clin. Microbiol. Infect.* **6:**303–307.

88. Sechi, L. A., A. Scanu, P. Molicotti, S. Canas, M. Mura, G. Dettori, G. Fadda, and S. Zanetti. 2005. Detection and isolation of *Mycobacterium avium* subsp. *paratuberculosis* from intestinal biopsies of patients with Crohn's disease. *Am. J. Gastroenterol.* **100:**1529–1536.

89. Sechi, L. A., M. Mura, E. Tanda, A. Lissia, G. Fadda, and S. Zanetti. 2004. *Mycobacterium avium* subsp. *paratuberculosis* in tissue samples of Crohn's disease patients. *New Microbiol.* **27:**75–77.

90. Sechi, L. A., M. Mura, F. Tanda, A. Lissia, A. Solinas, G. Fadda, and S. Zanetti. 2001. Identification of *Mycobacterium avium* subsp. *paratuberculosis* in biopsy specimens from patients with Crohn's disease identified by in situ hybridization. *J. Clin. Microbiol.* **39:**4514–4517.

91. Shafran, I., C. Piromalli, J. W. Decker, J. Sandoval, S. A. Naser, and F. A. El-Zaatari. 2002. Seroreactivities against *Saccharomyces cerevisiae* and *Mycobacterium avium* subsp. *paratuberculosis* p35 and p36 antigens in Crohn's disease patients. *Dig. Dis. Sci.* **47:**2079–2081.

92. Shafran, I., L. Kuqler, F. A. K. El-Zaatari, S. A. Naser, and J. Sandoval. 2002. Open clinical trial of rifabutin and clarithromycin in therapy in Crohn's disease. *Dig. Liver Dis.* **34:**22–28.

93. Suenaga, K., Y. Yokoyama, K. Okazaki, and Y. Yamamoto. 1995. Mycobacteria in the intestine of Japanese patients with inflammatory bowel disease. *Am. J. Gastroenterol.* **90:**76–80.

94. **Thorel, M. F., M. Krichevsky, and V. V. Levy-Frebault.** 1990. Numerical taxonomy of mycobactin-dependent mycobacteria, emended description of *Mycobacterium avium*, and description of *Mycobacterium avium* subsp. *avium* subsp. nov., *Mycobacterium avium* subsp. *paratuberculosis* subsp. nov., and *Mycobacterium avium* subsp. *silvaticum* subsp. nov. *Int. J. Syst. Bacteriol.* **40:**254–260.

95. **Van Kruiningen, H. J., M. Joossens, S. Vermeire, S. Joossens, S. Debeugny, C. Gower-Rousseau, A. Cortot, J. F. Colombel, P. Rutgeerts, and R. Vlietinck.** 2005. Environmental factors in familial Crohn's disease in Belgium. *Inflamm. Bowel Dis.* **11:**360–365.

96. **Van Kruiningen, H. J., R. J. Chiodini, W. R. Thayer, J. A. Coutu, R. S. Merkal, and P. L. Runnels.** 1986. Experimental disease in infant goats induced by a *Mycobacterium* isolated from a patient with Crohn's disease. *Dig. Dis. Sci.* **31:**1351–1360.

97. **Wall, S., Z. M. Kunze, S. Saboor, J. Soufleri, P. Seechurn, R. Chiodini, and J. J. McFadden.** 1993. Identification of spheroplast-like agents isolated from tissues of patients with Crohn's disease and control tissues by polymerase chain reaction. *J. Clin. Microbiol.* **31:**1241–1245.

98. **Winthrop, K. L., and J. N. Siegel.** 2004. Tuberculosis cases associated with infliximab and etanercept. *Clin. Infect. Dis.* **39:**1256–1257.

Emerging Infections 7
Edited by W. M. Scheld, D. C. Hooper, and J. M. Hughes
© 2007 ASM Press, Washington, D.C.

Chapter 14

Zygomycosis

Corina E. Gonzalez, Charalampos Antachopoulos, Shmuel Shoham, and Thomas J. Walsh

The term zygomycosis refers to a group of uncommon but frequently fatal mycoses caused by the filamentous fungi of the class Zygomycetes. Over the last decades, an increase in the reporting of zygomycosis among immunocompromised patients and other susceptible hosts has been observed (342). The class Zygomycetes is subdivided into two orders, the Mucorales and the Entomophthorales. Organisms of the order Mucorales cause the majority of human disease, characterized by a rapidly evolving course, tissue necrosis, and angioinvasion. Infections caused by the Entomophthorales have been mainly reported in tropical and subtropical areas, usually affecting immunocompetent hosts; they are characterized by an indolent course involving the subcutaneous, nasal, and sinus tissues (207, 208, 219, 337, 338, 381). Lately, however, reports of infections caused by Entomophthorales have involved a wider geographic distribution, spectrum of clinical manifestations, and range of affected hosts, including cases of fulminant presentation in immunocompromised hosts resembling infections caused by the Mucorales (51, 68, 100, 132, 176, 199, 285, 355, 404, 410). The taxonomic classification of the Zygomycetes is presented in Table 1. The results of phylogenetic analysis of nuclear small-subunit ribosomal-DNA sequences recently supported the suggestion that the order Entomophthorales should be divided into two phylogenetically distinct groups: the genus *Basidiobolus* should be classified in a new order, the Basidiobolales, while *Conidiobolus* appears to be closely related to the Mucorales and should form a distinct group (180, 181).

EPIDEMIOLOGY

The Zygomycetes grow rapidly, using virtually any carbohydrate substrate. Many of these organisms exhibit thermotolerance and are able to grow at temperatures above 37°C. They are commonly found in soil; in decaying organic matter, including plants and fruits; and in a variety of food items, including bread and seeds (207, 334, 335, 338).

Corina E. Gonzalez • Department of Pediatrics, Division of Pediatric Hematology-Oncology, Georgetown University Hospital, Washington, DC 20007. *Charalampos Antachopoulos and Thomas J. Walsh* • Pediatric Oncology Branch, National Cancer Institute, National Institutes of Health, Bethesda, MD 20892. *Shmuel Shoham* • Division of Infectious Diseases, Washington Hospital Center, Washington, DC 20010.

Table 1. Classification of organisms of the class Zygomycetes

Order	Family	Genus	Pathogenic species for humans
Mucorales	Mucoraceae	*Absidia*	*A. corymbifera*
		Apophysomyces	*A. elegans*
		Mucor	*M. circinelloides, M. ramosissimus, M. racemosus, M. hiemalis, M. rouxianus*
		Rhizomucor	*R. pusillus*
		Rhizopus	*R. oryzae (R. arrhizus), R. microsporus* var. *rhizopodiformis*
	Cunninghamellaceae	*Cunninghamella*	*C. bertholletiae*
	Mortierellaceae	*Mortierella*	—[a]
	Saksenaceae	*Saksenaea*	*S. vasiformis*
	Syncephalastraceae	*Syncephalastrum*	*S. racemosum*
	Thamnidaceae	*Cokeromyces*	*C. recurvatus*
Entomophthorales	Ancylistaceae	*Conidiobolus*	*C. coronatus, C. incongruus*
	Basidiobolaceae	*Basidiobolus*	*B. ranarum*

[a]None of the *Mortierella* species have been associated with human disease.

Zygomycosis is a rare mycosis, occurring approximately 10- to 50-fold less commonly than invasive *Candida* or *Aspergillus* infections. An incidence of 1.7 cases per million per year has been calculated for the United States (330). In a recent review of 929 reported cases of zygomycosis, the male-to-female ratio was approximately 2:1, suggesting a male predisposition (342). Unlike other filamentous fungi, which target mainly immunocompromised patients, the Zygomycetes cause disease in a wider and more heterogeneous population.

Among the underlying conditions favoring the development of invasive infection caused by the Mucorales, the most common is diabetes, both type I and type II (Table 2). A significant proportion of these patients have documented ketoacidosis; occasionally zygomycosis may present as the diabetes-defining illness. Other predisposing conditions include the presence of hematological malignancy and bone marrow or solid-organ transplantation. In these immunocompromised patient populations, risk factors associated with the development of zygomycosis have been reported to include prolonged neutropenia, corticosteroid use, and graft-versus-host disease. Prior deferoxamine therapy and injecting drug use also have been implicated in a significant number of zygomycosis cases (18, 19, 27, 89, 119, 123, 128, 154, 204, 206, 232, 250, 259, 276, 288, 297, 298, 332, 342, 360, 370, 409, 412). As mentioned above, the Entomophthorales commonly affect healthy hosts; invasive infections in immunocompromised hosts have been reported, however (207, 380, 410). Conversely, disease caused by agents of the order Mucorales has been reported in immunocompetent individuals with no identifiable risk factors (31, 58, 187, 209, 217, 329, 342, 371), as well as in employees of both the malt and lumber industries (289, 424).

Invasive infections caused by the Zygomycetes are not limited to hematology-oncology or diabetic patients (23, 64, 81, 87, 124, 131, 223, 297) but also occur in high-risk nurseries (14, 74, 191, 201, 264, 332, 419) and general surgery (57, 251, 298, 392), cardiac surgery (62, 195, 379), burn (278, 327), and trauma (143, 165, 198, 255, 291, 353) wards, underscoring the wide range of hosts susceptible to these organisms. The major mode of

Table 2. Common predisposing conditions with corresponding pathogenetic mechanisms
and clinical presentations for zygomycosis[a]

Predisposing condition	Pathogenetic mechanism	Most common presentation, by site
Diabetes (with/without ketoacidosis)	Dysfunction of neutrophils and monocytes/macrophages Increased availability of unbound serum iron	Sinus
Malignancy	Neutropenia, neutrophil dysfunction	Pulmonary
Solid-organ transplantation	Neutropenia, neutrophil dysfunction	Pulmonary
Bone marrow transplantation	Neutropenia, neutrophil dysfunction	Pulmonary
Deferoxamine therapy	Increased uptake of iron by the fungus	Pulmonary, sinus, disseminated
Injecting drug use	Direct inoculation of organisms	Cerebral
Trauma	Inoculation of organisms through skin breakdown	Cutaneous

[a]Based on a review of 929 reported cases of zygomycosis by Roden et al. (342).

acquisition of infection by the Zygomycetes is through inhalation of sporangiospores from environmental sources. The sporangiospores are presumably deposited in the nasal turbinates and may be inhaled into the pulmonary alveoli. Sporangiospore inhalation provides the exposure for the allergic interstitial pneumonitis or alveolitis syndrome seen in occupational disease (24, 138, 289, 424) and for the sinus and pulmonary forms seen in diabetic and immunocompromised patients (87, 107, 204, 217, 232, 257, 259). Percutaneous routes of exposure are also common in the development of zygomycosis. Traumatic implantation of sporangiospores has been reported in a number of patients (6, 53, 60, 67, 84, 143, 165, 170, 234, 240, 255, 270, 291, 305, 306, 317, 342, 353). Needle entry points (122, 155, 162, 177, 253, 349, 367, 390, 398, 430), catheter exit sites (119, 193, 194, 221, 288), and tattooing (301) have all been implicated in cases of cutaneous infection. The development of zygomycosis in areas of skin breakdown, most commonly surgical sites (298, 392) and burn wounds (48, 72, 278, 327, 384), has also been associated with the use of adhesive products and elastic bandages (38, 40, 90, 95, 128, 193, 251, 360). In addition, direct contact with contaminated tongue depressors, used for oropharyngeal examinations or as arm boards, has been associated with oropharyngeal disease in hematology-oncology patients and cutaneous zygomycosis in neonates, respectively (158, 218, 262, 397). The ingestion of contaminated milk, vegetables, or bread has been implicated in the development of gastrointestinal zygomycosis (214, 280). Sporangiospore-contaminated herbal remedies also have been linked to gastrointestinal and hepatic disease (292).

The percentage of patients with hematological malignancy or solid-organ or hematopoietic stem cell transplantation (HSCT) among all reported cases of zygomycosis has significantly increased since the 1980s (342). This has coincided with an increase in the incidence of zygomycosis in many large cancer centers during the same period (190, 204, 238, 297). The reason for this trend is not entirely clear. Potential explanations include an increase in the posttransplantation survival rate, changes in transplantation procedures, and more aggressive immunosuppressive regimens, particularly high-dose steroids (190, 204, 238). Since 2002, another phenomenon seems to have begun accounting for an even higher increase in the incidence of zygomycosis in HSCT recipients. There is now accumulating evidence that receipt of prophylaxis or treatment with voriconazole and the severity of the immunosuppression appear to work in conjunction to favor this phenomenon (171, 203, 242, 294, 365, 400). This increase in zygomycosis stands in contrast to prior reports of breakthrough infections seen when fluconazole or itraconazole was used for antifungal prophylaxis in HSCT recipients. The controlled trials of antifungal prophylaxis with these second-generation azoles were associated with either no cases or only an occasional case of zygomycosis. Typically, breakthrough fungal infections included aspergillosis and invasive candidiasis, mostly due to fluconazole-resistant *Candida* species (141, 190, 235, 366, 426). The inability of fluconazole to prevent aspergillosis, as well as the high morbidity and mortality associated with the infection, have prompted the use of voriconazole for prophylaxis in HSCT recipients, despite the fact that there are no reported controlled clinical trials showing its benefit. Voriconazole likely exerts selective pressure for the growth of resistant fungi, such as zygomycetes. A large, multicenter, blinded clinical trial comparing voriconazole with fluconazole for prophylaxis in HSCT recipients is ongoing and will likely define this issue (190).

PATHOGENESIS

In order to mount an effective host immune response following the inoculation of sporangiospores of Zygomycetes, adequate numbers of functional effector cells, including tissue macrophages and neutrophils, are required. The macrophages prevent the germination of sporangiospores into hyphae by phagocytosis and oxidative killing of the sporangiospores (222, 362). In case germination and progression to hypha formation occur, the presence of neutrophils is required for hyphal damage (94, 362).

Insufficient numbers of effector cells, as in the case of neutropenia secondary to myelosuppressive chemotherapy, or derangement of their phagocytic functions, as in the case of corticosteroid treatment or diabetes mellitus, increases the risk for development of zygomycosis (Table 2). In particular, in hosts with diabetes, the monocytes/macrophages fail to suppress the germination of sporangiospores (402, 403). Diabetic ketoacidosis is associated with impairment of various functions of neutrophils, such as chemotaxis, adherence, and oxidative burst (17, 52, 271, 361). Besides phagocytic dysfunction, an additional mechanism favoring the development of zygomycosis in the ketoacidotic state is increased availability of unbound serum iron (which can then be used by the fungus) in the presence of acidic pH (15, 20). Interestingly, besides diabetic ketoacidosis, there have been reports of zygomycosis in patients with metabolic acidosis secondary to other causes (110, 224).

The importance of iron availability in the pathogenesis of zygomycosis is underscored by the increased incidence of zygomycosis in patients on deferoxamine therapy or with iron overload (34, 236, 342). In contrast to humans, in whom deferoxamine is an iron chelator agent, in vitro studies with *Rhizopus* spp. suggested that for these fungi, deferoxamine acts as a siderophore by facilitating iron uptake (33, 86). Increased iron uptake was shown to correlate with growth of the fungus in serum (33). As opposed to deferoxamine, hydroxypyridinone iron chelators, which do not have siderophore activity for *Rhizopus* spp., did not increase host susceptibility to zygomycosis in animal studies (35).

A key feature of infections caused by the Mucorales in humans is the presence of angioinvasion, resulting in thrombosis and tissue necrosis. Recent in vitro studies have demonstrated the ability of pregerminated sporangiospores of *Rhizopus oryzae* to adhere to and subsequently damage human umbilical-vein endothelial cells. Endothelial-cell damage followed phagocytosis of *R. oryzae* by the endothelial cells and occurred even in the presence of nonviable organisms (169).

CLINICAL MANIFESTATIONS

Clinical manifestations of zygomycosis are varied and may be classified based upon the tissue site affected as sinus disease, localized or extended to the orbit and/or brain; pulmonary; cutaneous; gastrointestinal; miscellaneous; and disseminated infections. Sinus disease is the most common clinical manifestation (342). Interestingly, some of the clinical presentations of zygomycosis may occur with increased frequency in hosts with a particular underlying condition, such as sinus zygomycosis in diabetes patients or pulmonary zygomycosis in neutropenic hosts (342). There are no specific signs or symptoms of the disease; however, suggestive clinical manifestations in the right clinical setting should alert physicians to the possibility of zygomycosis.

Sinus Zygomycosis

Sinus disease is the most common form of zygomycosis (1, 42, 63, 188, 310, 328, 342, 433). It is estimated that about two-thirds of the cases of sinus zygomycosis occur in diabetic patients, often in the presence of diabetic ketoacidosis. It may still occur, however, in immunocompromised patients (87, 168, 175, 266, 281, 342, 356). The infection originates in the paranasal sinuses following inspiration of sporangiospores, and it may be confined to the paranasal sinuses or infiltrate the orbit (sino-orbital) and/or the brain parenchyma (rhinocerebral) (Fig. 1). It usually evolves rapidly, but occasionally progression may be slow, with extension to neighboring tissues (142). The nose, sinus, eye, and brain may be sequentially involved (111). Common symptoms at initial presentation include nasal congestion, dark blood-tinged rhinorrhea or epistaxis, sinus tenderness, retro-orbital headache, fever, and malaise (112, 114, 188, 260, 283). With progression of the disease, facial or periorbital swelling, blurred vision, lacrimation, chemosis, periorbital numbness, diplopia, proptosis, and loss of vision in the affected eye may be observed (30, 49, 129, 166, 281, 303, 416). Often, a painful black necrotic ulceration may develop on the hard palate, indicating extension of the infection from the sinuses into the mouth (188, 283, 303). Nasal endoscopy may reveal necrotic ulcers along the nasal mucosa or turbinates (112). The infectious process may expand to adjacent bone tissue and ultimately to the skull base (61, 303). Progression of the infection into the central nervous system may occur via the optic nerve or the venous drainage of ethmoid sinuses via the cavernous sinus. Alteration of mental status often heralds cerebral involvement (10, 73, 137, 139, 146, 293, 303, 359, 372, 399). Loss of vision, ophthalmoplegia, corneal anesthesia, and facial anhidrosis may signify cavernous-sinus thrombosis (368, 394, 399). Another complication could be thrombosis of the internal carotid artery, resulting in contralateral hemiplegia (9, 126, 231, 359). Consequently, signs and symptoms suggestive of sinus disease, acute onset of blurred vision, or diplopia in a diabetic or immunocompromised patient should prompt careful examination for early recognition of zygomycosis. Imaging studies are needed to determine the extent of disease in adjacent tissues. Plain films of the sinus may be helpful

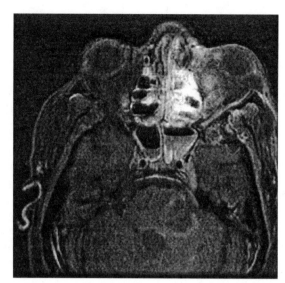

Figure 1. Rhinocerebral zygomycosis, demonstrating left ethmoidal infection, disruption of the lamina papyracea, invasion of the orbital compartment, proptosis of the globe of the eye, sphenoidal sinusitis, cavernous sinus involvement, and a cerebellar pontine infarct.

for initial study, but computerized tomography (CT) or magnetic resonance imaging provides more information with respect to the extent of infection and better guidance for surgical debridement. Opacification of the paranasal sinuses, fluid levels, bone destruction, and osteomyelitis are the main radiographic findings associated with sinus zygomycosis (91, 148, 215, 318, 320, 388).

Pulmonary Zygomycosis

Pulmonary disease commonly occurs in severely immunocompromised patients, including those with hematologic malignancies or bone marrow transplant recipients. In these patients, prolonged neutropenia, corticosteroid use, and graft-versus-host disease have been implicated in the development of zygomycosis (27, 37, 124, 145, 196, 204, 217, 252, 297, 341, 342, 396, 409). Less commonly, pulmonary disease develops in patients with diabetes, renal transplantation, or human immunodeficiency virus infection (47, 88, 197, 213, 256, 299, 304). It also may occur with concomitant sinus disease (sinopulmonary infection) or as part of a disseminated infection (204, 341). Pulmonary involvement may include solitary nodular (125, 245), segmental, or lobar consolidation or cavitary and bronchopneumonic lesions (43, 217, 257, 379, 411) (Fig. 2). The clinical presentation may in fact resemble pulmonary aspergillosis in immunocompromised hosts, with persistent fever and pulmonary infiltrates refractory to broad-spectrum antimicrobial agents (27, 208, 248). Rapid progression is the rule; rarely, chronic or spontaneously resolving lesions have been reported (125, 161, 256). Fungal invasion of the pulmonary vessels may result in thrombosis and subsequent infarcts in the lung parenchyma. Direct extension of the infection across planes to involve the chest wall, pericardium, myocardium, superior vena cava, and diaphragm has been described (68, 71, 147, 159, 331). Erosion and invasion of the pulmonary artery or aorta by the Zygomycetes may lead to fatal hemoptysis (98, 157, 200, 229, 274, 296, 414). A predilection for the upper lobes has

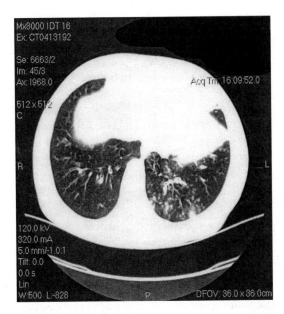

Figure 2. Pulmonary zygomycosis. The CT image demonstrates early pulmonary zygomycosis involving the left lower lobe, with multiple small nodular infiltrates, including a larger peripheral subpleural nodule surrounded by a delicate alveolar infiltrate.

been reported; however, any part of the lung may be involved, and bilateral disease is not uncommon (217). Invasion of the glottis or trachea and endobronchial disease associated with airway obstruction also may occur (11, 70, 101, 116, 357). Radiographic findings may be consistent with infiltrate, cavity, or consolidation. High-resolution CT is more sensitive than chest radiographs for early diagnosis of the infection and determination of the extent of pulmonary involvement. The air crescent and halo signs, which are recognized radiologic features of invasive aspergillosis, may also be observed in pulmonary zygomycosis (43, 178, 217, 249, 411).

Cutaneous Zygomycosis

Cutaneous infection may be confined to the cutaneous and subcutaneous tissue or extend into the adjacent fat, muscle, tendon, or bone structures. It may originate from primary inoculation or occur in the context of disseminated disease (22, 40, 50, 156, 177, 205, 258, 278, 298, 309, 340, 353, 384, 395, 428). Infection associated with primary cutaneous inoculation usually presents with acute inflammation, tissue swelling, induration, and necrosis (48, 50, 53, 60, 66, 67, 72, 93, 95, 128, 165, 183, 186, 194, 198, 221, 230, 251, 291, 298, 305, 319, 322, 327, 353, 360, 384, 392, 417, 418). The lesions initially appear red and indurated but often progress to necrotic eschars (4, 14, 56, 156, 160, 163, 432). Necrotic tissue may slough off and produce large ulcers (225, 298, 349, 419, 420, 423). Primary cutaneous disease may be very invasive locally, involving fat, muscle, and the fascial layers beneath (14, 59, 121, 179, 192, 225, 287, 291, 317, 385). It may be associated with necrotizing fasciitis (210, 244, 282). Direct extension to the adjacent bone has also been described (99, 253, 270, 315). When cutaneous disease is the result of disseminated infection, the lesions tend to be nodular with minimal destruction of the epidermis and may ulcerate (205, 258, 309, 395, 428). Biopsy of the lesions, with histopathological examination and fungal cultures, helps to establish the diagnosis.

Gastrointestinal Zygomycosis

Gastrointestinal disease is rare and usually occurs after ingestion of sporangiospores. The stomach, ileum, and large bowel are the most common sites involved; however, any part of the gastrointestinal tract may be affected. Most cases reported involve malnourished patients and premature neonates (8, 55, 57, 74, 79, 83, 103, 164, 184, 191, 214, 241, 264, 265, 312, 332, 364, 387, 425). Fungal invasion of the mucosa, submucosa, and vessels occurs, occasionally resulting in rupture of the intestinal wall and associated peritonitis (273, 375, 412). Clinical manifestations are nonspecific and include abdominal pain, distension, nausea, vomiting, diarrhea, fever, hematemesis, and hematochezia. The mortality rate is high; most of the reported cases were diagnosed postmortem.

Miscellaneous Zygomycoses

Miscellaneous zygomycoses may include different presentations, such as endocarditis and isolated cerebral, renal, or peritoneal infection. Endocarditis is rare and occurs particularly with prosthetic-valve placement or other cardiac surgery (16, 62, 108, 174, 195, 336, 350, 401, 408). The infection may extend to involve the myocardial wall and pericardium (279, 401). Formation of large vegetations on the valves may lead to embolic complications affecting major arteries. Endocarditis also has been reported in immunosuppressed patients, intravenous-heroin users, and patients treated with deferoxamine (176, 279, 401). Isolated cerebral zygomycosis commonly occurs in injecting drug users with and without human immunodeficiency virus infection (75, 122, 146, 154, 155, 162, 172, 314, 342, 430, 435) and less frequently in patients with open head trauma (84, 170, 234). Infection of the kidney is very rare and is usually observed in the presence of serious underlying pathology (65, 82, 120, 150, 153, 212, 233, 263, 313, 324, 352, 390, 398, 415, 422). In patients on peritoneal dialysis, isolated peritonitis caused by the Zygomycetes has rarely been reported (45, 113, 277).

Disseminated Zygomycosis

Disseminated infection refers to involvement of at least two noncontiguous sites. It commonly occurs in patients undergoing deferoxamine therapy but may also develop in severely immunocompromised patients. It is associated with poor outcome (25, 32, 34, 80, 117, 154, 172, 173, 202, 204, 228, 302, 323, 342, 351, 429). Hematogenous dissemination may originate from any of the primary sites of infection (74, 264, 276, 317, 350, 395, 401, 428, 432). Among the different sites, however, primary pulmonary infection is more frequently associated with disseminated zygomycosis (5, 29, 80, 104, 117, 140, 152, 173, 202, 204, 237, 275, 286, 302, 346, 351, 354, 358, 376, 429). In cases of disseminated infection, biopsy of skin nodules is relatively easy to perform and helps to establish the diagnosis.

DIAGNOSIS

The presenting signs, symptoms, and radiographic findings of zygomycosis are nonspecific and should be interpreted with respect to the underlying condition of the patient. Confirmation of the diagnosis requires direct morphologic identification of mycotic elements and/or recovery of Zygomycetes in culture from biopsy specimens obtained on the site of presumed involvement. Examination of wet mounts of sputum, paranasal sinus secretions, or bronchoalveolar-lavage fluid is frequently negative (386). However, the recovery of Zygomycetes from these specimens in the presence of predisposing conditions, such as severe immunosuppression, diabetes, or deferoxamine treatment, should not be disregarded as contamination but should rather be considered as strong evidence for development of zygomycosis in these patients (7, 27, 92, 135, 297, 421). Despite the fact that Zygomycetes are angioinvasive molds, blood cultures or urine cultures are rarely positive (140). Although histopathology is sensitive and reliable for establishing the diagnosis of zygomycosis, obtaining biopsy material from hematological patients may not always be feasible due to concomitant thrombocytopenia. Depending on the presentation of the disease, samples for histopathologic examination may be collected by radiographically guided fine-needle aspirates or core biopsies of approachable lesions in deep tissues, transbronchial biopsies of pulmonary lesions, samples from sinus tissue biopsies, or debridements, scrapings of necrotic mucocutaneous lesions, and open biopsies of deep-tissue lesions.

Direct Examination and Histopathology

Direct microscopic examination is usually done on all materials sent to the clinical laboratory. Where possible, tissue should also be submitted for histopathological examination. Infected specimens may exhibit the typical broad (6 to 16 μm in diameter), ribbon-like, irregular, nonseptate (coenocytic) or sparsely septated hyphae of the Zygomycetes, with branches often arising at perpendicular angles (207, 335, 338, 377) (Fig. 3). The morphology of zygomycetes is usually distinguishable in tissue from those of other filamentous fungi, such as *Aspergillus* spp., *Fusarium* spp., or *Pseudallescheria boydii*, or yeasts, such as *Candida* spp., that may cause similar clinical manifestations and/or angioinvasive

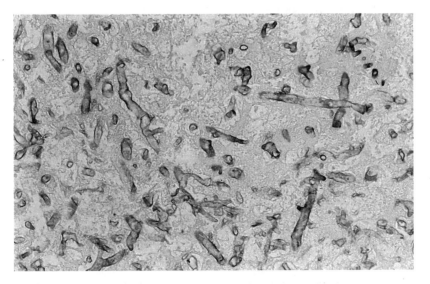

Figure 3. Histological characteristics of invasive zygomycosis. The isolate of *Rhizopus* in this excisional biopsy specimen of the kidney demonstrates broad, ribbon-like, sparsely septated hyphae with nondichotomous "right-angled" branching.

disease in the immunosuppressed host (334). The features differentiating the Zygomycetes from these other fungi are detailed in Table 3.

Microbiological Diagnosis

Identification of Zygomycetes to the species level is performed in culture and should be attempted whenever possible (338). Specimens are inoculated onto appropriate media, such as Sabouraud dextrose agar, and incubated at room temperature. Special care should be taken in preparing the specimen for plating in the culture medium. Specimen grinding or homogenization may result in the destruction of the delicate hyphae of the Zygomycetes, with consequent negative cultures (207, 335, 338, 377). The recovery rate of Zygomycetes in culture is enhanced if the tissue is sliced into small pieces. This is an important consideration for clinicians and infectious-disease specialists who need to alert the microbiologist to their clinical suspicion for proper handling of the specimen.

Zygomycetes typically grow rapidly within 24 to 48 h unless they are suppressed by residual antifungal agents, such as amphotericin B, in tissue. As with most medically important filamentous fungi, colony morphology serves as an adjunct to identification between Entomophthorales and Mucorales. Most mucoraceous species easily fill a petri dish within 3 to 5 days and demonstrate a grayish-white aerial mycelium with a woolly texture. The colonies are easy to separate from the agar surface. By contrast, the Entomophthorales grow in 3 to 5 days as flat, waxy-appearing colonies that often may develop radial groves and that are gray to pale-yellow in color. They are difficult to remove from the agar surface (334, 338).

To provide an accurate genus and species designation, Zygomycetes must be identified microscopically. Characteristic and distinctive fruiting structures serve to distinguish among genera and species within the genera (Fig. 4).

There are currently no identification kits, nucleic acid probes, or commercially available immunological or serological means to identify Zygomycetes, so the eye and a good reference text are necessary for proper identification.

Table 3. Differentiating morphological and histopathological features of the Zygomycetes compared to other filamentous fungi in tissue sections

Feature	Zygomycetes	*Aspergillus* spp. and other filamentous fungi[a]
Fungal elements	Hyphae	Hyphae
Hyphal characteristics		
Width	Broad (6–16 μm)	Narrow (4–5 μm)
Septations	Aseptate or sparsely septated	Distinctive septa
Walls	Irregular walls	Parallel walls
Branching	Frequently "right angled"	Frequently dichotomous and acute
Sporulation	Generally absent[b,c]	Absent[b]
Angioinvasion	Present	Present

[a]Including *Fusarium* spp. and *Scedosporium* spp.
[b]Sporulation may be present if the infected space communicates with air.
[c]Formation of chlamydoconidia in tissue has been rarely reported in zygomycosis (197).

TREATMENT AND PREVENTION

Despite the recent advances in antifungal therapy, zygomycosis continues to be one of the most fulminant mycoses in humans. Current therapy against zygomycosis involves a combined approach. This approach (Fig. 5) relies on prompt institution of therapy, reversal of the patient's underlying predisposing condition, administration of appropriate antifungal agents, and extensive surgical debridement of all devitalized tissue. The overall survival rate in zygomycosis approximates 70% for cases treated with antifungal therapy and surgery (342). However, we need to keep in mind that this figure represents a composite of the proportions of different predisposing conditions, sites, extents of infection, and treatments provided and is influenced by the tendency to report successful outcomes. Despite high overall mortality, an improvement in the survival rates in certain types of zygomycosis has been demonstrated in retrospective studies (30, 217, 386, 433).

Reversal of the Underlying Predisposing Condition

Correction of the patient's underlying condition that predisposes to zygomycosis is one of the cornerstones of successful management of this devastating infection. When this predisposing condition is a metabolic disturbance, such as hyperglycemia and metabolic acidosis due to diabetic ketoacidosis or other causes, rapid correction is usually feasible and should be pursued. The rationale for correction of the metabolic disarrangement is supported by in vivo studies and clinical observations. In experimental models of alloxan-induced diabetes in rabbits, susceptibility to Zygomycetes was highest in the presence of acidic pH (105, 333, 373). In the clinical setting, regulation of diabetes alone resulted in the resolution of zygomycosis of the ethmoid sinus and orbit in one reported case (19), while in a number of well-controlled diabetic patients, sinus zygomycosis remained a localized process and responded readily to treatment (257). Moreover, in a review of 145 cases of sinus zygomycosis in a heterogeneous population of patients with diabetes mellitus, renal failure, hematologic malignancies, or autoimmune diseases as predisposing conditions, the survival rate was highest among those with diabetes. The increased survival in these patients was attributed to the quick reversal of underlying hyperglycemia and/or ketoacidosis (433).

In immunocompromised patients with zygomycosis, rapid restoration of the host immune response is important in order to optimize the outcome. A therapeutic dilemma may arise in transplant recipients or patients with hematological malignancies who develop zygomycosis as to whether the immunosuppressive regimen for treatment of their underlying condition should be discontinued in order to be able to control the fungal infection. In view of the poor prognosis of zygomycosis in these patients, a reduction or temporary discontinuation of corticosteroids or other immunosuppressive agents should probably be considered until control of the infection is achieved. In patients with chemotherapy-induced neutropenia who developed zygomycosis, neutrophil recovery was associated with response to treatment and resolution of infection (140, 220, 297, 347). On the other hand, persistence of neutropenia may compromise the efficacy of antifungal therapy. In a review of 26 neutropenic ($\leq$500 cells/mm^3) patients with histologically documented disseminated zygomycosis that included reports from 1959 through 1994, the outcome for the patients was uniformly fatal, due to the rapid progression of the infection (140).

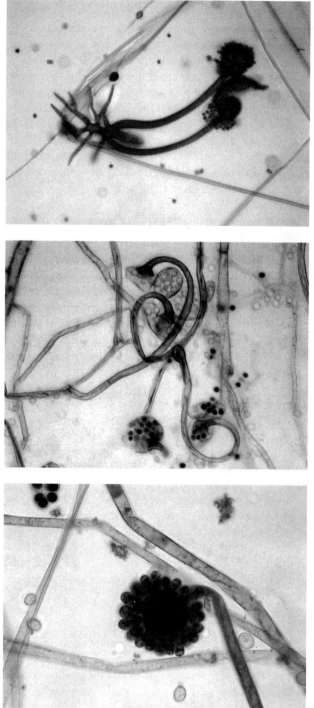

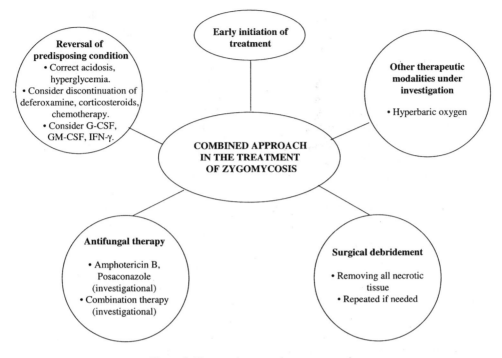

Figure 5. Therapeutic approach to zygomycosis.

Even with discontinuation of chemotherapy or corticosteroid treatment in patients with zygomycosis, spontaneous restoration of phagocytic activity or recovery from neutropenia is likely to occur after several days, during which time the infection may progress. Immune recovery, however, may be accelerated with the use of cytokines, such as granulocyte colony-stimulating factor (G-CSF), granulocyte-macrophage colony-stimulating factor (GM-CSF), and gamma interferon (IFN-γ). G-CSF and GM-CSF stimulate the production of neutrophils and/or monocytes and enhance the activities of these cells against fungal hyphae and conidia (226, 247, 343, 344, 369). IFN-γ also enhances the antifungal activity of host effector cells but in addition has an important regulatory role in the development of the protective Th1 response against fungal pathogens (345). Ex vivo incubation with G-CSF enhanced the impaired respiratory burst of neutrophils derived from transplant recipients

Figure 4. Photomicrographs of three medically important genera of Zygomycetes: *Rhizopus* (top), *Mucor* (middle), and *Cunninghamella* (bottom). (Top) The rhizoids, or root-like structures, of the genus *Rhizopus* arise from the base of the connection between the sporangiophores and stolon. The sporangia in this photomicrograph have opened to release their contents of sporangiospores (original magnification, ×200). (Middle) The genus *Mucor* is characterized by the absence of rhizoids at the junction between the sporangiophores and stolon. The curved sporangiophores in this photomicrograph are typical of *Mucor circinelloides* (original magnification, ×400). (Bottom) The sporangium of *Cunninghamella* is distinct in having sporangioles on the surface of the sporangium (original magnification, ×630). Sporangioles of *Cunninghamella* spp. are connected to the sporangium by short processes known as ostioles.

against *Rhizopus* conidia (325), while administration of GM-CSF and IFN-γ enhanced in vitro the activities of neutrophils against *R. oryzae* and other species of Zygomycetes (133).

The administration of G-CSF and GM-CSF to patients receiving myelosuppressive chemotherapy has reduced the degree and duration of neutropenia and diminished the frequency of infections (12, 13, 44, 267, 300, 434). In addition to these studies, several individual reports describing the use of G-CSF, GM-CSF, and/or IFN-γ as adjuvant therapy for zygomycosis have been published (2, 130, 140, 220, 291, 297, 347). Nevertheless, the efficacy and potential complications of cytokine use as adjunctive treatment for zygomycosis have not been evaluated through adequately powered randomized controlled trials (12, 300). In the absence of such studies, the use of cytokines for immunocompromised hosts with zygomycosis may be considered on an individual-patient basis.

Granulocyte transfusion is another approach for the acceleration of neutrophil recovery in neutropenic patients suffering from invasive fungal infections. The efficacy of this strategy in early studies, however, was compromised by limitations in collecting adequate doses of leukocytes from healthy steroid-mobilized donors. The use of G-CSF has markedly enhanced the yield of leukocytes from healthy donors, thus renewing interest in granulocyte transfusions (46). However, evidence of the efficacy of this intervention in patients with zygomycosis is limited (25, 27, 28, 90, 308, 354, 431), and potential complications have been reported with the treatment (431).

Whenever zygomycosis is diagnosed in patients receiving deferoxamine, it is recommended that the therapy be withheld, if possible, in order to discontinue its stimulating effect on fungal growth. In order to decrease the risk of developing zygomycosis in patients who require such therapy, lower doses of deferoxamine or its replacement by hydroxypyridinone chelators may be considered (34, 36, 316).

Antifungal Therapy

Amphotericin B is the drug of choice for treatment of zygomycosis. Its efficacy against the Zygomycetes has been demonstrated in both laboratory and clinical studies (106, 109, 290, 295, 311, 342, 393, 413). In a recent review of 929 reported cases of zygomycosis, survival was 61% for 532 patients treated with amphotericin B deoxycholate versus 69% for 116 patients treated with lipid formulations of amphotericin B ($P > 0.05$ between the deoxycholate and lipid formulations) versus 3% for 241 individuals who received no treatment. In a multivariate analysis of risk factors for mortality among cases, all forms of antifungal treatment and surgery were significantly associated with reduced risk of mortality (342). Apparent in vitro resistance, however, with elevated MICs of amphotericin B may still be observed among clinical isolates, especially among *Cunninghamella* species (76, 78, 261, 363, 382).

All lipid formulations of amphotericin B, including colloidal dispersion, lipid complex (ABLC), and liposomal, have been used in the treatment of zygomycosis; the most experience has been reported with the liposomal formulation and ABLC (41, 57, 95, 118, 130, 131, 136, 140, 167, 191, 216, 220, 223, 227, 246, 248, 253, 268, 272, 281, 291, 308, 347, 348, 376, 378, 391, 407, 415). The lipid formulations of amphotericin B appear to be at least as active as conventional amphotericin B for the treatment of invasive mycoses. In addition, they have been associated with less infusion-related toxicity and nephrotoxicity (41, 136, 227, 342, 405, 407, 419, 427). However, the efficacy of lipid formulations versus deoxycholate amphotericin B for the treatment of zygomycosis has not been evaluated in prospective randomized controlled studies.

For this rapidly evolving infection, the full dose of amphotericin B can be given from the beginning of treatment, and there is no need for dose escalation. No studies have been published to date investigating the optimal dosage of amphotericin B formulations for the treatment of zygomycosis. The use of ABLC at 5 mg/kg of body weight/day as salvage treatment in 24 cases of zygomycosis was associated with complete or partial response in 17 (71%) patients (407). In a maximum-tolerated-dose study of the safety, tolerance, and pharmacokinetics of liposomal amphotericin B in patients with invasive mycoses, no dose-limiting nephrotoxicity or infusion-related toxicity was demonstrated over a dose range of 7.5 to 15 mg/kg/day (406). The plasma concentrations of liposomal amphotericin B achieved their peak at 10 mg/kg/day and were not increased when higher dosages of 12.5 or 15 mg/kg/day were administered. Although the use of liposomal amphotericin B at 10 mg/kg/day for the treatment of zygomycosis has been reported (21), the efficacy of higher dosages of this lipid formulation in the treatment of zygomycosis, compared to the Food and Drug Administration-approved dosage of 3 to 5 mg/kg/day for aspergillosis, has not been systematically evaluated through randomized controlled studies. In the absence of such trials, for patients with zygomycosis who do not respond to liposomal amphotericin B at 5 mg/kg/day, an increase in dosage of liposomal amphotericin B to 7.5 or 10 mg/kg/day could be considered on an individual basis. Treatment with amphotericin B should be continued for as long as needed in order to control the infection and facilitate surgical debridement. Although the optimal duration has not been clearly defined, it seems prudent to continue therapy until complete resolution of signs and symptoms is achieved. Treatment should be individualized according to the patient's response and underlying condition. This is particularly important for the population of severely immunocompromised patients, including those receiving immunosuppressive therapy for an underlying malignancy or a transplant. In these patients, even after the infection has been brought under control, a chronic suppressive course with amphotericin B, such as alternate-day or three-times-a-week therapy, could be considered for as long as their immune responses are severely impaired.

In a number of cases of zygomycosis, amphotericin B has been administered by local irrigation in the paranasal sinuses, orbit, and lung (intracavitary/interstitial), as well as in the cerebrospinal fluid. Clinical evidence in support of this approach, however, is limited (3, 69, 130, 188, 239, 260, 291, 307, 368).

Of the azole agents, fluconazole and voriconazole have little or no activity against the Zygomycetes (39, 78, 96, 382). Itraconazole and the newer triazole ravuconazole have demonstrated variable in vitro activities against some of these filamentous fungi (78, 96, 261, 363, 382). In animal models of zygomycosis, itraconazole was not efficacious against *Rhizopus* or *Mucor* infection but demonstrated some activity in the treatment of *Absidia corymbifera* infection (77, 269, 383). There are few case reports of successful outcomes with the use of itraconazole for the treatment of *Basidiobolus*, *Rhizopus*, and cutaneous *Cunninghamella* infections (102, 243, 326). Another second-generation triazole, posaconazole, has been shown to exhibit promising activity against the Zygomycetes, both in vitro and in animal models (39, 77, 78, 96, 382, 383). Posaconazole has already been used in a number of case reports as salvage therapy for patients with zygomycosis refractory to or intolerant of amphotericin B treatment (97, 127, 134, 149, 389). The pharmacokinetics and pharmacodynamics of posaconazole in the treatment of zygomycosis, either as monotherapy or in combination with amphotericin B, however, needs to be evaluated further in laboratory animal studies and in carefully designed prospective randomized clinical trials versus deoxycholate amphotericin B or a lipid formulation of amphotericin B.

Given the rapid progression and high mortality of zygomycosis in susceptible hosts, administration of combination antifungal therapy has also been considered in an effort to improve outcomes. Although the echinocandin agents have no in vitro activity against the Zygomycetes (39, 295, 311), the combination of caspofungin plus amphotericin B lipid complex demonstrated synergy in a murine model of disseminated zygomycosis (374). However, neither this nor any other combination has been prospectively evaluated in clinical studies for the treatment of zygomycosis. The addition of other agents, such as flucytosine, rifampin, or even tetracycline, to amphotericin B in an attempt to obtain enhanced antifungal activity is controversial and is not recommended (10, 281, 284, 304, 328, 384).

Hyperbaric Oxygen

Hyperbaric oxygen is another therapeutic modality that has been used as adjunctive therapy in the treatment of zygomycosis. In a number of case reports, a favorable outcome was achieved with the use of hyperbaric oxygen in sinus and cutaneous/soft tissue zygomycosis in conjunction with surgery and amphotericin B (10, 26, 73, 85, 115, 130, 131, 182, 254, 291, 307, 321, 353, 359, 399). It is known that a lengthy exposure to high pressures (10 atmospheres absolute) of 100% oxygen is fungicidal for zygomycetes and other fungi in vitro (54, 189, 339). Shorter exposures and lower pressures at 100% oxygen also showed inhibition of growth, to the point that a fungistatic effect over *Rhizopus* spp. could be exerted with clinically relevant doses of hyperbaric oxygen. The selection of the therapeutic oxygen pressure involves a compromise between efficacy and toxicity. Potential side effects associated with hyperbaric oxygen include seizures, nausea, tinnitus, tunnel vision, and pneumothorax (144, 185). Most of the reported cases have been treated with 100% oxygen at 2 to 2.5 atmospheres absolute, pressures at which central nervous system oxygen toxicity manifestations are rare. The fungistatic and fungicidal effects of hyperbaric oxygen are thought to be related to the generation of oxygen-based free radicals. In addition, hyperbaric oxygen may be beneficial in reducing the tissue hypoxia and acidosis caused by the vascular invasion typical of zygomycosis and in increasing neutrophil function and fibroblastic collagen production. However, because of the uncontrolled nature of these observations, hyperbaric oxygen therapy cannot be routinely recommended for the treatment of zygomycosis.

Surgical Therapy

Surgical debridement is of critical importance for the successful management of zygomycosis. Eradicating Zygomycetes from the site of the infection with antifungal therapy alone is difficult, because vascular thrombosis secondary to the infection compromises the delivery of antifungal agents. Surgery should aim to remove all necrotic tissue, should be considered early in the course of treatment, and should be repeated if necessary; frozen-section guided debridement is preferable (211). Clinical evidence suggests the beneficial role of surgical debridement in the management of zygomycosis. A number of retrospective studies have demonstrated that the survival of patients treated with a combination of antifungal and surgical therapies was significantly higher than for those treated with antifungal therapy alone (1, 30, 151, 217, 310, 342, 386).

Prevention of Zygomycosis

Currently, there are no therapeutic regimens with proven value for the prevention of zygomycosis. Prevention may be feasible for a proportion of cases through adequate control of diabetes, judicious use of deferoxamine and corticosteroids, and appropriate environmental-control measures.

Rhizopus spp. have caused outbreaks of nosocomial infections associated with construction activity, contaminated elastic bandages, and tongue depressors (38, 40, 90, 95, 128, 158, 193, 206, 218, 251, 262, 360, 397). Construction activity can increase the number of airborne *Rhizopus* organisms in hospital air (87, 107, 223, 409). Control of environmental transmission during construction and renovation by applying floor-to-ceiling barriers, as well as periodic microbiologic monitoring of air conditioning and ventilation systems, should be established. HEPA filters used in hospital rooms for patients with profound immunosuppression have been shown to reduce the risks of aspergillosis and mucormycosis (37). However, due to high costs, many centers do not use HEPA filters in the routine care of these patients. Appropriate wound care and daily inspection of the portions of the skin covered by bandages or boards is also recommended.

CONCLUSIONS

Although rare in comparison with other opportunistic fungal infections, zygomycosis has been reported with increased incidence among immunocompromised patients over the last 2 decades. This increase seems to be explained in part by the introduction and use of novel antifungal agents, such as voriconazole, which are active against *Aspergillus* spp. but not against the Zygomycetes. Apart from pharmacologically immunocompromised patients, Zygomycetes cause disease in a number of susceptible hosts with different predisposing conditions, including surgery, burns, trauma, diabetes mellitus, and treatment with deferoxamine. The underlying mechanisms explaining the occurrence of zygomycosis in these patient populations are numerical or functional deficiencies of host phagocytic cells (neutrophils and monocytes/macrophages), as well as the increased availability of serum iron for the organisms. As zygomycosis may be rapidly fatal, early recognition of its different clinical presentations and prompt treatment with antifungal agents and surgical debridement are important for a favorable outcome.

Future areas of research should include appropriate trials evaluating the clinical efficacy of posaconazole in the treatment of zygomycosis, either as monotherapy or in combination with one of the amphotericin B formulations, and the optimal dosages of antifungal agents for this infection, as well as the efficacies of other adjunctive therapies, including cytokine treatment or hyperbaric oxygen. Also of particular importance will be increased understanding of pathogenesis and host defenses and the development of molecular or other methods with sufficient sensitivity and specificity for early detection of zygomycosis. This would enable the timely initiation of preemptive therapy for patients at risk for this devastating infection.

REFERENCES

1. **Abedi, E., A. Sismanis, K. Choi, and P. Pastore.** 1984. Twenty-five years' experience treating cerebro-rhino-orbital mucormycosis. *Laryngoscope* **94:**1060–1062.
2. **Abzug, M. J., and T. J. Walsh.** 2004. Interferon-gamma and colony-stimulating factors as adjuvant therapy for refractory fungal infections in children. *Pediatr. Infect. Dis. J.* **23:**769–773.
3. **Adler, D. E., T. H. Milhorat, and J. I. Miller.** 1998. Treatment of rhinocerebral mucormycosis with intravenous interstitial, and cerebrospinal fluid administration of amphotericin B: case report. *Neurosurgery* **42:** 644–649.
4. **Adriaenssens, K., P. G. Jorens, L. Meuleman, W. Jeuris, and J. Lambert.** 2000. A black necrotic skin lesion in an immunocompromised patient. Diagnosis: cutaneous mucormycosis. *Arch. Dermatol.* **136:** 1165–1170.
5. **Agh, F., S. Spanik, J. Gyarfas, J. Horvath, and V. Krcmery, Jr.** 1992. Three fatal cases of disseminated mucormycosis associated with respiratory distress syndrome and shock in patients with hematologic malignancies. *Infection* **20:**112.
6. **Ajello, L., D. F. Dean, and R. S. Irwin.** 1976. The zygomycete *Saksenaea vasiformis* as a pathogen of humans with a critical rewiew of the etiology of zygomycosis. *Mycologia* **68:**52–62.
7. **al-Abbadi, M. A., K. Russo, and E. J. Wilkinson.** 1997. Pulmonary mucormycosis diagnosed by bronchoalveolar lavage: a case report and review of the literature. *Pediatr. Pulmonol.* **23:**222–225.
8. **Amin, S. B., R. M. Ryan, L. A. Metlay, and W. J. Watson.** 1998. *Absidia corymbifera* infections in neonates. *Clin. Infect. Dis.* **26:**990–992.
9. **Anaissie, E. J., and A. H. Shikhani.** 1985. Rhinocerebral mucormycosis with internal carotid occlusion: report of two cases and review of the literature. *Laryngoscope* **95:**1107–1113.
10. **Anand, V. K., G. Alemar, and J. A. Griswold, Jr.** 1992. Intracranial complications of mucormycosis: an experimental model and clinical review. *Laryngoscope* **102:**656–662.
11. **Andrews, D. R., A. Allan, and R. I. Larbalestier.** 1997. Tracheal mucormycosis. *Ann. Thorac. Surg.* **63:** 230–232.
12. **Antachopoulos, C., and E. Roilides.** 2005. Cytokines and fungal infections. *Br. J. Haematol.* **129:**583–596.
13. **Antman, K. S., J. D. Griffin, A. Elias, M. A. Socinski, L. Ryan, S. A. Cannistra, D. Oette, M. Whitley, E. Frei III, and L. E. Schnipper.** 1988. Effect of recombinant human granulocyte-macrophage colony-stimulating factor on chemotherapy-induced myelosuppression. *N. Engl. J. Med.* **319:**593–598.
14. **Arisoy, A. E., E. S. Arisoy, A. Correa-Calderon, and S. L. Kaplan.** 1993. Rhizopus necrotizing cellulitis in a preterm infant: a case report and review of the literature. *Pediatr. Infect. Dis. J.* **12:**1029–1031.
15. **Artis, W. M., J. A. Fountain, H. K. Delcher, and H. E. Jones.** 1982. A mechanism of susceptibility to mucormycosis in diabetic ketoacidosis: transferrin and iron availability. *Diabetes* **31:**1109–1114.
16. **Atkinson, J. B., D. H. Connor, M. Robinowitz, H. A. McAllister, and R. Virmani.** 1984. Cardiac fungal infections: review of autopsy findings in 60 patients. *Hum. Pathol.* **15:**935–942.
17. **Bagdade, J. D.** 1976. Phagocytic and microbicidal function in diabetes mellitus. *Acta Endocrinol. Suppl.* **205:**27–34.
18. **Baker, R. D.** 1962. Leukopenia and therapy in leukemia as factors predisposing to fatal mycoses. Mucormycosis, aspergillosis, and cryptococcosis. *Am. J. Clin. Pathol.* **37:**358–373.
19. **Baker, R. D.** 1957. Mucormycosis; a new disease? *JAMA* **163:**805–808.
20. **Baldwin, D. A., D. M. De Sousa, and R. M. Von Wandruszka.** 1982. The effect of pH on the kinetics of iron release from human transferrin. *Biochim. Biophys. Acta* **719:**140–146.
21. **Barron, M. A., M. Lay, and N. E. Madinger.** 2005. Surgery and treatment with high-dose liposomal amphotericin B for eradication of craniofacial zygomycosis in a patient with Hodgkin's disease who had undergone allogeneic hematopoietic stem cell transplantation. *J. Clin. Microbiol.* **43:**2012–2014.
22. **Bearer, E. A., P. R. Nelson, M. Y. Chowers, and C. E. Davis.** 1994. Cutaneous zygomycosis caused by *Saksenaea vasiformis* in a diabetic patient. *J. Clin. Microbiol.* **32:**1823–1824.
23. **Beck-Sague, C., W. R. Jarvis, et al.** 1993. Secular trends in the epidemiology of nosocomial fungal infections in the United States, 1980–1990. *J. Infect. Dis.* **167:**1247–1251.
24. **Belin, L.** 1980. Clinical and immunological data on "wood trimmer's disease" in Sweden. *Eur. J. Respir. Dis. Suppl.* **107:**169–176.
25. **Benbow, E. W., I. W. Delamore, R. W. Stoddart, and H. Reid.** 1985. Disseminated zygomycosis associated with erythroleukaemia: confirmation by lectin stains. *J. Clin. Pathol.* **38:**1039–1044.

26. **Bentur, Y., A. Shupak, Y. Ramon, A. Abramovich, G. Wolfin, H. Stein, and N. Krivoi.** 1998. Hyperbaric oxygen therapy for cutaneous/soft-tissue zygomycosis complicating diabetes mellitus. *Plast. Reconstr. Surg.* **102:**822–824.

27. **Bhaduri, S., E. Kurrle, E. Vanek, and R. Spanel.** 1983. Mucormycosis in the immunocompromised host. *Infection* **11:**170–172.

28. **Bhatia, S., J. McCullough, E. H. Perry, M. Clay, N. K. Ramsay, and J. P. Neglia.** 1994. Granulocyte transfusions: efficacy in treating fungal infections in neutropenic patients following bone marrow transplantation. *Transfusion* **34:**226–232.

29. **Birchall, D., W. K. Leong, and W. McAuliffe.** 1999. Cerebral mucormycosis. *J. Neurol. Neurosurg. Psychiatry* **66:**404–405.

30. **Blitzer, A., W. Lawson, B. R. Meyers, and H. F. Biller.** 1980. Patient survival factors in paranasal sinus mucormycosis. *Laryngoscope* **90:**635–648.

31. **Blodi, F. C., F. T. Hannah, and J. A. Wadsworth.** 1969. Lethal orbito-cerebral phycomycosis in otherwise healthy children. *Am. J. Ophthalmol.* **67:**698–705.

32. **Bloxham, C. A., S. Carr, D. W. Ryan, P. J. Kesteven, R. S. Bexton, I. D. Griffiths, and J. Richards.** 1990. Disseminated zygomycosis and systemic lupus erythematosus. *Intensive Care Med.* **16:**201–207.

33. **Boelaert, J. R., M. de Locht, J. Van Cutsem, V. Kerrels, B. Cantinieaux, A. Verdonck, H. W. Van Landuyt, and Y. J. Schneider.** 1993. Mucormycosis during deferoxamine therapy is a siderophore-mediated infection. In vitro and in vivo animal studies. *J. Clin. Invest.* **91:**1979–1986.

34. **Boelaert, J. R., A. Z. Fenves, and J. W. Coburn.** 1991. Deferoxamine therapy and mucormycosis in dialysis patients: report of an international registry. *Am. J. Kidney Dis.* **18:**660–667.

35. **Boelaert, J. R., J. Van Cutsem, M. de Locht, Y. J. Schneider, and R. R. Crichton.** 1994. Deferoxamine augments growth and pathogenicity of *Rhizopus*, while hydroxypyridinone chelators have no effect. *Kidney Int.* **45:**667–671.

36. **Boelaert, J. R., G. F. van Roost, P. L. Vergauwe, J. J. Verbanck, C. de Vroey, and M. F. Segaert.** 1988. The role of desferrioxamine in dialysis-associated mucormycosis: report of three cases and review of the literature. *Clin. Nephrol.* **29:**261–266.

37. **Bogard, B. N.** 1972. Pulmonary mucormycosis. *N. Engl. J. Med.* **286:**606.

38. **Bottone, E. J., I. Weitzman, and B. A. Hanna.** 1979. *Rhizopus rhizopodiformis*: emerging etiological agent of mucormycosis. *J. Clin. Microbiol.* **9:**530–537.

39. **Boucher, H. W., A. H. Groll, C. C. Chiou, and T. J. Walsh.** 2004. Newer systemic antifungal agents: pharmacokinetics, safety and efficacy. *Drugs* **64:**1997–2020.

40. **Boyce, J. M., L. A. Lawson, W. R. Lockwood, and J. L. Hughes.** 1981. *Cunninghamella bertholletiae* wound infection of probable nosocomial origin. *South. Med. J.* **74:**1132–1135.

41. **Boyle, J. A.** 2000. Controlled trials of amphotericin B lipid complex. *Clin. Infect. Dis.* **31:**1117–1118.

42. **Bradley, R., B. R. Straatsma, and E. Lorenz.** 1962. Phycomycosis: a clinicopathologic study of fifty-one cases. *Lab. Investigo.* **11:**963–985.

43. **Bragg, G. D., and B. Janis.** 1973. The roentgenographic manifestations of pulmonary opportunistic infections. *Am. J. Roentgenol. Radium Ther. Nucl. Med.* **117:**798–809.

44. **Brandt, S. J., W. P. Peters, S. K. Atwater, J. Kurtzberg, M. J. Borowitz, R. B. Jones, E. J. Shpall, R. C. Bast, Jr., C. J. Gilbert, and D. H. Oette.** 1988. Effect of recombinant human granulocyte-macrophage colony-stimulating factor on hematopoietic reconstitution after high-dose chemotherapy and autologous bone marrow transplantation. *N. Engl. J. Med.* **318:**869–876.

45. **Branton, M. H., S. C. Johnson, J. D. Brooke, and J. A. Hasbargen.** 1991. Peritonitis due to *Rhizopus* in a patient undergoing continuous ambulatory peritoneal dialysis. *Rev. Infect. Dis.* **13:**19–21.

46. **Briones, M. A., C. D. Josephson, and C. D. Hillyer.** 2003. Granulocyte transfusion: revisited. *Curr. Hematol. Rep.* **2:**522–527.

47. **Brown, R. B., J. H. Johnson, J. M. Kessinger, and W. C. Sealy.** 1992. Bronchovascular mucormycosis in the diabetic: an urgent surgical problem. *Ann. Thorac. Surg.* **53:**854–855.

48. **Bruck, H. M., G. Nash, D. Foley, and B. A. Pruitt, Jr.** 1971. Opportunistic fungal infection of the burn wound with phycomycetes and *Aspergillus*. A clinical-pathologic review. *Arch. Surg.* **102:**476–482.

49. **Bullock, J. D., L. M. Jampol, and A. J. Fezza.** 1974. Two cases of orbital phycomycosis with recovery. *Am. J. Ophthalmol.* **78:**811–815.

50. **Burkitt, D. P., A. M. Wilson, and D. B. Jelliffe.** 1964. Subcutaneous phycomycosis: a review of 31 cases seen in Uganda. *Br. Med. J.* **i:**1669–1672.

51. **Busapakum, R., U. Youngchaiyud, S. Sriumpai, G. Segretain, and H. Fromentin.** 1983. Disseminated infection with *Conidiobolus incongruus. Sabouraudia* **21:**323–330.

52. **Bybee, J. D., and D. E. Rogers.** 1964. The phagocytic activity of polymorphonuclear leukocytes obtained from patients with diabetes mellitus. *J. Lab. Clin. Med.* **64:**1–13.

53. **Caceres, A. M., C. Sardinas, C. Marcano, R. Guevara, J. Barros, G. Bianchi, V. Rosario, R. Balza, M. Silva, M. C. Redondo, and M. Nunez.** 1997. *Apophysomyces elegans* limb infection with a favorable outcome: case report and review. *Clin. Infect. Dis.* **25:**331–332.

54. **Caldwell, J.** 1963. Effects of high partial pressures of oxygen on fungi. *Nature* **197:**772–774.

55. **Calle, S., and S. Klatsky.** 1966. Intestinal phycomycosis (mucormycosis). *Am. J. Clin. Pathol.* **45:**264–272.

56. **Carpenter, C. F., and A. K. Subramanian.** 1999. Images in clinical medicine. Cutaneous zygomycosis (mucormycosis). *N. Engl. J. Med.* **341:**1891.

57. **Carr, E. J., P. Scott, and J. D. Gradon.** 1999. Fatal gastrointestinal mucormycosis that invaded the postoperative abdominal wall wound in an immunocompetent host. *Clin. Infect. Dis.* **29:**956–957.

58. **Castelli, J. B., and J. L. Pallin.** 1978. Lethal rhinocerebral phycomycosis in a healthy adult: a case report and review of the literature. *Otolaryngology* **86:**696–703.

59. **Cefai, C., T. S. Elliott, R. W. Nutton, A. E. Lockett, and J. Pooley.** 1987. Zygomycetic gangrenous cellulitis. *Lancet* **ii:**1337–1338.

60. **Chakrabarti, A., P. Kumar, A. A. Padhye, L. Chatha, S. K. Singh, A. Das, J. D. Wig, and R. N. Kataria.** 1997. Primary cutaneous zygomycosis due to *Saksenaea vasiformis* and *Apophysomyces elegans. Clin. Infect. Dis.* **24:**580–583.

61. **Chan, L. L., S. Singh, D. Jones, E. M. Diaz, Jr., and L. E. Ginsberg.** 2000. Imaging of mucormycosis skull base osteomyelitis. *Am. J. Neuroradiol.* **21:**828–831.

62. **Chaudhry, R., P. Venugopal, and P. Chopra.** 1987. Prosthetic mitral valve mucormycosis caused by *Mucor* species. *Int. J. Cardiol.* **17:**333–335.

63. **Chetchotisakd, P., M. Boonma, and M. Sookprane.** 1991. Rhinocerebral mucormycosis: a report of eleven cases. *Southeast Asian J. Trop. Med. Public Health* **22:**268–271.

64. **Cho, S. Y., and H. Y. Choi.** 1979. Opportunistic fungal infection among cancer patients. A ten-year autopsy study. *Am. J. Clin. Pathol.* **72:**617–621.

65. **Chugh, K. S., V. Sakhuja, K. L. Gupta, V. Jha, A. Chakravarty, N. Malik, P. Kathuria, N. Pahwa, and O. P. Kalra.** 1993. Renal mucormycosis: computerized tomographic findings and their diagnostic significance. *Am. J. Kidney Dis.* **22:**393–397.

66. **Clark, R., D. L. Greer, T. Carlisle, and B. Carroll.** 1990. Cutaneous zygomycosis in a diabetic HTLV-I-seropositive man. *J. Am. Acad. Dermatol.* **22:**956–959.

67. **Cocanour, C. S., P. Miller-Crotchett, R. L. Reed II, P. C. Johnson, and R. P. Fischer.** 1992. Mucormycosis in trauma patients. *J. Trauma* **32:**12–15.

68. **Coelho Filho, J. C., J. Pereira, and A. Rabello, Jr.** 1989. Mediastinal and pulmonary entomophthoromycosis with superior vena cava syndrome: case report. *Rev. Inst. Med. Trop. Sao Paulo* **31:**430–433.

69. **Cohen, S. G., and M. S. Greenberg.** 1980. Rhinomaxillary mucormycosis in a kidney transplant patient. *Oral Surg. Oral Med. Oral Pathol.* **50:**33–38.

70. **Collins, D. M., T. A. Dillard, K. W. Grathwohl, G. N. Giacoppe, and B. F. Arnold.** 1999. Bronchial mucormycosis with progressive air trapping. *Mayo Clin. Proc.* **74:**698–701.

71. **Connor, B. A., R. J. Anderson, and J. W. Smith.** 1979. Mucor mediastinitis. *Chest* **75:**525–526.

72. **Cooter, R. D., I. S. Lim, D. H. Ellis, and I. O. Leitch.** 1990. Burn wound zygomycosis caused by *Apophysomyces elegans. J. Clin. Microbiol.* **28:**2151–2153.

73. **Couch, L., F. Theilen, and J. T. Mader.** 1988. Rhinocerebral mucormycosis with cerebral extension successfully treated with adjunctive hyperbaric oxygen therapy. *Arch. Otolaryngol. Head Neck Surg.* **114:**791–794.

74. **Craig, N. M., F. L. Lueder, J. M. Pensler, B. S. Bean, M. L. Petrick, R. B. Thompson, and L. R. Eramo.** 1994. Disseminated *Rhizopus* infection in a premature infant. *Pediatr. Dermatol.* **11:**346–350.

75. **Cuadrado, L. M., A. Guerrero, J. A. Garcia Asenjo, F. Martin, E. Palau, and D. Garcia Urra.** 1988. Cerebral mucormycosis in two cases of acquired immunodeficiency syndrome. *Arch. Neurol.* **45:**109–111.

76. **Dannaoui, E., J. Afeltra, J. F. Meis, and P. E. Verweij.** 2002. In vitro susceptibilities of zygomycetes to combinations of antimicrobial agents. *Antimicrob. Agents Chemother.* **46:**2708–2711.

77. **Dannaoui, E., J. F. Meis, D. Loebenberg, and P. E. Verweij.** 2003. Activity of posaconazole in treatment of experimental disseminated zygomycosis. *Antimicrob. Agents Chemother.* **47:**3647–3650.

78. **Dannaoui, E., J. Meletiadis, J. W. Mouton, J. F. Meis, and P. E. Verweij.** 2003. In vitro susceptibilities of zygomycetes to conventional and new antifungals. *J. Antimicrob. Chemother.* **51:**45–52.

79. **Dannheimer, I. P., W. Fouche, and C. Nel.** 1974. Gastric mucormycosis in a diabetic patient. *S. Afr. Med. J.* **48:**838–839.

80. **Dansky, A. S., C. M. Lynne, and V. A. Politano.** 1978. Disseminated mucormycosis with renal involvement. *J. Urol.* **119:**275–277.

81. **Darrisaw, L., G. Hanson, D. H. Vesole, and S. C. Kehl.** 2000. *Cunninghamella* infection post bone marrow transplant: case report and review of the literature. *Bone Marrow Transplant.* **25:**1213–1216.

82. **Davila, R. M., S. A. Moser, and L. E. Grosso.** 1991. Renal mucormycosis: a case report and review of the literature. *J. Urol.* **145:**1242–1244.

83. **Deal, W. B., and J. E. Johnson III.** 1969. Gastric phycomycosis. Report of a case and review of the literature. *Gastroenterology* **57:**579–586.

84. **Dean, D. F., L. Ajello, R. S. Irwin, W. K. Woelk, and G. J. Skarulis.** 1977. Cranial zygomycosis caused by *Saksenaea vasiformis*. Case report. *J. Neurosurg.* **46:**97–103.

85. **De La Paz, M. A., J. R. Patrinely, H. M. Marines, and W. D. Appling.** 1992. Adjunctive hyperbaric oxygen in the treatment of bilateral cerebro-rhino-orbital mucormycosis. *Am. J. Ophthalmol.* **114:**208–211.

86. **de Locht, M., J. R. Boelaert, and Y. J. Schneider.** 1994. Iron uptake from ferrioxamine and from ferrirhizoferrin by germinating spores of *Rhizopus microsporus. Biochem. Pharmacol.* **47:**1843–1850.

87. **del Palacio Hernanz, A., J. Fereres, S. Larregla Garraus, A. Rodriguez-Noriega, and F. Sanz Sanz.** 1983. Nosocomial infection by *Rhizomucor pusillus* in a clinical haematology unit. *J. Hosp. Infect.* **4:**45–49.

88. **Demirag, A., E. A. Elkhammas, M. L. Henry, E. A. Davies, R. P. Pelletier, G. L. Bumgardner, B. Dorner, and R. M. Ferguson.** 2000. Pulmonary *Rhizopus* infection in a diabetic renal transplant recipient. *Clin. Transplant.* **14:**8–10.

89. **Denning, D. W.** 1991. Epidemiology and pathogenesis of systemic fungal infections in the immunocompromised host. *J. Antimicrob. Chemother.* **28**(Suppl. B)**:**1–16.

90. **Dennis, J. E., K. H. Rhodes, and D. R. Cooney.** 1980. Nosocomial *Rhizopus* infection (zygomycosis) in children. *J. Pediatr.* **96:**824–828.

91. **deShazo, R. D., M. O'Brien, K. Chapin, M. Soto-Aguilar, L. Gardner, and R. Swain.** 1997. A new classification and diagnostic criteria for invasive fungal sinusitis. *Arch. Otolaryngol. Head Neck Surg.* **123:**1181–1188.

92. **Deshpande, A. H., and M. M. Munshi.** 2000. Rhinocerebral mucormycosis diagnosis by aspiration cytology. *Diagn. Cytopathol.* **23:**97–100.

93. **Diamond, H. J., R. G. Phelps, M. L. Gordon, E. Lambroza, H. Namdari, and E. J. Bottone.** 1992. Combined *Aspergillus* and zygomycotic (*Rhizopus*) infection in a patient with acquired immunodeficiency syndrome. Presentation as inflammatory tinea capitis. *J. Am. Acad. Dermatol.* **26:**1017–1018.

94. **Diamond, R. D., and R. A. Clark.** 1982. Damage to *Aspergillus fumigatus* and *Rhizopus oryzae* hyphae by oxidative and nonoxidative microbicidal products of human neutrophils in vitro. *Infect. Immun.* **38:**487–495.

95. **Dickinson, M., T. Kalayanamit, C. A. Yang, G. J. Pomper, C. Franco-Webb, and D. Rodman.** 1998. Cutaneous zygomycosis (mucormycosis) complicating endotracheal intubation: diagnosis and successful treatment. *Chest* **114:**340–342.

96. **Diekema, D. J., S. A. Messer, R. J. Hollis, R. N. Jones, and M. A. Pfaller.** 2003. Activities of caspofungin, itraconazole, posaconazole, ravuconazole, voriconazole, and amphotericin B against 448 recent clinical isolates of filamentous fungi. *J. Clin. Microbiol.* **41:**3623–3626.

97. **Dupont, B.** 2005. Pulmonary mucormycosis (zygomycosis) in a lung transplant recipient: recovery after posaconazole therapy. *Transplantation* **80:**544–545.

98. **Dykhuizen, R. S., K. N. Kerr, and R. L. Soutar.** 1994. Air crescent sign and fatal haemoptysis in pulmonary mucormycosis. *Scand. J. Infect. Dis.* **26:**498–501.

99. **Eaton, M. E., A. A. Padhye, D. A. Schwartz, and J. P. Steinberg.** 1994. Osteomyelitis of the sternum caused by *Apophysomyces elegans. J. Clin. Microbiol.* **32:**2827–2828.

100. **Eckert, H. L., G. H. Khoury, R. S. Pore, E. F. Gilbert, and J. R. Gaskell.** 1972. Deep *Entomophthora* phycomycotic infection reported for the first time in the United States. *Chest* **61:**392–394.

101. **Eckmann, D. M., I. Seligman, C. J. Cote, and J. W. Hussong.** 1998. Mucormycosis supraglottitis on induction of anesthesia in an immunocompromised host. *Anesth. Analg.* **86:**729–730.

102. **Eisen, D. P., and J. Robson.** 2004. Complete resolution of pulmonary *Rhizopus oryzae* infection with itraconazole treatment: more evidence of the utility of azoles for zygomycosis. *Mycoses* **47:**159–162.

103. **Eiser, A. R., R. F. Slifkin, and M. S. Neff.** 1987. Intestinal mucormycosis in hemodialysis patients following deferoxamine. *Am. J. Kidney Dis.* **10:**71–73.

104. **El-Ani, A. S., and V. Dhar.** 1982. Disseminated mucormycosis in a case of metastatic carcinoma. *Am. J. Clin. Pathol.* **77:**110–114.

105. **Elder, T. D., and R. D. Baker.** 1956. Pulmonary mucormycosis in rabbits with alloxan diabetes; increased invasiveness of fungus during acute toxic phase of diabetes. *AMA Arch. Pathol.* **61:**159–168.

106. **Eng, R. H., A. Person, C. Mangura, H. Chmel, and M. Corrado.** 1981. Susceptibility of zygomycetes to amphotericin B, miconazole, and ketoconazole. *Antimicrob. Agents Chemother.* **20:**688–690.

107. **England, A. C., III, M. Weinstein, J. J. Ellner, and L. Ajello.** 1981. Two cases of rhinocerebral zygomycosis (mucormycosis) with common epidemiologic and environmental features. *Am. Rev. Respir. Dis.* **124:**497–498.

108. **Erdos, M. S., K. Butt, and L. Weinstein.** 1972. Mucormycotic endocarditis of the pulmonary valve. *JAMA* **222:**951–953.

109. **Espinel-Ingroff, A.** 2001. In vitro fungicidal activities of voriconazole, itraconazole, and amphotericin B against opportunistic moniliaceous and dematiaceous fungi. *J. Clin. Microbiol.* **39:**954–958.

110. **Espinoza, C. G., and D. G. Halkias.** 1983. Pulmonary mucormycosis as a complication of chronic salicylate poisoning. *Am. J. Clin. Pathol.* **80:**508–511.

111. **Fairley, C., T. J. Sullivan, P. Bartley, T. Allworth, and R. Lewandowski.** 2000. Survival after rhino-orbital-cerebral mucormycosis in an immunocompetent patient. *Ophthalmology* **107:**555–558.

112. **Feeley, M. A., P. D. Righi, T. E. Davis, and A. Greist.** 1999. Mucormycosis of the paranasal sinuses and septum. *Otolaryngol. Head Neck Surg.* **120:**750.

113. **Fergie, J. E., D. S. Fitzwater, P. Einstein, and R. J. Leggiadro.** 1992. Mucor peritonitis associated with acute peritoneal dialysis. *Pediatr. Infect. Dis. J.* **11:**498–500.

114. **Ferguson, B. J.** 2000. Mucormycosis of the nose and paranasal sinuses. *Otolaryngol. Clin. N. Am.* **33:**349–365.

115. **Ferguson, B. J., T. G. Mitchell, R. Moon, E. M. Camporesi, and J. Farmer.** 1988. Adjunctive hyperbaric oxygen for treatment of rhinocerebral mucormycosis. *Rev. Infect. Dis.* **10:**551–559.

116. **Fermanis, G. G., K. S. Matar, and R. Steele.** 1991. Endobronchial zygomycosis. *Aust. N. Z. J. Surg.* **61:**391–393.

117. **Fingerote, R. J., S. Seigel, M. H. Atkinson, and R. M. Lewkonia.** 1990. Disseminated zygomycosis associated with systemic lupus erythematosus. *J. Rheumatol.* **17:**1692–1694.

118. **Fisher, E. W., A. Toma, P. H. Fisher, and A. D. Cheesman.** 1991. Rhinocerebral mucormycosis: use of liposomal amphotericin B. *J. Laryngol. Otol.* **105:**575–577.

119. **Fisher, J., C. U. Tuazon, and G. W. Geelhoed.** 1980. Mucormycosis in transplant patients. *Am. Surg.* **46:**315–322.

120. **Flood, H. D., A. M. O'Brien, and D. G. Kelly.** 1985. Isolated renal mucormycosis. *Postgrad. Med. J.* **61:**175–176.

121. **Foley, F. D., and J. M. Shuck.** 1968. Burn-wound infection with phycomycetes requiring amputation of hand. *JAMA* **203:**596.

122. **Fong, K. M., E. M. Seneviratne, and J. G. McCormack.** 1990. Mucor cerebral abscess associated with intravenous drug abuse. *Aust. N. Z. J. Med.* **20:**74–77.

123. **Fridkin, S. K., and W. R. Jarvis.** 1996. Epidemiology of nosocomial fungal infections. *Clin. Microbiol. Rev.* **9:**499–511.

124. **Funada, H., and T. Matsuda.** 1996. Pulmonary mucormycosis in a hematology ward. *Intern. Med.* **35:**540–544.

125. **Gale, A. M., and W. P. Kleitsch.** 1972. Solitary pulmonary nodule due to phycomycosis (mucormycosis). *Chest* **62:**752–755.

126. **Galetta, S. L., A. E. Wulc, H. I. Goldberg, C. W. Nichols, and J. S. Glaser.** 1990. Rhinocerebral mucormycosis: management and survival after carotid occlusion. *Ann. Neurol.* **28:**103–107.

127. **Garbino, J., I. Uckay, K. Amini, M. Puppo, M. Richter, and D. Lew.** 2005. Absidia posttraumatic infection: successful treatment with posaconazole. *J. Infect.* **51:**e135–e138.

128. **Gartenberg, G., E. J. Bottone, G. T. Keusch, and I. Weitzman.** 1978. Hospital-acquired mucormycosis (*Rhizopus rhizopodiformis*) of skin and subcutaneous tissue: epidemiology, mycology and treatment. *N. Engl. J. Med.* **299:**1115–1118.

129. **Gass, J. D.** 1961. Ocular manifestations of acute mucormycosis. *Arch. Ophthalmol.* **65:**226–237.

130. **Gaviria, J. M., L. A. Grohskopf, R. Barnes, and R. K. Root.** 1999. Successful treatment of rhinocerebral zygomycosis: a combined-strategy approach. *Clin. Infect. Dis.* **28:**160–161.

131. **Gaziev, D., D. Baronciani, M. Galimberti, P. Polchi, E. Angelucci, C. Giardini, P. Muretto, S. Perugini, S. Riggio, S. Ghirlanda, B. Erer, A. Maiello, and G. Lucarelli.** 1996. Mucormycosis after bone marrow transplantation: report of four cases in thalassemia and review of the literature. *Bone Marrow Transplant.* **17:**409–414.

132. **Gilbert, E. F., G. H. Khoury, and R. S. Pore.** 1970. Histopathological identification of *Entomophthora* phycomycosis. Deep mycotic infection in an infant. *Arch. Pathol.* **90:**583–587.

133. **Gil-Lamaignere, C., M. Simitsopoulou, E. Roilides, A. Maloukou, R. M. Winn, and T. J. Walsh.** 2005. Interferon-gamma and granulocyte-macrophage colony-stimulating factor augment the activity of polymorphonuclear leukocytes against medically important zygomycetes. *J. Infect. Dis.* **191:**1180–1187.

134. **Gilman, A. L., A. Serrano, J. Skelley, and D. Zwick.** 2005. Successful treatment of pulmonary zygomycosis with posaconazole in a recipient of a haploidentical donor stem cell transplant. *Pediatr. Blood Cancer.* Epub ahead of print.

135. **Glazer, M., S. Nusair, R. Breuer, J. Lafair, Y. Sherman, and N. Berkman.** 2000. The role of BAL in the diagnosis of pulmonary mucormycosis. *Chest* **117:**279–282.

136. **Gleissner, B., A. Schilling, I. Anagnostopolous, I. Siehl, and E. Thiel.** 2004. Improved outcome of zygomycosis in patients with hematological diseases? *Leuk. Lymphoma* **45:**1351–1360.

137. **Gokcil, Z., Z. Odabasi, Y. Kutukcu, H. Umudum, O. Vural, and M. Yardim.** 1998. Rhino-orbito-cerebral mucormycosis. *J. Neurol.* **245:**689–690.

138. **Goldstein, M. F., D. J. Dvorin, E. H. Dunsky, R. W. Lesser, P. J. Heuman, and J. H. Loose.** 1992. Allergic *Rhizomucor* sinusitis. *J. Allergy Clin. Immunol.* **90:**394–404.

139. **Gonis, G., and M. Starr.** 1997. Fatal rhinoorbital mucormycosis caused by *Saksenaea vasiformis* in an immunocompromised child. *Pediatr. Infect. Dis. J.* **16:**714–716.

140. **Gonzalez, C. E., D. R. Couriel, and T. J. Walsh.** 1997. Disseminated zygomycosis in a neutropenic patient: successful treatment with amphotericin B lipid complex and granulocyte colony-stimulating factor. *Clin. Infect. Dis.* **24:**192–196.

141. **Goodman, J. L., D. J. Winston, R. A. Greenfield, P. H. Chandrasekar, B. Fox, H. Kaizer, R. K. Shadduck, T. C. Shea, P. Stiff, D. J. Friedman, et al.** 1992. A controlled trial of fluconazole to prevent fungal infections in patients undergoing bone marrow transplantation. *N. Engl. J. Med.* **326:**845–851.

142. **Goodnight, J., P. Dulguerov, and E. Abemayor.** 1993. Calcified mucor fungus ball of the maxillary sinus. *Am. J. Otolaryngol.* **14:**209–210.

143. **Gordon, G., M. Indeck, J. Bross, D. A. Kapoor, and S. Brotman.** 1988. Injury from silage wagon accident complicated by mucormycosis. *J. Trauma* **28:**866–867.

144. **Gottlieb, S. F.** 1965. Hyperbaric oxygenation. *Adv. Clin. Chem.* **8:**69–139.

145. **Grauer, M. E., C. Bokemeyer, T. Welte, M. Freund, and H. Link.** 1993. Successful treatment of *Mucor* pneumonia in a patient with relapsed lymphoblastic leukemia after bone marrow transplantation. *Bone Marrow Transplant.* **12:**421.

146. **Graus, F., L. R. Rogers, and J. B. Posner.** 1985. Cerebrovascular complications in patients with cancer. *Medicine* (Baltimore) **64:**16–35.

147. **Green, W. R., and D. Bouchette.** 1986. Pleural mucormycosis (zygomycosis). *Arch. Pathol. Lab. Med.* **110:**441–442.

148. **Greenberg, M. R., S. M. Lippman, V. S. Grinnell, M. F. Colman, and J. E. Edwards, Jr.** 1985. Computed tomographic findings in orbital *Mucor. West. J. Med.* **143:**102–103.

149. **Greenberg, R. N., L. J. Scott, H. H. Vaughn, and J. A. Ribes.** 2004. Zygomycosis (mucormycosis): emerging clinical importance and new treatments. *Curr. Opin. Infect. Dis.* **17:**517–525.

150. **Guardia, J. A., J. Bourgoignie, and J. Diego.** 2000. Renal mucormycosis in the HIV patient. *Am. J. Kidney Dis.* **35:**e24.

151. **Gupta, A. K., S. B. Mann, V. K. Khosla, K. V. Sastry, and J. S. Hundal.** 1999. Non-randomized comparison of surgical modalities for paranasal sinus mycoses with intracranial extension. *Mycoses* **42:**225–230.

152. **Gupta, K. L., K. Joshi, B. J. Pereira, and K. Singh.** 1987. Disseminated mucormycosis presenting with acute renal failure. *Postgrad. Med. J.* **63:**297–299.

153. **Gupta, K. L., K. Joshi, K. Sud, H. S. Kohli, V. Jha, B. D. Radotra, and V. Sakhuja.** 1999. Renal zygomycosis: an under-diagnosed cause of acute renal failure. *Nephrol. Dial. Transplant.* **14:**2720–2725.

154. **Hagensee, M. E., J. E. Bauwens, B. Kjos, and R. A. Bowden.** 1994. Brain abscess following marrow transplantation: experience at the Fred Hutchinson Cancer Research Center, 1984–1992. *Clin. Infect. Dis.* **19:**402–408.

155. **Hameroff, S. B., J. W. Eckholdt, and R. Lindenberg.** 1970. Cerebral phycomycosis in a heroin addict. *Neurology* **20:**261–265.

156. **Hammond, D. E., and R. K. Winkelmann.** 1979. Cutaneous phycomycosis. Report of three cases with identification of *Rhizopus. Arch. Dermatol.* **115:**990–992.

157. **Harada, M., T. Manabe, K. Yamashita, and N. Okamoto.** 1992. Pulmonary mucormycosis with fatal massive hemoptysis. *Acta Pathol. Jpn.* **42:**49–55.

158. **Harper, J. J., C. Coulter, G. R. Lye, and G. R. Nimmo.** 1996. *Rhizopus* and tongue depressors. *Lancet* **348:**1250.

159. **Helenglass, G., J. A. Elliott, and N. P. Lucie.** 1981. An unusual presentation of opportunistic mucormycosis. *Br. Med. J.* **282:**108–109.

160. **Hicks, W. L., Jr., K. Nowels, and J. Troxel.** 1995. Primary cutaneous mucormycosis. *Am. J. Otolaryngol.* **16:**265–268.

161. **Hoffman, R. M.** 1987. Chronic endobronchial mucormycosis. *Chest* **91:**469.

162. **Hopkins, R. J., M. Rothman, A. Fiore, and S. E. Goldblum.** 1994. Cerebral mucormycosis associated with intravenous drug use: three case reports and review. *Clin. Infect. Dis.* **19:**1133–1137.

163. **Hopwood, V., D. A. Hicks, S. Thomas, and E. G. Evans.** 1992. Primary cutaneous zygomycosis due to *Absidia corymbifera* in a patient with AIDS. *J. Med. Vet. Mycol.* **30:**399–402.

164. **Hosseini, M., and J. Lee.** 1998. Gastrointestinal mucormycosis mimicking ischemic colitis in a patient with systemic lupus erythematosus. *Am. J. Gastroenterol.* **93:**1360–1362.

165. **Huffnagle, K. E., P. M. Southern, Jr., L. T. Byrd, and R. M. Gander.** 1992. *Apophysomyces elegans* as an agent of zygomycosis in a patient following trauma. *J. Med. Vet. Mycol.* **30:**83–86.

166. **Humphry, R. C., G. Wright, W. J. Rich, and R. Simpson.** 1989. Acute proptosis and blindness in a patient with orbital phycomycosis. *J. R. Soc. Med.* **82:**304–305.

167. **Hunstad, D. A., A. H. Cohen, and J. W. St Geme III.** 1999. Successful eradication of mucormycosis occurring in a pulmonary allograft. *J. Heart. Lung Transplant.* **18:**801–804.

168. **Hyatt, D. S., Y. M. Young, K. A. Haynes, J. M. Taylor, D. M. McCarthy, and T. R. Rogers.** 1992. Rhinocerebral mucormycosis following bone marrow transplantation. *J. Infect.* **24:**67–71.

169. **Ibrahim, A. S., B. Spellberg, V. Avanessian, Y. Fu, and J. E. Edwards, Jr.** 2005. *Rhizopus oryzae* adheres to, is phagocytosed by, and damages endothelial cells in vitro. *Infect. Immun.* **73:**778–783.

170. **Ignelzi, R. J., and G. D. VanderArk.** 1975. Cerebral mucormycosis following open head trauma. Case report. *J. Neurosurg.* **42:**593–596.

171. **Imhof, A., S. A. Balajee, D. N. Fredricks, J. A. Englund, and K. A. Marr.** 2004. Breakthrough fungal infections in stem cell transplant recipients receiving voriconazole. *Clin. Infect. Dis.* **39:**743–746.

172. **Inamasu, J., K. Uchida, K. Mayanagi, S. Suga, and T. Kawase.** 2000. Basilar artery occlusion due to mucormycotic emboli, preceded by acute hydrocephalus. *Clin. Neurol. Neurosurg.* **102:**18–22.

173. **Ingram, C. W., J. Sennesh, J. N. Cooper, and J. R. Perfect.** 1989. Disseminated zygomycosis: report of four cases and review. *Rev. Infect. Dis.* **11:**741–754.

174. **Iqbal, S. M., and R. L. Scheer.** 1986. Myocardial mucormycosis with emboli in a hemodialysis patient. *Am. J. Kidney Dis.* **8:**455–458.

175. **Iwen, P. C., M. E. Rupp, and S. H. Hinrichs.** 1997. Invasive mold sinusitis: 17 cases in immunocompromised patients and review of the literature. *Clin. Infect. Dis.* **24:**1178–1184.

176. **Jaffey, P. B., A. K. Haque, M. el-Zaatari, L. Pasarell, and M. R. McGinnis.** 1990. Disseminated *Conidiobolus* infection with endocarditis in a cocaine abuser. *Arch. Pathol. Lab. Med.* **114:**1276–1278.

177. **Jain, J. K., A. Markowitz, P. V. Khilanani, and C. B. Lauter.** 1978. Localized mucormycosis following intramuscular corticosteroid. Case report and review of the literature. *Am. J. Med. Sci.* **275:**209–216.

178. **Jamadar, D. A., E. A. Kazerooni, B. D. Daly, C. S. White, and B. H. Gross.** 1995. Pulmonary zygomycosis: CT appearance. *J. Comput. Assist. Tomogr.* **19:**733–738.

179. **Jantunen, E., E. Kolho, P. Ruutu, P. Koukila-Kahkola, M. Virolainen, E. Juvonen, and L. Volin.** 1996. Invasive cutaneous mucormycosis caused by *Absidia corymbifera* after allogeneic bone marrow transplantation. *Bone Marrow Transplant.* **18:**229–230.

180. **Jensen, A. B., and K. M. Dromph.** 2005. The causal agents of 'entomophthoramycosis' belong to two different orders: a suggestion for modification of the clinical nomenclature. *Clin. Microbiol. Infect.* **11:**249–250.

181. **Jensen, A. B., A. Gargas, J. Eilenberg, and S. Rosendahl.** 1998. Relationships of the insect-pathogenic order Entomophthorales (Zygomycota, Fungi) based on phylogenetic analyses of nuclear small subunit ribosomal DNA sequences (SSU rDNA). *Fungal Genet. Biol.* **24:**325–334.

182. **John, B. V., G. Chamilos, and D. P. Kontoyiannis.** 2005. Hyperbaric oxygen as an adjunctive treatment for zygomycosis. *Clin. Microbiol. Infect.* **11:**515–517.

183. **Josefiak, E. J., J. H. Foushee, and L. C. Smith.** 1958. Cutaneous mucormycosis. *Am. J. Clin. Pathol.* **30:**547–552.

184. **Kahn, L. B.** 1963. Gastric mucormycosis: report of a case with a review of the literature. *S. Afr. Med. J.* **37:**1265–1269.

185. **Kajs-Wyllie, M.** 1995. Hyperbaric oxygen therapy for rhinocerebral fungal infection. *J. Neurosci. Nurs.* **27:**174–181.

186. **Kamalam, A., and A. S. Thambiah.** 1980. Cutaneous infection by *Syncephalastrum. Sabouraudia* **18:** 19–20.

187. **Kamat, S. R., S. P. Shah, A. A. Mahashur, D. C. Shah, and A. P. Mehta.** 1982. Disseminated systemic mucormycosis (a case report). *J. Postgrad. Med.* **28:**229–232.

188. **Kaplan, A. L., A. R. Huerta, and S. J. Chiou.** 1981. Rhinocerebral mucormycosis. *West. J. Med.* **135:** 326–329.

189. **Karsner, H. T., and O. Saphir.** 1926. Influence of high partial pressures of oxygen on the growth of certain molds. *J. Infect. Dis.* **39:**231–236.

190. **Kauffman, C. A.** 2004. Zygomycosis: reemergence of an old pathogen. *Clin. Infect. Dis.* **39:**588–590.

191. **Kecskes, S., G. Reynolds, and G. Bennett.** 1997. Survival after gastrointestinal mucormycosis in a neonate. *J. Paediatr. Child Health* **33:**356–359.

192. **Kerr, P. G., H. Turner, A. Davidson, C. Bennett, and M. Maslen.** 1988. Zygomycosis requiring amputation of the hand: an isolated case in a patient receiving haemodialysis. *Med. J. Aust.* **148:**258–259.

193. **Keys, T. F., A. M. Haldorson, and K. H. Rhodes.** 1978. Nosocomial outbreak of *Rhizopus* infections associated with Elastoplast wound dressings. *Morb. Mortal. Wkly. Rep.* **27:**33–34.

194. **Khardori, N., S. Hayat, K. Rolston, and G. P. Bodey.** 1989. Cutaneous *Rhizopus* and *Aspergillus* infections in five patients with cancer. *Arch. Dermatol.* **125:**952–956.

195. **Khicha, G. J., R. B. Berroya, F. B. Escano, Jr., and C. S. Lee.** 1972. Mucormycosis in a mitral prosthesis. *J. Thorac. Cardiovasc. Surg.* **63:**903–905.

196. **Kiehn, T. E., F. Edwards, D. Armstrong, P. P. Rosen, and I. Weitzman.** 1979. Pneumonia caused by *Cunninghamella bertholletiae* complicating chronic lymphatic leukemia. *J. Clin. Microbiol.* **10:**374–379.

197. **Kimura, M., V. J. Schnadig, and M. R. McGinnis.** 1998. Chlamydoconidia formation in zygomycosis due to *Rhizopus* species. *Arch. Pathol. Lab. Med.* **122:**1120–1122.

198. **Kimura, M., M. B. Smith, and M. R. McGinnis.** 1999. Zygomycosis due to *Apophysomyces elegans*: report of 2 cases and review of the literature. *Arch. Pathol. Lab. Med.* **123:**386–390.

199. **King, D. S., and S. C. Jong.** 1976. Identity of the etiological agent of the first deep entomophthoraceous infection of man in the United States. *Mycologia* **68:**181–183.

200. **Kitabayashi, A., M. Hirokawa, A. Yamaguchi, H. Takatsu, and A. B. Miura.** 1998. Invasive pulmonary mucormycosis with rupture of the thoracic aorta. *Am. J. Hematol.* **58:**326–329.

201. **Kline, M. W.** 1985. Mucormycosis in children: review of the literature and report of cases. *Pediatr. Infect. Dis.* **4:**672–676.

202. **Kolbeck, P. C., R. G. Makhoul, R. R. Bollinger, and F. Sanfilippo.** 1985. Widely disseminated *Cunninghamella* mucormycosis in an adult renal transplant patient: case report and review of the literature. *Am. J. Clin. Pathol.* **83:**747–753.

203. **Kontoyiannis, D. P., M. S. Lionakis, R. E. Lewis, G. Chamilos, M. Healy, C. Perego, A. Safdar, H. Kantarjian, R. Champlin, T. J. Walsh, and I. I. Raad.** 2005. Zygomycosis in a tertiary-care cancer center in the era of *Aspergillus*-active antifungal therapy: a case-control observational study of 27 recent cases. *J. Infect. Dis.* **191:**1350–1360.

204. **Kontoyiannis, D. P., V. C. Wessel, G. P. Bodey, and K. V. Rolston.** 2000. Zygomycosis in the 1990s in a tertiary-care cancer center. *Clin. Infect. Dis.* **30:**851–856.

205. **Kramer, B. S., A. D. Hernandez, R. L. Reddick, and A. S. Levine.** 1977. Cutaneous infarction. Manifestation of disseminated mucormycosis. *Arch. Dermatol.* **113:**1075–1076.

206. **Krasinski, K., R. S. Holzman, B. Hanna, M. A. Greco, M. Graff, and M. Bhogal.** 1985. Nosocomial fungal infection during hospital renovation. *Infect. Control* **6:**278–282.

272   Gonzalez et al.

207. **Kwon-Chung, J. K., and J. E. Bennett.** 1992. Mucormycosis (physomycosis, zygomycosis), p. 524–559. *In* K. J. Kwon-Chung and J. E. Bennett (ed.), *Medical Mycology.* Lea & Febiger, Philadelphia, Pa.
208. **Kwon-Chung, K. J., R. C. Young, and M. Orlando.** 1975. Pulmonary mucormycosis caused by *Cunninghamella elegans* in a patient with chronic myelogenous leukemia. *Am. J. Clin. Pathol.* **64:**544–548.
209. **Lake, F. R., R. McAleer, and A. E. Tribe.** 1988. Pulmonary mucormycosis without underlying systemic disease. *Med. J. Aust.* **149:**323–326.
210. **Lakshmi, V., T. S. Rani, S. Sharma, V. S. Mohan, C. Sundaram, R. R. Rao, and G. Satyanarayana.** 1993. Zygomycotic necrotizing fasciitis caused by *Apophysomyces elegans. J. Clin. Microbiol.* **31:**1368–1369.
211. **Langford, J. D., D. L. McCartney, and R. C. Wang.** 1997. Frozen section-guided surgical debridement for management of rhino-orbital mucormycosis. *Am. J. Ophthalmol.* **124:**265–267.
212. **Langston, C., D. A. Roberts, G. A. Porter, and W. M. Bennett.** 1973. Renal phycomycosis. *J. Urol.* **109:**941–944.
213. **Latif, S., N. Saffarian, K. Bellovich, and R. Provenzano.** 1997. Pulmonary mucormycosis in diabetic renal allograft recipients. *Am. J. Kidney Dis.* **29:**461–464.
214. **Lawson, H. H., and A. Schmaman.** 1974. Gastric phycomycosis. *Br. J. Surg.* **61:**743–746.
215. **Lazo, A., H. I. Wilner, and J. J. Metes.** 1981. Craniofacial mucormycosis: computed tomographic and angiographic findings in two cases. *Radiology* **139:**623–626.
216. **Lee, E., Y. Vershvovsky, F. Miller, W. Waltzer, H. Suh, and E. P. Nord.** 2001. Combined medical surgical therapy for pulmonary mucormycosis in a diabetic renal allograft recipient. *Am. J. Kidney Dis.* **38:**e37.
217. **Lee, F. Y., S. B. Mossad, and K. A. Adal.** 1999. Pulmonary mucormycosis: the last 30 years. *Arch. Intern. Med.* **159:**1301–1309.
218. **Leeming, J. G., H. A. Moss, and T. S. Elliott.** 1996. Risk of tongue depressors to the immunocompromised. *Lancet* **348:**889.
219. **Lehrer, R. I.** 1980. Mucormycosis (UCL conference). *Ann. Intern. Med.* **93:**93–108.
220. **Leleu, X., B. Sendid, J. Fruit, H. Sarre, E. Wattel, C. Rose, F. Bauters, T. Facon, and J. Jouet.** 1999. Combined anti-fungal therapy and surgical resection as treatment of pulmonary zygomycosis in allogeneic bone marrow transplantation. *Bone Marrow Transplant.* **24:**417–420.
221. **Leong, K. W., B. Crowley, B. White, G. M. Crotty, D. S. O'Briain, C. Keane, and S. R. McCann.** 1997. Cutaneous mucormycosis due to *Absidia corymbifera* occurring after bone marrow transplantation. *Bone Marrow Transplant.* **19:**513–515.
222. **Levitz, S. M., M. E. Selsted, T. Ganz, R. I. Lehrer, and R. D. Diamond.** 1986. In vitro killing of spores and hyphae of *Aspergillus fumigatus* and *Rhizopus oryzae* by rabbit neutrophil cationic peptides and bronchoalveolar macrophages. *J. Infect. Dis.* **154:**483–489.
223. **Levy, V., B. Rio, A. Bazarbachi, M. Hunault, A. Delmer, R. Zittoun, V. Blanc, and M. Wolff.** 1996. Two cases of epidemic mucormycosis infection in patients with acute lymphoblastic leukemia. *Am. J. Hematol.* **52:**64–65.
224. **Lewis, L. L., H. K. Hawkins, and M. S. Edwards.** 1990. Disseminated mucormycosis in an infant with methylmalonicaciduria. *Pediatr. Infect. Dis. J.* **9:**851–854.
225. **Lidor, C., and J. A. Nunley.** 1997. Images in clinical medicine. Mucormycosis of the hand and forearm. *N. Engl. J. Med.* **337:**1511.
226. **Liles, W. C., J. E. Huang, J. A. van Burik, R. A. Bowden, and D. C. Dale.** 1997. Granulocyte colony-stimulating factor administered in vivo augments neutrophil-mediated activity against opportunistic fungal pathogens. *J. Infect. Dis.* **175:**1012–1015.
227. **Linden, P., P. Williams, and K. M. Chan.** 2000. Efficacy and safety of amphotericin B lipid complex injection (ABLC) in solid-organ transplant recipients with invasive fungal infections. *Clin. Transplant.* **14:**329–339.
228. **Liu, M. F., F. F. Chen, T. R. Hsiue, and C. C. Liu.** 2000. Disseminated zygomycosis simulating cerebrovascular disease and pulmonary alveolar haemorrhage in a patient with systemic lupus erythematosus. *Clin. Rheumatol.* **19:**311–314.
229. **Loevner, L. A., J. C. Andrews, and I. R. Francis.** 1992. Multiple mycotic pulmonary artery aneurysms: a complication of invasive mucormycosis. *Am. J. Roentgenol.* **158:**761–762.
230. **Lopes, J. O., D. V. Pereira, L. A. Streher, A. A. Fenalte, S. H. Alves, and J. P. Benevenga.** 1995. Cutaneous zygomycosis caused by *Absidia corymbifera* in a leukemic patient. *Mycopathologia* **130:**89–92.
231. **Lowe, J. T., Jr., and W. R. Hudson.** 1975. Rhinocerebral phycomycosis and internal carotid artery thrombosis. *Arch. Otolaryngol.* **101:**100–103.

232. **Lueg, E. A., R. H. Ballagh, and V. Forte.** 1996. Analysis of the recent cluster of invasive fungal sinusitis at the Toronto Hospital for Sick Children. *J. Otolaryngol.* **25:**366–370.
233. **Lussier, N., M. Laverdiere, K. Weiss, L. Poirier, and E. Schick.** 1998. Primary renal mucormycosis. *Urology* **52:**900–903.
234. **Mackenzie, D. W., J. F. Soothill, and J. H. Millar.** 1988. Meningitis caused by *Absidia corymbifera*. *J. Infect.* **17:**241–248.
235. **MacMillan, M. L., J. L. Goodman, T. E. DeFor, and D. J. Weisdorf.** 2002. Fluconazole to prevent yeast infections in bone marrow transplantation patients: a randomized trial of high versus reduced dose, and determination of the value of maintenance therapy. *Am. J. Med.* **112:**369–379.
236. **Maertens, J., H. Demuynck, E. K. Verbeken, P. Zachee, G. E. Verhoef, P. Vandenberghe, and M. A. Boogaerts.** 1999. Mucormycosis in allogeneic bone marrow transplant recipients: report of five cases and review of the role of iron overload in the pathogenesis. *Bone Marrow Transplant.* **24:**307–312.
237. **Mamlok, V., W. T. Cowan, Jr., and V. Schnadig.** 1987. Unusual histopathology of mucormycosis in acute myelogenous leukemia. *Am. J. Clin. Pathol.* **88:**117–120.
238. **Marr, K. A., R. A. Carter, F. Crippa, A. Wald, and L. Corey.** 2002. Epidemiology and outcome of mould infections in hematopoietic stem cell transplant recipients. *Clin. Infect. Dis.* **34:**909–917.
239. **Marr, T. J., H. S. Traismann, A. T. Davis, and D. Kernahan.** 1978. Rhinocerebral mucormycosis and juvenile diabetes mellitus: report of a case with recovery. *Diabetes Care* **1:**250–251.
240. **Marshall, D. H., S. Brownstein, W. B. Jackson, G. Mintsioulis, S. M. Gilberg, and B. F. al-Zeerah.** 1997. Post-traumatic corneal mucormycosis caused by *Absidia corymbifera*. *Ophthalmology* **104:**1107–1111.
241. **Martinez, E. J., M. R. Cancio, J. T. T. Sinnott, A. L. Vincent, and S. G. Brantley.** 1997. Nonfatal gastric mucormycosis in a renal transplant recipient. *South. Med. J.* **90:**341–344.
242. **Marty, F. M., L. A. Cosimi, and L. R. Baden.** 2004. Breakthrough zygomycosis after voriconazole treatment in recipients of hematopoietic stem-cell transplants. *N. Engl. J. Med.* **350:**950–952.
243. **Mathew, R., S. Kumaravel, S. Kuruvilla, R. G. Varghese, Shashikala, S. Srinivasan, and M. Z. Mani.** 2005. Successful treatment of extensive basidiobolomycosis with oral itraconazole in a child. *Int. J. Dermatol.* **44:**572–575.
244. **Mathews, M. S., A. Raman, and A. Nair.** 1997. Nosocomial zygomycotic post-surgical necrotizing fasciitis in a healthy adult caused by *Apophysomyces elegans* in south India. *J. Med. Vet. Mycol.* **35:**61–63.
245. **Matsushima, T., R. Soejima, and T. Nakashima.** 1980. Solitary pulmonary nodule caused by phycomycosis in a patient without obvious predisposing factors. *Thorax* **35:**877–878.
246. **Maury, S., T. Leblanc, M. Feuilhade, J. M. Molina, and G. Schaison.** 1998. Successful treatment of disseminated mucormycosis with liposomal amphotericin B and surgery in a child with leukemia. *Clin. Infect. Dis.* **26:**200–202.
247. **Mayer, P., E. Schutze, C. Lam, F. Kricek, and E. Liehl.** 1991. Recombinant murine granulocyte-macrophage colony-stimulating factor augments neutrophil recovery and enhances resistance to infections in myelosuppressed mice. *J. Infect. Dis.* **163:**584–590.
248. **Mazade, M. A., J. F. Margolin, S. N. Rossmann, and M. S. Edwards.** 1998. Survival from pulmonary infection with *Cunninghamella bertholletiae*: case report and review of the literature. *Pediatr. Infect. Dis. J.* **17:**835–839.
249. **McAdams, H. P., M. Rosado de Christenson, D. C. Strollo, and E. F. Patz, Jr.** 1997. Pulmonary mucormycosis: radiologic findings in 32 cases. *Am. J. Roentgenol.* **168:**1541–1548.
250. **McNulty, J. S.** 1982. Rhinocerebral mucormycosis: predisposing factors. *Laryngoscope* **92:**1140–1143.
251. **Mead, J. H., G. P. Lupton, C. L. Dillavou, and R. B. Odom.** 1979. Cutaneous *Rhizopus* infection. Occurrence as a postoperative complication associated with an elasticized adhesive dressing. *JAMA* **242:**272–274.
252. **Medoff, G., and G. S. Kobayashi.** 1972. Pulmonary mucormycosis. *N. Engl. J. Med.* **286:**86–87.
253. **Meis, J. F., B. J. Kullberg, M. Pruszczynski, and R. P. Veth.** 1994. Severe osteomyelitis due to the zygomycete *Apophysomyces elegans*. *J. Clin. Microbiol.* **32:**3078–3081.
254. **Melero, M., I. Kaimen Maciel, N. Tiraboschi, M. Botargues, and M. Radisic.** 1991. Adjunctive treatment with hyperbaric oxygen in a patient with rhino-sinuso-orbital mucormycosis. *Medicina* **51:**53–55.
255. **Melsom, S. M., and M. S. Khangure.** 2000. Craniofacial mucormycosis following assault: an unusual presentation of an unusual disease. *Australas. Radiol.* **44:**104–106.
256. **Mendoza-Ayala, R., R. Tapia, and M. Salathe.** 1999. Spontaneously resolving pulmonary mucormycosis. *Clin. Infect. Dis.* **29:**1335–1336.

257. **Meyer, R. D., and D. Armstrong.** 1973. Mucormycosis—changing status. *Crit. Rev. Clin. Lab. Sci.* **4:** 421–451.

258. **Meyer, R. D., M. H. Kaplan, M. Ong, and D. Armstrong.** 1973. Cutaneous lesions in disseminated mucormycosis. *JAMA* **225:**737–738.

259. **Meyer, R. D., P. Rosen, and D. Armstrong.** 1972. Phycomycosis complicating leukemia and lymphoma. *Ann. Intern. Med.* **77:**871–879.

260. **Meyers, B. R., G. Wormser, S. Z. Hirschman, and A. Blitzer.** 1979. Rhinocerebral mucormycosis: premortem diagnosis and therapy. *Arch. Intern. Med.* **139:**557–560.

261. **Minassian, B., E. Huczko, T. Washo, D. Bonner, and J. Fung-Tomc.** 2003. In vitro activity of ravuconazole against *Zygomycetes, Scedosporium* and *Fusarium* isolates. *Clin. Microbiol. Infect.* **9:**1250–1252.

262. **Mitchell, S. J., J. Gray, M. E. Morgan, M. D. Hocking, and G. M. Durbin.** 1996. Nosocomial infection with *Rhizopus microsporus* in preterm infants: association with wooden tongue depressors. *Lancet* **348:** 441–443.

263. **Mitwalli, A., G. H. Malik, J. al-Wakeel, H. Abu Aisha, S. al-Mohaya, A. al-Jaser, H. Assaf, and H. el Gamal.** 1994. Mucormycosis of the graft in a renal transplant recipient. *Nephrol. Dial. Transplant.* **9:** 718–720.

264. **Mooney, J. E., and A. Wanger.** 1993. Mucormycosis of the gastrointestinal tract in children: report of a case and review of the literature. *Pediatr. Infect. Dis. J.* **12:**872–876.

265. **Moore, M., A. D. Anderson, and H. H. Everett.** 1949. Mucormycosis of the large bowel. *Am. J. Pathol.* **25:**559–563.

266. **Morduchowicz, G., D. Shmueli, Z. Shapira, S. L. Cohen, A. Yussim, C. S. Block, J. B. Rosenfeld, and S. D. Pitlik.** 1986. Rhinocerebral mucormycosis in renal transplant recipients: report of three cases and review of the literature. *Rev. Infect. Dis.* **8:**441–446.

267. **Morstyn, G., L. Campbell, L. M. Souza, N. K. Alton, J. Keech, M. Green, W. Sheridan, D. Metcalf, and R. Fox.** 1988. Effect of granulocyte colony stimulating factor on neutropenia induced by cytotoxic chemotherapy. *Lancet* **i:**667–672.

268. **Moses, A. E., G. Rahav, Y. Barenholz, J. Elidan, B. Azaz, S. Gillis, M. Brickman, I. Polacheck, and M. Shapiro.** 1998. Rhinocerebral mucormycosis treated with amphotericin B colloidal dispersion in three patients. *Clin. Infect. Dis.* **26:**1430–1433.

269. **Mosquera, J., P. A. Warn, J. L. Rodriguez-Tudela, and D. W. Denning.** 2001. Treatment of *Absidia corymbifera* infection in mice with amphotericin B and itraconazole. *J. Antimicrob. Chemother.* **48:** 583–586.

270. **Mostaza, J. M., F. J. Barbado, J. Fernandez-Martin, J. Pena-Yanez, and J. J. Vazquez-Rodriguez.** 1989. Cutaneoarticular mucormycosis due to *Cunninghamella bertholletiae* in a patient with AIDS. *Rev. Infect. Dis.* **11:**316–318.

271. **Mowat, A., and J. Baum.** 1971. Chemotaxis of polymorphonuclear leukocytes from patients with diabetes mellitus. *N. Engl. J. Med.* **284:**621–627.

272. **Munckhof, W., R. Jones, F. A. Tosolini, A. Marzec, P. Angus, and M. L. Grayson.** 1993. Cure of *Rhizopus* sinusitis in a liver transplant recipient with liposomal amphotericin B. *Clin. Infect. Dis.* **16:**183.

273. **Munipalli, B., M. G. Rinaldi, and S. B. Greenberg.** 1996. *Cokeromyces recurvatus* isolated from pleural and peritoneal fluid: case report. *J. Clin. Microbiol.* **34:**2601–2603.

274. **Murray, H. W.** 1975. Pulmonary mucormycosis with massive fatal hemoptysis. *Chest* **68:**65–68.

275. **Myskowski, P. L., A. E. Brown, R. Dinsmore, T. Kiehn, F. Edwards, B. Wong, B. Safai, and D. Armstrong.** 1983. Mucormycosis following bone marrow transplantation. *J. Am. Acad. Dermatol.* **9:**111–115.

276. **Nagy-Agren, S. E., P. Chu, G. J. Smith, H. A. Waskin, and F. L. Altice.** 1995. Zygomycosis (mucormycosis) and HIV infection: report of three cases and review. *J. Acquir. Immune Defic. Syndr. Hum. Retrovirol.* **10:**441–449.

277. **Nakamura, M., W. B. Weil, Jr., and D. B. Kaufman.** 1989. Fatal fungal peritonitis in an adolescent on continuous ambulatory peritoneal dialysis: association with deferoxamine. *Pediatr. Nephrol.* **3:**80–82.

278. **Nash, G., F. D. Foley, M. N. Goodwin, Jr., H. M. Bruck, K. A. Greenwald, and B. A. Pruitt, Jr.** 1971. Fungal burn wound infection. *JAMA* **215:**1664–1666.

279. **Naumann, R., M. L. Kerkmann, U. Schuler, W. G. Daniel, and G. Ehninger.** 1999. *Cunninghamella bertholletiae* infection mimicking myocardial infarction. *Clin. Infect. Dis.* **29:**1580–1581.

280. **Neame, P., and D. Rayner.** 1960. Mucormycosis: a report of twenty-two cases. *Arch. Pathol.* **70:** 143–150.

281. **Nenoff, P., S. Kellermann, R. Schober, H. Nenning, M. Kubel, J. Winkler, and U. F. Haustein.** 1998. Rhinocerebral zygomycosis following bone marrow transplantation in chronic myelogenous leukaemia. Report of a case and review of the literature. *Mycoses* **41:**365–372.

282. **Newton, W. D., F. S. Cramer, and S. H. Norwood.** 1987. Necrotizing fasciitis from invasive Phycomycetes. *Crit. Care Med.* **15:**331–332.

283. **Ng, K. H., C. S. Chin, R. D. Jalleh, C. H. Siar, C. H. Ngui, and S. P. Singaram.** 1991. Nasofacial zygomycosis. *Oral Surg. Oral Med. Oral Pathol.* **72:**685–688.

284. **Ng, T. T., C. K. Campbell, M. Rothera, J. B. Houghton, D. Hughes, and D. W. Denning.** 1994. Successful treatment of sinusitis caused by *Cunninghamella bertholletiae*. *Clin. Infect. Dis.* **19:**313–316.

285. **Nguyen, B. D.** 2000. CT features of basidiobolomycosis with gastrointestinal and urinary involvement. *Am. J. Roentgenol.* **174:**878–879.

286. **Nimmo, G. R., R. F. Whiting, and R. W. Strong.** 1988. Disseminated mucormycosis due to *Cunninghamella bertholletiae* in a liver transplant recipient. *Postgrad. Med. J.* **64:**82–84.

287. **Nomura, J., J. Ruskin, F. Sahebi, N. Kogut, and P. M. Falk.** 1997. Mucormycosis of the vulva following bone marrow transplantation. *Bone Marrow Transplant.* **19:**859–860.

288. **Oberle, A. D., and R. L. Penn.** 1983. Nosocomial invasive *Saksenaea vasiformis* infection. *Am. J. Clin. Pathol.* **80:**885–888.

289. **O'Connell, M. A., J. L. Pluss, P. Schkade, A. R. Henry, and D. L. Goodman.** 1995. *Rhizopus*-induced hypersensitivity pneumonitis in a tractor driver. *J. Allergy Clin. Immunol.* **95:**779–780.

290. **Odds, F. C., F. Van Gerven, A. Espinel-Ingroff, M. S. Bartlett, M. A. Ghannoum, M. V. Lancaster, M. A. Pfaller, J. H. Rex, M. G. Rinaldi, and T. J. Walsh.** 1998. Evaluation of possible correlations between antifungal susceptibilities of filamentous fungi in vitro and antifungal treatment outcomes in animal infection models. *Antimicrob. Agents Chemother.* **42:**282–288.

291. **Okhuysen, P. C., J. H. Rex, M. Kapusta, and C. Fife.** 1994. Successful treatment of extensive posttraumatic soft-tissue and renal infections due to *Apophysomyces elegans*. *Clin. Infect. Dis.* **19:**329–331.

292. **Oliver, M. R., W. C. Van Voorhis, M. Boeckh, D. Mattson, and R. A. Bowden.** 1996. Hepatic mucormycosis in a bone marrow transplant recipient who ingested naturopathic medicine. *Clin. Infect. Dis.* **22:**521–524.

293. **Onerci, M., B. Gursel, S. Hosal, N. Gulekon, and A. Gokoz.** 1991. Rhinocerebral mucormycosis with extension to the cavernous sinus. A case report. *Rhinology* **29:**321–324.

294. **Oren, I.** 2005. Breakthrough zygomycosis during empirical voriconazole therapy in febrile patients with neutropenia. *Clin. Infect. Dis.* **40:**770–771.

295. **Otcenasek, M., and V. Buchta.** 1994. In vitro susceptibility to 9 antifungal agents of 14 strains of Zygomycetes isolated from clinical specimens. *Mycopathologia* **128:**135–137.

296. **Pagano, L., P. Ricci, A. Nosari, A. Tonso, M. Buelli, M. Montillo, L. Cudillo, A. Cenacchi, C. Savignana, L. Melillo, et al.** 1995. Fatal haemoptysis in pulmonary filamentous mycosis: an underevaluated cause of death in patients with acute leukaemia in haematological complete remission. A retrospective study and review of the literature. *Br. J. Haematol.* **89:**500–505.

297. **Pagano, L., P. Ricci, A. Tonso, A. Nosari, L. Cudillo, M. Montillo, A. Cenacchi, L. Pacilli, F. Fabbiano, A. Del Favero, et al.** 1997. Mucormycosis in patients with haematological malignancies: a retrospective clinical study of 37 cases. *Br. J. Haematol.* **99:**331–336.

298. **Paparello, S. F., R. L. Parry, D. C. MacGillivray, N. Brock, and D. L. Mayers.** 1992. Hospital-acquired wound mucormycosis. *Clin. Infect. Dis.* **14:**350–352.

299. **Papasian, C. J., C. M. Zarabi, L. H. Dall, J. F. Stanford, J. M. Galant, and J. R. Parker.** 1991. Invasive polymycotic pneumonia in an uncontrolled diabetic. *Arch. Pathol. Lab. Med.* **115:**517–519.

300. **Pappas, P. G.** 2004. Immunotherapy for invasive fungal infections: from bench to bedside. *Drug Resist. Updat.* **7:**3–10.

301. **Parker, C., G. Kaminski, and D. Hill.** 1986. Zygomycosis in a tattoo, caused by *Saksenaea vasiformis*. *Australas. J. Dermatol.* **27:**107–111.

302. **Parkhurst, G. F., and G. D. Vlahides.** 1967. Fatal opportunistic fungal disease. *JAMA* **202:**131–133.

303. **Parthiban, K., S. Gnanaguruvelan, C. Janaki, G. Sentamilselvi, and J. M. Boopalraj.** 1998. Rhinocerebral zygomycosis. *Mycoses* **41:**51–53.

304. **Passi, G. R., P. S. Menon, D. K. Gupta, and R. Lodha.** 1996. Recovery from pulmonary mucormycosis and candidiasis in diabetic ketoacidosis. *Indian Pediatr.* **33:**1047–1050.

305. **Patino, J. F., D. Castro, A. Valencia, and P. Morales.** 1991. Necrotizing soft tissue lesions after a volcanic cataclysm. *World J. Surg.* **15:**240–247.

306. **Patino, J. F., R. Mora, M. A. Guzman, and E. Rodriguez-Franco.** 1984. Mucormycosis: a fatal case by *Saksenaea vasiformis. World J. Surg.* **8:**419–422.

307. **Pelton, R. W., E. A. Peterson, B. C. Patel, and K. Davis.** 2001. Successful treatment of rhino-orbital mucormycosis without exenteration: the use of multiple treatment modalities. *Ophthal. Plast. Reconstr. Surg.* **17:**62–66.

308. **Penalver, F. J., R. Romero, R. Fores, R. Cabrera, J. L. Diez-Martin, C. Regidor, and M. N. Fernandez.** 1998. Rhinocerebral mucormycosis following donor leukocyte infusion: successful treatment with liposomal amphotericin B and surgical debridement. *Bone Marrow Transplant.* **22:**817–818.

309. **Penas, P. F., L. Rios, R. de la Camara, J. Fraga, and E. Dauden.** 1995. Cutaneous lesions as the first sign of disseminated mucormycosis. *Acta Derm. Venereol.* **75:**166–167.

310. **Peterson, K. L., M. Wang, R. F. Canalis, and E. Abemayor.** 1997. Rhinocerebral mucormycosis: evolution of the disease and treatment options. *Laryngoscope* **107:**855–862.

311. **Pfaller, M. A., F. Marco, S. A. Messer, and R. N. Jones.** 1998. In vitro activity of two echinocandin derivatives, LY303366 and MK-0991 (L-743,792), against clinical isolates of *Aspergillus, Fusarium, Rhizopus,* and other filamentous fungi. *Diagn. Microbiol. Infect. Dis.* **30:**251–255.

312. **Pickeral, J. J., III, J. F. Silverman, and C. D. Sturgis.** 2000. Gastric zygomycosis diagnosed by brushing cytology. *Diagn. Cytopathol.* **23:**51–54.

313. **Pickles, R., G. Long, and R. Murugasu.** 1994. Isolated renal mucormycosis. *Med. J. Aust.* **160:**514–516.

314. **Pierce, P. F., Jr., S. L. Solomon, L. Kaufman, V. F. Garagusi, R. H. Parker, and L. Ajello.** 1982. Zygomycetes brain abscesses in narcotic addicts with serological diagnosis. *JAMA* **248:**2881–2882.

315. **Pierce, P. F., M. B. Wood, G. D. Roberts, R. H. Fitzgerald, Jr., C. Robertson, and R. S. Edson.** 1987. *Saksenaea vasiformis* osteomyelitis. *J. Clin. Microbiol.* **25:**933–935.

316. **Porter, J. B., R. C. Hider, and E. R. Huehns.** 1990. Update on the hydroxypyridinone oral iron-chelating agents. *Semin. Hematol.* **27:**95–100.

317. **Potvliege, C., F. Crokaert, L. Hooghe, and A. De Mey.** 1983. Post-traumatic gangrene and systemic mucormycosis. *J. Infect.* **6:**277–278.

318. **Press, G. A., S. M. Weindling, J. R. Hesselink, J. W. Ochi, and J. P. Harris.** 1988. Rhinocerebral mucormycosis: MR manifestations. *J. Comput. Assist. Tomogr.* **12:**744–749.

319. **Prevoo, R. L., T. M. Starink, and P. de Haan.** 1991. Primary cutaneous mucormycosis in a healthy young girl. Report of a case caused by *Mucor hiemalis* Wehmer. *J. Am. Acad. Dermatol.* **24:**882–885.

320. **Price, D. L., E. R. Wolpow, and E. P. Richardson, Jr.** 1971. Intracranial phycomycosis: a clinicopathological and radiological study. *J. Neurol. Sci.* **14:**359–375.

321. **Price, J. C., and D. L. Stevens.** 1980. Hyperbaric oxygen in the treatment of rhinocerebral mucormycosis. *Laryngoscope* **90:**737–747.

322. **Pritchard, R. C., D. B. Muir, K. H. Archer, and J. M. Beith.** 1986. Subcutaneous zygomycosis due to *Saksenaea vasiformis* in an infant. *Med. J. Aust.* **145:**630–631.

323. **Prokopowicz, G. P., S. F. Bradley, and C. A. Kauffman.** 1994. Indolent zygomycosis associated with deferoxamine chelation therapy. *Mycoses* **37:**427–431.

324. **Prout, G. R., Jr., and A. R. Goddard.** 1960. Renal mucormycosis. Survival after nephrectomy and amphotericin B therapy. *N. Engl. J. Med.* **263:**1246–1248.

325. **Pursell, K., S. Verral, F. Daraiesh, N. Shrestha, A. Skariah, E. Hasan, and D. Pitrak.** 2003. Impaired phagocyte respiratory burst responses to opportunistic fungal pathogens in transplant recipients: in vitro effect of r-metHuG-CSF (Filgrastim). *Transpl. Infect. Dis.* **5:**29–37.

326. **Quinio, D., A. Karam, J. P. Leroy, M. C. Moal, B. Bourbigot, O. Masure, B. Sassolas, and A. M. Le Flohic.** 2004. Zygomycosis caused by *Cunninghamella bertholletiae* in a kidney transplant recipient. *Med. Mycol.* **42:**177–180.

327. **Rabin, E. R., G. D. Lundberg, and E. T. Mitchell.** 1961. Mucormycosis in severely burned patients. Report of two cases with extensive destruction of the face and nasal cavity. *N. Engl. J. Med.* **264:**1286–1289.

328. **Rangel-Guerra, R. A., H. R. Martinez, C. Saenz, F. Bosques-Padilla, and I. Estrada-Bellmann.** 1996. Rhinocerebral and systemic mucormycosis. Clinical experience with 36 cases. *J. Neurol. Sci.* **143:**19–30.

329. **Record, N. B., Jr., and D. R. Ginder.** 1976. Pulmonary phycomycosis without obvious predisposing factors. *JAMA* **235:**1256–1257.

330. **Rees, J. R., R. W. Pinner, R. A. Hajjeh, M. E. Brandt, and A. L. Reingold.** 1998. The epidemiological features of invasive mycotic infections in the San Francisco Bay area, 1992–1993: results of population-based laboratory active surveillance. *Clin. Infect. Dis.* **27:**1138–1147.

331. **Reich, J., and A. D. Renzetti, Jr.** 1970. Pulmonary phycomycosis. Report of a case of bronchocutaneous fistula formation and pulmonary arterial mycothrombosis. *Am. Rev. Respir. Dis.* **102:**959–964.

332. **Reimund, E., and A. Ramos.** 1994. Disseminated neonatal gastrointestinal mucormycosis: a case report and review of the literature. *Pediatr. Pathol.* **14:**385–389.

333. **Reinhardt, D. J., I. Licata, W. Kaplan, L. Ajello, F. W. Chandler, and J. J. Ellis.** 1981. Experimental cerebral zygomycosis in alloxan-diabetic rabbits: variation in virulence among zygomycetes. *Sabouraudia* **19:** 245–256.

334. **Ribes, J. A., C. L. Vanover-Sams, and D. J. Baker.** 2000. Zygomycetes in human disease. *Clin. Microbiol. Rev.* **13:**236–301.

335. **Richardson, M. D., and G. S. Shankland.** 1999. *Rhizopus, Rhizomucor, Absidia,* and other agents of systemic and subcutaneous zygomycosis, p. 1242–1258. *In* P. R. Murray, E. J. Baron, M. A. Pfaller, F. C. Tenover, and R. H. Yolken (ed.), *Manual of Clinical Microbiology,* 7th ed. ASM Press, Washington, D.C.

336. **Ridley, L., N. Karunaratne, S. Mann, and T. Solano.** 2000. Cardiac mucormycosis revealed on imaging. *Am. J. Roentgenol.* **174:**1469.

337. **Rinaldi, M. G.** 1989. Zygomycosis. *Infect. Dis. Clin. N. Am.* **3:**19–41.

338. **Rippon, J. W.** 1988. Zygomycosis, p. 681–713, *Medical Mycology: the Pathogenic Fungi and the Pathogenic Actinomycetes,* 3rd ed. WB Saunders Co., Philadelphia, Pa.

339. **Robb, S. M.** 1966. Reactions of fungi to exposure to 10 atmospheres pressure of oxygen. *J. Gen. Microbiol.* **45:**17–29.

340. **Roberts, H. J.** 1962. Cutaneous mucormycosis. Report of a case with survival. *Arch. Intern. Med.* **110:** 108–112.

341. **Robinson, B. E., M. T. Stark, T. L. Pope, F. M. Stewart, and G. R. Donowitz.** 1990. *Cunninghamella bertholletiae*: an unusual agent of zygomycosis. *South. Med. J.* **83:**1088–1091.

342. **Roden, M. M., T. E. Zaoutis, W. L. Buchanan, T. A. Knudsen, T. A. Sarkisova, R. L. Schaufele, M. Sein, T. Sein, C. C. Chiou, J. H. Chu, D. P. Kontoyiannis, and T. J. Walsh.** 2005. Epidemiology and outcome of zygomycosis: a review of 929 reported cases. *Clin. Infect. Dis.* **41:**634–653.

343. **Roilides, E., and P. A. Pizzo.** 1993. Biologicals and hematopoietic cytokines in prevention or treatment of infections in immunocompromised hosts. *Hematol. Oncol. Clin. N. Am.* **7:**841–864.

344. **Roilides, E., K. Uhlig, D. Venzon, P. A. Pizzo, and T. J. Walsh.** 1993. Enhancement of oxidative response and damage caused by human neutrophils to *Aspergillus fumigatus* hyphae by granulocyte colony-stimulating factor and gamma interferon. *Infect. Immun.* **61:**1185–1193.

345. **Romani, L.** 2004. Immunity to fungal infections. *Nat. Rev. Immunol.* **4:**1–23.

346. **Rozich, J., H. P. Holley, Jr., F. Henderson, J. Gardner, and F. Nelson.** 1988. Cauda equina syndrome secondary to disseminated zygomycosis. *JAMA* **260:**3638–3640.

347. **Sahin, B., S. Paydas, E. Cosar, K. Bicakci, and B. Hazar.** 1996. Role of granulocyte colony-stimulating factor in the treatment of mucormycosis. *Eur. J. Clin. Microbiol. Infect. Dis.* **15:**866–869.

348. **Saltoglu, N., Y. Tasova, S. Zorludemir, and I. H. Dundar.** 1998. Rhinocerebral zygomycosis treated with liposomal amphotericin B and surgery. *Mycoses* **41:**45–49.

349. **Sanchez, M. R., I. Ponge-Wilson, J. A. Moy, and S. Rosenthal.** 1994. Zygomycosis and HIV infection. *J. Am. Acad. Dermatol.* **30:**904–908.

350. **Sanchez-Recalde, A., J. L. Merino, F. Dominguez, I. Mate, J. L. Larrea, and J. A. Sobrino.** 1999. Successful treatment of prosthetic aortic valve mucormycosis. *Chest* **116:**1818–1820.

351. **Sands, J. M., A. M. Macher, T. J. Ley, and A. W. Nienhuis.** 1985. Disseminated infection caused by *Cunninghamella bertholletiae* in a patient with beta-thalassemia. Case report and review of the literature. *Ann. Intern. Med.* **102:**59–63.

352. **Santos, J., P. Espigado, C. Romero, J. Andreu, A. Rivero, and J. A. Pineda.** 1994. Isolated renal mucormycosis in two AIDS patients. *Eur. J. Clin. Microbiol. Infect. Dis.* **13:**430–432.

353. **Scalise, A., F. Barchiesi, M. A. Viviani, D. Arzeni, A. Bertani, and G. Scalise.** 1999. Infection due to *Absidia corymbifera* in a patient with a massive crush trauma of the foot. *J. Infect.* **38:**191–192.

354. **Scheld, W. M., D. Royston, S. A. Harding, C. E. Hess, and M. A. Sande.** 1979. Simultaneous disseminated aspergillosis and zygomycosis in a leukemic patient. *South. Med. J.* **72:**1325–1328.

355. **Schmidt, J. H., R. J. Howard, J. L. Chen, and K. K. Pierson.** 1986. First culture-proven gastrointestinal entermophthoromycosis in the United States: a case report and review of the literature. *Mycopathologia* **95:**101–104.

356. **Schmidt, J. M., and R. M. Poublon.** 1998. Rhinocerebral mycosis in immunocompromised patients. A case report and review of the literature. *Rhinology* **36:**90–93.

357. **Schwartz, J. R., M. G. Nagle, R. C. Elkins, and J. A. Mohr.** 1982. Mucormycosis of the trachea: an unusual cause of acute upper airway obstruction. *Chest* **81:**653–654.

358. **Severo, L. C., F. Job, and T. C. Mattos.** 1991. Systemic zygomycosis: nosocomial infection by *Rhizomucor pusillus*. *Mycopathologia* **113:**79–80.

359. **Shah, P. D., K. R. Peters, and P. D. Reuman.** 1997. Recovery from rhinocerebral mucormycosis with carotid artery occlusion: a pediatric case and review of the literature. *Pediatr. Infect. Dis. J.* **16:**68–71.

360. **Sheldon, D. L., and W. C. Johnson.** 1979. Cutaneous mucormycosis. Two documented cases of suspected nosocomial cause. *JAMA* **241:**1032–1034.

361. **Sheldon, W. H., and H. Bauer.** 1959. The development of the acute inflammatory response to experimental cutaneous mucormycosis in normal and diabetic rabbits. *J. Exp. Med.* **110:**845–852.

362. **Shoham, S., and S. M. Levitz.** 2005. The immune response to fungal infections. *Br. J. Haematol.* **129:**569–582.

363. **Singh, J., D. Rimek, and R. Kappe.** 2005. In vitro susceptibility of 15 strains of zygomycetes to nine antifungal agents as determined by the NCCLS M38-A microdilution method. *Mycoses* **48:**246–250.

364. **Singh, N., T. Gayowski, J. Singh, and V. L. Yu.** 1995. Invasive gastrointestinal zygomycosis in a liver transplant recipient: case report and review of zygomycosis in solid-organ transplant recipients. *Clin. Infect. Dis.* **20:**617–620.

365. **Siwek, G. T., K. J. Dodgson, M. de Magalhaes-Silverman, L. A. Bartelt, S. B. Kilborn, P. L. Hoth, D. J. Diekema, and M. A. Pfaller.** 2004. Invasive zygomycosis in hematopoietic stem cell transplant recipients receiving voriconazole prophylaxis. *Clin. Infect. Dis.* **39:**584–587.

366. **Slavin, M. A., B. Osborne, R. Adams, M. J. Levenstein, H. G. Schoch, A. R. Feldman, J. D. Meyers, and R. A. Bowden.** 1995. Efficacy and safety of fluconazole prophylaxis for fungal infections after marrow transplantation—a prospective, randomized, double-blind study. *J. Infect. Dis.* **171:**1545–1552.

367. **Smith, A. G., C. I. Bustamante, and G. D. Gilmor.** 1989. Zygomycosis (absidiomycosis) in an AIDS patient. Absidiomycosis in AIDS. *Mycopathologia* **105:**7–10.

368. **Smith, J. L., and D. A. Stevens.** 1986. Survival in cerebro-rhino-orbital zygomycosis and cavernous sinus thrombosis with combined therapy. *South. Med. J.* **79:**501–504.

369. **Smith, P. D., C. L. Lamerson, S. M. Banks, S. S. Saini, L. M. Wahl, R. A. Calderone, and S. M. Wahl.** 1990. Granulocyte-macrophage colony-stimulating factor augments human monocyte fungicidal activity for *Candida albicans*. *J. Infect. Dis.* **161:**999–1005.

370. **Smitherman, K. O., and J. E. Peacock, Jr.** 1995. Infectious emergencies in patients with diabetes mellitus. *Med. Clin. N. Am.* **79:**53–77.

371. **Solano, T., B. Atkins, E. Tambosis, S. Mann, and T. Gottlieb.** 2000. Disseminated mucormycosis due to *Saksenaea vasiformis* in an immunocompetent adult. *Clin. Infect. Dis.* **30:**942–943.

372. **Soloniuk, D. S., and D. B. Moreland.** 1988. Rhinocerebral mucormycosis with extension to the posterior fossa: case report. *Neurosurgery* **23:**641–643.

373. **Sondhi, J., and P. P. Gupta.** 2000. Effect of immunosuppression on the clinicopathological changes in experimental zygomycosis in rabbits. *Vet. Res. Commun.* **24:**213–227.

374. **Spellberg, B., Y. Fu, J. E. Edwards, Jr., and A. S. Ibrahim.** 2005. Combination therapy with amphotericin B lipid complex and caspofungin acetate of disseminated zygomycosis in diabetic ketoacidotic mice. *Antimicrob. Agents Chemother.* **49:**830–832.

375. **Stein, A., and A. Schmaman.** 1965. Rupture of the stomach due to mucormycosis. *S. Afr. J. Surg.* **3:**123–129.

376. **St-Germain, G., A. Robert, M. Ishak, C. Tremblay, and S. Claveau.** 1993. Infection due to *Rhizomucor pusillus*: report of four cases in patients with leukemia and review. *Clin. Infect. Dis.* **16:**640–645.

377. **St-Germain, G., and R. Summerbel.** 1996. Descriptions, p. 51–242. *In* G. St-Germain and R. Summerbel (ed.), *Identifying Filamentous Fungi: a Clinical Laboratory Handbook.* Star Publishing Co., Belmont, Calif.

378. **Strasser, M. D., R. J. Kennedy, and R. D. Adam.** 1996. Rhinocerebral mucormycosis. Therapy with amphotericin B lipid complex. *Arch. Intern. Med.* **156:**337–339.

379. **Studemeister, A. E., K. Kozak, E. Garrity, and F. R. Venezio.** 1988. Survival of a heart transplant recipient after pulmonary cavitary mucormycosis. *J. Heart Transplant.* **7:**159–161.

380. **Sugar, A. M.** 2000. Agents of mucormycosis and related species, p. 2685–2695. *In* G. L. Mandell, J. E. Bennett, and R. Dolin (ed.), *Principles and Practice of Infectious Diseases*, 5th ed. Churchil Livingstone, Philadelphia, Pa.
381. **Sugar, A. M.** 1992. Mucormycosis. *Clin. Infect. Dis.* **14**(Suppl. 1):S126–S129.
382. **Sun, Q. N., A. W. Fothergill, D. I. McCarthy, M. G. Rinaldi, and J. R. Graybill.** 2002. In vitro activities of posaconazole, itraconazole, voriconazole, amphotericin B, and fluconazole against 37 clinical isolates of zygomycetes. *Antimicrob. Agents Chemother.* **46**:1581–1582.
383. **Sun, Q. N., L. K. Najvar, R. Bocanegra, D. Loebenberg, and J. R. Graybill.** 2002. In vivo activity of posaconazole against *Mucor* spp. in an immunosuppressed-mouse model. *Antimicrob. Agents Chemother.* **46**:2310–2312.
384. **Tang, D., and W. Wang.** 1998. Successful cure of an extensive burn injury complicated with mucor wound sepsis. *Burns* **24**:72–73.
385. **Tanphaichitr, V. S., A. Chaiprasert, V. Suvatte, and P. Thasnakorn.** 1990. Subcutaneous mucormycosis caused by *Saksenaea vasiformis* in a thalassaemic child: first case report in Thailand. *Mycoses* **33**:303–309.
386. **Tedder, M., J. A. Spratt, M. P. Anstadt, S. S. Hegde, S. D. Tedder, and J. E. Lowe.** 1994. Pulmonary mucormycosis: results of medical and surgical therapy. *Ann. Thorac. Surg.* **57**:1044–1050.
387. **ter Borg, F., E. J. Kuijper, and H. van der Lelie.** 1990. Fatal mucormycosis presenting as an appendiceal mass with metastatic spread to the liver during chemotherapy-induced granulocytopenia. *Scand. J. Infect. Dis.* **22**:499–501.
388. **Terk, M. R., D. J. Underwood, C. S. Zee, and P. M. Colletti.** 1992. MR imaging in rhinocerebral and intracranial mucormycosis with CT and pathologic correlation. *Magn. Reson. Imaging* **10**:81–87.
389. **Tobon, A. M., M. Arango, D. Fernandez, and A. Restrepo.** 2003. Mucormycosis (zygomycosis) in a heart-kidney transplant recipient: recovery after posaconazole therapy. *Clin. Infect. Dis.* **36**:1488–1491.
390. **Torres-Rodriguez, J. M., M. Lowinger, J. M. Cerominas, N. Madrenys, and P. Saballs.** 1993. Renal infection due to *Absidia corymbifera* in an AIDS patient. *Mycoses* **36**:255–258.
391. **Tsaousis, G., A. Koutsouri, C. Gatsiou, O. Paniara, C. Peppas, and G. Chalevelakis.** 2000. Liver and brain mucormycosis in a diabetic patient type II successfully treated with liposomial amphotericin B. *Scand. J. Infect. Dis.* **32**:335–337.
392. **Vainrub, B., A. Macareno, S. Mandel, and D. M. Musher.** 1988. Wound zygomycosis (mucormycosis) in otherwise healthy adults. *Am. J. Med.* **84**:546–548.
393. **Van Cutsem, J., F. Van Gerven, J. Fransen, and P. A. Janssen.** 1989. Treatment of experimental zygomycosis in guinea pigs with azoles and with amphotericin B. *Chemotherapy* **35**:267–272.
394. **Van Johnson, E., L. B. Kline, B. A. Julian, and J. H. Garcia.** 1988. Bilateral cavernous sinus thrombosis due to mucormycosis. *Arch. Ophthalmol.* **106**:1089–1092.
395. **Veliath, A. J., R. Rao, M. R. Prabhu, and A. L. Aurora.** 1976. Cutaneous phycomycosis (mucormycosis) with fatal pulmonary dissemination. *Arch. Dermatol.* **112**:509–512.
396. **Ventura, G. J., H. M. Kantarjian, E. Anaissie, R. L. Hopfer, and V. Fainstein.** 1986. Pneumonia with *Cunninghamella* species in patients with hematologic malignancies. A case report and review of the literature. *Cancer* **58**:1534–1536.
397. **Verweij, P. E., A. Voss, J. P. Donnelly, B. E. de Pauw, and J. F. Meis.** 1997. Wooden sticks as the source of a pseudoepidemic of infection with *Rhizopus microsporus* var. *rhizopodiformis* among immunocompromised patients. *J. Clin. Microbiol.* **35**:2422–2423.
398. **Vesa, J., O. Bielsa, O. Arango, C. Llado, and A. Gelabert.** 1992. Massive renal infarction due to mucormycosis in an AIDS patient. *Infection* **20**:234–236.
399. **Vessely, M. B., R. P. Zitsch III, S. A. Estrem, and G. Renner.** 1996. Atypical presentations of mucormycosis in the head and neck. *Otolaryngol. Head Neck Surg.* **115**:573–577.
400. **Vigouroux, S., O. Morin, P. Moreau, F. Mechinaud, N. Morineau, B. Mahe, P. Chevallier, T. Guillaume, V. Dubruille, J. L. Harousseau, and N. Milpied.** 2005. Zygomycosis after prolonged use of voriconazole in immunocompromised patients with hematologic disease: attention required. *Clin. Infect. Dis.* **40**:e35–e37.
401. **Virmani, R., D. H. Connor, and H. A. McAllister.** 1982. Cardiac mucormycosis. A report of five patients and review of 14 previously reported cases. *Am. J. Clin. Pathol.* **78**:42–47.
402. **Waldorf, A. R., S. M. Levitz, and R. D. Diamond.** 1984. In vivo bronchoalveolar macrophage defense against *Rhizopus oryzae* and *Aspergillus fumigatus*. *J. Infect. Dis.* **150**:752–760.

403. **Waldorf, A. R., N. Ruderman, and R. D. Diamond.** 1984. Specific susceptibility to mucormycosis in murine diabetes and bronchoalveolar macrophage defense against *Rhizopus. J. Clin. Invest.* **74:**150–160.

404. **Walker, S. D., R. V. Clark, C. T. King, J. E. Humphries, L. S. Lytle, and D. E. Butkus.** 1992. Fatal disseminated *Conidiobolus coronatus* infection in a renal transplant patient. *Am. J. Clin. Pathol.* **98:** 559–564.

405. **Walsh, T. J., R. W. Finberg, C. Arndt, J. Hiemenz, C. Schwartz, D. Bodensteiner, P. Pappas, N. Seibel, R. N. Greenberg, S. Dummer, M. Schuster, J. S. Holcenberg, et al.** 1999. Liposomal amphotericin B for empirical therapy in patients with persistent fever and neutropenia. *N. Engl. J. Med.* **340:**764–771.

406. **Walsh, T. J., J. L. Goodman, P. Pappas, I. Bekersky, D. N. Buell, M. Roden, J. Barrett, and E. J. Anaissie.** 2001. Safety, tolerance, and pharmacokinetics of high-dose liposomal amphotericin B (AmBisome) in patients infected with *Aspergillus* species and other filamentous fungi: maximum tolerated dose study. *Antimicrob. Agents Chemother.* **45:**3487–3496.

407. **Walsh, T. J., J. W. Hiemenz, N. L. Seibel, J. R. Perfect, G. Horwith, L. Lee, J. L. Silber, M. J. DiNubile, A. Reboli, E. Bow, J. Lister, and E. J. Anaissie.** 1998. Amphotericin B lipid complex for invasive fungal infections: analysis of safety and efficacy in 556 cases. *Clin. Infect. Dis.* **26:**1383–1396.

408. **Walsh, T. J., G. M. Hutchins, B. H. Bulkley, and G. Mendelsohn.** 1980. Fungal infections of the heart: analysis of 51 autopsy cases. *Am. J. Cardiol.* **45:**357–366.

409. **Walsh, T. J., and P. A. Pizzo.** 1988. Nosocomial fungal infections: a classification for hospital-acquired fungal infections and mycoses arising from endogenous flora or reactivation. *Annu. Rev. Microbiol.* **42:** 517–545.

410. **Walsh, T. J., G. Renshaw, J. Andrews, J. Kwon-Chung, R. C. Cunnion, H. I. Pass, J. Taubenberger, W. Wilson, and P. A. Pizzo.** 1994. Invasive zygomycosis due to *Conidiobolus incongruus. Clin. Infect. Dis.* **19:**423–430.

411. **Walsh, T. J., M. R. Rinaldi, and P. A. Pizzo.** 1993. Zygomycosis of the respiratory tract, p. 149–170. *In* G. A. Sarosi and S. F. Davies (ed.), *Fungal Diseases of the Lung*, 2nd ed. Raven Press, Ltd., New York, N.Y.

412. **Watson, K. C.** 1957. Gastric perforation due to the fungus *Mucor* in a child with kwashiorkor. *S. Afr. Med. J.* **31:**99–101.

413. **Watson, K. C., and P. B. Neame.** 1960. In vitro activity of amphotericin B on strains of mucorales pathogenic to man. *J. Lab. Clin. Med.* **56:**251–257.

414. **Watts, W. J.** 1983. Bronchopleural fistula followed by massive fatal hemoptysis in a patient with pulmonary mucormycosis. A case report. *Arch. Intern. Med.* **143:**1029–1030.

415. **Weng, D. E., W. H. Wilson, R. Little, and T. J. Walsh.** 1998. Successful medical management of isolated renal zygomycosis: case report and review. *Clin. Infect. Dis.* **26:**601–605.

416. **Weprin, B. E., W. A. Hall, J. Goodman, and G. L. Adams.** 1998. Long-term survival in rhinocerebral mucormycosis. Case report. *J. Neurosurg.* **88:**570–575.

417. **West, B. C., K. J. Kwon-Chung, J. W. King, W. D. Grafton, and M. S. Rohr.** 1983. Inguinal abscess caused by *Rhizopus rhizopodiformis*: successful treatment with surgery and amphotericin B. *J. Clin. Microbiol.* **18:**1384–1387.

418. **West, B. C., A. D. Oberle, and K. J. Kwon-Chung.** 1995. Mucormycosis caused by *Rhizopus microsporus* var. *microsporus*: cellulitis in the leg of a diabetic patient cured by amputation. *J. Clin. Microbiol.* **33:** 3341–3344.

419. **White, C. B., P. J. Barcia, and J. W. Bass.** 1986. Neonatal zygomycotic necrotizing cellulitis. *Pediatrics* **78:**100–102.

420. **Wickline, C. L., T. G. Cornitius, and T. Butler.** 1989. Cellulitis caused by *Rhizomucor pusillus* in a diabetic patient receiving continuous insulin infusion pump therapy. *South. Med. J.* **82:**1432–1434.

421. **Williams, D., M. Yungbluth, G. Adams, and J. Glassroth.** 1985. The role of fiberoptic bronchoscopy in the evaluation of immunocompromised hosts with diffuse pulmonary infiltrates. *Am. Rev. Respir. Dis.* **131:** 880–885.

422. **Williams, J. C., A. R. Schned, J. R. Richardson, J. A. Heaney, M. R. Curtis, I. P. Rupp, and C. F. von Reyn.** 1995. Fatal genitourinary mucormycosis in a patient with undiagnosed diabetes. *Clin. Infect. Dis.* **21:**682–684.

423. **Wilson, C. B., G. R. Siber, T. F. O'Brien, and A. P. Morgan.** 1976. Phycomycotic gangrenous cellulitis. A report of two cases and a review of the literature. *Arch. Surg.* **111:**532–538.

424. **Wimander, K., and L. Belin.** 1980. Recognition of allergic alveolitis in the trimming department of a Swedish sawmill. *Eur. J. Respir. Dis. Suppl.* **107:**163–167.

425. **Winkler, S., S. Susani, B. Willinger, R. Apsner, A. R. Rosenkranz, R. Potzi, G. A. Berlakovich, and E. Pohanka.** 1996. Gastric mucormycosis due to *Rhizopus oryzae* in a renal transplant recipient. *J. Clin. Microbiol.* **34:**2585–2587.

426. **Winston, D. J., R. T. Maziarz, P. H. Chandrasekar, H. M. Lazarus, M. Goldman, J. L. Blumer, G. J. Leitz, and M. C. Territo.** 2003. Intravenous and oral itraconazole versus intravenous and oral fluconazole for long-term antifungal prophylaxis in allogeneic hematopoietic stem-cell transplant recipients. A multi-center, randomized trial. *Ann. Intern. Med.* **138:**705–713.

427. **Winston, D. J., and G. J. Schiller.** 2000. Controlled trials of amphotericin B lipid complex and other lipid-associated formulations. *Clin. Infect. Dis.* **30:**236–237.

428. **Wirth, F., R. Perry, A. Eskenazi, R. Schwalbe, and G. Kao.** 1997. Cutaneous mucormycosis with subsequent visceral dissemination in a child with neutropenia: a case report and review of the pediatric literature. *J. Am. Acad. Dermatol.* **36:**336–341.

429. **Wong, K. L., Y. T. Tai, S. L. Loke, E. K. Woo, W. S. Wong, M. K. Chan, and J. T. Ma.** 1986. Disseminated zygomycosis masquerading as cerebral lupus erythematosus. *Am. J. Clin. Pathol.* **86:**546–549.

430. **Woods, K. F., and B. J. Hanna.** 1986. Brain stem mucormycosis in a narcotic addict with eventual recovery. *Am. J. Med.* **80:**126–128.

431. **Wright, D. G., K. J. Robichaud, P. A. Pizzo, and A. B. Deisseroth.** 1981. Lethal pulmonary reactions associated with the combined use of amphotericin B and leukocyte transfusions. *N. Engl. J. Med.* **304:**1185–1189.

432. **Wu, C. L., W. H. Hsu, C. M. Huang, and C. D. Chiang.** 2000. Indolent cutaneous mucormycosis with pulmonary dissemination in an asthmatic patient: survival after local debridement and amphotericin B therapy. *J. Formos. Med. Assoc.* **99:**354–357.

433. **Yohai, R. A., J. D. Bullock, A. A. Aziz, and R. J. Markert.** 1994. Survival factors in rhino-orbital-cerebral mucormycosis. *Surv. Ophthalmol.* **39:**3–22.

434. **Yoshida, T., S. Nakamura, S. Ohtake, K. Okafuji, K. Kobayashi, K. Kondo, M. Kanno, S. Matano, T. Matsuda, M. Kanai, et al.** 1990. Effect of granulocyte colony-stimulating factor on neutropenia due to chemotherapy for non-Hodgkin's lymphoma. *Cancer* **66:**1904–1909.

435. **Zarei, M., J. Morris, V. Aachi, R. Gregory, C. Meanock, and F. Brito-Babapulle.** 2000. Acute isolated cerebral mucormycosis in a patient with high grade non-Hodgkins lymphoma. *Eur. J. Neurol.* **7:**443–447.

Emerging Infections 7
Edited by W. M. Scheld, D. C. Hooper, and J. M. Hughes
© 2007 ASM Press, Washington, D.C.

Chapter 15

Emerging Food- and Waterborne Protozoan Diseases

*Michael J. Arrowood, Ynes R. Ortega,
Lihua X. Xiao, and Ronald Fayer*

INTRODUCTION

In the past decade, the number of food-borne and waterborne disease outbreaks has increased significantly in the United States. This may be related to changes in the food supply and water sanitation systems and new parasite-diagnostic methodologies that are more specific and sensitive.

This chapter describes the most relevant features of protozoan agents of food- and waterborne disease, specifically, *Cryptosporidium* and *Cyclospora*, which cause diarrheal illness in humans, and *Toxoplasma*, which is associated with encephalitis, chorioretinitis, and abortion. *Cyclospora* has been associated more frequently with food-borne outbreaks, particularly with ingestion of imported raspberries, lettuce, and basil. *Cryptosporidium* has been associated with prepared foods, but it is more commonly recognized in various large waterborne outbreaks. *Toxoplasma* is a parasite that is present worldwide, and it can infect almost all warm-blooded animals, including humans. The seroprevalence of this parasite can vary from 35 to 80% in selected populations and geographical areas. However, waterborne outbreaks of toxoplasmosis involving a large number of individuals presenting with acute toxoplasmosis have been reported. These three parasites belong to the phylum Apicomplexa (with an apical complex generally consisting of a polar ring, micronemes, rhoptries, and subpellicular microtubules), class Sporozoasida, subclass Coccidiasina, order Eucoccidiorida (merogony present), and suborder Eimeriorina (macro- and microgametes develop independently).

Michael J. Arrowood and Lihua X. Xiao • Division of Parasitic Diseases, National Center for Infectious Diseases, Centers for Disease Control and Prevention, U.S. Department of Health and Human Services, Atlanta, GA 30341. *Ynes R. Ortega* • Center for Food Safety and Quality Enhancement, University of Georgia, 1109 Experiment Street, Griffin, GA 30223. *Ronald Fayer* • Environmental Microbial Safety Laboratory, Animal and Natural Resources Institute, Agricultural Research Service, U.S. Department of Agriculture, Beltsville, MD 20705.

Cryptosporidium

Cryptosporidium belongs to the family Cryptosporidiidae (62). The life cycle of *Cryptosporidium* spp. initiates when a susceptible host ingests oocysts in contaminated water or food. These oocysts excyst in the digestive tract, and sporozoites are released. The invasive sporozoites preferentially infect the epithelial cells of the ileum. Asexual multiplication (merogony) produces type I and II meronts, which contain eight or four merozoites, respectively. Asexual multiplication can continue repeatedly or differentiate into the sexual-stage male- and female-specific gamonts (gametogony). The microgametocyte fertilizes the macrogametocyte, and the product of this fertilization is a zygote, which upon maturation will form the oocyst. Two types of oocysts are produced: thin-walled oocysts that may autoinfect the host, and thick-walled oocysts, which upon excretion in the feces are immediately infectious. These oocysts can remain viable for an extended period in the environment until another susceptible host ingests them and the life cycle begins again (63, 222).

The parasite is contained in a parasitophorous vacuole within the host cell, a location considered intracellular but extracytoplasmic. A unique characteristic of *Cryptosporidium* is the presence of a feeding organelle at the junction between the parasite and the host cell. This organelle is thought to selectively control the uptake of nutrients to the parasitic vacuole and may play a role in conferring resistance to drug therapy. Recent studies suggest that this drug resistance may also be related to the absence of de novo pyrimidine synthesis by the parasite, which is compensated for by three salvage enzymes. Two of these salvage enzymes (uridine kinase-uracil phosphoribosyltransferase and thymidine kinase) are unique in *Cryptosporidium* (197).

There are 15 recognized species of *Cryptosporidium* in fish, reptiles, birds, and mammals. *Cryptosporidium hominis* (previously known as *Cryptosporidium parvum* genotype 1, the "human" or anthroponotic genotype) (167) and *C. parvum* are the species that most commonly infect humans. *Cryptosporidium meleagridis* (of birds), *Cryptosporidium felis* (of cats), and *Cryptosporidium canis* (of dogs) have also been identified in humans. *Cryptosporidium muris*, *Cryptosporidium suis*, and the *Cryptosporidium* cervine genotype have rarely been found in humans (216–218). Recent studies suggested that *Cryptosporidium* may fit better in the gregarine group of parasites than with the coccidian parasites (53, 109), but a more extensive DNA sequence study did not reinforce this hypothesis (136). Studies are under way to further clarify the taxonomy of *Cryptosporidium*.

Cyclospora

Cyclospora belongs to the family Eimeriidae (172). The life cycle of *Cyclospora* spp. initiates when a susceptible host ingests oocysts (or possibly free sporocysts) in contaminated water or food. Sporocysts released from sporulated oocysts excyst in the gut to release sporozoites that infect cells of the intestinal epithelium. Information obtained from biopsies of infected individuals suggests that the ileum is preferentially colonized. Asexual multiplication (merogony) occurs within the vertebrate host, and subsequent sexual multiplication (gametogony) occurs. Upon gamete fertilization, immature oocysts are formed and excreted into the environment in the feces of the infected individual. Approximately 7 to 15 days are required for the oocysts to differentiate and mature, forming two sporocysts, each with two potentially infectious sporozoites (173). Molecular phylogenetic studies using the 18S ribosomal DNA demonstrated that *Cyclospora cayetanensis* is most closely related to *Eimeria* species (184).

There are 14 additional morphologically different species of *Cyclospora* that infect insectivores, rodents, and snakes. Three *Cyclospora* species that are morphologically similar to *C. cayetanensis*, but phylogenetically different, have been described as infecting nonhuman primates (80). *Cyclospora cayetanensis* seems to be exclusively anthroponotic (infecting humans) (81).

Toxoplasma

Toxoplasma belongs to the family Sarcocystidae, subfamily Toxoplasmatinae. *Toxoplasma* can infect a large variety of animals. It infects felines (definitive host) and nearly any warm-blooded animal (intermediary hosts). Cats excrete environmentally resistant oocysts in their feces. A susceptible host acquires the infection by ingestion of contaminated food or water containing oocysts, by ingestion of animal tissues containing cystic forms (bradyzoites), or by congenital transfer during gestation (74).

Immature oocysts excreted in feces require 24 h outside the host to differentiate and become infectious. When an intermediate host ingests oocysts, the oocyst and sporocyst walls rupture, releasing the sporozoites, which then invade epithelial cells and rapidly multiply asexually, producing tachyzoites. Tachyzoites multiply by endodyogeny (daughter cells are produced by "internal budding" within a mother cell). Eventually, the tachyzoites encyst in the brain, liver, skeletal muscle, and cardiac muscle. These cysts contain bradyzoites, which are slowly multiplying forms. The cysts persist for the duration of the life of the host.

When animal tissues containing cysts are ingested by felines, proteolytic enzymes digest the cyst wall, and the bradyzoites are released. The bradyzoites infect and multiply in the intestinal epithelial cells, transforming into tachyzoites, and disperse via blood and lymph. The enteroepithelial cycle initiates, and gametocytes are produced. Sexual multiplication occurs when the microgametocyte fertilizes the macrogametocyte, forming the zygote, which later differentiates into an oocyst. Unsporulated oocysts are then excreted in the feces (77).

Three major genotypes of *Toxoplasma gondii* have been identified: I, II, and III (117). Other strains have been described as recombinant and are closely related to the dominant types, particularly I and III, and are exotic. The association between these genotypes and the clinical presentation is still being investigated. In humans, type II predominates in AIDS and congenital infections (encephalitis, pneumonitis, or disseminated infections) and in about 75 to 80% of AIDS and non-AIDS immunocompromised patients. In Spain, however, it appears that genotype I is more prevalent in congenital infections (90). Type I or IV or novel types have been identified in adults with severe chorioretinitis, which is a common sequela of congenital toxoplasmosis, but can remain dormant for years (138). Infections with type I strains are characterized by severe ocular toxoplasmosis and have been described in waterborne outbreaks in Canada and Brazil (47).

CLINICAL PRESENTATION AND EPIDEMIOLOGY

Prevalence, Geographic Distribution, and Demographics

In developing countries, human cryptosporidiosis and cyclosporiasis occur most frequently in children. The peak age-associated occurrence differs between *Cryptosporidium* and *Cyclospora*. *Cryptosporidium* has the highest prevalence in children less than 2 years of age (42–44, 154, 170), whereas *Cyclospora* has relatively constant infection rates among children 1 to 9 years of age (42–44, 154, 170). In South America, *Cyclospora* has the highest prevalence in warm months, whereas *Cryptosporidium* peaks during the rainy season (42, 43).

In developed countries, children tend to acquire *Cryptosporidium* infections later in life than in developing countries, probably due to more limited exposure to contaminated environments, a result of better sanitation and hygiene (198). Children in developed countries frequently acquire *Cryptosporidium* infection from another infected child attending the same day care or school (2, 135, 200, 201). Cryptosporidiosis is also common in elderly individuals attending nursing homes, where person-to-person transmission probably also plays a major role in the spread of *Cryptosporidium* infections (169). In rural areas, zoonotic infections acquired via direct or indirect contact with farm animals have been reported many times, but the relative importance of direct zoonotic transmission of cryptosporidiosis is not entirely clear (64, 162). The prevalence of sporadic, non-outbreak-associated *Cyclospora* infections in the general population is generally low in developed nations. A substantial number of adults in these areas are probably susceptible to both *Cryptosporidium* and *Cyclospora* infections, as sporadic *Cryptosporidium* infections occur in all age groups in the United States and the United Kingdom, and traveling to developing countries and consumption of contaminated food or water can frequently lead to the occurrence of cryptosporidiosis and cyclosporiasis (69, 70, 94, 124, 190). While *Cryptosporidium* is common worldwide, endemic *Cyclospora* may be restricted to those communities that lack adequate water treatment (e.g., filtration) and sanitation (sewage treatment). The delay required for *Cyclospora* oocyst maturation makes it vulnerable to treatment processes (primarily removal or inactivation), but in their absence, it can lead to contamination of water supplies and, consequently, agricultural products.

Hemodialysis patients with chronic renal failure are also frequently infected with *Cryptosporidium* and *Cyclospora* (1, 58, 206, 207).

The prevalence of *T. gondii* infection varies geographically and increases with age. In the United States and the United Kingdom, it is estimated that 16 to 40% of the population become infected, whereas in Central and South America and continental Europe, infection estimates reach 50 to 80% (73, 165).

Diseases and Clinical Presentations

In children, frequent symptoms of both cryptosporidiosis and cyclosporiasis include diarrhea, abdominal cramps, vomiting, headache, fatigue, and low-grade fever (79, 171). The diarrhea can be voluminous and watery for cryptosporidiosis but usually resolves within 1 to 2 weeks without treatment. Not all infected children have diarrhea or other gastrointestinal symptoms, and the occurrence of diarrhea in children with cryptosporidiosis and cyclosporiasis can be as low as 23 to 33% in community-based studies (43, 215). The likelihood of having infection-associated diarrhea decreases with a child's age for *Cryptosporidium* but remains constant for *Cyclospora* (43). Even subclinical cryptosporidiosis exerts a significant adverse effect on a child's growth, as infected children with subclinical or no clinical symptoms experience growth faltering, both in weight and in height (55, 56, 123). The growth retardation observed in *Cryptosporidium*-infected children may never be completely compensated for by "catch-up" growth (55, 163). Children can have multiple episodes of cryptosporidiosis and cyclosporiasis, implying that the acquired anti-*Cryptosporidium* or anti-*Cyclospora* immunity in children is short-lived or incomplete (42, 43, 170, 215). Nevertheless, the association of these infections with diarrhea decreases with each episode of infection with both parasites (43). Cryptosporidiosis has been associated with increased child mortality in developing countries (205).

Unlike in developing countries, immunocompetent persons with sporadic cryptosporidiosis or cyclosporiasis in industrialized nations usually have diarrhea (6, 33, 59, 67, 94, 124, 186, 203). The median number of stools per day during the worst period of *Cryptosporidium* infection is 7 to 9.5 in Australia (186). The duration of illness includes a mean of 12 days in Finland and medians of 9 days in the United Kingdom and 15 to 21 days in Australia (94, 127, 186), with a median 5 days of missed work or study (186). Other common symptoms include abdominal pain (in 72.4 to 91.7% of patients), vomiting (in 55.2 to 70.9% of patients), and low-grade fever (in 38.1 to 48.5% of patients) (94, 127, 186). In the United States, the United Kingdom, and Australia, 14.4 to 17.4%, 8.5 to 22.1%, and 7 to 11.9%, respectively, of patients with sporadic cryptosporidiosis require hospitalization (70, 94, 186).

Cryptosporidiosis is common in immunocompromised persons, such as AIDS patients, persons with primary immunodeficiency, and cancer and transplant patients undergoing immunosuppressive therapy (108, 120, 158). It is frequently associated with chronic, life-threatening diarrhea (87, 108, 120). In human immunodeficiency virus-positive (HIV+) persons, the occurrence of cryptosporidiosis increases as the $CD4^+$ lymphocyte counts fall, especially below 200 cells/ml (87, 168, 180). Manabe and colleagues described four clinical syndromes of cryptosporidiosis in the United States: chronic diarrhea (36% of patients), cholera-like disease (33%), transient diarrhea (15%), and relapsing illness (15%) (152). Sclerosing cholangitis and other biliary involvement, however, are also very common in AIDS patients with cryptosporidiosis (57, 89, 100, 157, 202, 208). Symptoms of cryptosporidiosis in AIDS patients vary in severity, duration, and response to drug treatment (88, 96, 152, 157). Much of this variation can be explained by the degree of immunosuppression (87, 157). In addition, variation in the site of infection (gastric, proximal small intestine, or ileocolonic versus panenteric infection) has been seen in AIDS patients with cryptosporidiosis (60, 130, 146, 209), and this anatomic variation may also contribute to differences in disease severity and survival (60, 146). Cryptosporidiosis in AIDS patients is associated with increased mortality and shortened survival times (61, 152).

Cyclosporiasis is also common in AIDS patients (68, 214). Its clinical presentation is similar to that of cryptosporidiosis (176); however, the median duration for diarrhea is over 3 months (193). Biliary involvement is common in *Cyclospora* infection in AIDS patients. Patients may present with acalculous cholecystitis (193, 221).

Toxoplasmosis can vary from asymptomatic self-limiting infection to fatal disease. In immunocompetent persons, the primary infection normally results in transient cervical or occipital lymphadenopathy associated with "flu-like" symptoms, such as fever, malaise, fatigue, muscle pain, sore throat, and headache. Chorioretinitis is sometimes also seen in primary *Toxoplasma* infection. In immunocompromised patients, reactivated *Toxoplasma* infection often involves the central nervous system, causing diffuse encephalopathy, meningoencephalitis, or cerebral mass lesions. Underlying immunosuppressive conditions associated with toxoplasmosis include various types of malignancies, organ transplants, and HIV infection. Of HIV patients seropositive for *T. gondii*, 27% develop encephalitis, and the median survival time from diagnosis of *Toxoplasma* encephalitis is 9 months (92). Over 50% of AIDS patients with toxoplasmosis have alterations in mental status, motor impairment, seizures, abnormal reflexes, and other neurological symptoms (30). *Toxoplasma* encephalitis is life threatening among AIDS patients (177). Encephalitis occurs in 50% of AIDS patients and in more than 90% of fatal cases. Of these, only 10% present circulating antibodies to *Toxoplasma* (73, 165).

In the United States, approximately 85% of women of childbearing age are susceptible to acute infection with *T. gondii*. Acute infections in pregnant women may cause serious health problems when the organism is transmitted to the fetus (congenital toxoplasmosis), including mental retardation, seizures, blindness, and death of the fetus. Toxoplasmosis is one of the most common causes of primary chorioretinitis in children. Manifestations of congenital toxoplasmosis may not become apparent until the second or third decade of life (128).

Laboratory Detection

Cryptosporidium and *Cyclospora* oocysts are readily detected in clinical (stool) samples using bright-field or fluorescent microscopy (31, 82). *Cryptosporidium* oocysts are mostly 4.5 to 5 μm in diameter, while *Cyclospora* oocysts are approximately 8 to 10 μm in diameter. Modified acid-fast stains are most commonly used, but a hot-safranin staining technique has advantages for *Cyclospora*, since it is variably acid-fast (some oocysts do not stain well or at all) (82). Commercial immunofluorescence assays are available for *Cryptosporidium* detection and are considered the "gold standard" for routine identification. *Cyclospora* oocysts are autofluorescent and are easily identified as bright, blue-white spheres in wet-mount preparations under UV illumination (typically a narrow- or wideband, 340- to 380-nm excitation filter; 400-nm dichroic mirror; 420-nm barrier filter). Oocyst numbers in stool for both parasites may be variable, especially as infections wane, and concentration methods may be of use. The formalin-ethyl acetate sedimentation method is widely used to concentrate and/or reduce background debris before wet-mount or staining methods are used (32). Note that *Cyclospora* oocysts are not sporulated when shed in stool. If stool is collected into buffered formalin, oocysts will be killed before sporulation can occur. To demonstrate sporulation, stool samples are preferentially stored in 2.5% potassium dichromate for 1 to 2 weeks at room temperature. Oocysts will contain two sporocysts, but the number of sporozoites per sporocyst is not easily discerned unless the sporocysts are excysted. Like those of *Cyclospora*, *Toxoplasma* oocysts are highly autofluorescent (10- to 12-μm diameter), but since humans are intermediate hosts, oocysts are not produced in the stool.

Alternatives to microscopical methods are available for *Cryptosporidium*, including commercial enzyme immunoassays (31). Molecular biological methods (e.g., PCR) are available as research tools for all three parasites but are not routinely used in diagnostic laboratories.

Clinical diagnosis of toxoplasmosis is generally accomplished by immunoassay (detection of *Toxoplasma*-reactive antibody in serum) (128, 213). Numerous commercial assays are available for the detection of immunoglobulin G (IgG), IgM, and/or IgA (the last primarily in newborns suspected to have congenital toxoplasmosis).

Treatment

Numerous pharmaceutical compounds have been screened for anti-*Cryptosporidium* activities in vitro or in laboratory animals. Some of those showing promise have been used in the experimental treatment of cryptosporidiosis in humans, but few have been effective in controlled clinical trials (120). Oral or intravenous rehydration is used whenever severe diarrhea is associated with *Cryptosporidium* infection (114). Nitazoxanide (NTZ) is the only FDA-approved drug for the treatment of pediatric cryptosporidiosis. It has also been recently approved for the treatment of giardiasis in adult patients. Clinical trials have demonstrated that NTZ can shorten clinical disease and reduce the parasite load (3, 188). Since most immunocompetent individuals recover from infections without specific drug therapy, it is not always clear that drug therapy contributes to infection resolution. NTZ is not yet approved for the treatment of *Cryptosporidium* infections in immunodeficient people, even though it may be partially effective (71, 189). For this population, paromomycin and spiramycin have been used in the treatment of some patients, but their efficacies remain unproven (107). Thus, rehydration is still the major supportive treatment in AIDS patients (114).

In industrialized nations, the most effective treatment and prophylaxis for cryptosporidiosis in AIDS patients is the use of highly active antiretroviral therapy (HAART) (52, 160). Nonetheless, it is believed that parasite eradication and prevention of infection are directly related to the replenishment of CD4$^+$ cells in treated persons rather than the antiparasitic activities of these drugs (52), even though some of the protease inhibitors used in HAART, such as indinavir, nelfinavir, and ritonavir, have been shown to have anticryptosporidial activities in vitro and in laboratory animals (115, 159). Relapse of cryptosporidiosis is common in AIDS patients who have stopped taking HAART (52, 150).

Both cyclosporiasis and toxoplasmosis can be treated effectively with "sulfa" drugs. Cyclosporiasis is usually treated with a 7-day course of oral trimethoprim-sulfamethoxazole (153). The most common treatment for toxoplasmosis in the United States is the combination of pyrimethamine, sulfadiazine, and folinic acid. Primary toxoplasmosis is usually not treated, but if necessary, can be treated with the drug combination for 4 to 6 weeks. Infection in pregnancy should be treated until term. The treatment duration of congenital toxoplasmosis and infections in immunocompromised persons is typically extended (165).

TRANSMISSION VIA DRINKING WATER

Based on the 3,016 cases of cryptosporidiosis reported in the United States in 2002 and extrapolating from the number of cases reported for salmonellosis, another diarrheal disease for which only 1 to 5% of cases are reported, the annual cryptosporidiosis disease burden in the United States has been estimated to be between 60,320 and 301,000 cases (110). While recognition of *Cryptosporidium* spp. as a cause of gastrointestinal illness continues to increase, the most common intestinal parasite identified by public health laboratories in the United States is *Giardia intestinalis* (syn. *Giardia lamblia* and *Giardia duodenalis*) (111). In comparison to cryptosporidiosis, the total numbers of reported cases of giardiasis were 24,226 for 1998, 19,708 for 2001, and 21,300 for 2002 (111). Although giardiasis cases occur sporadically, outbreaks are well documented. Between 1991 and 2000, *Giardia* was identified as the causal agent in 16.2% (21 of 130) of reported drinking-water-associated outbreaks of gastroenteritis of known or suspected infectious etiology (111).

Cryptosporidium oocysts and *Giardia* cysts have been identified worldwide in surface waters, including streams, rivers, estuaries, lakes, ponds, irrigation ditches, and reservoirs, as well as in untreated wastewater, filtered secondarily treated wastewater, activated sludge effluent, sewer overflows, groundwater, and treated drinking water (83, 126, 187, 204). *Toxoplasma* oocysts have been linked only by epidemiologic evidence to a jungle pond, a reservoir, and unfiltered drinking water (36, 41, 48).

Contamination of surface source waters with *Cryptosporidium* oocysts has been reported from at least 11 countries (83). A summary of studies of drinking-water treatment plants in North America that used conventional filtration found that *Cryptosporidium* oocysts were detected in finished water 3.8 to 33.3% of the time at concentrations from 0.1 to 48 oocysts per 100 liters (187). These oocyst contamination levels provide a basis for daily exposure for persons using tap water. In 1988, surface water was used by over 155 million people in 6,000 community water systems in the United States, 23% of which provided unfiltered water to 21 million people (U.S. Census, 1995 [23]).

The viability, species, and sources of *Cryptosporidium* oocysts found in tap water have not been well studied. The public health significance of oocysts found in tap water is unclear, because species identification is not conducted routinely. Although sporadic cases of waterborne cryptosporidiosis are difficult to document, outbreaks of cryptosporidiosis linked to drinking water (Table 1) clearly confirm that oocysts enter and pass through drinking-water purification processes while retaining their infectivity.

Cryptosporidiosis

One of the first reports of a waterborne outbreak of diarrhea in which *Cryptosporidium* was found to be the etiologic agent by detection of oocysts in stools and by serologic tests occurred in the summer of 1984 in Braun Station, a suburb of about 5,900 persons located 32 km from San Antonio, Tex. (66). A survey found an attack rate of 34% of 100 homes. Unfiltered artesian well water that supplied all 1,791 homes in the community was contaminated with fecal coliforms. Although dye placed in the sewage system was traced to the well water, providing circumstantial evidence of the route of contamination, oocysts were not detected.

In 1987, an outbreak of gastroenteritis among college students affected approximately 13,000 of the 64,900 residents in Carroll County, Ga. (101). *Cryptosporidium* oocysts were identified in effluent from the water treatment plant, dead water mains, and streams above the plant. Dye added to a sewage overflow reached the treatment plant within 6 h, indicating the probable source of contamination. However, failures within the plant included the removal of mechanical agitators from the flocculation basins, impaired filtration, and use of filters that were not back washed.

A 1993 outbreak affecting an estimated 403,000 persons in the greater Milwaukee, Wis., area was the largest documented waterborne epidemic in the United States (147). Within days after the health department was notified that gastrointestinal illness had resulted in high absenteeism of hospital employees, students, and teachers, (i) oocysts were identified in residents' stools, (ii) treated water from the southern treatment plant that obtained water from Lake Michigan was found to be highly turbid, (iii) a "boil

Table 1. Cryptosporidiosis: drinking-water outbreaks

Date	Location	Estimated no. of cases	Source of contamination	Reference(s)
1983	Surrey, England	16	Contaminated spring	38
1984	Texas	2,006	Sewage-contaminated community well	66
1986	New Mexico	78	Untreated surface water?	5
1986	Great Yarmouth, United Kingdom	36	Unknown	50
1986	Hull, England	16	River?	97
1987	Georgia	12,960	Treatment plant deficiency (river water)	101
1988	Ayrshire, Scotland	27	Treatment deficiency (spring water)	194
1989	Oxfordshire, England	516	Treatment deficiency (river water)	185
1990	Loch Lomond, Scotland	442	Treatment deficiency (loch water)	38
1990–1991	Isle of Thanet, United Kingdom	47	Treatment deficiency (river water)	129
1991	Pennsylvania	551	Contaminated well water	166
1991	South London, England	44	Treatment deficiency (tap water)	151
1992	Jackson County, Oreg.	15,000	Treatment deficiency (spring/river water)	140, 166
1992	South Devon, England	?	Municipal water	27
1992	Northwest United Kingdom	42	Contaminated drinking water	91
1992	Northwest United Kingdom	63	Contaminated drinking water	91
1992	Southwest United Kingdom	108	Contaminated drinking water	91
1992	Bradford, Yorkshire, England	125	Contaminated tap water	34, 91
1992	Mersey, England	47	Contaminated tap water	91
1992	Warrington, England	47	Contaminated tap water	49
1993	Wisconsin	403,000	Treatment plant failure (lake water)	147, 149, 179
1993	Washington	7	Well contaminated by surface water	132
1993	Minnesota	27	Resort lake water	132
1993	Las Vegas, Nev.	103	Community water system from lake	95, 132
1993	Wessex, England	40	Contaminated tap water	91
1993	Wessex, England	27	Contaminated tap water	91
1993	Northern United Kingdom	5	Contaminated water at university	91
1993	Yorkshire, England	97	Contaminated tap water	91
1994	Kanagawa, Japan	461	Contaminated drinking water	134
1994	Walla Walla, Wash.	134	Sewage-contaminated well	78, 132

(Table continues)

Table 1. *Continued*

Date	Location	Estimated no. of cases	Source of contamination	Reference(s)
1994	Southwest Thames, Wessex, Oxford, England	224	Contaminated tap water	91
1994	Trent, England	33	Contaminated tap water	91
1995	Gainesville, Fla.	77	Outdoor faucet	15
1995	South and West Devon, England	575	Contaminated tap water	91, 99, 178
1995	Northern Italy	294	Treatment deficiency (tap water)	180
1995	Ireland	13	Farm animal-contaminated water	192
1996	Kelowna, British Columbia, Canada	1,136	Contaminated drinking water	11
1996	Cranbrook, British Columbia, Canada	>2,000	Contaminated tap water from reservoir	25
1996	Ogose, Japan	10,000	Contaminated municipal water	219
1996	Collingwood, Ontario, Canada	182	Contaminated spring	28
1996	Wirrel Peninsula, Wales	52	Contaminated river water	121
1997	Shoal Lake, Ontario, Canada	100	Lake	12
1997	North Thames, England	345	Contaminated borehole	178, 212
1997	England and Wales	>4,321	Multiple outbreaks and sources	21, 26
1997	Italy	293	Contaminated water tank	180
1998	New Mexico	32	Group home well	39
1998	Brushy Creek, Tex.	1,400	Contaminated community well	39
1998	Chilliwack, British Columbia, Canada	30	Unknown	4
1999	Hawke's Bay, New Zealand	20	Unknown	10
1999	Northwest England	360	Unfiltered surface water	13
2000	Florida	5	Community well	137
2000	Clitheroe, Lancashire, England	45	Unfiltered community water from reservoir	16, 116
2000	Northern Ireland	97	Community water supply	17
2001	Burgundy, France	31	Public water supply	65
2001	Indiana	10	Household well	46

water" advisory was issued, and (iv) the treatment plant was closed. Possible causes of the treatment plant failure included insufficient quantities of polyaluminum chloride or alum coagulant to reduce the high turbidity and recycling of filter backwash water that may have increased the number of oocysts in the finished water. Heavy rains washing cattle manure from fields into the watershed, dumping of abattoir waste, and sewage overflow were all suspected sources of the parasite. However, when oocysts from infected persons failed to infect laboratory animals and molecular testing demonstrated they were the major species of human origin, the most likely source became sewage overflow (179).

Cattle and sheep have been suspected of being sources of waterborne outbreaks outside the United States but have not been conclusively identified (by genotyping) as the source of any waterborne outbreak. The outbreak in Cranbrook, British Columbia, is one of the earlier waterborne outbreaks in North America in which oocysts of *Cryptosporidium parvum* have been identified (179). However, this zoonotic species, prevalent in unweaned cattle but less frequently found in weaned cattle (86, 191), has also been reported to infect several other species of mammals (85).

Most reports of waterborne outbreaks come from North America and the United Kingdom (Table 1). Most epidemiologic investigations have detected a combination of causes with patterns similar to those mentioned above, including contaminated source water, high turbidity, and failures at treatment plants. Where *Cryptosporidium* oocysts or *Giardia* cysts were detected by microscopy, only a few studies actually used molecular methods to identify the species or genotype.

Toxoplasmosis

Although transmission of *Toxoplasma* by water has been implicated based on epidemiological evidence, infectious oocysts have never been detected in suspect waters. The first potentially waterborne outbreak of toxoplasmosis was reported for 31 army recruits on a jungle exercise in Panama who filled their canteens with drinking water from a jungle pond (41). A community-wide outbreak in western Canada involved 100 acute cases and 12 congenital cases of infection with *Toxoplasma gondii* (48). A cluster of cases was detected in central greater Victoria, British Columbia. Eighty-three of 94 persons residing in the greater Victoria area with acute infections lived in an area that received its water from a treatment plant that provided unfiltered water that it received from its source, the Humpback Reservoir. When drinking water was identified as a likely source of infection, a method was adopted to recover and identify *T. gondii* oocysts based on a method used to detect waterborne *Cryptosporidium* oocysts, but water collected from the reservoir failed to infect mice used as biological indicators (122). When multivariate analysis was performed, drinking unfiltered water was identified as a risk factor for increased seropositivity for the lower and middle socioeconomic populations in Campos dos Goytacazes, northern Rio de Janeiro State, Brazil, where uveitis consistent with toxoplasmosis was studied in 1997 to 1999 (36).

TRANSMISSION VIA RECREATIONAL WATER

Swimming and other water-related recreational activities are very popular worldwide. More than 350 million swimming-related person-events take place annually in the United States alone (U.S. Census, 1995 [23]). In the past 17 years of reporting, outbreaks of cryptosporidiosis related to recreational waters affected over 16,600 people (Table 2). Frequent fecal contamination coupled with oocyst resistance to chlorine (51), a low infectious dose, and high bather densities have facilitated transmission of *Cryptosporidium*. Between 1991 and 2000, *Giardia* was identified as a causal agent of 9.4% (10 of 106) of reported recreational-water-associated outbreaks of gastroenteritis (111). While *Giardia* cysts are

Table 2. Cryptosporidiosis: recreational-water outbreaks

Date	Location	Estimated no. of cases	Source	Reference(s)
1988	California	44	Private pool	195
1988	Doncaster, United Kingdom	79	Sports center pool	125
1990	British Columbia, Canada	89	Community pool complex	40
1992	Gloucestershire, England	12	Pool	119
1992	Idaho	22	Water slide	166
1992	Oregon	500	Wave pool	166
1992	Oregon	55	Wave pool	156
1993	Wisconsin	65	2 community pools	7
1993	Florida	51	Hotel pool	148
1993	Wisconsin	51	Motel pool	132
1993	Wisconsin	5	Community pool	132
1993	Wisconsin	54	Community pool	132
1993	Wisconsin	64	Motel pool	132
1994	Missouri	101	Motel pool	132
1994	New South Wales, Australia	70	Pool	141
1994	Missouri	101	Motel pool	211
1994	New Jersey	2,070	State park lake	133
1995	Georgia	5,449	Pool	142
1996	Indiana	8	Lake	142
1996	California	3,000	Water park	142
1996	Florida	22	Wading pool	142
1996	Florida	17	Children's wading pool	142
1996	Andover, England	8	Pool	199
1997	Minnesota	369	Zoo sprinkler fountain	14
1998	Hutt Valley, New Zealand	175	Public pool	37
1998	Brisbane, Australia	52	Pool complex	196
1997–1998	New South Wales, Australia	1,060	Public pools	181
1998	Victoria, Australia	125	7 pools	103
1998	Minnesota	26	Pool	143
1999	Minnesota	10	Trailer park pool	137
1999	Wisconsin	10	Municipal pool	137
1999	Florida	6	Home pool	137
1999	Florida	38	Beach park fountain	137
2000	Colorado	112	Municipal pool	137
2000	Florida	3	Apartment pool	137
2000	Ohio	>700	Swim club pool	24, 155
2000	Nebraska	225	2 swim club pools	24, 137
2000	Florida	5	Country club pool	137
2000	Florida	19	Resort pool	137
2000	Florida	5	Condominium pool	137
2000	Georgia	36	Community pool	137
2000	Minnesota	220	Lake	137
2000	Minnesota	7	Day camp pool	137
2000	Minnesota	6	Hotel pool	137
2000	Minnesota	4	Municipal pool	137
2000	South Carolina	26	Community pool	137
2001	Illinois	358	Water park pool	220
2001	Nebraska	157	Community pools	220
2001	Nebraska	21	Community pool	220
2001	Wyoming	2	State park pool	220

Table 2. *Continued*

Date	Location	Estimated no. of cases	Source	Reference(s)
2002	Georgia	3	Wading pool at child care center	220
2002	Massachusetts	767	Sports club pool	220
2002	Minnesota	52	Health club pool	220
2002	Minnesota	41	Hotel pool	220
2002	Minnesota	16	Resort pool	220
2002	Texas	54	Hotel wading pool	220
2002	Wyoming	3	Lake	220
2003	Surrey, England	16	Pool complex	145

more resistant to disinfection than most bacterial and viral pathogens (hence the frequent association with recreational-water outbreaks), the much more resistant (and smaller) oocysts of *Cryptosporidium* contribute significantly to its potential as an agent of gastrointestinal illness in recreational-water settings.

TRANSMISSION VIA FOOD

Cryptosporidiosis

Reports of food-related infections by *Cryptosporidium* are few, difficult to document, and probably greatly underreported, with individual cases and small-group outbreaks unlikely to be recognized. A small number of food-borne outbreaks of cryptosporidiosis have been reported (Table 3).

Because molluscan shellfish filter large quantities of water, extracting tiny particles that remain on their gills, they are excellent biological indicators of pathogens found in the water. They also become potential sources of those pathogens if eaten raw. Oocysts of

Table 3. Cryptosporidiosis: food-borne outbreaks

Date	Location	No. of cases[a]	Venue	Implicated vehicle (source)	Reference
October 1993	Maine	160	County fair	Apple cider (unpasteurized)	161
September 1995	Minnesota	15	Catered meal	Chicken salad (caterer)	9
September 1995	Yorkshire, United Kingdom	50	School	Milk (contaminated pasteurizer)	93
October 1996	New York	31	Fair	Apple cider (unpasteurized)	22
December 1997	Washington	54	Banquet	Fresh vegetables (food handler?)	8
September–October 1998	Washington, D.C.	92	University	Fresh fruit and vegetables (cafeteria food worker)	182
August–September 2001	Queensland, Australia	8	School	Milk (unpasteurized)	98

[a]Numbers of cases are based on laboratory-confirmed and clinically defined cases.

Cryptosporidium have been identified by molecular methods in oysters, clams, and mussels from coastal waters of Ireland, the United States, Canada, the United Kingdom, Spain, Portugal, and Italy (84). Although consumption of shellfish has not been linked to outbreaks of cryptosporidiosis, repeated outbreaks of viral and bacterial illness associated with ingestion of raw shellfish serve as a warning of the potential risk of illness from all waterborne pathogens.

Of waters used to irrigate vegetables in the United States and Central American countries, 60% tested positive for *Giardia* cysts and 36% tested positive for *Cryptosporidium* oocysts (204). Oocysts have been found on the surfaces of raw vegetables purchased at markets. In Costa Rica, oocysts were found on cilantro leaves and roots, lettuce, radishes, tomatoes, cucumbers, and carrots (164). Oocysts found on basil, cabbage, celery, cilantro, green onions, ground green chili, leeks, lettuce, parsley, and yerba buena from several markets near Lima, Peru, were identified by restriction fragment length polymorphism (RFLP) analysis as *C. parvum* (175). Detecting oocysts washed from foods can be difficult. Under controlled laboratory conditions, only 1% of oocysts added to fruit and vegetables were recovered (45).

A cryptosporidiosis outbreak involving milk from a local, small-scale producer using an on-farm pasteurizer affected 50 schoolchildren (93). Environmental-health officers found that the pasteurizer was not working properly at the time of the outbreak.

Two outbreaks of cryptosporidiosis were associated with drinking fresh, unpasteurized apple cider in the United States. In Maine, apples collected from the ground near a cattle pasture were used for cider at an agricultural fair where 160 people acquired cryptosporidiosis (161). Oocysts from the attendees had genetic characteristics implicating the zoonotic species *C. parvum* (179). In New York, the apples may have been washed with well water contaminated with feces (22).

Chicken salad was associated with an outbreak affecting 15 of 50 people at a catered social event (9). The food handler who prepared the chicken salad also operated a home day care facility where earlier that day she had changed a baby's diaper.

Uncooked green onions were eaten by 51 of 54 affected persons who attended a catered banquet and became ill 3 to 9 days later (8). Between 3 and 4 weeks after the banquet, two of the food preparers were positive for *Cryptosporidium*; one had been symptomatic at the time of the banquet.

Raw fruits and vegetables were eaten by 88 students and 4 university cafeteria employees who were diagnosed with cryptosporidiosis (182). A food handler who cut up vegetables and fruit and became ill approximately 3 days before the food was served may have acquired cryptosporidiosis from a child in his family. RFLP analysis of PCR products, as well as DNA sequencing, identified all positive specimens as *Cryptosporidium hominis*; all were identical and linked to the food handler.

Cyclosporiasis

Early reports of cyclosporiasis were linked to water (54, 118, 183), but it is clear that most outbreaks involve contaminated food as the primary vehicle for transmission (Table 4). During the mid- to late 1990s, large outbreaks occurred throughout North America (the United States and Canada) and were linked to imported fruit and vegetables, especially raspberries and leafy green produce, including basil and mesclun lettuce (104). Attempts

Table 4. Cyclosporiasis: food-borne and waterborne outbreaks

Date	Seasonality[a]	Location	No. of cases[b]	Implicated vehicle (source)	Reference
1990	June or July	Illinois	21	Water or food	118
1994	June	Nepal	12	Water (local river or municipal supply)	183
1995	May–June	New York	32	Water or food, including berries	54
1995	May	Florida	38[c]	Raspberries? (Guatemala?)	131
1996	May–June	United States and Canada	1,465[c]	Raspberries (Guatemala)	105
1997	March–April	Florida	NR	Mesclun lettuce (Peru or United States)	29
1997	April–May	United States and Canada	1,012[c]	Raspberries (Guatemala)	106
1997	June–July	Washington, D.C.	341[c]	Basil (multiple sources)	18
1997	September	Virginia	21	Fruit, including raspberries	104
1997	December	Florida	12	Salad, mesclun (Peru?)	104
1998	May	Ontario	315[c]	Raspberries (Guatemala)	19
1998	May	Georgia	17	Fruit (undetermined)	104
1999	May	Ontario	104	Dessert, including berries (Guatemala, Chile, U.S. sources)	102
1999	May	Florida	94	Fruit, including berries	104
1999	July	Missouri	64	Basil (Mexico or United States)	144
2000	June	Pennsylvania	54	Raspberries (Guatemala)	112
2001	May	British Columbia	17	Basil (United States)	113
2001	April	Mexico	101	Watercress (Mexico)	35
2004	June–July	Pennsylvania	96[c]	Snow peas (Guatemala)	20

[a]With two exceptions, all outbreaks and sporadic cases occurred in the late spring or early summer.
[b]Numbers of cases are based on laboratory-confirmed and clinically defined cases.
[c]Multiple outbreaks/clusters.

to isolate the parasite from epidemiologically implicated food items were unsuccessful until 1999, when microscopical and PCR assays of a sample of chicken pasta salad (containing basil) verified the presence of small numbers of the parasite (144). Despite attempts in several laboratories to develop methods for detecting the parasite in food, relevant samples have rarely been available for analysis (most perishable food has been consumed or discarded by the time an outbreak is recognized). PCR methods clearly showed their value in an outbreak associated with consumption of a wedding cake containing a cream filling (with imported raspberries) (112). Limited surveys of produce samples have yielded positive samples (174); however, contamination levels can be quite low. Assuming the infectious dose is small (as is true for *Cryptosporidium* and *Toxoplasma*) and the food portions consumed are relatively modest, the estimated numbers of *Cyclospora* oocysts contaminating implicated food may be quite small (<100 oocysts/serving). Unlike *Cryptosporidium*, no compelling evidence supports immediate person-to-person contact or direct contamination of a food item by a food handler as a mechanism for disease transmission. This is consistent with the requirement for sporulation of oocysts before they become infectious. Consequently, food items must be contaminated with sporulated oocysts or must have sufficient storage time at room temperature for the oocysts to sporulate before consumption in order to be infectious.

Toxoplasmosis

Toxoplasma gondii, a zoonotic protozoan found worldwide, is probably the most common human parasite in Europe. Felids are the only hosts that excrete oocysts in their feces. Humans and a wide range of wild and domesticated animal species ingest sporulated oocysts and serve as intermediate hosts, becoming chronic carriers of tissue cysts. Humans and animals also can be infected by eating undercooked or raw meat containing the tissue cysts. Pork and mutton are important sources of *T. gondii* infection for humans. In a national survey of 11,842 pigs in the United States, 23.1% of market hogs and 41.4% of breeding stock had antibodies to *T. gondii* (76). Infected meat from wild animals also represents risks for human infection (72). Viable cysts of *T. gondii* have been demonstrated in the muscles of roe deer (*Capreolus capreolus*), red deer (*Cervus elaphus*), mule deer (*Odocoileus hemionus*), pronghorn (*Antilocapra americana*), and moose (*Alces alces*) (reviewed in reference 210). In Norway, for example, large populations of wild cervids are hunted for human consumption. In 2001, a total of 37,300 moose, 23,600 red deer, and 7,000 wild reindeer (*Rangifer tarandus*) were shot, along with an estimated 30,000 to 40,000 roe deer (210). Thus, wild cervids constitute an important part of the meat consumption for many Norwegian households. Vikoren et al. (210) reported that sera from 4,339 wild cervids collected in Norway were tested for antibodies against *Toxoplasma gondii*. Positive titers were found in 33.9% of 760 roe deer, 12.6% of 2,142 moose, 7.7% of 571 red deer, and 1.0% of 866 reindeer.

Although molecular methods have been used to identify *T. gondii* genotypes in humans, few studies have identified *T. gondii* isolates from meat animals. Most isolates of *T. gondii* have been grouped into three genetic lineages. In a study of asymptomatic chickens from an area of Rio de Janeiro, Brazil, where human infection is highly endemic, 48 isolates of *T. gondii* were genotyped; 70% were type I, and 27% were type III (75). Transmission of *T. gondii* on a pig farm in New England was investigated using genetic and ecological methods (139). Genetic characterization of 25 *T. gondii* isolates from market pigs identified three distinct strains based on RFLP assays at the *SAG2* locus with no evidence of recombinants, implying that three distinct exposure events occurred during the lifespans of the pigs. The presence of the two most common *T. gondii* genotypes in eight isolates from free-ranging chickens on this farm corroborated the role of cats, because the chickens were probably infected through ingestion of oocysts in the soil.

CONCLUSIONS

Cryptosporidium, Cyclospora, and *Toxoplasma* represent classic examples of emerging and opportunistic infectious agents. *Cryptosporidium* was unrecognized as a human pathogen before 1976 but gained notoriety as a serious opportunistic pathogen in HIV-infected AIDS patients in the early 1980s and as a common agent of gastrointestinal disease among healthy individuals. *Cyclospora*, though occasionally observed in sporadic infections, was not recognized as a significant (though unnamed) pathogen until the mid- to late 1980s in HIV-infected patients. In the mid- to late 1990s, *Cyclospora* was associated with widespread, multistate outbreaks of gastrointestinal illness associated with imported produce, a harbinger of the potential risks associated with the globalization of agricultural products. *Toxoplasma*, though known as a human pathogen since the early 20th century, was usually considered benign, except in congenital infections or in patients with chorioretinitis, until the emergence of HIV and the AIDS epidemic. All three parasites have revealed sinister potential among immunocompromised patients when the patient's immune system cannot assist in the resolution of infection and efficacious drug therapies fail. Whether the risks are associated with improper water or sewage treatment, improper or inadequate food preparation or agricultural practices, or simply hygiene failures leading to person-to-person transmission, our efforts to control these opportunistic parasites will continue to be a challenge.

Acknowledgment. The findings and conclusions in this chapter are those of the authors and do not necessarily represent the views of the Centers for Disease Control and Prevention.

REFERENCES

1. **Ali, M. S., L. A. Mahmoud, B. E. Abaza, and M. A. Ramadan.** 2000. Intestinal spore-forming protozoa among patients suffering from chronic renal failure. *J. Egypt. Soc. Parasitol.* **30:**93–100.
2. **Alpert, G., L. M. Bell, C. E. Kirkpatrick, L. D. Budnick, J. M. Campos, H. M. Friedman, and S. A. Plotkin.** 1984. Cryptosporidiosis in a day-care center. *N. Engl. J. Med.* **311:**860–861.
3. **Amadi, B., M. Mwiya, J. Musuku, A. Watuka, S. Sianongo, A. Ayoub, and P. Kelly.** 2002. Effect of nitazoxanide on morbidity and mortality in Zambian children with cryptosporidiosis: a randomised controlled trial. *Lancet* **360:**1375–1380.
4. **Anonymous.** 1998. Cases in British Columbia prompt boil water alert. *Cryptosporidium Capsule* **3:**3.
5. **Anonymous.** 1987. Cryptosporidiosis—New Mexico, 1986. *Morb. Mortal. Wkly. Rep.* **36:**561–563.
6. **Anonymous.** 1990. Cryptosporidiosis in England and Wales—prevalence and clinical and epidemiological features. Public Health Laboratory Service Study. *Br. Med. J.* **300:**774–777.
7. **Anonymous.** 1994. *Cryptosporidium* infections associated with swimming pools—Dane county, Wisconsin, 1993. *Morb. Mortal. Wkly. Rep.* **43:**561–563.
8. **Anonymous.** 1998. Foodborne outbreak of cryptosporidiosis—Spokane, Washington, 1997. *Morb. Mortal. Wkly. Rep.* **47:**565–567.
9. **Anonymous.** 1996. Foodborne outbreak of diarrheal illness associated with *Cryptosporidium parvum*—Minnesota, 1995. *Morb. Mortal. Wkly. Rep.* **45:**783–784.
10. **Anonymous.** 1999. Increase in cases in New Zealand. *Cryptosporidium Capsule* **4:**1.
11. **Anonymous.** 1996. Kelowna outbreak spreads to neighboring areas in British Columbia. *Cryptosporidium Capsule* **1:**1–2.
12. **Anonymous.** 1997. Outbreak at a first nation community on Shoal Lake, Ontario, Canada. *Cryptosporidium Capsule* **2:**2–3.
13. **Anonymous.** 1999. Outbreak in NW England—water samples found positive. *Cryptosporidium Capsule* **4:**1.
14. **Anonymous.** 1998. Outbreak of cryptosporidiosis associated with a water sprinkler fountain—Minnesota, 1997. *Morb. Mortal. Wkly. Rep.* **47:**856–860.
15. **Anonymous.** 1996. Outbreak of cryptosporidiosis at a day camp—Florida, July-August 1995. *Morb. Mortal. Wkly. Rep.* **45:**442–444.
16. **Anonymous.** 2000. Outbreak of cryptosporidiosis in Lancashire. *Commun. Dis. Rep. CDR Wkly.* **10:**115.
17. **Anonymous.** 2000. Outbreak of cryptosporidiosis in Northern Ireland. *Commun. Dis. Rep. CDR Wkly.* **10:** 323, 326.
18. **Anonymous.** 1997. Outbreak of cyclosporiasis—northern Virginia-Washington, D.C.-Baltimore, Maryland, metropolitan area, 1997. *Morb. Mortal. Wkly. Rep.* **46:**689–691.
19. **Anonymous.** 1998. Outbreak of cyclosporiasis—Ontario, Canada, May 1998. *Morb. Mortal. Wkly. Rep.* **47:**806–809.
20. **Anonymous.** 2004. Outbreak of cyclosporiasis associated with snow peas—Pennsylvania, 2004. *Morb. Mortal. Wkly. Rep.* **53:**876–878.
21. **Anonymous.** 1998. Outbreaks in England and Wales: first half of 1997. *Cryptosporidium Capsule* **3:**4.

22. **Anonymous.** 1997. Outbreaks of *Escherichia coli* O157:H7 infection and cryptosporidiosis associated with drinking unpasteurized apple cider—Connecticut and New York, October 1996. *Morb. Mortal. Wkly. Rep.* **46:**4–8.

23. **Anonymous.** 2000, posting date. Population estimates. U.S. Census Bureau. [Online.] http://www.census.gov/popest/.

24. **Anonymous.** 2001. Protracted outbreaks of cryptosporidiosis associated with swimming pool use—Ohio and Nebraska, 2000. *Morb. Mortal. Wkly. Rep.* **50:**406–410.

25. **Anonymous.** 1996. Report released on outbreak in Cranbrook, British Columbia. *Cryptosporidium Capsule* **2:**6.

26. **Anonymous.** 1998. Reported cases in England and Wales for 1997. *Cryptosporidium Capsule* **3:**6.

27. **Anonymous.** 1998. Reports released on 1992 and 1995 outbreaks in South Devon. *Cryptosporidium Capsule* **3:**7–8.

28. **Anonymous.** 1996. Update on outbreak in Collingwood, Ontario. *Cryptosporidium Capsule* **1:**4.

29. **Anonymous.** 1997. Update: outbreaks of cyclosporiasis—United States and Canada, 1997. *Morb. Mortal. Wkly. Rep.* **46:**521–523.

30. **Arendt, G., H. J. von Giesen, H. Hefter, E. Neuen-Jacob, H. Roick, and H. Jablonowski.** 1999. Long-term course and outcome in AIDS patients with cerebral toxoplasmosis. *Acta Neurol. Scand.* **100:**178–184.

31. **Arrowood, M. J.** 1997. Diagnosis, p. 43–64. *In* R. Fayer (ed.), *Cryptosporidium and Cryptosporidiosis*. CRC Press, Boca Raton, Fla.

32. **Ash, L. R., and T. C. Orihel.** 1987. Parasites: a guide to laboratory procedures and identification. American Society of Clinical Pathologists Press, Chicago. Ill.

33. **Assadamongkol, K., M. Gracey, D. Forbes, and W. Varavithya.** 1992. *Cryptosporidium* in 100 Australian children. *Southeast Asian J. Trop. Med. Public Health* **23:**132–137.

34. **Atherton, F., C. P. Newman, and D. P. Casemore.** 1995. An outbreak of waterborne cryptosporidiosis associated with a public water supply in the UK. *Epidemiol. Infect.* **115:**123–131.

35. **Ayala-Gaytan, J. J., C. Diaz-Olachea, P. Riojas-Montalvo, and C. Palacios-Martinez.** 2004. Cyclosporidiosis: clinical and diagnostic characteristics of an epidemic outbreak. *Rev. Gastroenterol. Mex.* **69:**226–229.

36. **Bahia-Oliveira, L. M., J. L. Jones, J. Azevedo-Silva, C. C. Alves, F. Orefice, and D. G. Addiss.** 2003. Highly endemic, waterborne toxoplasmosis in north Rio de Janeiro state, Brazil. *Emerg. Infect. Dis.* **9:**55–62.

37. **Baker, M., N. Russell, C. Roseveare, J. O'Hallahan, S. Palmer, and A. Bichan.** 1998. Outbreak of cryptosporidiosis linked to Hutt Valley swimming pool. *N. Z. Public Health Rep.* **5:**41–45.

38. **Barer, M., and A. Wright.** 1990. A review: *Cryptosporidium* and water. *Lett. Appl. Microbiol.* **11:**271–277.

39. **Barwick, R. S., D. A. Levy, G. F. Craun, M. J. Beach, and R. L. Calderon.** 2000. Surveillance for waterborne-disease outbreaks—United States, 1997–1998. *Morb. Mortal. Wkly. Rep. CDC Surveill. Summ.* **49:**1–21.

40. **Bell, A., R. Guasparini, D. Meeds, R. G. Mathias, and J. D. Farley.** 1993. A swimming pool-associated outbreak of cryptosporidiosis in British Columbia. *Can. J. Public Health* **84:**334–337.

41. **Benenson, M. W., E. T. Takafuji, S. M. Lemon, R. L. Greenup, and A. J. Sulzer.** 1982. Oocyst-transmitted toxoplasmosis associated with ingestion of contaminated water. *N. Engl. J. Med.* **307:**666–669.

42. **Bern, C., B. Hernandez, M. B. Lopez, M. J. Arrowood, A. M. De Merida, and R. E. Klein.** 2000. The contrasting epidemiology of *Cyclospora* and *Cryptosporidium* among outpatients in Guatemala. *Am. J. Trop. Med. Hyg.* **63:**231–235.

43. **Bern, C., Y. Ortega, W. Checkley, J. M. Roberts, A. G. Lescano, L. Cabrera, M. Verastegui, R. E. Black, C. Sterling, and R. H. Gilman.** 2002. Epidemiologic differences between cyclosporiasis and cryptosporidiosis in Peruvian children. *Emerg. Infect. Dis.* **8:**581–585.

44. **Bhattacharya, M. K., T. Teka, A. S. Faruque, and G. J. Fuchs.** 1997. *Cryptosporidium* infection in children in urban Bangladesh. *J. Trop. Pediatr.* **43:**282–286.

45. **Bier, J. W.** 1991. Isolation of parasites on fruits and vegetables. *Southeast Asian J. Trop. Med. Public Health* **22:**144–145.

46. **Blackburn, B. G., G. F. Craun, J. S. Yoder, V. Hill, R. L. Calderon, N. Chen, S. H. Lee, D. A. Levy, and M. J. Beach.** 2004. Surveillance for waterborne-disease outbreaks associated with drinking water—United States, 2001–2002. *Morb. Mortal. Wkly. Rep.* **53:**23–45.

47. **Boothroyd, J. C., and M. E. Grigg.** 2002. Population biology of *Toxoplasma gondii* and its relevance to human infection: do different strains cause different disease? *Curr. Opin. Microbiol.* **5:**438–442.

48. **Bowie, W. R., A. S. King, D. H. Werker, J. L. Isaac-Renton, A. Bell, S. B. Eng, and S. A. Marion.** 1997. Outbreak of toxoplasmosis associated with municipal drinking water. *Lancet* **350:**173–177.

49. **Bridgman, S. A., R. M. Robertson, Q. Syed, N. Speed, N. Andrews, and P. R. Hunter.** 1995. Outbreak of cryptosporidiosis associated with a disinfected groundwater supply. *Epidemiol. Infect.* **115:**555–566.

50. **Brown, E. A., D. P. Casemore, A. Gerken, and I. F. Greatorex.** 1989. Cryptosporidiosis in Great Yarmouth—the investigation of an outbreak. *Public Health* **103:**3–9.

51. **Carpenter, C., R. Fayer, J. Trout, and M. J. Beach.** 1999. Chlorine disinfection of recreational water for *Cryptosporidium parvum. Emerg. Infect. Dis.* **5:**579–584.

52. **Carr, A., D. Marriott, A. Field, E. Vasak, and D. A. Cooper.** 1998. Treatment of HIV-1-associated microsporidiosis and cryptosporidiosis with combination antiretroviral therapy. *Lancet* **351:**256–261.

53. **Carreno, R. A., D. S. Martin, and J. R. Barta.** 1999. *Cryptosporidium* is more closely related to the gregarines than to coccidia as shown by phylogenetic analysis of apicomplexan parasites inferred using small-subunit ribosomal RNA gene sequences. *Parasitol. Res.* **85:**899–904.

54. **Carter, R. J., F. Guido, G. Jacquette, and M. Rapoport.** 1996. Outbreak of cyclosporiasis associated with drinking water. *Abstr. 36th Intersci. Conf. Antimicrob. Agents Chemother.,* abstr. K52. American Society for Microbiology, Washington, D.C.

55. **Checkley, W., L. D. Epstein, R. H. Gilman, R. E. Black, L. Cabrera, and C. R. Sterling.** 1998. Effects of *Cryptosporidium parvum* infection in Peruvian children: growth faltering and subsequent catch-up growth. *Am. J. Epidemiol.* **148:**497–506.

56. **Checkley, W., R. H. Gilman, L. D. Epstein, M. Suarez, J. F. Diaz, L. Cabrera, R. E. Black, and C. R. Sterling.** 1997. Asymptomatic and symptomatic cryptosporidiosis: their acute effect on weight gain in Peruvian children. *Am. J. Epidemiol.* **145:**156–163.

57. **Chen, X. M., and N. F. LaRusso.** 2002. Cryptosporidiosis and the pathogenesis of AIDS-cholangiopathy. *Semin. Liver Dis.* **22:**277–289.

58. **Chieffi, P. P., Y. A. Sens, M. A. Paschoalotti, L. A. Miorin, H. G. Silva, and P. Jabur.** 1998. Infection by *Cryptosporidium parvum* in renal patients submitted to renal transplant or hemodialysis. *Rev. Soc. Bras. Med. Trop.* **31:**333–337.

59. **Chmelik, V., O. Ditrich, R. Trnovcova, and J. Gutvirth.** 1998. Clinical features of diarrhoea in children caused by *Cryptosporidium parvum. Folia Parasitol.* **45:**170–172.

60. **Clayton, F., T. Heller, and D. P. Kotler.** 1994. Variation in the enteric distribution of cryptosporidia in acquired immunodeficiency syndrome. *Am. J. Clin. Pathol.* **102:**420–425.

61. **Colford, J. M., Jr., I. B. Tager, A. M. Hirozawa, G. F. Lemp, T. Aragon, and C. Petersen.** 1996. Cryptosporidiosis among patients infected with human immunodeficiency virus. Factors related to symptomatic infection and survival. *Am. J. Epidemiol.* **144:**807–816.

62. **Corliss, J. O.** 1994. An interim utilitarian ('user-friendly') hierarchical classification and characterization of the protists. *Acta Protozool.* **33:**1–51.

63. **Current, W. L., and P. H. Bick.** 1989. Immunobiology of *Cryptosporidium* spp. *Pathol. Immunopathol. Res.* **8:**141–160.

64. **Current, W. L., N. C. Reese, J. V. Ernst, W. S. Bailey, M. B. Heyman, and W. M. Weinstein.** 1983. Human cryptosporidiosis in immunocompetent and immunodeficient persons. Studies of an outbreak and experimental transmission. *N. Engl. J. Med.* **308:**1252–1257.

65. **Dalle, F., P. Roz, G. Dautin, M. Di-Palma, E. Kohli, C. Sire-Bidault, M. G. Fleischmann, A. Gallay, S. Carbonel, F. Bon, C. Tillier, P. Beaudeau, and A. Bonnin.** 2003. Molecular characterization of isolates of waterborne *Cryptosporidium* spp. collected during an outbreak of gastroenteritis in South Burgundy, France. *J. Clin. Microbiol.* **41:**2690–2693.

66. **D'Antonio, R. G., R. E. Winn, J. P. Taylor, T. L. Gustafson, W. L. Current, M. M. Rhodes, G. W. Gary, and R. A. Zajac.** 1985. A waterborne outbreak of cryptosporidiosis in normal hosts. *Ann. Intern. Med.* **103:**886–888.

67. **Daoud, A. S., M. Zaki, R. N. Pugh, G. al-Mutairi, F. al-Ali, and Q. el-Saleh.** 1990. *Cryptosporidium* gastroenteritis in immunocompetent children from Kuwait. *Trop. Geogr. Med.* **42:**113–118.

68. **Deodhar, L., J. K. Maniar, and D. G. Saple.** 2000. *Cyclospora* infection in acquired immunodeficiency syndrome. *J. Assoc. Physicians India* **48:**404–406.

69. **Dietz, V., D. Vugia, R. Nelson, J. Wicklund, J. Nadle, K. G. McCombs, and S. Reddy.** 2000. Active, multisite, laboratory-based surveillance for *Cryptosporidium parvum. Am. J. Trop. Med. Hyg.* **62:**368–372.

70. **Dietz, V. J., and J. M. Roberts.** 2000. National surveillance for infection with *Cryptosporidium parvum*, 1995–1998: what have we learned? *Public Health Rep.* **115:**358–363.

71. **Doumbo, O., J. F. Rossignol, E. Pichard, H. A. Traore, T. M. Dembele, M. Diakite, F. Traore, and D. A. Diallo.** 1997. Nitazoxanide in the treatment of cryptosporidial diarrhea and other intestinal parasitic infections associated with acquired immunodeficiency syndrome in tropical Africa. *Am. J. Trop. Med. Hyg.* **56:**637–639.

72. **Dubey, J. P.** 1994. Toxoplasmosis. *J. Am. Vet. Med. Assoc.* **205:**1593–1598.

73. **Dubey, J. P.** 2004. Toxoplasmosis—a waterborne zoonosis. *Vet. Parasitol.* **126:**57–72.

74. **Dubey, J. P., and C. P. Beattie.** 1988. *Toxoplasmosis of Animals and Man.* CRC Press, Boca Raton, Fla.

75. **Dubey, J. P., D. H. Graham, D. S. da Silva, T. Lehmann, and L. M. Bahia-Oliveira.** 2003. *Toxoplasma gondii* isolates of free-ranging chickens from Rio de Janeiro, Brazil: mouse mortality, genotype, and oocyst shedding by cats. *J. Parasitol.* **89:**851–853.

76. **Dubey, J. P., J. C. Leighty, V. C. Beal, W. R. Anderson, C. D. Andrews, and P. Thulliez.** 1991. National seroprevalence of *Toxoplasma gondii* in pigs. *J. Parasitol.* **77:**517–521.

77. **Dubey, J. P., D. S. Lindsay, and C. A. Speer.** 1998. Structures of *Toxoplasma gondii* tachyzoites, bradyzoites, and sporozoites and biology and development of tissue cysts. *Clin. Microbiol. Rev.* **11:**267–299.

78. **Dworkin, M. S., D. P. Goldman, T. G. Wells, J. M. Kobayashi, and B. L. Herwaldt.** 1996. Cryptosporidiosis in Washington State: an outbreak associated with well water. *J. Infect. Dis.* **174:**1372–1376.

79. **Eberhard, M. L., and M. J. Arrowood.** 2002. *Cyclospora* spp. *Curr. Opin. Infect. Dis.* **15:**519–522.

80. **Eberhard, M. L., A. J. da Silva, B. G. Lilley, and N. J. Pieniazek.** 1999. Morphologic and molecular characterization of new *Cyclospora* species from Ethiopian monkeys: *C. cercopitheci* sp.n., *C. colobi* sp.n., and *C. papionis* sp.n. *Emerg. Infect. Dis.* **5:**651–658.

81. **Eberhard, M. L., Y. R. Ortega, D. E. Hanes, E. K. Nace, R. Q. Do, M. G. Robl, K. Y. Won, C. Gavidia, N. L. Sass, K. Mansfield, A. Gozalo, J. Griffiths, R. Gilman, C. R. Sterling, and M. J. Arrowood.** 2000. Attempts to establish experimental *Cyclospora cayetanensis* infection in laboratory animals. *J. Parasitol.* **86:**577–582.

82. **Eberhard, M. L., N. J. Pieniazek, and M. J. Arrowood.** 1997. Laboratory diagnosis of *Cyclospora* infections. *Arch. Pathol. Lab. Med.* **121:**792–797.

83. **Fayer, R.** 2004. *Cryptosporidium*: a water-borne zoonotic parasite. *Vet. Parasitol.* **126:**37–56.

84. **Fayer, R., J. P. Dubey, and D. S. Lindsay.** 2004. Zoonotic protozoa: from land to sea. *Trends Parasitol.* **20:**531–536.

85. **Fayer, R., U. Morgan, and S. J. Upton.** 2000. Epidemiology of *Cryptosporidium*: transmission, detection and identification. *Int. J. Parasitol.* **30:**1305–1322.

86. **Fayer, R., M. Santin, and L. Xiao.** 2005. *Cryptosporidium bovis* n. sp. (Apicomplexa: Cryptosporidiidae) in cattle, *Bos taurus*. *J. Parasitol.* **91:**624–629.

87. **Flanigan, T., C. Whalen, J. Turner, R. Soave, J. Toerner, D. Havlir, and D. Kotler.** 1992. *Cryptosporidium* infection and CD4 counts. *Ann. Intern. Med.* **116:**840–842.

88. **Flanigan, T. R., and R. Graham.** 1990. Extended spectrum of symptoms in cryptosporidiosis. *Am. J. Med.* **89:**252.

89. **French, A. L., L. M. Beaudet, D. A. Benator, C. S. Levy, M. Kass, and J. M. Orenstein.** 1995. Cholecystectomy in patients with AIDS: clinicopathologic correlations in 107 cases. *Clin. Infect. Dis.* **21:**852–858.

90. **Fuentes, I., J. M. Rubio, C. Ramirez, and J. Alvar.** 2001. Genotypic characterization of *Toxoplasma gondii* strains associated with human toxoplasmosis in Spain: direct analysis from clinical samples. *J. Clin. Microbiol.* **39:**1566–1570.

91. **Furtado, C., G. K. Adak, J. M. Stuart, P. G. Wall, H. S. Evans, and D. P. Casemore.** 1998. Outbreaks of waterborne infectious intestinal disease in England and Wales, 1992–5. *Epidemiol. Infect.* **121:**109–119.

92. **Garly, M. L., E. Petersen, C. Pedersen, J. D. Lundgren, and J. Gerstoft.** 1997. Toxoplasmosis in Danish AIDS patients. *Scand. J. Infect. Dis.* **29:**597–600.

93. **Gelletlie, R., J. Stuart, N. Soltanpoor, R. Amstrong, and G. Nichols.** 1997. Cryptosporidiosis associated with school milk. *Lancet* **350:**1005–1006.

94. **Goh, S., M. Reacher, D. P. Casemore, N. Q. Verlander, R. Chalmers, M. Knowles, J. Williams, K. Osborn, and S. Richards.** 2004. Sporadic cryptosporidiosis, North Cumbria, England, 1996–2000. *Emerg. Infect. Dis.* **10:**1007–1015.

95. **Goldstein, S. T., D. D. Juranek, O. Ravenholt, A. W. Hightower, D. G. Martin, J. L. Mesnik, S. D. Griffiths, A. J. Bryant, R. R. Reich, and B. L. Herwaldt.** 1996. Cryptosporidiosis: an outbreak associated with drinking water despite state-of-the-art water treatment. *Ann. Intern. Med.* **124:**459–468.

96. **Goodgame, R. W., R. M. Genta, A. C. White, and C. L. Chappell.** 1993. Intensity of infection in AIDS-associated cryptosporidiosis. *J. Infect. Dis.* **167:**704–709.

97. **Grime, J. S.** 1987. Investigation of an outbreak of cryptosporidiosis in Hull. *Community Med.* **9:**310–311.

98. **Harper, C. M., N. A. Cowell, B. C. Adams, A. J. Langley, and T. D. Wohlsen.** 2002. Outbreak of *Cryptosporidium* linked to drinking unpasteurised milk. *Commun. Dis. Intell.* **26:**449–450.

99. **Harrison, S. L., R. Nelder, L. Hayek, I. F. Mackenzie, D. P. Casemore, and D. Dance.** 2002. Managing a large outbreak of cryptosporidiosis: how to investigate and when to decide to lift a 'boil water' notice. *Commun. Dis. Public Health* **5:**230–239.

100. **Hashmey, R., N. H. Smith, S. Cron, E. A. Graviss, C. L. Chappell, and A. C. White, Jr.** 1997. Cryptosporidiosis in Houston, Texas. A report of 95 cases. *Medicine* **76:**118–139.

101. **Hayes, E. B., T. D. Matte, T. R. O'Brien, T. W. McKinley, G. S. Logdson, J. B. Rose, B. L. P. Ungar, D. M. Word, P. F. Pinsky, M. L. Cummings, M. A. Wilson, E. G. Long, W. S. Hurwitz, and D. D. Juranek.** 1989. Large community outbreak of cryptosporidiosis due to contamination of a filtered public water supply. *N. Engl. J. Med.* **320:**1372–1376.

102. **Health and Social Services Committee of the Regional Municipality of York Ontario Canada.** 2000. The 1999 outbreak of *Cyclospora* in York region 1. Regional Municipality of York, York, Canada.

103. **Hellard, M. E., M. I. Sinclair, C. K. Fairley, R. M. Andrews, M. Bailey, J. Black, S. C. Dharmage, and M. D. Kirk.** 2000. An outbreak of cryptosporidiosis in an urban swimming pool: why are such outbreaks difficult to detect? *Aust. N. Z. J. Public Health* **24:**272–275.

104. **Herwaldt, B. L.** 2000. *Cyclospora cayetanensis*: a review, focusing on the outbreaks of cyclosporiasis in the 1990s. *Clin. Infect. Dis.* **31:**1040–1057.

105. **Herwaldt, B. L., and M. L. Ackers.** 1997. An outbreak in 1996 of cyclosporiasis associated with imported raspberries. *N. Engl. J. Med.* **336:**1548–1556.

106. **Herwaldt, B. L., M. J. Beach, et al.** 1999. The return of *Cyclospora* in 1997: another outbreak of cyclosporiasis in North America associated with imported raspberries. *Ann. Intern. Med.* **130:**210–220.

107. **Hewitt, R. G., C. T. Yiannoutsos, E. S. Higgs, J. T. Carey, P. J. Geiseler, R. Soave, R. Rosenberg, G. J. Vazquez, L. J. Wheat, R. J. Fass, Z. Antoninievic, A. L. Walawander, T. P. Flanigan, J. F. Bender, et al.** 2000. Paromomycin: no more effective than placebo for treatment of cryptosporidiosis in patients with advanced human immunodeficiency virus infection. *Clin. Infect. Dis.* **31:**1084–1092.

108. **Heyworth, M. F.** 1996. Parasitic diseases in immunocompromised hosts. Cryptosporidiosis, isosporiasis, and strongyloidiasis. *Gastroenterol. Clin. N. Am.* **25:**691–707.

109. **Hijjawi, N. S., B. P. Meloni, U. M. Ryan, M. E. Olson, and R. C. Thompson.** 2002. Successful in vitro cultivation of *Cryptosporidium andersonii*: evidence for the existence of novel extracellular stages in the life cycle and implications for the classification of *Cryptosporidium*. *Int. J. Parasitol.* **32:**1719–1726.

110. **Hlavsa, M. C., J. C. Watson, and M. J. Beach.** 2005. Cryptosporidiosis surveillance—United States 1999–2002. *Morb. Mortal. Wkly. Rep.* **54:**1–8.

111. **Hlavsa, M. C., J. C. Watson, and M. J. Beach.** 2005. Giardiasis surveillance—United States, 1998–2002. *Morb. Mortal. Wkly. Rep.* **54:**9–16.

112. **Ho, A. Y., A. S. Lopez, M. G. Eberhart, R. Levenson, B. S. Finkel, A. J. da Silva, J. M. Roberts, P. A. Orlandi, C. C. Johnson, and B. L. Herwaldt.** 2002. Outbreak of cyclosporiasis associated with imported raspberries, Philadelphia, Pennsylvania, 2000. *Emerg. Infect. Dis.* **8:**783–788.

113. **Hoang, L. M., M. Fyfe, C. Ong, J. Harb, S. Champagne, B. Dixon, and J. Isaac-Renton.** 2005. Outbreak of cyclosporiasis in British Columbia associated with imported Thai basil. *Epidemiol. Infect.* **133:**23–27.

114. **Hoepelman, A. I.** 1996. Current therapeutic approaches to cryptosporidiosis in immunocompromised patients. *J. Antimicrob. Chemother.* **37:**871–880.

115. **Hommer, V., J. Eichholz, and F. Petry.** 2003. Effect of antiretroviral protease inhibitors alone, and in combination with paromomycin, on the excystation, invasion and in vitro development of *Cryptosporidium parvum*. *J. Antimicrob. Chemother.* **52:**359–364.

116. **Howe, A. D., S. Forster, S. Morton, R. Marshall, K. S. Osborn, P. Wright, and P. R. Hunter.** 2002. *Cryptosporidium* oocysts in a water supply associated with a cryptosporidiosis outbreak. *Emerg. Infect. Dis.* **8:**619–624.

117. **Howe, D. K., and L. D. Sibley.** 1995. *Toxoplasma gondii* comprises three clonal lineages: correlation of parasite genotype with human disease. *J. Infect. Dis.* **172:**1561–1566.

118. **Huang, P., J. T. Weber, D. M. Sosin, P. M. Griffin, E. G. Long, J. J. Murphy, F. Kocka, C. Peters, and C. Kallick.** 1995. The first reported outbreak of diarrheal illness associated with *Cyclospora* in the United States. *Ann. Intern. Med.* **123:**409–414.

119. **Hunt, D. A., S. Sebugwawo, S. G. Edmondson, and D. P. Casemore.** 1994. Cryptosporidiosis associated with a swimming pool complex. *Commun. Dis. Rep. CDR Rev.* **4:**R20–R22.

120. **Hunter, P. R., and G. Nichols.** 2002. Epidemiology and clinical features of *Cryptosporidium* infection in immunocompromised patients. *Clin. Microbiol. Rev.* **15:**145–154.

121. **Hunter, P. R., and C. Quigley.** 1998. Investigation of an outbreak of cryptosporidiosis associated with treated surface water finds limits to the value of case control studies. *Commun. Dis. Public Health* **1:**234–238.

122. **Isaac-Renton, J., W. R. Bowie, A. King, G. S. Irwin, C. S. Ong, C. P. Fung, M. O. Shokeir, and J. P. Dubey.** 1998. Detection of *Toxoplasma gondii* oocysts in drinking water. *Appl. Environ. Microbiol.* **64:** 2278–2280.

123. **Janoff, E. N., P. S. Mead, J. R. Mead, P. Echeverria, L. Bodhidatta, M. Bhaibulaya, C. R. Sterling, and D. N. Taylor.** 1990. Endemic *Cryptosporidium* and *Giardia lamblia* infections in a Thai orphanage. *Am. J. Trop. Med. Hyg.* **43:**248–256.

124. **Jelinek, T., M. Lotze, S. Eichenlaub, T. Loscher, and H. D. Nothdurft.** 1997. Prevalence of infection with *Cryptosporidium parvum* and *Cyclospora cayetanensis* among international travellers. *Gut* **41:**801–804.

125. **Joce, R. E., J. Bruce, D. Kiely, N. D. Noah, W. B. Dempster, R. Stalker, P. Gumsley, P. A. Chapman, P. Norman, J. Watkins, H. V. Smith, T. J. Price, and D. Watts.** 1991. An outbreak of cryptosporidiosis associated with a swimming pool. *Epidemiol. Infect.* **107:**497–508.

126. **Johnson, D. C., K. A. Reynolds, C. P. Gerba, I. L. Pepper, and J. B. Rose.** 1995. Detection of *Giardia* and *Cryptosporidium* in marine waters. *Water Sci. Technol.* **31:**439–442.

127. **Jokipii, L., and A. M. Jokipii.** 1986. Timing of symptoms and oocyst excretion in human cryptosporidiosis. *N. Engl. J. Med.* **315:**1643–1647.

128. **Jones, J., A. Lopez, and M. Wilson.** 2003. Congenital toxoplasmosis. *Am. Fam. Physician* **67:**2131–2138.

129. **Joseph, C., G. Hamilton, M. O'Connor, S. Nicholas, R. Marshall, R. Stanwell-Smith, R. Sims, E. Ndawula, D. Casemore, P. Gallagher, and P. Harnett.** 1991. Cryptosporidiosis in the Isle of Thanet; an outbreak associated with local drinking water. *Epidemiol. Infect.* **107:**509–519.

130. **Kelly, P., F. A. Makumbi, S. Carnaby, A. E. Simjee, and M. J. Farthing.** 1998. Variable distribution of *Cryptosporidium parvum* in the intestine of AIDS patients revealed by polymerase chain reaction. *Eur. J. Gastroenterol. Hepatol.* **10:**855–858.

131. **Koumans, E. H., D. J. Katz, J. M. Malecki, S. Kumar, S. P. Wahlquist, M. J. Arrowood, A. W. Hightower, and B. L. Herwaldt.** 1998. An outbreak of cyclosporiasis in Florida in 1995: a harbinger of multistate outbreaks in 1996 and 1997. *Am. J. Trop. Med. Hyg.* **59:**235–242.

132. **Kramer, M. H., B. L. Herwaldt, G. F. Craun, R. L. Calderon, and D. D. Juranek.** 1996. Surveillance for waterborne-disease outbreaks—United States, 1993–1994. *Morb. Mortal. Wkly. Rep.* **45:**1–33.

133. **Kramer, M. H., F. E. Sorhage, S. T. Goldstein, E. Dalley, S. P. Wahlquist, and B. L. Herwaldt.** 1998. First reported outbreak in the United States of cryptosporidiosis associated with a recreational lake. *Clin. Infect. Dis.* **26:**27–33.

134. **Kuroki, T., Y. Watanabe, Y. Asai, S. Yamai, T. Endo, S. Uni, I. Kimata, and M. Iseki.** 1996. An outbreak of waterborne cryptosporidiosis in Kanagawa, Japan. *Kansenshogaku Zasshi* **70:**132–140.

135. **Lacroix, C., M. Berthier, G. Agius, D. Bonneau, B. Pallu, and J. L. Jacquemin.** 1987. *Cryptosporidium* oocysts in immunocompetent children: epidemiologic investigations in the day care centers of Poitiers, France. *Eur. J. Epidemiol.* **3:**381–385.

136. **Leander, B. S., R. E. Clopton, and P. J. Keeling.** 2003. Phylogeny of gregarines (Apicomplexa) as inferred from small-subunit rDNA and beta-tubulin. *Int. J. Syst. Evol. Microbiol.* **53:**345–354.

137. **Lee, S. H., D. A. Levy, G. F. Craun, M. J. Beach, and R. L. Calderon.** 2002. Surveillance for waterborne-disease outbreaks—United States, 1999–2000. *Morb. Mortal. Wkly. Rep.* **51:**1–47.

138. **Lehmann, T., C. R. Blackston, S. F. Parmley, J. S. Remington, and J. P. Dubey.** 2000. Strain typing of *Toxoplasma gondii*: comparison of antigen-coding and housekeeping genes. *J. Parasitol.* **86:**960–971.

139. **Lehmann, T., D. H. Graham, E. Dahl, C. Sreekumar, F. Launer, J. L. Corn, H. R. Gamble, and J. P. Dubey.** 2003. Transmission dynamics of *Toxoplasma gondii* on a pig farm. *Infect. Genet. Evol.* **3:**135–141.

140. **Leland, D., J. McAnulty, W. Keene, and G. Stevens.** 1993. A cryptosporidiosis outbreak in a filtered water supply. *J. Am. Water Works Assoc.* **85:**34–37.

141. **Lemmon, J. M., J. M. McAnulty, and J. Bawden-Smith.** 1996. Outbreak of cryptosporidiosis linked to an indoor swimming pool. *Med. J. Aust.* **165:**613–616.

142. **Levy, D. A., M. S. Bens, G. F. Craun, R. L. Calderon, and B. L. Herwaldt.** 1998. Surveillance for waterborne-disease outbreaks—United States, 1995–1996. *Morb. Mortal. Wkly. Rep.* **47:**1–34.

143. **Lim, L. S., P. Varkey, P. Giesen, and L. Edmonson.** 2004. Cryptosporidiosis outbreak in a recreational swimming pool in Minnesota. *J. Environ. Health* **67:**16–20, 27, 28, 31, 32.

144. **Lopez, A. S., D. R. Dodson, M. J. Arrowood, P. A. Orlandi, Jr., A. J. da Silva, J. W. Bier, S. D. Hanauer, R. L. Kuster, S. Oltman, M. S. Baldwin, K. Y. Won, E. M. Nace, M. L. Eberhard, and B. L. Herwaldt.** 2001. Outbreak of cyclosporiasis associated with basil in Missouri in 1999. *Clin. Infect. Dis.* **32:**1010–1017.

145. **Louie, K., L. Gustafson, M. Fyfe, I. Gill, L. MacDougall, L. Tom, Q. Wong, and J. Isaac-Renton.** 2004. An outbreak of *Cryptosporidium parvum* in a Surrey pool with detection in pool water sampling. *Can. Commun. Dis. Rep.* **30:**61–66.

146. **Lumadue, J. A., Y. C. Manabe, R. D. Moore, P. C. Belitsos, C. L. Sears, and D. P. Clark.** 1998. A clinicopathologic analysis of AIDS-related cryptosporidiosis. *AIDS* **12:**2459–2466.

147. **MacKenzie, W. R., N. J. Hoxie, M. E. Proctor, M. S. Gradus, K. A. Blair, D. E. Peterson, J. J. Kazmierczak, D. G. Addiss, K. R. Fox, J. B. Rose, et al.** 1994. A massive outbreak in Milwaukee of *Cryptosporidium* infection transmitted through the public water supply. *N. Engl. J. Med.* **331:**161–167.

148. **MacKenzie, W. R., J. J. Kazmierczak, and J. P. Davis.** 1995. An outbreak of cryptosporidiosis associated with a resort swimming pool. *Epidemiol. Infect.* **115:**545–553.

149. **MacKenzie, W. R., W. L. Schell, K. A. Blair, D. G. Addiss, D. E. Peterson, N. J. Hoxie, J. J. Kazmierczak, and J. P. Davis.** 1995. Massive outbreak of waterborne *Cryptosporidium* infection in Milwaukee, Wisconsin: recurrence of illness and risk of secondary transmission. *Clin. Infect. Dis.* **21:**57–62.

150. **Maggi, P., A. M. Larocca, M. Quarto, G. Serio, O. Brandonisio, G. Angarano, and G. Pastore.** 2000. Effect of antiretroviral therapy on cryptosporidiosis and microsporidiosis in patients infected with human immunodeficiency virus type 1. *Eur. J. Clin. Microbiol. Infect. Dis.* **19:**213–217.

151. **Maguire, H. C., E. Holmes, J. Hollyer, J. E. Strangeways, P. Foster, R. E. Holliman, and R. Stanwell-Smith.** 1995. An outbreak of cryptosporidiosis in south London: what value the *P* value? *Epidemiol. Infect.* **115:**279–287.

152. **Manabe, Y. C., D. P. Clark, R. D. Moore, J. A. Lumadue, H. R. Dahlman, P. C. Belitsos, R. E. Chaisson, and C. L. Sears.** 1998. Cryptosporidiosis in patients with AIDS: correlates of disease and survival. *Clin. Infect. Dis.* **27:**536–542.

153. **Mansfield, L. S., and A. A. Gajadhar.** 2004. *Cyclospora cayetanensis*, a food- and waterborne coccidian parasite. *Vet. Parasitol.* **126:**73–90.

154. **Mata, L.** 1986. *Cryptosporidium* and other protozoa in diarrheal disease in less developed countries. *Pediatr. Infect. Dis.* **5:**S117–S130.

155. **Mathieu, E., D. A. Levy, F. Veverka, M. K. Parrish, J. Sarisky, N. Shapiro, S. Johnston, T. Handzel, A. Hightower, L. Xiao, Y. M. Lee, S. York, M. Arrowood, R. Lee, and J. L. Jones.** 2004. Epidemiologic and environmental investigation of a recreational water outbreak caused by two genotypes of *Cryptosporidium parvum* in Ohio in 2000. *Am. J. Trop. Med. Hyg.* **71:**582–589.

156. **McAnulty, J. M., D. W. Fleming, and A. H. Gonzalez.** 1994. A community-wide outbreak of cryptosporidiosis associated with swimming at a wave pool. *JAMA* **272:**1597–1600.

157. **McGowan, I., A. S. Hawkins, and I. V. Weller.** 1993. The natural history of cryptosporidial diarrhoea in HIV-infected patients. *AIDS* **7:**349–354.

158. **McLauchlin, J., C. F. Amar, S. Pedraza-Diaz, G. Mieli-Vergani, N. Hadzic, and E. G. Davies.** 2003. Polymerase chain reaction-based diagnosis of infection with *Cryptosporidium* in children with primary immunodeficiencies. *Pediatr. Infect. Dis. J.* **22:**329–335.

159. **Mele, R., M. A. Gomez Morales, F. Tosini, and E. Pozio.** 2003. Indinavir reduces *Cryptosporidium parvum* infection in both in vitro and in vivo models. *Int. J. Parasitol.* **33:**757–764.

160. **Miao, Y. M., F. M. Awad-El-Kariem, C. Franzen, D. S. Ellis, A. Muller, H. M. Counihan, P. J. Hayes, and B. G. Gazzard.** 2000. Eradication of cryptosporidia and microsporidia following successful antiretroviral therapy. *J. Acquir. Immun. Defic. Syndr.* **25:**124–129.

161. **Millard, P. S., K. F. Gensheimer, D. G. Addiss, D. M. Sosin, G. A. Beckett, A. Houck-Jankoski, and A. Hudson.** 1994. An outbreak of cryptosporidiosis from fresh-pressed apple cider. *JAMA* **272:**1592–1596.

162. **Miron, D., J. Kenes, and R. Dagan.** 1991. Calves as a source of an outbreak of cryptosporidiosis among young children in an agricultural closed community. *Pediatr. Infect. Dis. J.* **10:**438–441.

163. **Molbak, K., M. Andersen, P. Aaby, N. Hojlyng, M. Jakobsen, M. Sodemann, and A. P. da Silva.** 1997. *Cryptosporidium* infection in infancy as a cause of malnutrition: a community study from Guinea-Bissau, West Africa. *Am. J. Clin. Nutr.* **65:**149–152.

164. **Monge, R., and M. L. Arias.** 1996. Presence of various pathogenic microorganisms in fresh vegetables in Costa Rica. *Arch. Latinoam. Nutr.* **46:**292–294.

165. **Montoya, J. G., and O. Liesenfeld.** 2004. Toxoplasmosis. *Lancet* **363:**1965–1976.

166. **Moore, A. C., B. L. Herwaldt, G. F. Craun, R. L. Calderon, A. K. Highsmith, and D. D. Juranek.** 1993. Surveillance for waterborne disease outbreaks—United States, 1991–1992. *Morb. Mortal. Wkly. Rep.* **42:**1–22.

167. **Morgan-Ryan, U. M., A. Fall, L. A. Ward, N. Hijjawi, I. Sulaiman, R. Fayer, R. C. Thompson, M. Olson, A. Lal, and L. Xiao.** 2002. *Cryptosporidium hominis* n. sp. (Apicomplexa: Cryptosporidiidae) from *Homo sapiens. J. Eukaryot. Microbiol.* **49:**433–440.

168. **Navin, T. R., R. Weber, D. J. Vugia, D. Rimland, J. M. Roberts, D. G. Addiss, G. S. Visvesvara, S. P. Wahlquist, S. E. Hogan, L. E. Gallagher, D. D. Juranek, D. A. Schwartz, C. M. Wilcox, J. M. Stewart, S. E. Thompson III, and R. T. Bryan.** 1999. Declining CD4$^+$ T-lymphocyte counts are associated with increased risk of enteric parasitosis and chronic diarrhea: results of a 3-year longitudinal study. *J. AIDS Hum. Retrovir.* **20:**154–159.

169. **Neill, M. A., S. K. Rice, N. V. Ahmad, and T. P. Flanigan.** 1996. Cryptosporidiosis: an unrecognized cause of diarrhea in elderly hospitalized patients. *Clin. Infect. Dis.* **22:**168–170.

170. **Newman, R. D., C. L. Sears, S. R. Moore, J. P. Nataro, T. Wuhib, D. A. Agnew, R. L. Guerrant, and A. A. Lima.** 1999. Longitudinal study of *Cryptosporidium* infection in children in northeastern Brazil. *J. Infect. Dis.* **180:**167–175.

171. **Nimri, L. F., and S. S. Hijazi.** 1994. *Cryptosporidium.* A cause of gastroenteritis in preschool children in Jordan. *J. Clin. Gastroenterol.* **19:**288–291.

172. **Ortega, Y. R., R. H. Gilman, and C. R. Sterling.** 1994. A new coccidian parasite (Apicomplexa: Eimeriidae) from humans. *J. Parasitol.* **80:**625–629.

173. **Ortega, Y. R., R. Nagle, R. H. Gilman, J. Watanabe, J. Miyagui, H. Quispe, P. Kanagusuku, C. Roxas, and C. R. Sterling.** 1997. Pathologic and clinical findings in patients with cyclosporiasis and a description of intracellular parasite life-cycle stages. *J. Infect. Dis.* **176:**1584–1589.

174. **Ortega, Y. R., C. R. Roxas, R. H. Gilman, N. J. Miller, L. Cabrera, C. Taquiri, and C. R. Sterling.** 1997. Isolation of *Cryptosporidium parvum* and *Cyclospora cayetanensis* from vegetables collected in markets of an endemic region in Peru. *Am. J. Trop. Med. Hyg.* **57:**683–686.

175. **Ortega, Y. R., R. R. Sheehy, V. A. Cama, K. K. Oishi, and C. R. Sterling.** 1991. Restriction fragment length polymorphism analysis of *Cryptosporidium parvum* isolates of bovine and human origin. *J. Protozool.* **38:**S40–S41.

176. **Pape, J. W., R. I. Verdier, M. Boncy, J. Boncy, and W. D. Johnson.** 1994. *Cyclospora* infection in adults infected with HIV: clinical manifestations, treatment, and prophylaxis. *Ann. Intern. Med.* **121:**654–657.

177. **Passos, L. N., O. F. Araujo Filho, and H. F. Andrade, Jr.** 2000. *Toxoplasma* encephalitis in AIDS patients in Sao Paulo during 1988 and 1991. A comparative retrospective analysis. *Rev. Inst. Med. Trop. São Paulo* **42:**141–145.

178. **Patel, S., S. Pedraza-Diaz, J. McLauchlin, D. P. Casemore, et al.** 1998. Molecular characterisation of *Cryptosporidium parvum* from two large suspected waterborne outbreaks. *Commun. Dis. Public Health* **1:**231–233.

179. **Peng, M. M., L. Xiao, A. R. Freeman, M. J. Arrowood, A. A. Escalante, A. C. Weltman, C. S. Ong, W. R. MacKenzie, A. A. Lal, and C. B. Beard.** 1997. Genetic polymorphism among *Cryptosporidium parvum* isolates: evidence of two distinct human transmission cycles. *Emerg. Infect. Dis.* **3:**567–573.

180. **Pozio, E., G. Rezza, A. Boschini, P. Pezzotti, A. Tamburrini, P. Rossi, M. Di Fine, C. Smacchia, A. Schiesari, E. Gattei, R. Zucconi, and P. Ballarini.** 1997. Clinical cryptosporidiosis and human immunodeficiency virus (HIV)-induced immunosuppression: findings from a longitudinal study of HIV-positive and HIV-negative former injection drug users. *J. Infect. Dis.* **176:**969–975.

181. **Puech, M. C., J. M. McAnulty, M. Lesjak, N. Shaw, L. Heron, and J. M. Watson.** 2001. A statewide outbreak of cryptosporidiosis in New South Wales associated with swimming at public pools. *Epidemiol. Infect.* **126:**389–396.

182. **Quiroz, E. S., C. Bern, J. R. MacArthur, L. Xiao, M. Fletcher, M. J. Arrowood, D. K. Shay, M. E. Levy, R. I. Glass, and A. Lal.** 2000. An outbreak of cryptosporidiosis linked to a food handler. *J. Infect. Dis.* **181:**695–700.

183. **Rabold, J. G., C. W. Hoge, D. R. Shlim, C. Kefford, R. Rajah, and P. Echeverria.** 1994. *Cyclospora* outbreak associated with chlorinated drinking water. *Lancet* **344:**1360–1361.

184. **Relman, D. A., T. M. Schmidt, A. Gajadhar, M. Sogin, J. Cross, K. Yoder, O. Sethabutr, and P. Echeverria.** 1996. Molecular phylogenetic analysis of *Cyclospora*, the human intestinal pathogen, suggests that it is closely related to *Eimeria* species. *J. Infect. Dis.* **173:**440–445.

185. **Richardson, A. J., R. A. Frankenberg, A. C. Buck, J. B. Selkon, J. S. Colbourne, J. W. Parsons, and R. T. Mayon-White.** 1991. An outbreak of waterborne cryptosporidiosis in Swindon and Oxfordshire. *Epidemiol. Infect.* **107:**485–495.

186. **Robertson, B., M. I. Sinclair, A. B. Forbes, M. Veitch, M. Kirk, D. Cunliffe, J. Willis, and C. K. Fairley.** 2002. Case-control studies of sporadic cryptosporidiosis in Melbourne and Adelaide, Australia. *Epidemiol. Infect.* **128:**419–431.

187. **Rose, J. B., and M. LeChevallier.** 1997. Waterborne cryptosporidiosis: incidence, outbreaks, and treatment strategies, p. 93–110. *In* R. Fayer (ed.), *Cryptosporidium* and cryptosporidiosis. CRC Press, Boca Raton, Fla.

188. **Rossignol, J. F., A. Ayoub, and M. S. Ayers.** 2001. Treatment of diarrhea caused by *Cryptosporidium parvum*: a prospective randomized, double-blind, placebo-controlled study of Nitazoxanide. *J. Infect. Dis.* **184:**103–106.

189. **Rossignol, J. F., H. Hidalgo, M. Feregrino, F. Higuera, W. H. Gomez, J. L. Romero, J. Padierna, A. Geyne, and M. S. Ayers.** 1998. A double-'blind' placebo-controlled study of nitazoxanide in the treatment of cryptosporidial diarrhoea in AIDS patients in Mexico. *Trans. R. Soc. Trop. Med. Hyg.* **92:**663–666.

190. **Roy, S. L., S. M. DeLong, S. A. Stenzel, B. Shiferaw, J. M. Roberts, A. Khalakdina, R. Marcus, S. D. Segler, D. D. Shah, S. Thomas, D. J. Vugia, S. M. Zansky, V. Dietz, and M. J. Beach.** 2004. Risk factors for sporadic cryptosporidiosis among immunocompetent persons in the United States from 1999 to 2001. *J. Clin. Microbiol.* **42:**2944–2951.

191. **Santin, M., J. M. Trout, L. Xiao, L. Zhou, E. Greiner, and R. Fayer.** 2004. Prevalence and age related variation of *Cryptosporidium* species and genotypes in dairy calves. *Vet. Parasitol.* **122:**103–117.

192. **Sayers, G. M., M. C. Dillon, E. Connolly, L. Thornton, E. Hyland, E. Loughman, M. A. O'Mahony, and K. M. Butler.** 1996. Cryptosporidiosis in children who visited an open farm. *Commun. Dis. Rep. CDR Rev.* **6:**R140–R144.

193. **Sifuentes-Osornio, J., G. Porras-Cortés, R. P. Bendall, F. Morales-Villarreal, G. Reyes-Terán, and G. M. Ruiz-Palacios.** 1995. *Cyclospora cayetanensis* infection in patients with and without AIDS: biliary disease as another clinical manifestation. *Clin. Infect. Dis.* **21:**1092–1097.

194. **Smith, H. V., W. J. Patterson, R. Hardie, L. A. Greene, C. Benton, W. Tulloch, R. A. Gilmour, R. W. A. Girdwood, J. C. M. Sharp, and G. I. Forbes.** 1989. An outbreak of waterborne cryptosporidiosis caused by post-treatment contamination. *Epidemiol. Infect.* **103:**703–715.

195. **Sorvillo, F. J., K. Fujioka, B. Nahlen, M. P. Tormey, R. Kebabjian, and L. Mascola.** 1992. Swimming-associated cryptosporidiosis. *Am. J. Public Health* **82:**742–744.

196. **Stafford, R., G. Neville, C. Towner, and B. McCall.** 2000. A community outbreak of *Cryptosporidium* infection associated with a swimming pool complex. *Commun. Dis. Intell.* **24:**236–239.

197. **Striepen, B., A. J. Pruijssers, J. Huang, C. Li, M. J. Gubbels, N. N. Umejiego, L. Hedstrom, and J. C. Kissinger.** 2004. Gene transfer in the evolution of parasite nucleotide biosynthesis. *Proc. Natl. Acad. Sci. USA* **101:**3154–3159.

198. **Sulaiman, I. M., P. R. Hira, L. Zhou, F. M. Al-Ali, F. A. Al-Shelahi, H. M. Shweiki, J. Iqbal, N. Khalid, and L. Xiao.** 2005. Unique endemicity of cryptosporidiosis in children in Kuwait. *J. Clin. Microbiol.* **43:**2805–2809.

199. **Sundkvist, T., M. Dryden, R. Gabb, N. Soltanpoor, D. Casemore, and J. Stuart.** 1997. Outbreak of cryptosporidiosis associated with a swimming pool in Andover. *Commun. Dis. Rep. CDR Rev.* **7:**R190–R192.

200. **Tangermann, R. H., S. Gordon, P. Wiesner, and L. Kreckman.** 1991. An outbreak of cryptosporidiosis in a day-care center in Georgia. *Am. J. Epidemiol.* **133:**471–476.

201. **Taylor, J. P., J. N. Perdue, T. Dingley, T. L. Gustafson, M. Patterson, and L. A. Reed.** 1985. Cryptosporidiosis outbreak in a day-care center. *Am. J. Dis. Child.* **139:**1023–1025.

202. **Teixidor, H. S., T. A. Godwin, and E. A. Ramirez.** 1991. Cryptosporidiosis of the biliary tract in AIDS. *Radiology* **180:**51–56.

203. **Thomson, M. A., J. W. Benson, and P. A. Wright.** 1987. Two year study of *Cryptosporidium* infection. *Arch. Dis. Child.* **62:**559–563.

204. **Thurston-Enriquez, J. A., P. Watt, S. E. Dowd, R. Enriquez, I. L. Pepper, and C. P. Gerba.** 2002. Detection of protozoan parasites and microsporidia in irrigation waters used for crop production. *J. Food Prot.* **65:**378–382.

205. **Tumwine, J. K., A. Kekitiinwa, N. Nabukeera, D. E. Akiyoshi, S. M. Rich, G. Widmer, X. Feng, and S. Tzipori.** 2003. *Cryptosporidium parvum* in children with diarrhea in Mulago Hospital, Kampala, Uganda. *Am. J. Trop. Med. Hyg.* **68:**710–715.

206. **Turkcapar, N., S. Kutlay, G. Nergizoglu, T. Atli, and N. Duman.** 2002. Prevalence of *Cryptosporidium* infection in hemodialysis patients. *Nephron* **90:**344–346.

207. **Udgiri, N., M. Minz, R. Kashyap, M. Heer, C. S. Gupta, K. Mohandas, R. W. Minz, and N. Malla.** 2004. Intestinal cryptosporidiasis in living related renal transplant recipients. *Transplant Proc.* **36:**2128–2129.

208. **Vakil, N. B., S. M. Schwartz, B. P. Buggy, C. F. Brummitt, M. Kherellah, D. M. Letzer, I. H. Gilson, and P. G. Jones.** 1996. Biliary cryptosporidiosis in HIV-infected people after the waterborne outbreak of cryptosporidiosis in Milwaukee. *N. Engl. J. Med.* **334:**19–23.

209. **Ventura, G., R. Cauda, L. M. Larocca, M. E. Riccioni, M. Tumbarello, and M. B. Lucia.** 1997. Gastric cryptosporidiosis complicating HIV infection: case report and review of the literature. *Eur. J. Gastroenterol. Hepatol.* **9:**307–310.

210. **Vikoren, T., J. Tharaldsen, B. Frederiksen, and K. Handeland.** 2003. Prevalence of *Toxoplasma gondii* antibodies in wild red deer, roe deer, moose and reindeer from Norway. *Vet. Parasitol.* **120:**159–169.

211. **Wilberschied, L.** 1995. A swimming-pool-associated outbreak of cryptosporidiosis. *Kans. Med.* **96:**67–68.

212. **Willocks, L., A. Crampin, L. Milne, C. Seng, M. Susman, R. Gair, M. Moulsdale, S. Shafi, R. Wall, R. Wiggins, N. Lightfoot, et al.** 1998. A large outbreak of cryptosporidiosis associated with a public water supply from a deep chalk borehole. *Commun. Dis. Public Health* **1:**239–243.

213. **Wilson, M., and J. B. McAuley.** 1991. Laboratory diagnosis of toxoplasmosis. *Clin. Lab. Med.* **11:**923–939.

214. **Wittner, M., H. B. Tanowitz, and L. M. Weiss.** 1993. Parasitic infections in AIDS patients. Crypto-sporidiosis, isoporiasis, microsporidiosis, cyclosporiasis. *Infect. Dis. Clin. N. Am.* **7:**569–586.

215. **Xiao, L., C. Bern, J. Limor, I. Sulaiman, J. Roberts, W. Checkley, L. Cabrera, R. H. Gilman, and A. A. Lal.** 2001. Identification of 5 types of *Cryptosporidium* parasites in children in Lima, Peru. *J. Infect. Dis.* **183:**492–497.

216. **Xiao, L., C. Bern, I. M. Sulaiman, and A. A. Lal.** 2003. Molecular epidemiology of human cryp-tosporidiosis, p. 121–146. *In* R. C. A. Thompson, A. Armson, and U. M. Ryan (ed.), Cryptosporidium: *from Molecules to Disease.* Elsevier, Amsterdam, The Netherlands.

217. **Xiao, L., R. Fayer, U. Ryan, and S. J. Upton.** 2004. *Cryptosporidium* taxonomy: recent advances and im-plications for public health. *Clin. Microbiol. Rev.* **17:**72–97.

218. **Xiao, L., and U. M. Ryan.** 2004. Cryptosporidiosis: an update in molecular epidemiology. *Curr. Opin. Infect. Dis.* **17:**483–490.

219. **Yamazaki, T., N. Sasaki, S. Takahashi, A. Satomi, G. Hashikita, F. Oki, A. Itabashi, K. Hirayama, and E. Hori.** 1997. Clinical features of Japanese children infected with *Cryptosporidium parvum* during a mas-sive outbreak caused by contaminated water supply. *Kansenshogaku Zasshi* **71:**1031–1036.

220. **Yoder, J. S., B. G. Blackburn, G. F. Craun, V. Hill, D. A. Levy, N. Chen, S. H. Lee, R. L. Calderon, and M. J. Beach.** 2004. Surveillance for waterborne-disease outbreaks associated with recreational water—United States, 2001–2002. *Morb. Mortal. Wkly. Rep.* **53:**1–22.

221. **Zar, F. A., E. El-Bayoumi, and M. M. Yungbluth.** 2001. Histologic proof of acalculous cholecystitis due to *Cyclospora cayetanensis. Clin. Infect. Dis.* **33:**e140–e141.

222. **Zu, S. X., and R. L. Guerrant.** 1993. Cryptosporidiosis. *J. Trop. Pediatr.* **39:**132–136.

Emerging Infections 7
Edited by W. M. Scheld, D. C. Hooper, and J. M. Hughes
© 2007 ASM Press, Washington, D.C.

Chapter 16

Multidrug-Resistant *Acinetobacter* Infections in U.S. Military Personnel, 2003 to 2005

Kepler A. Davis and Kimberly A. Moran

Multidrug-resistant (MDR) *Acinetobacter* species are important nosocomial pathogens. They are causative organisms in many hospital outbreaks and demonstrate extensive antimicrobial resistance (5, 6, 23, 32, 40). In early 2003, with the onset of military action in Iraq, an outbreak of severe infections in wounded personnel caused by these organisms began. Separate from these infections, the military campaign in Iraq has demonstrated an increase in the ratio of wounded to fatal casualties compared to previous operations in the Persian Gulf, Vietnam, and Korea (13). Military personnel are surviving what previously might have been fatal injuries due to use of body armor and far-forward advanced medical care that frequently is available within minutes of the time of injury. The most common injuries are severe extremity trauma wounds, which occur as a result of proximate-blast explosions. At times, these wounds develop infection. *Acinetobacter* species have been a substantial and challenging cause of serious wound infection, osteomyelitis, and bacteremia in these casualties (10, 12). The precise epidemiology of these infections has not been clearly demonstrated and has generated debate among those investigating and treating casualties involved in this outbreak.

The number of casualties with infections caused by *Acinetobacter* spp. was initially somewhat unexpected and novel to military medical facilities treating these patients. Prior to receiving casualties with these infections, *Acinetobacter* spp. were rarely encountered in military medical facilities, and with the exception of Tong's report of U.S. Marines wounded during the Vietnam War (35), there were limited data reporting the microbiology of war wounds. In Tong's report, organisms now recognized as *Acinetobacter* spp., previously placed in the *Mimeae* group, were the most frequent gram-negative bacteria isolated from combat-associated extremity wounds and the second most common organism causing bloodstream infections in these individuals (35). After the previous experience of Tong was considered, the current incidence of combat-associated infections caused by *Acinetobacter* spp. was not as surprising, yet it did pose major challenges to the military medical and research communities. After differentiating infection from colonization, the foremost

Kepler A. Davis • Infectious Disease Service, D. D. Eisenhower Army Medical Center, 300 Hospital Rd., Fort Gordon, GA 30905. *Kimberly A. Moran* • Infectious Disease Service, Walter Reed Army Medical Center, 6900 Georgia Ave. NW, Washington, DC 20307.

challenge was determining appropriate therapy for these MDR infections with limited institutional and historical experience for guidance. In addition, the increased prevalence of this MDR gram-negative organism in military medical facilities mandated new infection control procedures to limit nosocomial transmission at all levels of military medical care. This included field treatment facilities, the airmobile medical evacuation system, and fixed medical treatment facilities in the United States; essentially, wherever these MDR isolates were identified and the management of casualties took place. Finally, the reservoir for these infections was unclear and generated much debate. Recent investigation has suggested that these are nosocomial infections, similar to those causing outbreaks in civilian medical centers; however, the exact source remains to be definitively determined.

This chapter discusses the military's clinical experience with severe infection caused by MDR *Acinetobacter* spp. in wounded personnel. We report general microbiologic experience, including the species identified and antimicrobial susceptibility patterns, along with more specific clinical experience with wound infection, osteomyelitis, and bloodstream infections. We also comment on preventive measures taken to limit nosocomial transmission and investigation into the reservoir for these infections.

EPIDEMIOLOGY

Acinetobacter is a ubiquitous organism and an opportunistic pathogen. It has been identified as the most common gram-negative bacterium colonizing the skin of hospital personnel (24). The genus *Acinetobacter* has evolved through a number of taxonomic changes over the past decades. In 1971, major clarification of the genus took place. Prior to this, the genus underwent multiple transitions, particularly those based on newly recognized nutritional differences, including oxidase activity, which clearly separates *Acinetobacter* from oxidase-positive bacteria, such as *Moraxella*. At least 15 different names have been used to describe bacteria currently belonging to the genus *Acinetobacter* (7). Today, the genus *Acinetobacter* includes gram-negative coccobacilli that are strictly aerobic, nonmotile, catalase positive, oxidase negative, and nonfermentative. There are at least 17 different *Acinetobacter* genomic species, and 7 have been given formal species names (Table 1) (14).

Species identification is a continuing challenge. DNA fingerprinting, which can be cumbersome and time-consuming, is the preferred method of species identification. Although there has been some success using phenotypic studies to differentiate *Acinetobacter* species, as yet, there is no rapid and reliable method of identification. As a result,

Table 1. *Acinetobacter* genomic species

Name	Number
Acinetobacter calcoaceticus	1
Acinetobacter baumannii	2
Acinetobacter haemolyticus	4
Acinetobacter junii	5
Acinetobacter johnsonii	7
Acinetobacter lwoffii	8
Acinetobacter radioresistens	12

grouping of phenotypically similar genospecies is required for clinical application. For example, the *Acinetobacter calcoaceticus-Acinetobacter baumannii* complex is composed of species 1, 2, 3, and 13 (17).

The ability of *Acinetobacter* to survive for prolonged periods on dry surfaces contributes to the challenge of controlling an outbreak situation. In vitro studies have demonstrated the bacterium's ability to survive up to 4 months on hospital environmental surfaces (45). Survival time differences between outbreak and nonoutbreak strains have not been elucidated. However, one study of an outbreak strain of *Acinetobacter baumannii* using an alternative method of detection revealed that a minority of bacteria may survive as long as 329 days in a dry environment (43). Environmental surface surveillance cultures performed at Walter Reed Army Medical Center (WRAMC) have grown *Acinetobacter* despite patient rooms having undergone a cleaning protocol for MDR pathogens (J. Fishbain, personal communication). Further study is required to determine the longevity of bacteria despite disinfecting procedures. In Southwest Asia, environmental samples, including soil, medical-facility equipment and surfaces, and clinical samples, have been collected for analysis by pulsed-field gel electrophoresis. Preliminary data have linked field hospital environmental isolates of *Acinetobacter baumannii* to patient isolates, including both surveillance and clinical specimens, which is evidence for possible nosocomial transmission (P. T. Scott, personal communication).

Acinetobacter has limited virulence in the healthy host. Despite the characteristics mentioned above, it possesses limited virulence factors. There is no known cytotoxin production; however, there is a cell wall lipopolysaccharide, with possible endotoxin production, and the capsule, resulting in evasion of phagocytosis (4) and bacteriocin production (3). Although rarely responsible for causing serious disease in the immunocompetent population, these factors are capable of promoting life-threatening *Acinetobacter* infection in the immunocompromised host.

The incidence of nosocomial transmission and outbreaks of *Acinetobacter* infection has increased markedly in the past decade (40). The outbreak in U.S. military personnel has led to a significant rise in nosocomial infections in military medical facilities. Prior to the start of the war in Southwest Asia, the incidence of *Acinetobacter* bloodstream infection (BSI) was two per year at WRAMC. From May 2003 to May 2005, there have been 53 documented instances of nosocomial transmission of MDR *Acinetobacter* at WRAMC (34 civilians and 19 active-duty personnel). They included 13 BSIs, 21 respiratory infections, 9 urinary tract infections, and 18 skin or wound infections (F. Leach, personal communication). Nosocomial transmission has resulted in four fatalities, all in immunocompromised patients, directly attributable to *Acinetobacter* infection. In addition, review of all clinical cultures at Brooke Army Medical Center (BAMC) in San Antonio, Tex., demonstrated a 300% increase in the rate of positive cultures from which *Acinetobacter* was recovered after the onset of military action in Iraq (K. A. Davis, unpublished data).

The increase in nosocomial infections in U.S. military medical facilities mirrors the increase in civilian hospitals. Villegas and Hartstein reviewed 51 published reports of *Acinetobacter* outbreaks from 1977 to 2000 (40). More than half of the reports (27 reports) were published in the past 10 years. All of the reports described nosocomial outbreaks, with 75% of the reports related to the intensive-care unit (ICU). The review emphasizes the concern about increasing resistance to multiple classes of antibiotics, including carbapenems. Multivariate analysis of data from a study of 118 patients with MDR *Acinetobacter* infections in Israel revealed risk factors for MDR *Acinetobacter* infection, including male sex, cardiovascular disease, mechanical ventilation, and exposure to antimicrobial drugs (1). A study of 15 inpatients at the Cleveland Clinic Foundation with nosocomial pneumonia caused by MDR *Acinetobacter baumannii* revealed an association with prior ceftazidime use by univariate analysis (20). Other studies have revealed additional risk factors for nosocomial *Acinetobacter* infection, including length of hospital stay, previous infection, surgery, wounds, admission to an intensive-care unit, parenteral nutrition, indwelling catheters (27), and fecal colonization with *Acinetobacter* (11). To date, risk factors for service member acquisition of *Acinetobacter* colonization and/or infection have not been determined. Clarifying colonization versus infection is challenging in this population, due to the nature of traumatic injury, particularly in the case of skin and soft tissue infection. Further studies are needed to identify pertinent risk factors in these individuals.

DIAGNOSIS

Acinetobacter spp. can be readily grown on common laboratory media, producing smooth, sometimes mucoid, pale-yellow to grayish-white colonies. These organisms are nonfermenting, strictly aerobic, short, plump, gram-negative rods during logarithmic growth but are more coccoid during the stationary phase. This duality, in addition to difficulty in destaining, at times leads to initial misidentification. As mentioned above, a characteristic differentiating them from other nonfermenting bacteria is the negative oxidase test (7, 30).

As the outbreak has progressed, specific definitions have been developed and refined into the current standards, which have been used to diagnose infection versus colonization with *Acinetobacter* in military treatment facilities.

> Primary bloodstream infection: recovery of the organism from one or more routine blood cultures without a related infection at another site.

> Secondary bloodstream infection: culture-confirmed bloodstream infection, along with a related *Acinetobacter* infection at a second site.

> Osteomyelitis: diagnosed if one of the following conditions is met.

1. Bone tissue collected during surgical procedures (primarily open debridements, but also including placement of external or internal fixators or bone grafting) was positive for *Acinetobacter* spp. on routine culture (26, 44).
2. Sampled bone tissue demonstrated histological evidence for infection, along with both of the following: (i) recovery of organisms from routine blood cultures and (ii) radiographic evidence for infection, e.g., abnormal findings on X ray, computed-tomography scan, magnetic resonance imaging, or radiolabel scan (gallium, technetium, etc).
3. Open fractures or exposed bone demonstrated gross findings of infection (purulence, necrotic tissue, or environmental contamination with exposed bone), clinical evidence of infection (fever of $\geq$100.5°F; white blood cell count of >12,000/mm^3), and *Acinetobacter* spp. identified on routine culture from samples of

deep-wound soft tissue, excluding bone, obtained intraopera-
tively (25).

Wound infection: samples of deep-wound soft tissue are positive for
Acinetobacter spp. on routine culture, along with the previously described gross findings and clinical evidence of infection but without
exposed bone or fracture. Associated bone tissue cultures and histological examination of bone are negative for infection.

Colonization: identification of microorganisms on routine culture of
skin, mucous membranes, open wounds, excretions, or secretions
without associated adverse clinical signs or symptoms.

CLINICAL FEATURES

Wars have always had a major impact on military medicine, and the conflict in Southwest Asia is no exception. Colonization and infection of war wounds with *Acinetobacter*
bacteria have resulted in significant management challenges, not only for battlefield casualties, but also for other hospitalized patients who are at risk for nosocomial transmission
of the organism.

General Infections Caused by *Acinetobacter*

The *Acinetobacter calcoaceticus-Acinetobacter baumannii* complex is responsible for
the majority of clinically significant infections (8). Any organ system can be involved, resulting in bacteremia, respiratory or urinary tract infections, meningitis, wound infections,
osteomyelitis, or, rarely, eye infections or endocarditis. The respiratory tract has been reported to be the most common site of infection (18). *Acinetobacter* is primarily associated
with nosocomial infections, accounting for 1% of nosocomial BSIs and 3% of nosocomial
pneumonias in U.S. hospitals, according to the Centers for Disease Control and Prevention
National Nosocomial Infection Surveillance report (31). Although nosocomial outbreaks
with *Acinetobacter* are more commonly described, community acquisition and infection
do exist. Up to 20% of healthy adults are colonized with *Acinetobacter* spp. on their skin,
and a small percentage of the healthy population has colonization of the oral cavity and
respiratory tract (2). Risk factors associated with community-acquired infection, particularly in cases of pneumonia and bacteremia, include alcoholism, cigarette smoking,
chronic obstructive lung disease, and diabetes mellitus (4).

Acinetobacter Infection in Military Personnel

U.S. active-duty military members suffering from *Acinetobacter* infections represent a
unique population. They are generally healthy adults who experience traumatic injuries
and subsequently become colonized or infected, likely due to nosocomial exposure to the
MDR pathogen. The majority of infections have involved wounds and osteomyelitis.
There have also been a number of cases of bacteremia and a few isolated cases of pneumonia, empyema, peritonitis, urinary tract infections, sinusitis, and meningitis. Some of these
infections may be prevented by identifying modifiable risk factors in this population. It is

likely that the young age and healthy status of these individuals at the time of injury are somewhat protective.

Treatment of *Acinetobacter* infections in personnel stationed in or returning from Southwest Asia has become a major challenge. In a report published in November 2004, there were 102 patients with *Acinetobacter baumannii* BSI hospitalized in military medical treatment facilities, including WRAMC, the Landstuhl Regional Medical Center (LRMC), BAMC, the National Naval Medical Center, and the U.S. Navy hospital ship *Comfort* between 1 January 2002 and 31 August 2004 (10). The majority (78) of these infections were reported from LRMC and WRAMC and were primarily in males who sustained traumatic injuries in the Iraq/Kuwait region. In 67% of the LRMC patients and 40% of the WRAMC patients, the BSIs were detected from cultures obtained within 48 h of hospital admission. Antimicrobial susceptibility testing performed by microdilution of 33 isolates from LRMC and 45 isolates from WRAMC indicated extensive resistance to the most common antibiotics used to treat *Acinetobacter* infections. Thirteen of the WRAMC isolates were susceptible to imipenem alone, and two were resistant to all antimicrobials tested. Due to extensive resistance observed in clinical isolates, supplemental susceptibility tests using disk diffusion and the Etest are being implemented at WRAMC. To date, 87 and 97% of clinical isolates remain susceptible to colistin and polymixin B, respectively.

It is not surprising that the increase in *Acinetobacter* colonization and infection has resulted in an increased rate of osteomyelitis caused by this organism in personnel serving in Southwest Asia. We described 18 soldiers diagnosed with *Acinetobacter baumannii* osteomyelitis, in addition to 2 with burn infections and 3 with deep-wound infections, admitted to BAMC from March 2003 through May 2004 (12). Twenty-nine of 38 cultures from the 23 patients revealed MDR *Acinetobacter*, defined as resistance to three or more classes of antimicrobials. All but four of the isolates were susceptible to imipenem. The majority of these patients received directed antimicrobial therapy (based on susceptibilities) for an average of 6 weeks. The patients were followed for up to 23 months, with none suffering recurrent infection. Despite the fact that the majority (15 of 23) of these infections were caused by MDR *Acinetobacter*, all of the patients did well, regardless of the antibiotic regimen selected, including one who received no antibiotic therapy and one who received gentamicin alone. These results support the low virulence of this organism in young, healthy hosts without comorbidities.

THERAPY

Acinetobacter multidrug resistance is an increasing problem throughout the world. Most strains are resistant to penicillins and cephalosporins, while ceftazidime, piperacillin, and carbapenems are the β-lactam antibiotics that may remain effective (39). Recently, increased resistance to carbapenems, aminoglycosides, and fluoroquinolones has been reported (15, 34, 39). Descriptions of isolates resistant to all antimicrobials tested continue to increase. Identified mechanisms of resistance include β-lactamase production, porin protein mutations, alteration in the affinities of penicillin-binding proteins, aminoglycoside-modifying enzymes, structural alteration of DNA gyrase and topoisomerase IV, and alteration of the influx or efflux mechanism (21, 39). Patterns of resistance vary based on the geographic region and the species identified. *Acinetobacter baumannii* remains more resistant than other clinically significant *Acinetobacter* species (41).

The majority of *Acinetobacter calcoaceticus-A. baumannii* complex infections in returning military personnel are caused by MDR isolates. In 2003 and 2004, 409 clinical isolates underwent susceptibility testing at WRAMC. The majority of isolates were resistant to ampicillin, cefepime, ceftazidime, cefotaxime, ciprofloxacin, levofloxacin, gentamicin, tobramycin, piperacillin, and trimethoprim-sulfamethoxazole. Fifty-eight percent of the isolates were susceptible to amikacin, 51% to ampicillin-sulbactam, and 75% to imipenem (Table 2). In contrast, clinical isolates of *Acinetobacter* collected in 2002 at WRAMC were mostly susceptible to the antimicrobials traditionally used to treat infection caused by this organism. As the prevalence of MDR isolates increases, our available treatment options decrease. Susceptibility testing should be expanded to include less commonly used antimicrobials, such as polymyxin and colistin, as well as newer agents, such as tigecycline, to allow directed therapy based on the agent most likely to be effective.

Combination Antimicrobials

There are limited prospective clinical data demonstrating optimal therapy for MDR *Acinetobacter* infections. Marques et al. tested for synergy in vitro using checkerboard titration against 14 nosocomial *Acinetobacter baumannii* isolates with nine different antimicrobial combinations (imipenem plus ciprofloxacin, amikacin, or tobramycin; ampicillin-sulbactam plus amikacin or tobramycin; piperacillin-tazobactam plus amikacin or tobramycin; and ticarcillin-clavulanate plus amikacin or tobramycin) (29). Synergy was demonstrated with one or more combinations against 9 of 14 isolates, while partial synergy was detected with one or more combinations against all 14 isolates. No antagonism was detected with any combination. Imipenem with amikacin or tobramycin demonstrated synergy or partial synergy against all 14 isolates. The significance of these findings is unclear, given the lack of clinical data.

A study of 237 clinical *Acinetobacter baumannii* isolates determined susceptibilities by the agar dilution MIC method (41). Imipenem and meropenem had the lowest MICs,

Table 2. Susceptibilities of 409 clinical *Acinetobacter* isolates collected in 2003 and 2004 at WRAMC

Antimicrobial	% Susceptible
Amikacin	58
Ampicillin	1
Ampicillin-sulbactam	51
Cefepime	30
Ceftazidime	29
Cefotaxime	9
Ciprofloxacin	28
Gentamicin	14
Imipenem	75
Levofloxacin	23
Piperacillin	12
Piperacillin-tazobactam	27
Tobramycin	36
Trimethoprim-sulfamethoxazole	25

ampicillin-sulbactam was the most active combination therapy tested, and sulbactam alone was more active than clavulanate or tazobactam. The activity of the β-lactam/β-lactamase inhibitor combinations was likely due to the β-lactamase inhibitor alone.

Although the data are primarily found in in vitro studies, it is not unreasonable to use combination therapy in severely ill or immunocompromised patients with *Acinetobacter* infections. For mild to moderate infections, monotherapy is likely to be effective, particularly for patients with no underlying medical disease.

Treatment of Injured Soldiers

As mentioned above, mortality directly attributable to *Acinetobacter* infection among our active-duty military members, despite a variety of infections, has been low. The study described above involving patients with osteomyelitis or wound infection demonstrated that both monotherapy and combination therapy were effective in this population. However, follow-up has been limited, and only time will tell if these patients suffer recurrent or chronic infections. Our current recommendation for treatment of active-duty personnel with *Acinetobacter* infections is directed based on susceptibility testing. Outcomes based on combination versus monotherapy require further study.

Alternative Therapies

We have found polymyxin B and colistin to be useful alternative therapies in our active-duty population with MDR *Acinetobacter* infections. The majority of isolates tested to date at WRAMC have remained susceptible to these agents. Potential toxicity associated with the agents, including nephrotoxicity and prolonged neuromuscular blockade, must be weighed against the severity of infection. A prospective study of 35 episodes of ventilator-associated pneumonia due to MDR *Acinetobacter baumannii* found intravenous colistin to be as effective for carbapenem-resistant strains as imipenem for carbapenem-susceptible strains (16). Nineteen percent of patients who received colistin and 43% of those who received imipenem developed renal failure. There was no evidence of neuromuscular blockade. Another study evaluating the safety and efficacy of colistin therapy in ICU patients revealed no difference in outcome or rates of renal dysfunction in the colistin-treated patients (55 patients) versus those not treated with colistin (130 patients) (33). Treatment with nebulized colistin has also reportedly been successful for the treatment of pneumonia caused by MDR *Acinetobacter* (22). Additional studies are needed to confirm the traditionally described toxicities associated with these antimicrobials.

As the number of infections with MDR *Acinetobacter* continues to rise, the lack of newer, effective agents against resistant gram-negative bacteria has become a pressing concern. Ultimately, we are relying on antimicrobials that have not been routinely used in decades. The development of resistance to these agents is unavoidable and has already been reported (37).

PREVENTION AND INVESTIGATION

The outbreak of infections with MDR *Acinetobacter* in military personnel has resulted in the institution of new infection control standards in military medical centers caring for these casualties. All casualties admitted to military medical facilities pose possible infection control risks. If not infected with these organisms, many soldiers are colonized with similar multidrug-resistant strains. As previously described, these organisms are able to survive for prolonged periods on hospital surfaces and are resistant to drying, both characteristics that increase the probability of nosocomial transmission (6, 9, 25). There have been multiple reports of environmental persistence of these organisms during similar outbreaks of MDR *Acinetobacter* in other facilities (6, 9, 40), in addition to their becoming endemic to hospitals (23, 28). These reports underscore the importance of limiting transmission of the organism in military medical facilities.

New infection control standards in our facilities mirror experience from previously reported outbreaks. Some of these procedures were illustrated during an 18-month-long outbreak of MDR *Acinetobacter* infection which occurred in an ICU (42). Isolation and cohorting of infected or colonized patients, improved hand hygiene, and disinfection of hospital surfaces led to the eventual termination of this outbreak. However, others have demonstrated that these types of procedures have not had any impact on halting outbreaks. Improved infection control procedures during a 3-month outbreak of MDR *Acinetobacter* infection in a 16-bed medical-surgical ICU included isolation procedures, accelerated staff education on infection control, and antibiotic usage restriction (6). None of these procedures had any impact on the outbreak. The investigators conducted hospital environmental sampling and found that 40% of the samples were positive for *Acinetobacter baumannii*. After decontamination of the ICU with hypochlorite-based disinfectants, repeat environmental sampling revealed no organisms, and the authors concluded that environmental contamination was the primary reason for the continuing outbreak. However, only 7% of the environmental *Acinetobacter baumannii* strains in this investigation were found to have the same biotype and antibiotic susceptibility pattern as the outbreak strain. Another outbreak was initially terminated in a 20-bed medical-surgical ICU by improved hand hygiene (9). A later occurrence of the outbreak strain, 4 months after the initial outbreak, was theorized to be due to environmental contamination, specifically hospital bed rails. Environmental decontamination was important in terminating this secondary outbreak.

The specific infection control procedures implemented have varied with each military medical center, but the elements of each hospital's procedures are essentially the same. BAMC and WRAMC implemented two key strategies. The first was active surveillance for *Acinetobacter* sp. colonization at admission, while the second was isolation of patients who were either colonized or infected with these organisms. Surveillance cultures are completed on all soldiers admitted to the hospital who were medically evacuated from Afghanistan or Iraq. Sterile culture swabs are used to sample both nares and both axillae at BAMC or the axillae and groin at WRAMC. Contact precautions are implemented for these soldiers at admission pending the results of these cultures. Soldiers with positive surveillance cultures for *Acinetobacter* spp. remain in contact isolation until they have two negative surveillance cultures separated by 5 days. In addition, those with wound infections, osteomyelitis, ventilator-associated pneumonia, or bacteremia with *Acinetobacter* are kept in contact isolation until appropriate antibiotics are started and all wounds are closed. At all times, strict hand hygiene is required, not only of health care workers exposed to these patients, but of all health care workers in these facilities. The health care staff has received specific education regarding these procedures, and patients and their families are informed of these issues by patient safety flyers distributed throughout the facility.

In addition to the strategies implemented at fixed military medical facilities, changes were made to infection control policies at deployed medical facilities located in Iraq. In one deployed medical unit, the primary strategy was to ensure 100% compliance with hand hygiene and use of gloves for every patient encounter (36). In addition, improved environmental-decontamination procedures were implemented as far as the limits of practicing in a field environment allowed. Furthermore, a standardized antibiotic prophylactic treatment regimen for battlefield wounds was drafted for all wounds sustained in the theater of operations (Table 3). These guidelines recommended specific antibiotics based on the location of the injury, with an emphasis on diagnosis of infection caused by *Acinetobacter* spp. In implementing these guidelines, the goal was to limit the development of multidrug-resistant organisms by minimizing the application of broad-spectrum antimicrobials (36).

Despite these precautions, there have been a number of suspected nosocomial transmissions of MDR *Acinetobacter* during this outbreak. The reasons for this may be the aforementioned characteristics of the organism itself, in addition to difficulty with adherence to implemented infection control procedures. Over a 15-month period, there have been multiple episodes of nosocomially acquired *Acinetobacter* infection at BAMC, with 53 occurrences over a 20-month period at WRAMC (as mentioned above) (36). Of the episodes at WRAMC, 40 occurred in patients who had not been deployed to Iraq. As the number of soldiers infected or colonized with MDR *Acinetobacter* has increased in military medical centers located in the continental United States, the incidence of nosocomial transmission has also increased.

As mentioned above, antibiotic restriction guidelines have been drafted with the goal of decreasing the incidence of MDR infections in soldiers injured in Iraq. Antibiotic restrictions have been successful in limiting or terminating outbreaks of MDR *Acinetobacter* in other facilities (19, 30, 38, 40). There has been speculation that liberal use of broad-spectrum antimicrobials in field military medical facilities contributed to the current MDR *Acinetobacter* outbreak; however, a definite causative relationship has not been demonstrated. Nonetheless, the current guidelines for antimicrobial prophylaxis for battlefield wounds stress the importance of narrow-spectrum antimicrobials based on the location of the wound and the potential causative pathogens of infection (36). Recommendations are further broken down by treatment location, i.e., far-forward deployed medical stations, which have a more limited antimicrobial formulary and employ "tactical antibiotics," versus larger combat support hospitals with expanded resources (C. K. Murray, personal communication). Military physicians practicing in theater utilize these guidelines, which limit use of broad-spectrum antimicrobials, specifically imipenem and meropenem, for prolonged periods.

Developing guidelines for antibiotic prophylaxis of battlefield wounds was one measure established in an attempt to control this outbreak. The exact cause of the outbreak has not been elicited and continues to generate debate. There have been multiple hypotheses, which have evolved to the current hypothesis that this outbreak is nosocomial in origin, similar to reports of nosocomial outbreaks of MDR *Acinetobacter* spp. in civilian medical centers. Initially it was theorized that colonized military personnel themselves were the reservoir for MDR *Acinetobacter* and that this colonization was obtained from the environment. This hypothesis was based on two facts. First, these organisms are ubiquitous in the environment (7, 30), and inoculation of these organisms during traumatic blast, shrapnel, or projectile injuries seemed to be a plausible method for introduction into war

Table 3. Antimicrobial prophylaxis of battlefield wounds[a]

Injury[b]	Potential pathogens[c]	Tactical antibiotic	MTF[d] antibiotic	MTF alternatives
Abdominal, pelvic, upper thigh, gluteal region, HEENT wound or chest wound crossing mouth/esophageal/sinus mucosa	Gram positive (*Streptococcus* spp., *Staphylococcus* spp.) Gram negative (*E. coli*, Enterobacteriaceae) Anaerobes (*Bacteroides* spp., *Clostridium* spp.)	Cefotetan[e,f] (1–2 g i.m./i.v. every 12 h) or gatifloxacin (400 mg p.o. every 24 h)	Cefotetan[f] (1–2 g i.m./i.v. every 12 h) or ampicillin-sulbactam[e,f] (1–2 g i.v. every 6 h) or ertapenem[e,f] (1 g i.m./i.v. every 24 h)	Fluoroquinolone[g] with metronidazole infusion (500 mg i.v. or p.o. every 6 h or 1 g every 12 h)[e]
Extremity wound[h] or HEENT wound or chest wound not crossing mouth/esophageal mucosa; penetrating brain injury	Gram positive (*Streptococcus* spp., *Staphylococcus* spp., group A and anaerobic streptococci) Gram-positive anaerobes (*Clostridium perfringens*, *Clostridium tetani*) If water exposure, consider *Pseudomonas* spp., *Aeromonas* spp.	Cefotetan[e,f] (1–2 g i.m./i.v. every 12 h) or gatifloxacin (400 mg p.o. every 24 h)	Cefazolin[e,f] (1–2 g i.v. push)[h], followed by oral fluoroquinolone or oral or i.v. fluoroquinolone[g]	Clindamycin[e] (300–600 mg orally every 6 h or 450–900 mg i.v. every 8 h)

[a]Courtesy of Clint Murray (36). These recommendations are for empiric therapy for those with acute battlefield wounds and do not apply to wound infections that develop in personnel receiving long-term medical care at echelon III facilities. Abbreviations: i.m., intramuscularly; i.v., intravenously; p.o., orally. Duration of therapy: intracranial involvement, 5 days; open fracture, 72 h after the time of injury or not more than 24 h after coverage of wound; perforated gastrointestinal tract, continue for only 24 h after surgery in the presence of injury to any hollow viscus (if no hollow-viscus involvement, a single preoperative dose is adequate); oral cavity, 5 days.

[b]HEENT, head, eyes, ears, nose, throat.

[c]Bacteria isolated at the 31st CSH (2004) from wounds occurring in 49 U.S. military personnel (61 wounds) near the time of battlefield injury were 32 coagulase-negative staphylococci, 4 *Staphylococcus aureus* isolates;1 micrococcus, 1 *Pseudomonas stutzeri* isolate, 1 *Escherichia coli* isolate, and 1 *Chryseobacterium meningosepticum* isolate.

[d]MTF, medical treatment facility.

[e]Does not cover *Pseudomonas* spp. or *Acinetobacter* spp. Imipenem-cilastatin or meropenem is required to cover these organisms. Ciprofloxacin may be effective against *Pseudomonas*.

[f]Not for use in a casualty known to have a severe β-lactam allergy due to potential cross-reaction.

[g]Gatifloxacin, 400 mg orally once a day; moxifloxacin, 400 mg orally once a day; or levofloxacin, 500 mg orally once a day.

[h]Consider addition of enhanced coverage of gram-negative bacteria (fluoroquinolone or aminoglycoside) for grade III open fractures due to possible excess infection.

wounds. In addition, organisms that would now be classified as *Acinetobacter* spp. had previously been described as common pathogens in war wounds (35). However, this hypothesis has not been supported by evidence, as soil sampling in Iraq has not revealed it as a source for *Acinetobacter*. There were only 5 soil samples, out of 53 taken from various locations in the theater, that demonstrated *Acinetobacter* on routine culture. Interestingly, all five of these samples were associated with deployed combat support hospitals (CSHs) in Iraq. One was isolated from a soil sample taken immediately adjacent to a CSH deployed in Iraq, while the remaining four positive samples were collected adjacent to an environmental control unit outside a CSH. However, multiple positive samples have been taken from within deployed medical treatment facilities in Iraq (36). They included swab samples of beds, sinks, and medical equipment within the CSHs. These data support the CSHs themselves as the reservoir for this organism, which is consistent with recently reported outbreaks in civilian hospitals. The final outcome of this investigation awaits further analysis.

In addition, there have been supporting clinical data for the nosocomial nature of these infections. *Acinetobacter* spp. have not been identified in war wounds close to the time of injury (C. K. Murray, personal communication). The wounds of 49 casualties were evaluated for bacterial contamination at the time of presentation to a combat support hospital in Iraq. Only 49% of the samples revealed any organisms, and the predominate organisms isolated were gram positive (93%), mostly commensal skin bacteria. Only three gram-negative organisms were identified, none of which demonstrated significant drug resistance. Despite the small sample size of this study, it did not support the theory of traumatic inoculation of MDR *Acinetobacter* spp. at the time of injury. However, the sampling methods limit the power of this study. It is possible that the density of *Acinetobacter* organisms may have been below the limits of detection of random culture swabs and not of tissue samples. In addition, the patients evaluated in this study were not longitudinally followed to assess the future development of wound infection. Soldiers have also been evaluated for *Acinetobacter* colonization prior to deployment to Iraq. Griffith et al. completed surveillance cultures of the forehead, nares, axillae, fingers, and toe webs of a group of soldiers prior to deployment to Iraq (M. Griffith, personal communication). Seventeen percent of these soldiers harbored *Acinetobacter* spp. from forehead or foot cultures only, but none of these isolates matched samples of clinical *Acinetobacter baumannii* pathogens recovered from wounded soldiers receiving treatment at BAMC by susceptibility profile or molecular assessment. In this study, Griffith et. al. have refuted the likelihood of the U.S. Army soldier being the possible reservoir of these MDR organisms.

CONCLUSIONS

The outbreak of MDR *Acinetobacter* infection in military medical facilities represents a significant increase in the incidence of infection with *Acinetobacter* compared to past military experience with this organism. Military medical centers that treat casualties evacuated from Iraq and Afghanistan have observed up to a threefold increase in blood, wound, and urine cultures positive for *Acinetobacter* spp. since the onset of Operation Iraqi Freedom and Operation Enduring Freedom (12). This increase, and the influx of severe extremity infections due to MDR *Acinetobacter*, challenged the military medical community to determine appropriate therapy, limit transmission, and determine the etiology of these infections. Nosocomial transmission and primary infection with the organism have been the principal challenges. Four deaths of nondeployed patients have been attributed to cross-infection with MDR *Acinetobacter*, and it is possible that the organism is becoming endemic to deployed combat support hospitals in the same manner that it has become endemic to certain civilian hospitals.

MDR *Acinetobacter* is an important nosocomial pathogen that has complicated the care of personnel wounded in Operation Iraqi Freedom and Operation Enduring Freedom. The data on nosocomial transmission during this outbreak can be tempered by the generally positive clinical response that these infections, including osteomyelitis and wound infection, have demonstrated to selected treatment regimens. Osteomyelitis caused by MDR *Acinetobacter* seems to initially respond to a multifaceted approach, including appropriate surgical debridement, carefully selected antimicrobial therapy based on susceptibility patterns, and careful follow-up. It is troubling, however, that there are few antibiotic options currently available for infections caused by MDR gram-negative organisms, with none soon to be released. The increasing prevalence of these infections highlights the necessity for newer antimicrobials with activity against these organisms.

Acknowledgments. We thank Clint Murray (Brooke Army Medical Center) for his technical advice and data on the microbiology of war wounds, Matthew Griffith for his data on colonization of soldiers prior to deployment, and Joel Fishbain and Paul Scott for their technical advice.

The views expressed herein are those of the authors and do not reflect the official policy or position of the Department of the Army, the Department of Defense, or the U.S. government.

REFERENCES

1. **A. Abbo, S. Navon-Venezia, O. Hammer-Muntz, T. Krichali, Y. Siegman-Igra, and Y. Carmeli.** 2005. Multidrug-resistant *Acinetobacter baumannii. Emerg. Infect. Dis.* **11:**22–29.

2. **Al-Khoja, M. S., and J. H. Darrell.** 1979. The skin as the source of *Acinetobacter* and *Moraxella* species occurring in blood cultures. *J. Clin. Pathol.* **32:**497–499.

3. **Andrews, H. J.** 1986. *Acinetobacter* bacteriocin typing. *J. Hosp. Infect.* **7:**169–175.

4. **Anstey, N. M., B. J. Currie, and K. M. Withnall.** 1992. Community-acquired *Acinetobacter* pneumonia in the Northern Territory of Australia. *Clin. Infect. Dis.* **20:**790–796.

5. **Ayan, M., R. Durmaz, E. Aktas, and B. Durmaz.** 2003. Bacteriological, clinical, and epidemiological characteristics of hospital acquired *Acinetobacter baumannii* infection in a teaching hospital. *J. Hosp. Infect.* **54:**39–45.

6. **Aygun, G., O. Demirkirian, T. Utku, B. Mete, S. Urkmez, M. Yilmaz, H. Yasar, Y. Dikmen, and R. Ozturk.** 2002. Environmental contamination during a carbapenem-resistant *Acinetobacter baumannii* outbreak in an intensive care unit. *J. Hosp. Infect.* **52:**259–262.

7. **Berezin, E. B., and K. J. Towner.** 1996. *Acinetobacter* spp. as nosocomial pathogens: microbiological, clinical, and epidemiological features. *Clin. Microbiol. Rev.* **9:**148–165.

8. **Bouvet, P. J., and P. A. Grimont.** 1987. Identification and biotyping of clinical isolates of *Acinetobacter. Ann. Inst. Pasteur Microbiol.* **138:**569–578.

9. **Catalano, M., L. S. Quelle, P. E. Jeric, A. DiMartino, and S. M. Maimone.** 1999. Survival of *Acinetobacter baumannii* on bed rails during an outbreak and during sporadic cases. *J. Hosp. Infect.* **42:**27–35.

10. **Centers for Disease Control and Prevention.** 2004. *Acinetobacter baumannii* infections among patients at military medical facilities treating injured U.S. service members, 2002–2004. *Morb. Mortal. Wkly. Rep.* **53:**1063–1066.

11. **Corbella, X., M. Pujol, J. Ayats, M. Sendra, C. Ardanuy, M. A. Dominguez, J. Linares, J. Ariza, and F. Gudiol.** 1996. Relevance of digestive tract colonization in the epidemiology of nosocomial infections due to multiresistant *Acinetobacter baumannii. Clin. Infect. Dis.* **23:**329–334.

12. **Davis, K. A., K. A. Moran, C. K. McAllister, and P. J. Gray.** 2005. Multidrug-resistant *Acinetobacter* extremity infections in soldiers. *Emerg. Infect. Dis.* **11:**1218–1224.

13. **Department of Defense, Directorate for Information Operations and Reports.** 18 April 2005. Military casualty information. [Online.] http://siadapp.dior.whs.mil/personnel/CASUALTY/castop.htm.

14. **Dijkshoorn, L., and J. van der Toorn.** 1992. *Acinetobacter* species: which do we mean? *Clin. Infect. Dis.* **15:**748–749.

15. **Gales, A. C., R. N. Jones, K. R. Forward, J. Linares, H. S. Sader, and J. Verhoef.** 2001. Emerging importance of multidrug-resistant *Acinetobacter* species and *Stenotrophomonas maltophilia* as pathogens in seriously ill patients: geographic patterns, epidemiological features, and trends in the SENTRY Antimicrobial Surveillance Program (1997–1999). *Clin. Infect. Dis.* **32**(Suppl. 2)**:**S104–S113.

16. **Garnacho-Montero, J., C. Ortiz-Leyba, F. J. Jimenez-Jimenez, A. E. Barrero-Almodovar, J. L. Garcia-Garmendia, M. Bernabeu-Wittell, S. L. Gallego-Lara, and J. I. Madrazo-Osuna.** 2003. Treatment of multidrug-resistant *Acinetobacter baumannii* ventilator-associated pneumonia (VAP) with intravenous colistin: a comparison with imipenem-susceptible VAP. *Clin. Infect. Dis.* **36:**1111–1118. (First published 14 April 2003.)

17. **Gerner-Smidt, P., I. Tjernberg, and J. Ursing.** 1991. Reliability of phenotypic tests for identification of *Acinetobacter* species. *J. Clin. Microbiol.* **29:**277–282.

18. **Glew, R. H., R. C. Moellering, Jr., and L. J. Kunz.** 1977. Infections with *Acinetobacter calcoaceticus* (*Herellea vaginicola*): clinical laboratory studies. *Medicine* **56:**79–97.

19. **Go, E. S., C. Urban, J. Burns, B. Kreiswirth, W. Eisner, N. Mariano, K. Mosinka-Snipas, and J. J. Rahal.** 1994. Clinical and molecular epidemiology of *Acinetobacter* infections sensitive only to polymyxin B and sulbactam. *Lancet* **344:**1329–1332.

20. **Husni, R. N., L. S. Goldstein, A. C. Arroliga, G. S. Hall, C. Fatica, J. K. Stoller, and S. M. Gordon.** 1999. Risk factors for an outbreak of multi-drug-resistant *Acinetobacter* nosocomial pneumonia among intubated patients. *Chest* **115:**1378–1382.

21. **Jain, R., and L. H. Danziger.** 2004. Multidrug-resistant *Acinetobacter* infections: an emerging challenge to clinicians. *Ann. Pharmacother.* **38:**1449–1459. (First published 27 July 2004.)

22. **Kwa, A. L., C. Loh, J. G. Low, A. Kurup, and V. H. Tam.** 2005. Nebulized colistin in the treatment of pneumonia due to multidrug-resistant *Acinetobacter baumannii* and *Pseudomonas aeruginosa*. *Clin. Infect. Dis.* **41:**754–757. (First published 20 July 2005.)

23. **Landman, D., J. M. Quale, D. Mayorga, A. Adedeji, K. Vangala, J. Ravishankar, C. Flores, and S. Brooks.** 2002. Citywide clonal outbreak of multiresistant *Acinetobacter baumannii* and *Pseudomonas aeruginosa* in Brooklyn, NY. The preantibiotic era has returned. *Arch. Intern. Med.* **162:**1515–1520.

24. **Larson, E. L.** 1981. Persistent carriage of gram-negative bacteria on hands. *Am. J. Infect. Control.* **9:**112–119.

25. **Lazzarini, L., J. T. Mader, and J. H. Calhoun.** 2004. Osteomyelitis in long bones. *J. Bone Joint Surg. Am.* **86:**2305–2318.

26. **Lew, D. P., and F. A. Waldvogel.** 2004. Osteomyelitis. *Lancet* **364:**369–379.

27. **Lortholary, O., J. Y. Fagon, A. B. Hoi, M. A. Slama, J. Pierre, P. Giral, R. Rosenzweig, L. Gutmann, M. Safar, and J. Acar.** 1995. Nosocomial acquisition of multi-resistant *Acinetobacter baumannii*: risk factors and prognosis. *Clin. Infect. Dis.* **20:**790–796.

28. **Manikal, V. M., D. Landman, G. Saurina, E. Oydna, H. Lal, and J. Quale.** 2000. Endemic carbapenem-resistant *Acinetobacter* species in Brooklyn, New York: citywide prevalence, interinstitutional spread, and relation to antibiotic usage. *Clin. Infect. Dis.* **31:**101–106.

29. **Marques, M. B., E. S. Brookings, S. A. Moser, P. B. Sonke, and K. B. Waites.** 1997. Comparative in vitro antimicrobial susceptibilities of nosocomial isolates of *Acinetobacter baumannii* and synergistic activities of nine antimicrobial combinations. *Antimicrob. Agents Chemother.* **41:**881–885.

30. **McDonald, L. C.** 2001. Understanding and controlling the threat of multidrug-resistant *Acinetobacter* spp. *Semin. Infect. Control* **1:**191–201.

31. **National Nosocomial Infections Surveillance System.** 1998. National Nosocomial Infections Surveillance System (NNIS) report, data summary from October 1986–April 1998, issued June 1998. *Am. J. Infect. Control* **26:**522–533.

32. **Rahal, J. J., C. Urban, and S. Segal-Maurer.** 2002. Nosocomial antibiotic resistance in multiple gram-negative species: experience at one hospital with squeezing the resistance balloon at multiple sites. *Clin. Infect. Dis.* **34:**499–503.

33. **Reina, R., E. Estenssoro, G. Saenz, H. S. Canales, R. Gonzalvo, G. Vidal, G. Martins, A. Das Neves, O. Santander, and C. Ramos.** 2005. Safety and efficacy of colistin in *Acinetobacter* and *Pseudomonas* infections: a prospective cohort study. *Intensive Care Med.* **31:**1058–1065. (First published 28 June 2005.)
34. **Scaife, W., H. K. Young, R. H. Paton, and S. G. Amyes.** 1995. Transferable imipenem-resistance in *Acinetobacter* species from a clinical source. *J. Antimicrob. Chemother.* **36:**585–586.
35. **Tong, M. J.** 1972. Septic complications of war wounds. *JAMA* **219:**1044–1047.
36. **U.S. Army Center for Health Promotion and Preventive Medicine.** 2005. *Investigating Acinetobacter baumannii Infections at U.S. Army Military Treatment Facilities, 27 August 2004 to 27 May 2005.* Epidemiological consultation no. 12-HA-01JK-04.
37. **Urban, C., N. Mariano, J. J. Rahal, et al.** 2001. Polymyxin B-resistant *Acinetobacter baumannii* clinical isolates susceptible to recombinant BPI21 and cecropin P1. *Antimicrob. Agents Chemother.* **45:**994–995.
38. **Urban, C., S. Segal-Maurer, and J. J. Rahal.** 2003. Considerations in control and treatment of nosocomial infections due to multidrug-resistant *Acinetobacter baumannii*. *Clin. Infect. Dis.* **36:**1268–1274.
39. **Van Looveren, M., H. Goossens, and the ARPAC Steering Group.** 2004. Antimicrobial resistance of *Acinetobacter* spp. in Europe. *Clin. Microbiol. Infect.* **10:**684–704.
40. **Villegas, M. V., and A. I. Hartstein.** 2003. *Acinetobacter* outbreaks, 1977–2000. *Infect. Control* **24:**284–295.
41. **Visalli, M. A., M. R. Jacobs, T. D. Moore, F. A. Renzi, and P. C. Appelbaum.** 1997. Activities of β-lactams against *Acinetobacter* genospecies as determined by agar dilution and E-test MIC methods. *Antimicrob. Agents Chemother.* **41:**767–770.
42. **Wagenvoort, J. H. T., E. I. G. B. DeBrauwer, H. M. J. Toenbreker, and C. J. van der Linden.** 2002. Epidemic *Acinetobacter baumannii* strain with MRSA-like behaviour carried by healthcare staff. *Eur. J. Clin. Microbiol. Infect. Dis.* **21:**326–327.
43. **Wagenvoort, J. H. T., and E. J. A. J. Joosten.** 2002. An outbreak of *Acinetobacter baumannii* that mimics MRSA in its environmental longevity. *J. Hosp. Infect.* **52:**226–227.
44. **Waldvogel, F. A., and H. Vasey.** 1980. Osteomyelitis: the past decade. *N. Engl. J. Med.* **303:**360–370.
45. **Wendt, C., B. Dietze, E. Dietz, and H. Ruden.** 1997. Survival of *Acinetobacter baumannii* on dry surfaces. *J. Clin. Microbiol.* **35:**1394–1397.

Emerging Infections 7
Edited by W. M. Scheld, D. C. Hooper, and J. M. Hughes
© 2007 ASM Press, Washington, D.C.

Chapter 17

Leishmaniasis in American Soldiers: Parasites from the Front

Naomi E. Aronson

Leishmaniasis is caused by a protozoan parasite of the genus *Leishmania* and is associated with several clinical syndromes: visceral (the most serious), mucosal (the most disfiguring), and cutaneous (the most common). The actual disease within these syndromes can be quite heterogeneous and varies over wide geographic areas of the world. Transmission usually occurs by the bite of an infected female sand fly; transmission via blood transfusion/needle sharing and perinatal and sexual transmission have rarely been reported in association with visceral leishmaniasis (VL).

The library of King Ashurbanipal of Assyria in Ninewa (the part of Iraq which includes the Mosul area) provided what some believe may be the first record of cutaneous leishmaniasis (CL), describing a common, painless skin ulcer. This information probably came from early Akkadian writings from the second or third millennium B.C. (53). Pringle, in 1949 to 1951, did house-to-house leishmaniasis surveys for skin scars or active ulcers, and the highest rate (50%) was found in Mosul, Iraq (38). During the war between the Islamic Republic of Iran and Iraq, thousands of CL cases appeared in the first 2 years along the front in southwest Iran (34). During the Persian Gulf War in 1990 and 1991, few cases of cutaneous leishmaniasis in coalition forces were reported from a winter-spring incursion into Iraq; however, with the current global war on terrorism (Operation Iraqi Freedom [Iraq] and Operation Enduring Freedom [Afghanistan]) placing large numbers of nonimmune U.S. ground forces in a region of endemicity over leishmaniasis transmission season, more than a thousand cases of cutaneous leishmaniasis have been confirmed among U.S. military forces (12, 23, 25, 26). This emerging population with a chronic infectious disease that is only rarely found in border areas of Texas in the United States presents challenges in diagnosis, treatment, and prevention for North American health care providers (30).

Naomi E. Aronson • Department of Medicine, Infectious Diseases Division, Uniformed Services University of the Health Sciences, Bethesda, MD 20814.

EPIDEMIOLOGY

In March 2003, in support of Operation Iraqi Freedom, many American soldiers deployed to one of the regions of the world where leishmaniasis is most endemic. In April 2003, the first *Leishmania*-infected sand fly was trapped in southern Iraq by military entomologists (R. Coleman, D. Burkett, B. Jennings, V. Sherwood, J. Caci, L. Hochberg, E. Rowton, J. Raymond, J. Dennett, K. Blount, J. McAvin, H. Ploch, G. Hopkins, R. Hadley, S. Gordon, D. Strickman, and P. Weina, *Abstr. 7th Force Health Prot. Conf.*, abstr. 625, 2004). From March 2003 to June 2005, 0.23% of deployed American ground forces (army and marines) were reported to have a diagnosis of leishmaniasis (data provided by the Army Medical Surveillance Activity, June 2005). The epidemiology of the observed CL infections supports the themes of seasonality and focality of transmission (Fig. 1).

Leishmaniasis is a vector-borne protozoan infection with intracellular parasites of the genus *Leishmania*. There are various clinical illnesses called leishmaniasis, depending on the infecting species of *Leishmania*, the geography, the local mammalian reservoir, the sand fly vector, and the host immune response. Human CL starts when people intrude upon the usual zoonotic habitat. In Iraq, where 98% of recent cases among American soldiers have been acquired, *Leishmania major*, a frequent cause of zoonotic CL, has a reservoir of burrow-dwelling rodents and is enzootically transmitted by the sand fly, *Phlebotomus papatasi*. In contrast, *Leishmania tropica* is reported from urban areas, such as Kabul, Afghanistan; humans are the reservoir (anthroponotic CL) and *Phlebotomus sergenti* is the vector (40). An infected female *Phlebotomus* sand fly, requiring a blood meal for ovulation, bites an exposed area of human skin in a probing, blood pool-feeding behavior and then regurgitates *Leishmania* promastigotes into the wound. Generally, sand flies are night feeders and poor fliers and have small mouthparts, so clothing may impede effective transmission. Among 375 CL patients seen at Walter Reed Army Medical Center (WRAMC), Washington, D.C., the locations of the leishmanial lesions were arms > legs > trunk > face. In an Army unit (*n* = "approximately 20,000") returning from deployment in northwest Iraq, 181 patients were reported with confirmed CL lesions that were distributed on the face (4%), on the extremities or trunk (90%), and over joints (30%) (60).

Over 300 patients with laboratory-confirmed CL who were being treated with sodium stibogluconate at WRAMC completed a risk factor survey during 2003 and 2004. Of those, 41% reported that they slept wearing a T shirt, 27% wearing shorts, 35% in battle dress uniform, and 24% in underwear. The most common sleeping places were outdoors (50%), in a building (23%), in a tent (20%), and in a vehicle (20%). Sixty-seven percent reported never or rarely sleeping under a bed net, and of those who slept under a bed net, only 14% pretreated the bed net with permethrin (W. Porter and N. Aronson, *Abstr. 7th Force Health Prot. Conf.*, abstr. 714, 2004). These data establish that in the fluid combat movement of the first year of deployment to Iraq, among the patients who contracted cutaneous leishmaniasis, there were evening exposures that could have facilitated leishmaniasis transmission.

Entomological surveillance expertise was included with preventive-medicine support in theater. In general, the vectors in the region are the sand flies *Phlebotomus alexandri* for *Leishmania infantum*, *P. papatasi* for *L. major*, and *P. sergenti* for *L. tropica* infections. Using light traps, many sand flies could be collected overnight (approximately 1,200 sand

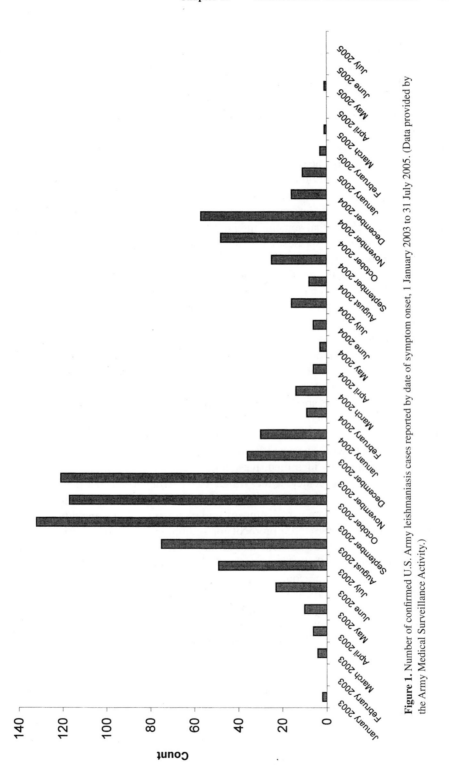

Figure 1. Number of confirmed U.S. Army leishmaniasis cases reported by date of symptom onset, 1 January 2003 to 31 July 2005. (Data provided by the Army Medical Surveillance Activity.)

flies per trap), with frequent fluctuations noted with weather conditions (especially wind) (12). More than 30% of the sand flies were seeking hosts between midnight and 2 a.m., with the rest trapped between 8 p.m. and 4 a.m. In 2003, the peak activity in southern Iraq (as measured by numbers of sand flies collected) was in September (D. Burkett, R. Coleman, V. Sherwood, C. McMeans, J. Caci, J. Swaby, K. Blount, S. Wolf, D. Teig, J. Dennett, R. Knight, E. Rowton, B. Jennings, R. Cushing, and C. Long, *Abstr. 7th Force Health Prot. Conf.*, abstr. 774, 2004; D. Burkett, USAF research in pest management—CY 2003 [unclassified military briefing]; 31). Pools of 1 to 15 female phlebotomine sand flies were tested using a 16S rRNA sequence target (genus level) fluorogenic PCR assay, with some areas having rates of *Leishmania*-infected sand flies of over 2% (12, 18, 61). Subsequently, positive sand fly pools were tested with PCR that permitted species level identification, and *L. major*, *L. tropica*, and *L. infantum/Leishmania donovani* were all identified. Recent exploratory work suggests that some of the pools contained sand flies that were infected with *Leishmania tarentolae*, a species that is not considered to be a human pathogen (R. Coleman, personal communication, 2005).

In most of the area, the gerbil *Rhombomys opimus* is thought to be the reservoir host for *L. major*, with other areas having the sand rat, *Psammomys obesus*, as the reservoir. Extensive burrows under tents were noted by preventive-medicine units, with descriptions of many rodent-like animals in the camp area.

Overwhelmingly, localized CL due to *L. major* has been identified in soldiers returning from Iraq. It has been found focally in units in specific areas of Iraq, predominantly army units. To date, only five cases of visceral leishmaniasis have been reported, with three cases from Operation Enduring Freedom and two acquired during Operation Iraqi Freedom. Consistent with the species of *Leishmania* present in the region, no mucosal leishmaniasis has been identified.

The army policy for management of CL at the beginning of Operation Iraqi Freedom was that all patients with suspected leishmaniasis would undergo a diagnostic procedure, and if leishmaniasis was identified, the patient would be evacuated to the sole military leishmaniasis treatment center at the Walter Reed Army Medical Center (as of March 2004, a second center was opened at Brooke Army Medical Center in San Antonio, Tex.). These centers provided complete diagnostic and treatment options, including access to the Investigational New Drug (IND) protocol for sodium stibogluconate, a pentavalent antimonial agent. When it became clear that *L. major* was the species associated with most cases from Iraq and that this type of skin infection was commonly self-healing, the diagnosis and treatment of Iraq-acquired CL were decentralized.

Using the Defense Medical Surveillance System, all reportable medical events, hospitalizations, and ambulatory visits to military treatment facilities coded with the diagnosis of leishmaniasis (ICD-9, 085.0 to 085.9) were searched. This data set did not require confirmation of diagnosis. In 2003, there were 400 incident reports of leishmaniasis among the U.S. Armed Forces. Restricted to active service components, there was an overall incident in 2003 of 40.9 per 100,000 person-years. This can be compared to 1990 and 1991 (Operation Desert Storm), when 41 diagnoses of leishmaniasis were attributed to hospitalized U.S. service members (the number diagnosed and treated as outpatients was not recorded, but during 1990, sodium stibogluconate was administered only in the inpatient setting) (25). In 2004, among the active components of the armed forces, the annual incidence of leishmaniasis was 24.4 per 100,000 person-years (26).

A harbinger of what lay ahead arrived with an observation by U.S. physicians in southern Iraq in April 2003. In a 6-week period, 46% of the soldiers in one infantry unit reported to sick call for sand fly bites (R. Coleman, personal communication, 2005) (Color Plate 3A [see color insert]). These were no ordinary arthropod assaults, but profuse pruritic bites, hundreds to thousands in some patients. There appeared to be immunological potentiation with subsequent bites.

Infection rates were focal among army units. Three military units produced 86% of the patients. The leishmaniasis attack rate in one squadron was 211/1,000, with the associated division having an attack rate of 12/1,000. (The rates were estimated using authorized unit strength data provided by the U.S. Army Force Management Support Agency.) In another division, one regiment had an attack rate of 9.6/1,000, with an overall division attack rate of 4.2/1,000. One combat engineer unit had an attack rate of 45/1,000. The squadron with the highest attack rate deployed during peak transmission months near the Iranian border in the Diyala Governate (Porter and Aronson, *Abstr. 7th Force Health Prot. Conf.*). The unifying exposure for most of the other patients, repeated in the 2004–2005 deployment cycle, was a base west of Mosul in the Ninewa Governate.

Review of the demographic information collected for 375 patients treated at WRAMC in 2003 and 2004 compared to the demographics of the active army (in parentheses) showed that 73% (64%) were Caucasian, 15% (25%) were African-American, 8% were Hispanic, and 2% were Asian (active-army demographic information was provided from the DMED program, Defense Medical Surveillance System, 25 May 2004). Ninety-eight percent (85%) of leishmaniasis patients were male, and 99% (75%) were in the army. The median age was 26 years (range, 19 to 57 years). The average duration of skin lesions at the time of treatment was 4 months. The median number of skin lesions was 4 (range, 1 to 47), and the median size of a lesion was 13 mm (range, 3 to 90 mm). Using data from the risk factor survey described above, the common military occupations represented among patients with CL were armor/cavalry (22%), supply (7%), and infantry, maintenance, fuel/cargo, combat engineer, and medical (each 4 to 5%).

CLINICAL PRESENTATION

The major clinical syndromes of leishmaniasis are cutaneous, mucosal, and visceral leishmaniasis. Cutaneous leishmaniasis is a chronic skin condition, often ulceronodular in presentation. Mucosal leishmaniasis is a granulomatous condition of the naso- or oropharynx, usually associated with New World leishmaniasis, occurring either simultaneously with or years after the skin lesion. Visceral leishmaniasis is a systemic infection that can vary from asymptomatic to subclinical to fully manifest. In advanced infection, symptoms and signs include fever, wasting, hepatosplenomegaly, hypergammaglobulinemia, and pancytopenia.

In practice in Iraq, a person from a region where leishmaniasis is not endemic (such as the United States) with a nonhealing progressive skin lesion that lasts 3 to 4 weeks and does not respond to broad-spectrum antibiotics is likely to have cutaneous leishmaniasis. The principal differential diagnosis, depending on the geographic region, may be pyoderma and allergic reactions to arthropod assault (e.g., lichen simplex chronicus). In some areas of Iraq, livestock myiasis has also been noted (caused by *Chrysomyia bezziana*, the Old World screwworm), peaking in late autumn to early winter and dispersed along the main rivers, where median dense vegetation may be found (47). A misdiagnosis made in

Iraq by American providers is spider bite, since the desert camel spider is quite notable. Reports of epidemic spider bites are often found to be cases of cutaneous leishmaniasis. Among hundreds of skin samples submitted for a clinical possibility of leishmaniasis reviewed by members of the Division of Infectious and Tropical Diseases Pathology at the Armed Forces Institute of Pathology, other nonleishmaniasis diagnoses that have been made include pyoderma gangrenosum, sarcoidosis, lupus, basal cell carcinoma, various melanocytic lesions, dermatofibroma, fibrous histiocytoma, contact dermatitis, arthropod reactions, pyoderma, lichen planus, prurigo nodularis, eccrine acrospiroma, and lichen simplex chronicus (24a).

The CL lesion starts as a papule that resembles an infected insect bite, which instead of resolving actually enlarges and then softens centrally and generally ulcerates. The typical volcaniform lesion may vary in size from 1 to 6 cm, and in Old World CL (OWCL), the ulcer is frequently covered with a hyperkeratotic eschar. The borders of the ulcer are indurated, and the lesion is remarkably painless. Pruritus is unusual. Secondary bacterial infection occurred often in 2003 and 2004, generally found to be due to *Staphylococcus aureus*, except among combat engineers, who sometimes had gram-negative bacterial secondary infections with water- or soil-type organisms. During the 2003–2004 deployment, access to water for bathing was sparse, and infected leishmanial sores developed purulence and tenderness of the lesion. These findings, often combined with localized cellulitis, were unlikely to be due solely to leishmaniasis. Secondary infection of leishmanial lesions contributed to the rapid expansion of small ulcers. Complicated CL includes lymphocutaneous extension, in which small, shotty, mobile nodules form, often in chains; gradually enlarge up to 1 cm in size; develop erythema over them; and eventually ulcerate. This sporotrichoid spread occurs proximally to the lesion. Small daughter, or satellite, papules may form around the initial lesion. *L. major* acquired near an airfield in northern Afghanistan was noted to be very reactogenic, with edema, phlebitic-appearing limbs, local cellulitis, prolific lymphocutaneous involvement, and large ragged ulcers (M. Bailey, A. Caddy, K. McKinnon, J. Bailey, T. O'Dempsey, and N. Beeching, *Abstr. Third World Congr. on Leishmaniosis*, p. 109, 2005). Regional lymphadenopathy is commonly seen in *L. infantum* cutaneous infections (including the so-called bubonic form) but less commonly with *L. major* infections in Iraq (9). Other complications include healing that results in a hyperpigmented, depressed, generally atrophic scar (or keloid in those predisposed). When this scarring occurs on cosmetically evident areas, such as the eyelids, ear pinna, lip, or nose, it has the potential to be a permanently disfiguring process. Some soldiers have been dissatisfied with the cosmesis of their scars at 12 months after treatment, even with shallow cicatrices. In female patients in areas of endemicity, facial disfigurement due to leishmaniasis has been associated with psychiatric and social complications (62).

The natural history of *L. major* is to heal without intervention in 6 to 12 months, with *L. tropica* CL taking longer. However, there are exceptions to this, as some lesions persist for many years (3, 14). The distribution of the skin lesions, often aligned with the skin creases and clustered where the sand fly repeatedly probed, may be clinically helpful. Common lesions are ulcerative, papular, nodular, ulceronodular, and plaques (Color Plate 3B to F). An unusual presentation, noted in several soldiers, was large tender psoriaform plaques with a small ulcer (2 mm) located over the elbow with underlying olecranon bursitis. Among a series of >1,000 patients with localized CL in Iran, lesions with less common appearances were described, such as zosteriform, erysipeloid, sporotrichoid, eczematoid, and verrucous (14). We have seen all of these in our soldiers. In Sudan, unusual *L. major* presentations included activation in the border of a scar (recidivans-like), mycetoma, crusted lesions, and a 5-cm subcutaneous mass without ulceration (leishmanoma) (15).

The interval from sand fly bite to lesion onset usually ranges from 2 to 8 weeks. The time in our population from self-reported onset until diagnosis was 9 ± 5 weeks.

Figure 1 shows the number of U.S. Army cases of leishmaniasis reported to the Defense Medical Surveillance System by date of symptom onset. This demonstrates a seasonal variation with a consistent peak in the fall and shows the effects of an extensive prevention effort during the second season of deployment, as fewer cases were reported.

DIAGNOSIS

The first step is to consider the diagnosis of leishmaniasis in a patient with a chronic skin sore and a history of recent travel to an area of endemicity (for Iraq, if travel was during the transmission season, May to September). Diagnosis currently requires parasitologic confirmation of *Leishmania* using tissue for evaluation by tissue smear or touch preparations, histology, parasite culture (in vitro or animal inoculation), or detection of parasite nucleic acids using assays, such as PCR. The serologic tests that are commercially available are not helpful, since they are neither sensitive nor specific for cutaneous infection. In some parts of the world, crude skin test antigens (usually derived from killed parasite extracts) are used to assess a delayed hypersensitivity response to *Leishmania*. No leishmaniasis skin test is FDA approved in the United States, and like the tuberculin skin test, a positive response may persist after acute infection.

Since most infection is cutaneous among U.S. forces, our procedure was to obtain some skin lesion samples for analysis. Many sores were ulcerative and could be easily accessed by lifting off any crust and scraping the ulcer bed. Recent *L. major* infections tend to have many parasites, whereas nearly healed or chronic lesions tend to have far fewer amastigotes. The scraping method has been well described in recent reviews (28, 58). If the lesion was not ulcerative, then a punch skin biopsy would be performed.

We prefer skin scraping as the initial method, since it is simple and quick and can be done with limited training. In patients with multiple lesions, we usually select one of the more recent ulcerative lesions for sampling and avoid those that appear secondarily bacterially infected. Obtaining a good-quality sample is paramount, avoiding bleeding, which may obscure reading of the slide. The tissue form of *Leishmania*, the amastigote, is an oval to round organism 1.5 to 4 mm in diameter, with a distinct cell membrane, an internal nucleus, a rod-shaped kinetoplast (containing the mitochondrial DNA), and cytoplasm. Giemsa stain is typically used (Fig. 2), and with this stain, the cytoplasm appears blue, the nucleus appears violet-blue, and the kinetoplast stains red to violet. A tissue Gram stain is the most useful stain to highlight the kinetoplast of amastigotes in tissue biopsy sections. A Giemsa stain provides no additional utility over a hematoxylin and eosin stain for tissue sections (P. McEvoy, personal communication, 2004).

Punch skin biopsies can be useful when other diagnoses are considered, when the lesion is not suitable for scraping (e.g., nodular, plaque-like, or not ulcerative, although in these cases aspiration or a slit skin smear could be performed in lieu of scraping), or when the diagnosis after scraping is not revealing but clinical concern about a leishmaniasis diagnosis remains high. Generally, about 4 mm of tissue is needed, either two 2- to 3-mm biopsy specimens or a larger sample bisected for histology, culture, and PCR. Histologically, cutaneous

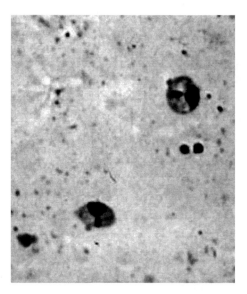

Figure 2. Amastigotes seen in a skin scraping; the stain is Diff-Quik (Dade-Behring, Newark, Del.). Magnification, ×300. (Photograph courtesy of R. Neafie, Armed Forces Institute of Pathology.)

leishmaniasis (with hematoxylin and eosin stain) is characterized by dermal chronic inflammation with lymphocytes, macrophages, and plasma cells, and sometimes with necrotizing granulomas. Parasites are often found in macrophages in the upper dermis.

If a skin lesion consistent with leishmaniasis is healing (completely epithelialized after a noduloulcerative period of growth) and the lesion was acquired in the Old World, then it is reasonable to observe the lesion and not sample it. Because OWCL is generally self-healing without visceralizing complications, the expected course would be for the lesion to continue to heal, eventually scarifying. Follow-up observations should be done to ensure that this occurs; otherwise, a biopsy to assess other chronic skin conditions is recommended.

The U.S. Army provides diagnostic support free of charge for samples from those who served in a military capacity when the infection was likely acquired. The military Leishmania Diagnostics Laboratory (Walter Reed Army Institute of Research, Silver Spring, Md.) can be reached by calling (301) 319-9956; further details regarding sample collection and processing can be found at the website (http://www.pdhealth.mil/leish.asp). The services offered include expert review of tissue sections (by the Armed Forces Institute of Pathology), rK39 serology for diagnosis of visceral leishmaniasis, parasite culture of fresh tissue samples with isoenzyme speciation, and *Leishmania* PCR genus and species level assays on fresh (tissue submitted in 70 to 100% ethanol) or paraffin-embedded samples. The Centers for Disease Control and Prevention (CDC) (Atlanta, Ga.) also provide diagnostic services for leishmaniasis to requesting health care providers. The CDC laboratory can be reached by calling (770) 488-4475; information is available on the website as well (http://www.dpd.cdc.gov/dpdx/HTML/DiagnosticProcedures.htm).

How well do our diagnostic tests work? Among 237 soldiers who returned from Iraq with a clinical diagnosis of cutaneous leishmaniasis, 181 had laboratory-confirmed cases (histology or PCR), 156 using the skin smear technique and 25 by skin biopsy. *Leishmania* PCR was positive in 185 samples. In no case was microscopy positive and PCR not positive; PCR was reactive in 37 persons who were microscopy negative, suggesting that it offers increased diagnostic sensitivity (60). Among 291 American service members referred to WRAMC who had expert microscopy, parasite culture, and *Leishmania* PCR performed on their samples using a "gold standard" of at least two positive assays, it was found that PCR identified 98%, culture 91%, and microscopy 89% (L. Hochberg, N. Aronson, R. Neafie, P. McEvoy, L. Gilmore, J. Fishbain, C. Hawkes, P. Weina, and G. Wortmann, *Abstr. 44th Intersci. Conf. Antimicrob. Agents Chemother.*, abstr. P-429, p. 453, 2004).

TREATMENT

The infecting parasite species is critical to planning treatment. Ninety-nine percent of the culture-positive skin samples in soldiers returning from Iraq were found to be infected by *L. major* (58). *L. major* has a benign clinical course with few complications in an immunocompetent host, and infection usually resolves without intervention in 6 to 12 months (3, 14, 32). Treatment decisions need to include the wishes of the patient (often cosmetic), the resources available, the potential for long-lasting cosmetic or functional limitations (scarring over small joints, chronic open skin lesions on hands or feet in occupations where keeping ulcers clean and dry would be difficult, or facial/eyelid/ear/nose lesions, and lesions which would be considered of more medical concern, such as ear lesions [which have been noted to often be more recalcitrant to therapy], many lesions, very large lesions, or lesions with lymphocutaneous dissemination), as well as the immune status of the patient and the infecting species of *Leishmania*. A consensus opinion on the best OWCL treatment awaits more well-controlled, definitive clinical trials. A treatment algorithm for Old World cutaneous leishmaniasis is provided in Fig. 3.

Local care and treatment of secondary bacterial infections, if present, are the first steps for ulceronodular lesions. Good wound care with careful cleaning and covering in the field environment may be helpful. Intriguing data from ongoing trials of an army paromomycin/gentamicin ointment suggest that the use of an occlusive dressing with daily cleaning is useful (50; A. Ben Salah, P. Buffet, H. Louzir, G. Morizot, A. Zaatour, N. Ben Alaya, N. Bel Hajhmida, Z. Elahmadi, S. Chlif, E. Lehnert, S. Doughty, K. Dellagi, and M. Grogl, *Abstr. Third World Congr. Leishmaniosis*, p. 17, 2005). Anecdotal reports in regions of endemicity suggest the use of silver nitrate cautery (52), but others have queried whether surgical cautery may be associated with lymphatic dissemination (19).

In Old World cutaneous leishmaniasis, *L. tropica* infections have a greater tendency to chronicity (in excess of 12 months) and relapse (leishmaniasis recidivans) (14). They also have the potential for mucosal involvement (contiguous involvement); associated viscerotropic infection; less responsiveness to therapy, including azoles, paromomycin, and sodium stibogluconate; and the potential for an anthroponotic cycle (e.g., in Kabul, Afghanistan) (29, 40, 48, 52). Because of these factors, infection with *L. tropica* is more aggressively treated in our center.

For *L. major* infections, localized therapy is initially preferred and can often be provided at a primary-care level. The methods of treatment currently employed for OWCL include physical methods, topical therapy, and systemic therapy. Physical methods have included cauterization, heat application, liquid nitrogen cryotherapy, and surgical excision. We have seen significant enlargement of leishmaniasis lesions along broken-down suture lines and discourage excision as a treatment modality. Thermotherapy capitalizes on the heat sensitivity of *Leishmania* (10).

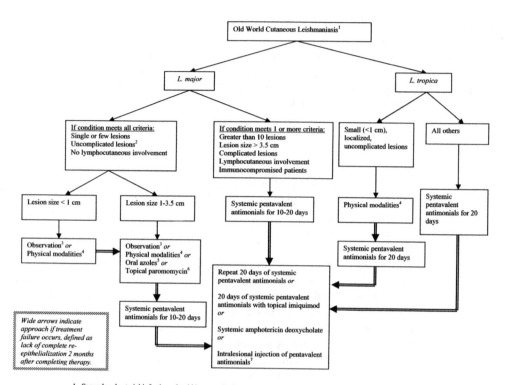

Figure 3. Treatment algorithm for Old World cutaneous leishmaniasis.

1. Secondary bacterial infections should be treated prior to using any physical methods.
2. Lesions are considered "complicated" if they are located on the hands, feet, over joints, or in cosmetically important areas. Also consider if located above a bursa, sporotrichoid extension with subcutaneous nodules, multiple daughter nodules, or regional adenopathy > 1 cm in size.
3. Depending on patient wishes. *L. major* typically resolves within one year if left untreated.
4. Physical modalities include heat (ThermoMed) or cryotherapy (liquid nitrogen) on anesthetized skin. Regimen used for cryotherapy is two 30-second freeze-thaw cycles. Can be used in pregnancy; use with care in dark-skinned individuals (particularly cryotherapy) due to risk of permanent hypopigmentation. Avoid treatment directly over blood vessels and nerves, implanted metal, or in those with a pacemaker (specifically, ThermoMed).
5. Ketoconazole, itraconazole, and fluconazole have all been used.
6. In the U.S., paromomycin capsules can be compounded into a topical formulation.
7. In some circumstances, pentavalent antimonials may be directly injected into skin lesions.

Cryotherapy is frequently employed by dermatologists in North America for a variety of indications. For cutaneous leishmaniasis, liquid nitrogen has been applied with a swab or spray on the lesion and extending into the normal-appearing surrounding skin to cause frosting for 20 to 30 seconds, followed by a slow thaw and retreatment (2). Patients are then observed after 2 weeks, and repeat treatment can be considered if needed. Localized heat therapy was used by the military with the FDA-cleared device ThermoMed (ThermoSurgery Technologies, Phoenix, Ariz.), which delivers localized radiofrequency-generated heat to the lesion via prongs placed in a gridlike pattern over the lesion and into the surrounding normal-appearing skin. A controlled trial ($n = 401$) of a single ThermoMed treatment compared to intralesional or intramuscular pentavalent antimony in presumed *L. tropica* infection found a shorter time to complete epithelialization (median, 53 days) in thermotherapy, with an intention-to-treat cure rate of 54% (with a high rate of cases lost to follow-up); the thermotherapy per-protocol cure rate was 69% (41). In a retrospective clinical experience of

L. major cutaneous leishmaniasis in U.S. soldiers, 26 patients were treated with one Ther-moMed treatment, followed by dressing changes and topical gentamicin (11, 60). Eighty-five percent of the patients were reported to have a clinical cure. One patient had a complication of secondary local bacterial infection. Among the 54 treated lesions, no ex-aggerated scarring or permanent pigmentary changes were noted (60). At WRAMC, a ran-domized clinical trial ($n = 56$) comparing one treatment session of ThermoMed to 10 days of systemic sodium stibogluconate, 20 mg/kg of body weight/day (excluding facial le-sions), had preliminary 6-month results of 93% cure in the sodium stibogluconate group compared to 73% of patients in the ThermoMed group (N. Aronson, G. Wortmann, W. Byrne, K. Kester, W. Bernstein, M. Marovich, I. Yoon, M. Polhemus, and P. Benson, *Abstr. 44th Intersci. Conf. Antimicrob. Agents Chemother.*, abstr. P-428, p. 452, 2004). The cost of the devices is high (>$20,000 each), but they are portable, battery operated, and simple to use. Local anesthetic is required, and treatment of multiple lesions can take more than 1 h, with additional daily time for dressing changes for 7 to 10 days.

Skin-deep treatments for OWCL include ointments and intralesional injections. Topi-cal use of the aminoglycoside paromomycin has been widely used in the Middle East ("P-ointment," or Leshcutan; Teva Pharmaceutical Industries, Jerusalem, Israel), com-pounded with 12% methylbenzethonium in soft white paraffin. Topical-paromomycin tri-als have used various study designs, endpoints, and products with varying results that are difficult to compare. Fifteen percent paromomycin and 12% or 5% methylbenzethonium chloride in paraffin used for treatment of *L. major* in Israel was associated with a cure rate of 74% after 10 to 20 days (16). In Turkey and Iran, controlled trials of 15% paro-momycin, 10% urea in white paraffin showed no clear clinical benefit (5, 36). In the United States, no topical paromomycin preparation is FDA approved or commercially available. Since a capsular form of paromomycin (Humatin) is approved in the United States, a compounding pharmacy can prepare a topical formulation with a prescription from a physician for an individual patient.

For cost containment, fewer side effects, and reported good efficacy, intralesional pen-tavalent antimony injection in various regimens and frequencies has been used (1, 46). This use of antimony is not currently permitted under the IND protocols for sodium sti-bogluconate in the United States, but its use is widespread in regions of endemicity, and it has recently been proposed as first-line management in the British military for OWCL (7). Reportedly, the injections can be somewhat painful and are associated with the complica-tion of vascular compromise if used on the face or digits.

Systemic agents for the treatment of OWCL include the azoles and pentavalent antimo-nial compounds. Ketoconazole, itraconazole, and fluconazole have all been studied in *L. major* infection (3, 32, 35, 43). A controlled trial of fluconazole, 200 mg per day for 6 weeks, was compared to a placebo in Saudi Arabia (for *L. major*) and showed greater healing at 3 months (59% versus 22%), and time to complete healing was 3 weeks shorter in the fluconazole arm (3). In the experience of OWCL with U.S. soldiers, 4 of 15 persons treated with oral fluconazole, 200 mg for 6 weeks, had clinical failure, including one pa-tient who had sporotrichoid lymphocutaneous spread occur while on azole therapy (60). Anecdotally, perhaps due to referral bias, our WRAMC experience with multiple flucona-zole failures has led us to consider it a modest therapy, albeit well tolerated and easily available. Miltefosine (hexadecylphosphocholine) is an oral agent that warrants considera-tion in the treatment of OWCL, although there are no published clinical trial data. A recent case report of disseminated *L. major* infection in a human immunodeficiency virus-infected patient showed a dramatic response to miltefosine after failure of pentavalent antimonial and amphotericin (45). A controlled trial of miltefosine for cutaneous leishmaniasis is ongoing in Afghanistan.

Systemic (intravenous or intramuscular) agents for OWCL include the pentavalent antimonials (e.g., sodium stibogluconate and meglumine antimoniate). Pentamidine has also been used, although most published studies are for New World cutaneous leishmaniasis (22, 51). Candidates for systemic antimonial treatment include patients with ear or facial lesions, local dissemination/lymphocutaneous extension, large lesions, lesions where scarring could effect future functionality, and cutaneous infections with OWCL species that have been associated with visceral disease *(L. tropica, L. infantum,* and *L. donovani),* as well as immunosuppressed hosts (e.g., those infected with human immunodeficiency virus). Antimonials have been used to treat leishmaniasis for nearly a century, but sodium stibogluconate is the only antimonial available for leishmaniasis treatment in the United States; as it has not been submitted for FDA approval, it must be given under an IND protocol. The U.S. military has such a protocol, which permits outpatient treatment at one of two sites: Walter Reed Army Medical Center, Washington, D.C. [(202) 782-1663 or -8691], and Brooke Army Medical Center, San Antonio, Tex. [(210) 916-5554] (43). The CDC provides sodium stibogluconate to requesting physicians through its own IND protocol. Interested physicians should contact the CDC Parasitic Drug Service at (404) 639-3670.

VISCERAL LEISHMANIASIS

VL is primarily a pediatric illness in Iraq, with a reported 2001 case rate of 10.9 cases per 100,000 persons (54, 59a). Few VL cases (23) have been reported as acquired in Afghanistan since the 1980s (13). In VL, parasites replicate in the reticuloendothelial system (the spleen, liver, and bone marrow). In the Old World, VL is caused by infection with *L. infantum* or *L. donovani.* During the Persian Gulf War (Operation Desert Storm), a syndrome called viscerotropic leishmaniasis, reportedly associated with *L. tropica,* was described among U.S. soldiers, with mild chronic symptomatology (29). The symptomatic expression of visceral leishmaniasis (known as kala-azar) includes fever, cachexia, pancytopenia, hepatosplenomegaly, and hypergammaglobulinemia with hypoalbuminemia. During World War II, 50 to 75 Allied soldiers were estimated to have VL, and only two deaths were noted (33). Visceral leishmaniasis can be asymptomatic, subclinical, symptomatic, or very severe (6, 20, 37, 49). In those who are malnourished, immunocompromised, or at the extremes of age, VL can be a fatal infection if it is not diagnosed and treated.

The highest rates of VL in Iraq have been described by the World Health Organization (WHO) to be in Baghdad and central Iraq, but since 1991, the area of endemicity has extended south to the Thi Qar, Muthanna, Missan, and Basrah Governates (58). Five U.S. military members have been diagnosed with VL acquired during Operation Iraqi Freedom and Operation Enduring Freedom (Afghanistan) (13, 21). Table 1 provides some clinical details of these cases. Notably, none of the patients had skin lesions; rather, they manifested fever, cytopenias, elevated-liver-associated enzymes, and splenomegaly, and often hepatomegaly and weight loss. All responded well to treatment. The Oman- and Afghanistan-acquired VL cases were pauciparasitic presentations, with PCR and expert detailed review of the histopathology leading to an eventual diagnosis. The Iraq-acquired cases had amastigotes

Table 1. Clinical summary of VL cases among American military personnel, 2002 to 2005

Parameter	Value for patient:				
	A (19)	B (31)	C (31)	D	E
Age (yr)	37	31	39	23	35
Race	Black	White	Black	Black	Black
Country where acquired	Oman	Afghanistan	Afghanistan	Iraq	Iraq
Symptom onset date	June 2002	December 2003	December 2003	March 2004	August 2004
Time since leaving an area of endemicity (mo)	3	3	14	11 in country	7
Symptoms					
Cytopenias	No	Yes	Yes	Yes	Yes
Hepatosplenomegaly	Yes	Yes	Yes	Yes	Yes
Fever	Yes	Yes	Yes	Yes	Yes
Weight loss (lb)	18	13	25	21	37
Elevated liver tests	Yes	Yes	Yes	Yes	Yes
Tissue biopsied	Bone marrow, positive	Bone marrow, negative Liver, positive	Bone marrow, negative Liver, positive	Bone marrow, positive	Bone marrow, positive
Method of parasitologic diagnosis	PCR, positive	Amastigotes seen	Amastigotes seen PCR, positive	Amastigotes seen Culture, positive (*L. donovani*)	Amastigotes seen PCR, positive
rK39 serology	Positive	Positive	Positive	Positive	Positive
Treatment	Liposomal amphotericin[a]	Liposomal amphotericin	ABLC[b]	Liposomal amphotericin	Liposomal amphotericin
Treatment outcome	Good response	Good response	Failed	Good response	Good response

[a]FDA-approved regimen: Ambisome, 3 mg/kg/day, days 1 to 5, day 14, and day 21.

[b]Patient developed chest pain with the first dose of liposomal amphotericin; changed to amphotericin lipid complex (Abelcet [ABLC]), 30 mg/kg, days 1 to 5 and 15. The patient then relapsed and therefore was treated with sodium stibogluconate with good response.

easily found on review of the bone marrow biopsy specimen, associated with foamy macrophages. In all cases, the recombinant *Leishmania chagasi* kinesin-associated antigen rK39 serology using the Kalazar Detect assay (Inbios International, Seattle, Wash.) was reactive.

It is anticipated that VL may become clinically manifest up to 2 years after an individual leaves a region of endemicity and that infection may often be asymptomatic or subclinical. In asymptomatic Mediterranean blood donors, parasitemia has been found to be present at low levels (27, 42). Blood donation by Iraq- and Afghanistan-deployed military personnel is deferred for 1 year with the guidance that any person who is diagnosed with leishmaniasis be deferred lifelong (http://www.militaryblood.dod.mil/library/policies/downloads/03-08.pdf).

In the United States, liposomal amphotericin B (Ambisome; Gilead Sciences [Fujisawa Healthcare], San Dimas, Calif.) is FDA approved for the treatment of VL. Conventional amphotericin B has more toxicity and requires a longer duration of dosing but also has an efficacy of >95% (55). The pentavalent antimonials (with the course extended to 28 days) have been an effective treatment, although regional resistance (e.g., in Bihar, India) has been reported (56). Miltefosine has been approved in India and Germany for the treatment of VL, with a reported efficacy of >95% (24, 57). Systemic paromomycin has also been effective for VL treatment in various countries (20).

PREVENTION

There are no approved medications or vaccine in the U.S. for prevention of leishmaniasis. Rahim and Tatar noted that "a lifelong immunity to reinfection seems to be the rule after recovery for cutaneous leishmaniasis in Iraq. We have noted only two cases of reinfection" (39). As our military forces repeatedly deploy back to areas of endemicity in Iraq and Afghanistan, it can be anticipated that some degree of immunity should be present among those subclinically or overtly infected during previous tours of duty. Leishmanization (intentional infection with viable *Leishmania*) is used in some parts of this region but has been associated with persistent infection (34).

The U.S. Army has a system of prevention for vector-borne diseases which includes covering the body with a uniform, environmental control, risk communication efforts, permethrin-treated uniforms and bed nets, *n*-diethyl-*m*-toluamide (DEET) topical repellent, and reservoir controls. A detailed 30-question survey was administered (individually or in small groups) to all patients with confirmed leishmaniasis cases who were enrolled in a sodium stibogluconate treatment protocol at WRAMC. Of 334 respondents in 2003 and 2004, only 33% had slept under a bed net, and of those who had used a bed net, only 23% used permethrin-treated nets. Eighty percent recalled a predeployment medical briefing, but only 6% remembered that leishmaniasis or a disease transmitted by biting flies was included; 12% received that information after arriving in theater. Overall, 82% reported that they had used insect repellent at any time after they deployed. The primary reasons given for not using repellent were as follows: 45% characterized access to military repellents as difficult or impossible, 5% felt it did not work, 4% were concerned about potential harm from it, and 14% did not note insect bites and so did not use it. Of those reporting using insect repellent, 54% used military issue DEET, 43% used a civilian product, 7% used animal flea collars, and 6% chewed matches (Porter and Aronson, *Abstr. 7th Force Health Prot.*

Conf.). During the following deployment cycle, a survey of U.S. military forces passing through Kuwait was administered to 1,200 persons waiting in line for a meal. There was a 73% response rate, and among the respondents, 36% had received DEET, 48% had received permethrin, and >78% recalled a medical threat briefing (59).

After the first year of deployment, partially due to security and military operational requirements, changes were instituted that have resulted in fewer cases (Fig. 1). Few troops were assigned to the area in the Diyala Governate where many cases had been acquired the prior year. Better housing, including hard structures with air conditioning, decreased evening exposure to sand flies, and pre- and post-deployment leishmaniasis briefings advised soldiers of risk and personal protective measures, including DEET, permethrin, and covering the body at night. Vector control was guided by sampling sand flies and targeting areas with higher rates of infected sand flies collected.

By June 2003, reports of PCR testing of pooled infected sand flies were being returned to preventive-medicine teams in Iraq. Measures to control the vector included using residual insecticides on tents (e.g., cyhalothrin), dusting fences and tree lines with Carbaryl, and nighttime fogging off trucks. These efforts were frustratingly ineffective in decreasing the number of captured sand flies, although anecdotally, soldiers reported fewer bites after treatments (Burkett et al., *Abstr. 7th Force Health Prot. Conf.*). Efforts to destroy sand fly and rodent habitats by bulldozing all around the camps had little impact on sand fly numbers (Burkett, unclassified military briefing). At one of the camps where leishmaniasis was more prevalent, during earth-moving operations, engineers reported that "the sky was black with insects." Reservoir control of small rodents was also extremely difficult, with burrows noted directly under tent platforms.

Prevention of infection remained at the individual level, including wearing long sleeves and trousers at night or sleeping inside an air-conditioned structure, application of 30 to 35% DEET to all exposed skin, and noting that high temperatures may reduce the duration of repellent effect (17). If a bed net is used, a mesh of at least 18 holes to the inch is needed, and all nets should be treated with permethrin before use. In areas where the infected vector is highly endemic, the vector and reservoir can be very focal, so when military circumstances allow, moving away from foci of high transmission by miles can decrease case rates significantly. No anthroponotic transmission of *L. major* has been noted, and none of the U.S. sand flies are known to be sufficient vectors (44).

It is estimated that the 2003 cost of an individual personal-protective-measure system was $81.00, while the cost associated with a 20-day course of sodium stibogluconate treatment in Washington, D.C., was about $11,000 per patient (D. West, personal communication, 2004). Leishmaniasis was estimated to account for 25,500 lost man-days during the first year of Operation Iraqi Freedom (J. Caci, *Abstr. 7th Force Health Prot. Conf.*, abstr. 781, 2004).

CONCLUSIONS

In the social chaos of wartime Afghanistan and Iraq, the incidence of OWCL is seemingly on the rise; reflecting that increase is the emergence of >1,000 cases of cutaneous leishmaniasis among U.S. military personnel since 2003. Fortunately, visceral leishmaniasis has manifested in few of our deployed soldiers, although the number of subclinical infections cannot easily be estimated without a sensitive screening test (which is not currently available). Active investigation has led to new advances in diagnostic devices (such as PCR and rK39 serology) and treatments (e.g., miltefosine and the accelerated pace of controlled trials to delineate the best clinical approach to treatment of OWCL). While the OWCL described in U.S. military personnel is generally benign, the impact of VL on the global poorest of the poor can be associated with high mortality and is estimated by the WHO to be in excess of 500,000 cases per year (56). Much remains to be done; the most effective treatments are expensive and generally challenging to administer, drug resistance is developing, and the prevalence of concomitant immunocompromising conditions is increasing.

Acknowledgments. The epidemiologic and prevention risk factor survey data among U.S. military leishmaniasis patients came from a joint project and were collected and analyzed by William D. Porter, Fort Hood, Tex. The treatment algorithm (Fig. 3) was derived from consensus opinion by myself, Andrew Werchniak (Brigham and Women's Hospital, Boston, Mass.), Denise Aaron and Sidney Klaus (Dartmouth-Hitchcock Medical Center, Dartmouth, N.H.), and Scott Norton (Walter Reed Army Medical Center, Washington, D.C.).

The views expressed in this chapter are those of the author and do not reflect the official position of the Department of the Army, Department of Defense, or U.S. government.

REFERENCES

1. **Alkhawajah, A., A. E. Larbi, Y. Al-Gindan, A. Abahussein, and S. Jain**. 1997. Treatment of cutaneous leishmaniasis with antimony: intramuscular vs. intralesional administration. *Ann. Trop. Med. Parasitol.* **91:** 899–905.
2. **Al-Majali, O., H. Routh, O. Abuloham, K. Bhowmik, M. Muhsen, and H. Hebeheba**. 1997. A two year study of liquid nitrogen therapy in cutaneous leishmaniasis. *Int. J. Dermatol.* **36:**460–462.
3. **Alrajhi, A., E. Ibrahim, E. de Vol, M. Khairat, R. Faris, and J. Maguire**. 2002. Fluconazole for the treatment of cutaneous leishmaniasis caused by *Leishmania major. N. Engl. J. Med.* **346:**891–895.
4. **Aronson, N. E., G. W. Wortmann, S. C. Johnson, J. E. Jackson, R. A. Gasser, Jr., A. J. Magill, T. P. Endy, P. E. Coyne, M. Grogl, P. M. Benson, J. S. Beard, J. D. Tally, J. M. Gambel, R. D. Kreutzer, and C. N. Oster**. 1998. Safety and efficacy of intravenous sodium stibogluconate in the treatment of leishmaniasis: recent U.S. military experience. *Clin. Infect. Dis.* **27:**1457–1464.
5. **Asilian, A., T. Jalayer, M. Nilforooshzadeh, R. Ghassemi, R. Peto, S. Wayling, P. Olliaro, and F. Modabber**. 2003. Treatment of cutaneous leishmaniasis with aminosidine (paromomycin) ointment: double-blind, randomized trial in the Islamic Republic of Iran. *Bull. W. H. O.* **81:**353–359.
6. **Badaro, R., T. Jones, E. Carvalho, D. Sampaio, S. Reed, A. Barral, R. Teixeira, and W. Johnson**. 1986. New perspectives on a subclinical form of visceral leishmaniasis. *J. Infect. Dis.* **154:**1003–1011.
7. **Bailey, M., A. Green, C. Ellis, T. O'Dempsey, N. Beeching, D. Lockwood, P. Chiodini, and A. Bryceson**. 2005. Clinical guidelines for the management of cutaneous leishmaniasis in British military personnel. *J. R. Army Med. Corps* **151:**73–80.
8. **Ben Salah, A., H. Zakraoui, A. Zaatour, A. Ftaiti, B. Zaafouri, A. Garraoui, P. L. Olliaro, K. Dellagi, and R. Ben Ismail**. 1995. A randomized, placebo-controlled trial in Tunisia treating cutaneous leishmaniasis with paromomycin ointment. *Am. J. Trop. Med. Hyg.* **53:**162–166.
9. **Berger, T., M. Meltzer, and C. Oster**. 1985. Lymph node involvement in leishmaniasis. *J. Am. Acad. Dermatol.* **12:**993–996.
10. **Berman, J. D., and F. A. Neva**. 1981. Effect of temperature on multiplication of *Leishmania* amastigotes within human monocyte-derived macrophages *in vitro. Am. J. Trop. Med. Hyg.* **30:**318–321.
11. **Carter, K. C., J. Alexander, and A. J. Baillie**. 1989. Studies on the topical treatment of experimental cutaneous leishmaniasis: the therapeutic effect of methyl benzethonium chloride and the aminoglycosides, gentamicin and paromomycin. *Ann. Trop. Med. Parasitol.* **83:**233–239.
12. **CDC**. 2003. Cutaneous leishmaniasis in U.S. military personnel—Southwest/Central Asia, 2002–3. *Morb. Mortal. Wkly. Rep.* **52:**1009–1012.
13. **CDC**. 2004. Two cases of visceral leishmaniasis in U.S. military personnel—Afghanistan, 2002–4. *Morb. Mortal. Wkly. Rep.* **53:**265–267.
14. **Dowlati, Y.** 1996.Cutaneous leishmaniasis: clinical aspects. *Clin. Dermatol.* **14:**425–431.

15. **Elamin, E. M., S. Guerbouj, A. M. Musa, I. Guizani, E. A. Khalil, M. M. Mukhtar, A. M. Elkadaro, H. S. Mohamed, M. E. Ibrahim, M. M. Abdel Hamid, M. El Azhari, and A. M. El Hassan.** 2005. Uncommon clinical presentations of cutaneous leishmaniasis in Sudan. *Trans. R. Soc. Trop. Med. Hyg.* **99:**803–808.

16. **El-On, J., S. Halevy, M. Grunwald, and L. Weinrauch.** 1992. Topical treatment of Old World cutaneous leishmaniasis caused by *Leishmania major*; a double-blind control study. *J. Am. Acad. Dermatol.* **27:**227–231.

17. **Fradin, M.** 1998. Mosquitoes and mosquito repellents: a clinician's guide. *Ann. Intern. Med.* **128:**931–940.

18. **Gómez-Saladín, E., C. W. Doud, and M. Maroli.** 2005. Short report: surveillance of *Leishmania* species among sand flies in Sicily (Italy) using a fluorogenic real-time polymerase chain reaction. *Am. J. Trop. Med. Hyg.* **72:**138–141.

19. **Griffiths, W., and S. Croft.** 1980. Cutaneous leishmaniasis. *Postgrad. Doctor MidEast* **3:**388–394.

20. **Guerin, P., P. Olliaro, S. Sundar, M. Boelaert, S. Croft, P. Desjeux, M. Wasunna, and A. Bryceson.** 2002. Visceral leishmaniasis: current status of control, diagnosis, and treatment, and a proposed research and development agenda. *Lancet Infect. Dis.* **2:**494–501.

21. **Halsey, E., M. Bryce, G. Wortmann, P. Weina, J. Ryan, and C. Dewitt.** 2004. Visceral leishmaniasis in a soldier returning from Operation Enduring Freedom. *Mil. Med.* **9:**699–701.

22. **Hellier, I., O. Dereure, I. Tournillac, F. Pratlong, B. Guillot, J. Dedet, and J. Guilhou.** 2000. Treatment of Old World cutaneous leishmaniasis by pentamidine isothionate. An open study of 11 patients. *Dermatology* **200:**120–123.

23. **Hyams, K. C., K. Hanson, F. S. Wignall, J. Escamilla, and E. C. Oldfield III.** 1995. The impact of infectious diseases on the health of U.S. troops deployed to the Persian Gulf during Operation Desert Shield/Desert Storm. *Clin. Infect. Dis.* **20:**1497–1504.

24. **Jha, T., S. Sundar, C. Thakur, P. Bachmann, J. Karbwang, C. Fischer, A. Voss, and J. Berman.** 1999. Miltefosine, an oral agent, for the treatment of Indian visceral leishmaniasis. *N. Engl. J. Med.* **341:**1795–1800.

24a. **Klassen-Fischer, M., J. Hallman, and R. Neafie.** 2006. Pathologic diagnoses of cutaneous diseases clinically mimicking leishmaniasis. *Mod. Pathol.* **19**(Suppl. 1):256A.

25. **Lay, J. C.** 2004. Leishmaniasis, US Armed Forces, 2003. *Med. Surveill. Mon. Rep.* **10**(1):2–5.

26. **Lay, J. C.** 2004. Leishmaniasis among U.S. Armed Forces, January 2003–November 2004. *Med. Surveill. Mon. Rep.* **10**(6):2–5.

27. **Le Fichoux, Y., J.-F. Quaranta, J.-P. Aufeuvre, A. Lelievre, P. Marty, I. Suffia, D. Rousseau, and J. Kubar.** 1999. Occurrence of *Leishmania infantum* parasitemia in asymptomatic blood donors living in an area of endemicity in southern France. *J. Clin. Microbiol.* **37:**1953–1957.

28. **Magill, A.** 2005. Cutaneous leishmaniasis in the returning traveler. *Infect. Dis. Clin. N. Am.* **19:**241–266.

29. **Magill, A., M. Grogl, R. Gasser, W. Sun, and C. Oster.** 1993. Visceral infection caused by *Leishmania tropica* in veterans of Operation Desert Storm. *N. Engl. J. Med.* **328:**1383–1387.

30. **McHugh, C., P. Melby, and S. LaFon.** 1996. Leishmaniasis in Texas; epidemiology and clinical aspects of human cases. *Am. J. Trop. Med. Hyg.* **55:**547–555.

31. **Mohsen, Z.** 1983. Biting activity, physiological age and vector potential of *Phlebotomus papatasi scopoli* (Diptera: *Phlebotomidae*) in central Iraq. *J. Biol. Sci.* **14:**79–94.

32. **Momeni, A., T. Jalayer, M. Emamjomeh, N. Bashardost, R. Ghassemi, M. Meghdadi, A. Javadi, and M. Aminjavaheri.** 1996. Treatment of cutaneous leishmaniasis with itraconazole. Randomized double-blind study. *Arch. Dermatol.* **132:**784–786.

33. **Most, H., and P. Lavietes.** 1947. Kala azar in American military personnel. *Medicine* **26:**221–284.

34. **Nadim, A., E. Javadian, and M. Mohebali.** 1997. The experience of leishmanization in the Islamic Republic of Iran. *East Medit. Health J.* **3:**284–289.

35. **Nassiri-Kashani, M., A. Firozze, A. Khamesipour, F. Mojtahed, M. Nilforoushzadeh, H. Hejazi, N. Bouzari, and Y. Dowlati.** 2005. A randomized, double-blind, placebo-controlled clinical trial of itraconazole in the treatment of cutaneous leishmaniasis. *J. Eur. Acad. Dermatol. Venereol.* **19:**80–83.

36. **Ozgoztasi, O., and I. Baydar.** 1997. A randomized clinical trial of topical paromomycin versus oral ketoconazole for treating cutaneous leishmaniasis in Turkey. *Int. J. Dermatol.* **36:**61–63.

37. **Pampiglione, S., P. Manson-Bahr, F. Guingi, G. Giuhti, A. Parenti, and G. Canesti Trotti.** 1974. Studies on Mediterranean leishmaniasis. 2. Asymptomatic cases of visceral leishmaniasis. *Trans. R. Soc. Trop. Med. Hyg.* **68:**447–453.

38. **Pringle, G.** 1957. Oriental sore in Iraq; historical and epidemiological problems. *Bull. Endem. Dis.* (Baghdad) **2:**41–76.

39. **Rahim, G. F., and I. Tatar.** 1966. Oriental sore in Iraq. *Bull. Endem. Dis.* (Baghdad) **8:**29–54.

40. **Reithinger, R., M. Mohsen, K. Aadil, M. Sidiqi, P. Erasmus, and P. Coleman.** 2003. Anthroponotic cutaneous leishmaniasis, Kabul, Afghanistan. *Emerg. Infect. Dis.* **9:**727–729.

41. **Reithinger, R., M. Mohsen, M. Wahid, M. Bismullah, R. J. Quinnell, C. R. Davies, J. Kolaczinski, and J. R. David.** 2005. Efficacy of thermotherapy to treat cutaneous leishmaniasis caused by *Leishmania tropica* in Kabul, Afghanistan: a randomized, controlled trial. *Clin. Infect. Dis.* **40:**1148–1155.

42. **Riera, C., R. Fisa, M. Udina, M. Gallego, and M. Portus.** 2004. Detection of *Leishmania infantum* cryptic infection in asymptomatic blood donors living in an endemic area (Eivissa, Balearic Islands, Spain) by different diagnostic methods. *Trans. R. Soc. Trop. Med. Hyg.* **98:**102–110.

43. **Salmanpour, R., F. Handjani, and M. Nouhpisheh.** 2001. Comparative study of the efficacy of oral ketoconazole with intra-lesional meglumine antimoniate (glucantime) for the treatment of cutaneous leishmaniasis. *J. Dermatol. Treat.* **12:**159–162.

44. **Schlein, Y., and R. Jacobson.** 1996. Why is man an unsuitable reservoir for the transmission of *Leishmania major? Exp. Parasitol.* **82:**298–305.

45. **Schraner, C., B. Hasse, U. Hasse, D. Baumann, A. Faeh, G. Burg, F. Grimm, A. Mathis, R. Weber, and H. Gunthard.** 2005. Successful treatment with miltefosine of disseminated cutaneous leishmaniasis in a severely immunocompromised patient infected with HIV-1. *Clin. Infect. Dis.* **40:**e120–e124.

46. **Sharquie, K., R. Najim, and I. Farjou.** 1997. A comparative controlled trial of intralesionally administered zinc sulfate, hypertonic sodium chloride and pentavalent antimony compound against acute cutaneous leishmaniasis. *Clin. Exp. Dermatol.* **22:**169–173.

47. **Siddig, A., S. Al Jowary, M. Al Izzi, J. Hopkins, M. Hall, and J. Slingenbergh.** 2005. Seasonality of Old World screwworm myiasis in the Mesopotamia Valley in Iraq. *Med. Vet. Entomol.* **19:**140–150.

48. **Singh, S., R. Singh, and S. Sundar.** 1995. Failure of ketoconazole treatment in cutaneous leishmaniasis. *Int. J. Dermatol.* **34:**120–121.

49. **Singh, S., V. Kumari, and N. Singh.** 2002. Predicting kala-azar disease manifestations in asymptomatic patients with latent *Leishmania donovani* infection by detection of antibody against recombinant K39 antigen. *Clin. Diagn. Lab. Immunol.* **9:**568–572.

50. **Soto, J. M., J. T. Toledo, P. Gutierrez, M. Arboleda, R. S. Nicholls, J. R. Padilla, J. D. Berman, C. K. English, and M. Grogl.** 2002. Treatment of cutaneous leishmaniasis with topical antileishmanial drug (WR 279396): phase 2 pilot study. *Am. J. Trop. Med. Hyg.* **66:**147–151.

51. **Soto-Mancipe, J., M. Grogl, and J. Berman.** 1993. Evaluation of pentamidine for the treatment of cutaneous leishmaniasis in Colombia. *Clin. Infect. Dis.* **16:**417–425.

52. **Storer, E., and J. Wayte.** 2005. Cutaneous leishmaniasis in Afghani refugees. *Australas. J. Dermatol.* **46:**80–83.

53. **Sukkar, F.** 1985. Leishmaniasis in the Middle East, p. 394–411. *In* K.-P. Chang and R. Bray (ed.), *Leishmaniasis.* Elsevier Science Publisher, Amsterdam, The Netherlands.

54. **Sukkar, F.** 1976. Some epidemiological and clinical aspects of kala-azar in Iraq. *Bull. Endem. Dis.* (Baghdad) **17:**53–62.

55. **Sundar, S., H. Mehta, A. Suresh, S. Singh, M. Rai, and H. Murray.** 2004. Amphotericin B treatment for Indian visceral leishmaniasis: conventional versus lipid formulations. *Clin. Infect. Dis.* **38:**377–383.

56. **Sundar, S.** 2001. Drug resistance in Indian visceral leishmaniasis. *Trop. Med. Int. Health* **6:**849–854.

57. **Sundar, S., T. Jha, C. Thakur, J. Engel, H. Sindermann, C. Fischer, K. Junge, A. Bryceson, and J. Berman.** 2002. Oral miltefosine for Indian visceral leishmaniasis. *N. Engl. J. Med.* **347:**1739–1746.

58. **Weina, P., R. Neafie, G. Wortmann, M. Polhemus, and N. Aronson.** 2004. Old World leishmaniasis: an emerging infection among deployed U.S. military and civilian workers. *Clin. Infect. Dis.* **39:**1674–1680.

59. **White, D., P. Davin, and M. Walter.** 2005. Survey of repellent use by service members arriving in Kuwait for Operation Iraqi Freedom. *Mil. Med.* **170:**496–500.

59a. **WHO.** 2003. *Visceral Leishmaniasis in the Lower South, 2003.* Basrah office report. WHO, Geneva, Switzerland.

60. **Willard, R., A. Jeffcoat, P. Benson, and D. Walsh.** 2005. Cutaneous leishmaniasis in soldiers from Ft. Campbell, KY returning from Operation Iraqi Freedom highlights diagnostic and therapeutic options. *J. Am. Acad. Dermatol.* **52:**977–987.

61. **Wortmann, G., C. Sweeney, H. Houng, N. Aronson, J. Stiteler, J. Jackson, and C. Ockenhouse.** 2001. Rapid diagnosis of leishmaniasis by fluorogenic polymerase chain reaction. *Am. J. Trop. Med. Hyg.* **65:**583–587.

62. **Yanik, M., M. Gurel, Z. Simsek, and M. Kati.** 2004. The psychological impact of cutaneous leishmaniasis. *Clin. Exp. Dermatol.* **29:**464–467.

Emerging Infections 7
Edited by W. M. Scheld, D. C. Hooper, and J. M. Hughes
© 2007 ASM Press, Washington, D.C.

Chapter 18

Smallpox Vaccination: a Review of Adverse Events for Contemporary Health Care Providers

Vincent A. Fulginiti

One would think that smallpox vaccination need not be a topic about which current health care workers should be concerned. Smallpox was eliminated as a naturally occurring disease in 1977, and routine smallpox vaccination in the United States was discontinued in 1972 and in most of the world by 1995 (11, 17). Why, then, should this chapter be written? The events of 11 September 2001, the use of martyrdom in terrorism, and the possibility that stocks of variola virus, the virus causing smallpox, exist in various places in the world have raised the specter of reintroduction of this disease as a bioterrorism agent. Recently, smallpox vaccination was instituted for the armed forces and electively for health care personnel and "first responders" (2; http://www.smallpox.army.mil/event/SPsafetysum.asp, http://www.cdc.gov). If smallpox is reintroduced, smallpox vaccination will become necessary for some, if not all, of the citizens in the country of introduction, and perhaps worldwide. However, current health care workers who have entered the field recently have not used smallpox vaccine and are unaware of the ways in which it differs from other commonly employed vaccines. They may be equally unaware of the potential complications from use of the vaccine.

For these reasons, it is prudent that we review the disease and the vaccine that resulted in its elimination. This chapter will deal with the vaccine, its benefits, its risks, and the current state of its use.

THE VIRUS AND THE VACCINES

Vaccinia virus describes a variety of viruses, many believed to be derived from Jenner's original strain or subsequent isolates, although the actual origins of most vaccinia virus strains are obscure, if not unknown (17). Dixon described the various possibilities for the origin of this agent, ranging from an original derivation from smallpox to cowpox transmitted over the centuries (7). In the United States, the vaccine stored at the CDC and currently used for vaccination, and the seed virus for new batches of vaccine being produced, is the New York City Board of Health strain (2, 12, 17).

Vincent A. Fulginiti • University of Colorado Health Sciences Center, Denver, Colo., and University of Arizona, Tucson, Ariz.

A number of attenuated strains have been produced, none of which are currently available (12, 17). Most promising is the Ankara strain, passed through chicken embryo fibroblasts more than 500 times. Studies are under way to evaluate this strain relative to the New York City Board of Health Strain derivatives. Other strains may also appear as attempts are made to reduce reactivity while maintaining antigenicity and, hopefully, protection against smallpox.

Vaccinia virus is one of the orthopoxviruses, a group which includes variola (smallpox) virus, molluscum contagiosum virus, and monkeypox virus, camelpox virus, cowpox virus, and other species-specific poxviruses. It has a distinct DNA genome, although it shares some characteristics and antigens with other members of the group to various degrees. It is *not* smallpox virus, but this myth occasionally results in irrational fear of the use of the vaccine.

Vaccinia virus infects by replication within the cytoplasm of cells and then migrates cell to cell though microtubules. This accounts for the localization of vaccination in a circumferential pattern, as the virus expands its infectious area until it is contained by the immune response. Accumulations of virus in the cytoplasm result in eosinophilic inclusions (Guarnieri bodies), which are visible microscopically.

Vaccinia virus variants have been investigated as host vectors for immunization against other viral diseases, e.g., rabies and human immunodeficiency virus infection (4). The concept is that the large amount of DNA permits the insertion of genes for antigens of these other agents, and following vaccination by various routes, specific antibodies directed against those agents are evoked.

The currently available vaccine (Dryvax; Wyeth Laboratories) was produced in 1970 and has been stored at the CDC since that time (2, 17). The vaccine is derived from calf skin infection, with the New York City Board of Health strain as the seed virus. When reconstituted from the dry state, it has a potency of approximately 100 million live virus particles per ml. Enough vaccine has been stored to immunize the entire U.S. population if diluted appropriately. Additional stores of vaccine produced by Aventis-Pasteur have been added to the national stockpile.

To ensure the future availability of appropriate amounts of smallpox vaccine, the U.S. government has funded the manufacture of tissue culture vaccine; the most likely candidate is an Acambis/Baxter Laboratories' product, grown in Vero monkey kidney cell culture.

VACCINATION

Screening

Before employing the actual technique of vaccination, it is important to identify individuals who should not be vaccinated if there is no immediate threat of exposure to smallpox. These instances are fully described below after the vaccination procedure is presented.

Technique

The earlier vaccination technique utilized a single sterile needle at a 45° angle to place multiple punctures in the skin through a drop of vaccine, usually delivered via a single-dose capillary tube. In some instances of mass vaccination, mechanical devices were used to introduce the vaccine into the skin (compressed-air pressure forced the vaccine into the skin via a "gunlike" device).

However, during the eradication effort that resulted in the complete elimination of smallpox, a technique for administering smallpox vaccine was developed which has been adopted for current use (11). In this technique, a bifurcated needle with the capacity to retain 0.25 ml of viable vaccine solution when dipped into a multidose container is used to puncture the skin (Fig. 1). The loaded needle is placed perpendicular to the site of vaccination, and rapid strokes are made to produce a trace of blood or serum at the site of inoculation (Fig. 2). The insertions should be made within a 0.5-cm circle to confine the vaccination site. Tissue culture vaccines currently being produced may be delivered in different containers; the information for these products, when they become available, should be consulted for the proper procedure.

For primary vaccination in a vaccinia-naive person, 15 insertions are made, resulting in 30 minute skin punctures inserting the vaccine into the deeper layers of the skin. For revaccination, only three insertions (six skin punctures) are used. The purpose of both insertions is to maximally ensure that infection occurs, and in experienced hands, they result in approximately 98% successful vaccinations (2, 11, 12, 17).

After the vaccination, there are several recommended methods for covering the site to avoid spread of the virus. A successful vaccination may exude liquid material on the surface. The simplest cover is a sterile cotton square loosely applied to the area. For those who may have close contact with potentially susceptible persons (such as health care workers in contact with patients), a semipermeable membrane covering has been shown to reduce or eliminate spread of the virus.

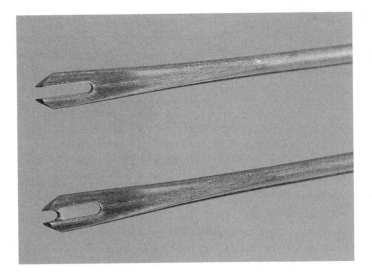

Figure 1. Bifurcated needle for smallpox vaccination; note the vaccine trapped in the bifurcation. Copyright © Logical Images, Inc.

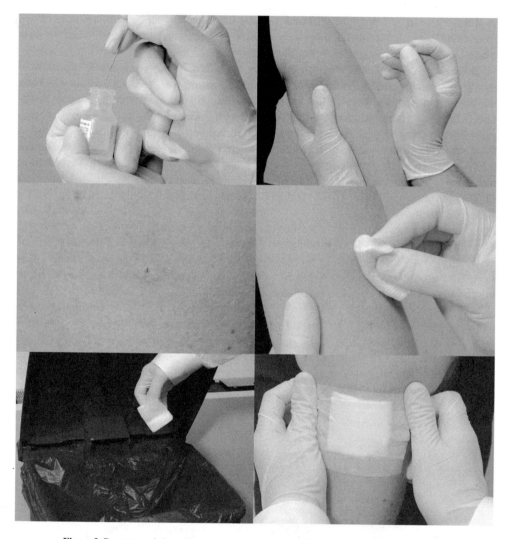

Figure 2. Recommended smallpox vaccination technique. Copyright © Logical Images, Inc.

TIMING OF VACCINATION AND IMMUNITY TO SMALLPOX

Prior to Jennerian vaccination, it was known that recovery from smallpox rendered the individual immune to further disease, even with extensive exposure (7). Early attempts at immunization mimicked this natural state by scarification and insertion of pustular material from a smallpox patient (called "variolation"). This practice resulted in significant protection, but it had the potential for lethal infection in a small number of recipients. Once Jenner demonstrated the success of "vaccination," the practice of variolation gradually disappeared.

A successful vaccination is an indication of immunity to smallpox. Mack reported a dramatic reduction in death from smallpox in those who had been vaccinated within

10 years prior to exposure and disease (24). There was a significant reduction even 30 years or more after primary vaccination. However, long-term protection against disease is uncertain, although most studies have shown dramatic differences between vaccinated and unvaccinated individuals.

Following vaccination, more than 95% of recipients develop circulating neutralizing antibody and strong virus-specific CD8 cytotoxic T lymphocytic responses. Based on our experience with vaccinia virus, it appears that T-cell immunity accounts for both recovery from smallpox infection and limitation of vaccinia virus infection after vaccination. The antibody appears to function as an inhibitor of viremia and may be a marker for protection against disease, although this is uncertain. Recent immunologic studies have suggested that antibody and T-cell immunity, as measured in the laboratory, last a great deal longer than previously suspected, but a definitive statement as to the duration of protection against disease based on these parameters cannot be made, since there is no exposure today (17). When the disease was rampant, our immunologic methods were not as refined as they are now, so we have no definitive surrogates for protection based on antibody level or degree of T-cell immune responsiveness to vaccinia.

Routine vaccination should not be carried out prior to the first birthday. This precaution is based on the assumption that most immunologic defects will be identified by then and by the historical occurrence of progressive vaccinia, a lethal adverse event, in young infants who had severe combined immunodeficiency, unidentified at the time of vaccination.

In epidemic circumstances, age is not a factor, and smallpox vaccine has historically been used even in early infancy. Exposure to smallpox or the potential for such exposure will dictate the timing, by age, of vaccination should an outbreak occur.

Older individuals who have never been vaccinated will be subject to vaccination in the event of an outbreak, but certain precautions will be necessary for unexposed adults. These are related to the vulnerabilities discussed below.

Revaccination can occur at any time after primary vaccination but historically was performed at 7- to 10-year intervals. Some experts suggest that immunity lasts from 3 to 5 years and wanes thereafter (17). Recent immunologic evidence suggests that immunity may be sustained for a very long time, and only a wide experience with clinical vaccination efforts will determine the exact intervals for protection after primary vaccination and revaccination. Unless there is introduction of smallpox, this issue will not be resolved.

NORMAL, EXPECTED REACTIONS AT THE SITE OF VACCINATION

In the past, many sites were used for vaccination. It is now recommended that the deltoid area of the nondominant arm be used (2, 12, 17). Sites that are exposed to moisture or tight confinement by clothing should be avoided, as this might lead to exacerbation of normal reactions, possible bacterial contamination, and increased propensity for some adverse reactions.

For primary vaccination, it is anticipated that at 6 to 8 days a well-formed pustule will result. The sequence of infection is illustrated in Fig. 3. A small papule first appears, surrounded quickly by erythema and edema of the vaccination site. The papule undergoes central necrosis and umbilication, scabs over, and eventually leaves a circular scar. Most individuals have modest erythema and local edema without much in the way of systemic reaction.

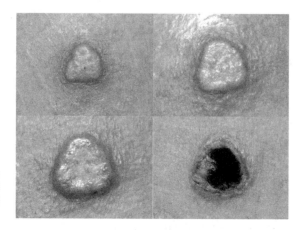

Figure 3. Appearance of primary vaccination site on days 6 (upper left), 8 (upper right), 10 (lower left), and 14 (lower right). Copyright © Logical Images, Inc.

In a small and variable number of individuals, a more robust reaction occurs, with florid erythema and massive edema of the surrounding tissues (Fig. 4). These are normal reactions and are not considered adverse events. In addition, a few individuals experience a lymphatic track leading from the vaccination site toward regional lymph nodes, which may also be manifest as enlarged tender masses. These reactions are also normal variants and not adverse events, and they are also depicted in Fig. 4.

Almost all vaccinees, regardless of the degree of local reaction, experience itching or local "discomfort," often described as awareness of the vaccination site. In some instances, the itching is severe and persistent and requires symptomatic treatment with either an antipruritic or an antihistamine.

Those experiencing robust reactions may also have systemic symptoms; fever, myalgia, and lethargy may be present. In addition, these individuals may have more severe local sensations of pain and/or intense itching.

In a very few individuals, some "satellite" lesions may occur within an inch of the primary vaccination (Fig. 4). The cause of these additional primary lesions is not known for

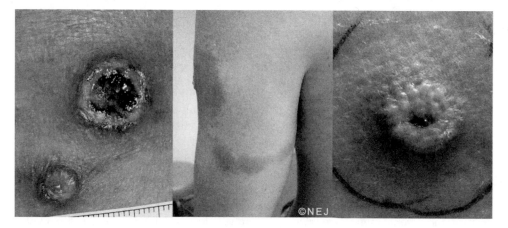

Figure 4. Normal robust vaccination reactions. Copyright © Logical Images, Inc.

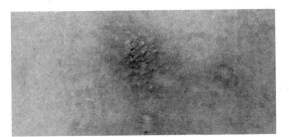

Figure 5. Example of a major reaction after revaccination. Copyright © Logical Images, Inc.

certain. It is my belief that they are caused either by minor abrasions in the skin not noticed originally, which become infected as a result of overflow of the vaccine fluid, or inadvertent punctures by the vaccinator outside the usual 0.5-cm area that is recommended. These reactions are also considered to be within the normal spectrum of expected reactions and are not adverse events.

In revaccinees, a positive take (called a major reaction) is manifested by any pustule, vesicle, or evidence of inflammation at 6 to 8 days (Fig. 5). This reaction involutes more quickly than does a primary vaccination. However, even an erythematous reaction is considered by experts to be evidence of a successful "take" in revaccinees. The presence of ulceration, induration, or a scab is even stronger evidence of a successful take. Transient erythema that appears soon after revaccination but is gone by 6 to 8 days probably reflects a hypersensitivity reaction and does not equate with immunity.

The lack of any reaction at the site does not indicate immunity, as is commonly believed. Rather, it implies unsuccessful vaccination procedure or inadequate vaccine. In such instances, revaccination with great care to use proper technique and with vaccine known to produce takes in others is required. Revaccinees rarely experience robust forms of reaction unless a very long time has elapsed since the primary vaccination.

TRUE ADVERSE EVENTS

It is critical to emphasize that the vast majority of vaccinees (nearly all) undergo vaccination without serious complications. Because the nature of adverse reactions to smallpox vaccine is often dramatic and is so different from most health workers' experience with vaccines, there is a tendency to fear this vaccine and to believe that it is very "dangerous." In fact, it is a very safe vaccine. For a few individuals, normal robust reactions are expected; for even fewer, moderate reactions will occur, which are either self-limited or treatable. For the rare vaccinee, more severe and potentially lethal adverse events may occur.

However, in contrast to other vaccines in common use, smallpox vaccine results in visible infectious lesions on the surface of the skin. This is a critical difference between smallpox vaccine and other viral vaccines. As a result of abundant virus on the skin, the opportunity for unique types of adverse events exists, as for no other vaccine. In common with other viral vaccines, however, this live agent has a propensity for producing adverse events in certain immunologically susceptible individuals.

There are some medical conditions that predispose to complications. Knowledge of these precursors to adverse events stems from experience in the 1960s and beyond. Some more recent experience has added to the list of conditions that might predispose to adverse events. I will describe these here, as it is necessary to exclude persons from receiving vaccine if they are present, and such screening is part of the vaccination protocol.

POTENTIAL PREDISPOSING CONDITIONS THAT MIGHT PREDICT ADVERSE EVENTS IN THE VACCINEE AND/OR CLOSE CONTACTS AFTER VACCINATION

As pointed out above, persons presenting for vaccination may have unique susceptibilities to some adverse events. Thus, all potential vaccinees should be screened for these susceptibilities.

If smallpox is not present, or if the individual has not been exposed to smallpox in the event of a bioterrorist introduction of the disease, then the following conditions are contraindications to the use of vaccine in that individual. However, if smallpox is present and the individual with these conditions is exposed, smallpox vaccination needs to be considered. The dilemma for the clinician in the latter instance is that both the disease and the vaccination may result in serious, even lethal, outcomes under some circumstances. I will attempt to deal with this dilemma under each of the specific categories. Suffice it to say that the current expert recommendations insist on vaccinating smallpox-exposed susceptible individuals regardless of predisposing vulnerabilities.

The potential vulnerabilities to adverse events after smallpox vaccination are listed in Table 1.

Allergy to Vaccine Components

Current vaccinia vaccines may contain the antibiotic polymyxin B, streptomycin, or chlortetracycline, and anyone sensitive to these agents should not receive the vaccine. If a person has experienced an allergic reaction to smallpox vaccine in the past, he or she should not receive the vaccine. Of course, if there is exposure to smallpox, then vaccine can be administered with antiallergic medications, with the risk of disease versus that of reaction carefully examined and explained.

Table 1. Potential vulnerabilities after smallpox vaccination

Allergy to vaccine components
Prior adverse reaction to smallpox vaccine
Age under 1 yr
Pregnancy
Breastfeeding
Inflammatory eye disease (caution only)
Atopic dermatitis
Darier's disease
Extensive skin disruption
T-cell deficiency (condition, disease, or treatment induced)
Cardiac conditions (see the text for CDC recommendations)

Pregnancy and Breast-Feeding

Precautions during pregnancy and breast-feeding are based on the potential threat, not on actual experience. There have been very few reported instances of fetal infection if a pregnant woman is vaccinated. The risk to the fetus of early termination of pregnancy or complications other than direct infection have varied in studies examining this issue. Regardless of the data or lack of a definitive definition of risk, it is deemed prudent not to vaccinate pregnant women. Virus may enter breast milk, and hence, this precaution is justified.

Atopic Dermatitis and Other Skin Afflictions

There is clear evidence that true atopic dermatitis poses a risk to the vaccinee; prior to the use of effective treatment, mortality was estimated at between 12 and 30%. The atopic individual, with or without current active skin lesions, is at risk because of the innate immunologic defect in modulating the immune response. As a result, the vaccine virus establishes infection in areas of current or past skin lesions. These are often massive and accompanied by systemic manifestations. Thus, no person with atopic dermatitis, regardless of whether disruptive skin lesions are present and regardless of age, should receive smallpox vaccine.

In the past, patients were deemed to have "eczema," a diagnosis that encompassed a variety of skin disorders, and not all of these patients had the same susceptibility as persons with atopic dermatitis. This has confused the exclusionary criteria. Further, burns or traumatic or surgical wounds pose an indefinable risk of vaccinia infections in the affected skin. Each situation must be considered individually and is further discussed below [see "Eczema Vaccinatum (Contact Vaccinia in Atopic Individuals)"].

Children under the Age of 1 Year

The exclusion of children under the age of 1 year is based solely on the need to be certain that young children are not immunodeficient and do not have another contraindication to vaccination. The presumption is that such conditions would be discovered by the first birthday.

T-Cell and Other Immunodeficiencies

Experience in the era when smallpox vaccination was routine demonstrated that true T-cell-deficient individuals were subject to progressive infection with vaccinia virus, most often with a lethal outcome. Other immunodeficiencies were less well known, and thus, we cannot be certain about the susceptibility of those with non-T-cell immunodeficiencies. It is important to remember that at that time both immunologic knowledge and laboratory determinations were not as sophisticated as they are today. As a result, much of what was known was empiric and based on cruder estimates of immunodeficiency. We do know that many patients with hypogammaglobulinemia but with intact T-cell function underwent smallpox vaccination without incident, presumably because their T-cell immunity was sufficient to contain the virus and to rid the body of infected skin cells, preventing further spread to other areas of the body. We also know that a few individuals with progressive vaccinia virus infection had a lack of T-cell function but intact antibody capacity to various degrees. These individuals had lesser degrees of progression, often without viremic spread. Because of our lack of knowledge of the degree of susceptibility, if any, of individuals

with non-T-cell immunodeficiencies, the recommendation has evolved to exclude such individuals from elective smallpox vaccination.

T-cell deficiencies include all those primary immunodeficiencies in which T-cell function is absent or impaired. We do not know the specific level of T cells that is sufficient for
protection. This becomes a critical issue for patients receiving immunosuppressive drugs
and for those who are infected with human immunodeficiency virus. In both groups, the
degree of T-cell deficiency is variable, not absent. For elective vaccination, all such persons should be excluded; individual judgments must be made if the potential vaccinee is
exposed to smallpox.

Cardiovascular Precautions

The CDC has recommended that persons fulfilling the following criteria should not receive smallpox vaccine (http://www.cdc.gov).

> Diagnosed by a doctor as having a heart condition, with or without
> symptoms, including conditions such as previous myocardial infarc-
> tion (heart attack), angina (chest pain caused by lack of blood flow to
> the heart), congestive heart failure, cardiomyopathy (the heart muscle
> becomes inflamed and does not work as well as it should), stroke or
> transient ischemic attack (a "ministroke" that produces stroke-like
> symptoms but not lasting damage), chest pain or shortness of breath
> with activity (such as walking upstairs), or other heart conditions
> being treated by a doctor

> Three or more of the following risk factors: high blood pressure diag-
> nosed by a doctor; high blood cholesterol diagnosed by a doctor, dia-
> betes or high blood sugar diagnosed by a doctor, a first-degree relative
> (for example, mother, father, brother, or sister) who had a heart condi-
> tion before the age of 50, and current cigarette smoking

While this may be a temporary exclusion, these people should not get the vaccine while
the conditions are present.

Darier's Disease

Darier's disease (keratosis follicularis) is a rare dermatitis, usually beginning in adoles-
cence and caused by the presence of a dominant abnormal gene (*ATP2A2* on chromosome
12). The rash affects the seborrheic areas, neck, and torso. Flexural rash predominates. The
nature of the rash and the potential immunologic susceptibility that accompanies it render
the patient susceptible to infection with vaccinia virus and other dermatotropic viruses.

Inflammatory Eye Disease

Inflammatory eye disease (allergic or mechanical conjunctivitis) has two characteristics
that favor implantation of vaccinia virus. The irritability of the lesion causes the patient to
rub the eyes repeatedly, and the disrupted mucosa permits implantation if the hands are
contaminated with vaccinia virus from the patient's own lesion or that of another. I saw this

most often in mothers tending young infants who had received a primary vaccination; the infant's lesion was touched by the mother when she was bathing or otherwise tending the child, and then the mother touched her eye.

TYPES OF ADVERSE EVENTS AFTER SMALLPOX VACCINATION

There are a number of ways to classify adverse reactions to smallpox vaccine. I have chosen to divide the reactions by the degree of severity, as this is the most critical factor that the clinician must consider in evaluating the diagnosis, treatment, and prognosis of a given event. The divisions are listed in Table 2.

Minimal Adverse Reactions

Minimal adverse reactions are generally mild, short-lived, and without serious implications for health. Rarely, some of these reactions may develop into more serious complications;

Table 2. Classification by severity of adverse events after smallpox vaccination

Event	Type
Minimal	
Noninfectious rashes (erythema multiforme)	Macular
	Vesicular
	Pustular
	Urticarial
	Mixed
Bacterial infection	Staphylococcal
	Streptococcal
	Other
Contact (inoculation; accidental)	Autoinoculation
	Transferred to contact
Generalized vaccinia	Single occurrence
	Few or no systemic symptoms
Moderate, severe, and life threatening (in ascending degrees of severity)	
Erythema multiforme	Stevens-Johnson syndrome
Generalized vaccinia	Severe symptoms
Cardiac	Myopericarditis
Contact	Vaccinia keratitis
	Eczema vaccinatum
Postvaccinal encephalitis	Only one form, with variable severity
Congenital vaccinia	Systemic, lethal infection
Progressive vaccinia	In congenitally T-cell-deficient individuals
	In antibody-deficient individuals (rare)
	In any disorder that suppresses T-cell function (e.g., cancer, HIV/AIDS)
	Accompanying T-cell-suppressive therapy (e.g. high-dose steroids, some forms of chemotherapy)

these are highlighted in the individual descriptions below. The minimal reactions are split into noninfectious consequences of smallpox vaccination and infectious complications.

Noninfectious Rashes

Noninfectious rashes are common and defy accurate classification because of the variety of types of rashes and the fact that the historical literature describes them in terms that are sometimes arcane and sometimes inaccurate (e.g., using "eczema" in an inexact way). Also, noninfectious rashes that were not recognized decades ago surfaced in the vaccination efforts since 2000, adding additional confusion to historical classifications. Finally, individual reporters and investigators have used the definition "generalized vaccinia" in a nonspecific way when most experienced clinicians and investigators have more narrowly defined this adverse event. Thus, the literature is confusing, but the fact remains that these rashes are common, are almost always benign, and are of uncertain etiology in each instance.

"Erythema multiforme." I prefer the use of the term erythema multiforme, but purists declare that it is too nondescript. For me, this category encompasses a host of rashes that occur within a week or two after vaccination, take many forms, are almost always intensely erythematous, and are associated with pruritis, often to a great degree (Color Plate 4 [see color insert]). A variety of individual lesions can be seen, and the extent of the rash is variable. The rash is often symmetrical, can involve the palms and soles, often appears as typical "target" lesions, may be flat or raised, and has intense erythema, either of the rash itself or surrounding individual lesions.

Most of these rashes were seen in infants and young children in the 1960s and earlier. This is not surprising, as routine primary vaccination was performed either in the first year of life or shortly after the first birthday. The precise frequency of these rashes is not known with certainty. Their benign nature, the fact that they occurred 1 to 2 weeks postvaccination and might have been ascribed to other causes, and the lack of reporting all contribute to uncertainty about their actual incidence. Two studies attempted to quantify the occurrence of generalized rashes with variable results (Table 3).

Subsequent to initial vaccination in infancy, older children, adolescents, and adults were reimmunized at various intervals (the usual recommendation was for revaccination every 7 to 10 years in that era). These older revaccinees did not experience the same frequency of rash as did primary vaccinees.

The course of erythema multiforme is almost always benign, with healing within a few days to 1 week. Because most of these patients experience pruritis, an antipruritic or

Table 3. Estimated rates of adverse events postvaccination[a]

Adverse event	Rate (per million primary vaccinations)
Death	0.5–5[b] (greater at extremes of age)
Postvaccinal encephalitis	2–6 (infants and adults at greatest risk)
Progressive vaccinia	0.5–10[b]
Eczema vaccinatum	14–44
Generalized rashes	140–9,600
Contact vaccinia	371–606

[a]Based on references 20, 21, 25, and 26.
[b]Higher rates than originally, based on the increased number of vulnerable individuals in the present population.

antihistamine given over 2 or 3 days suffices to control symptoms as the lesions clear. Rarely, the rash may increase in severity, affect the mucous membranes and the cornea, and behave as typical Stevens-Johnson syndrome. In these instances, the course may not be benign, and more aggressive therapy with steroid preparations may become necessary.

Vaccinia folliculitis. During the vaccination campaigns that occurred after the 11 September terrorist attacks, Talbot et al. from Vanderbilt University noted a different type of rash occurring after smallpox vaccination (30). Of 148 volunteers who were vaccinated, 4 developed generalized eruptions and 11 noted focal eruptions. All recovered completely without scarring. The lesions were papulovesicular, and microscopic evaluation revealed suppurative folliculitis. Vaccinia virus was not recovered from biopsy specimens. To the authors, it appeared that these extended the range of noninfectious rashes previously known to occur following smallpox vaccination.

Infectious Adverse Events

Bacterial infections at the vaccination site. An uncommon complication is bacterial superinfection of the vaccination site (7, 13). Historically, these infections ranged from very serious (tetanus, syphilis, etc.) to mild (staphylococcus or streptococcus infections). In modern times, with care taken to use sterile equipment and vaccine, bacterial infection has been uncommon. When infants and young children were the primary vaccinees, common organisms, such as streptococci and staphylococci, occasionally caused complications of vaccination, since these organisms were ubiquitous in that age group and it was difficult to control touching of the vaccination site (Fig. 6). On even rarer occasions, a bacterial infection occurred at the vaccination site with no viral replication apparent. Presumably, this was due to contaminated vaccine or improper sterile technique. In recent use of smallpox vaccine, bacterial infection has not been noted.

Contact vaccinia or inadvertent inoculation. Given that the vaccinia virus is abundant on the skin of a vaccinee and that it can easily be spread by hand contact to other parts of the vaccinee's body or to other individuals, it is not surprising that the second most common adverse event is contact vaccinia. Contact vaccinia or inadvertent inoculation is most often benign but rarely may be more serious, even life threatening [see

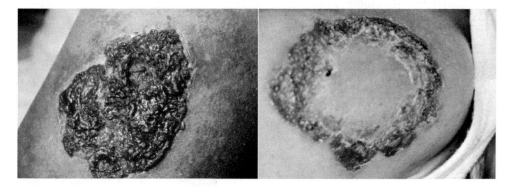

Figure 6. Bacterial superinfection of vaccination site. (Left) streptococcal infection (stained with mercurochrome); (right) staphylococcal impetiginous infection. Copyright © Logical Images, Inc.

"Eczema Vaccinatum (Contact Vaccinia in Atopic Individuals)" and "Progressive Vaccinia" below].

Somewhat more surprising is the spread of vaccinia to other sites on the body in apparently healthy individuals, called generalized vaccinia. Presumably, inapparent viremia leads to this type of spread. This is a benign condition in almost all individuals who experience it.

Characteristics of contact vaccinia. Vaccinia virus can be transmitted from the site of vaccination by direct or indirect contact (13, 27). Lesions may develop in the vaccinee at sites other than the primary vaccination or in other individuals by spread from the vaccinee. Virus titers at the surface of the vaccination site are very high, and the exudate that forms serves as a vehicle for transmission, although even dry lesions can yield sufficient virus for transmission to occur. Since most vaccinees experience pruritis at the primary site, there is great temptation to touch or rub the developing vaccination, particularly in infants and children. In this fashion, virus can be transmitted by hand contact. Direct skin-to-skin contact can also occur, and it is suspected that some fomites, such as bed sheets or clothing, may lead to inadvertent transmission.

Lesions form at the distant sites or on the skin of contacts within 3 to 7 days and follow the usual pattern of a primary vaccination in most instances (Fig. 7). They may be isolated or massive, depending on the amount of virus transferred and the extent of skin infected. In healthy individuals, the lesions are usually few and bothersome but are not associated with serious symptoms or life-threatening complications. More serious contact vaccinia is discussed below.

In the past, vaccinia immune globulin (VIG) was used almost routinely in all instances of contact vaccinia (13, 18, 27; http://www.bt.cdc.gov/training/smallpoxvaccine/reactions/vig.html). However, some individuals were not treated and healed spontaneously, suggesting that mild contact vaccinia need not be treated with VIG.

Generalized vaccinia. In apparently healthy individuals, new lesions may appear throughout the body, presumably from viremic spread (13). These lesions resemble primary vaccination and can be numerous (Fig. 8). These individuals usually have no or few systemic symptoms, and the lesions resolve rapidly, more rapidly than primary lesions, and heal completely, most often without scars. On occasion, patients may have more significant systemic symptoms but recover with symptomatic treatment. Antiviral therapy is not indicated.

There is a significant problem with the term "generalized vaccinia." I have used it in the strictest sense, describing the clinical syndrome listed above. Reports in the literature have used this term to describe contact vaccinia in patients with atopic dermatitis (so-called

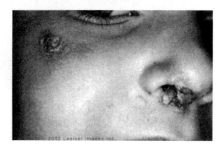

Figure 7. Autoinoculation. The photograph shows vaccinia transferred to the nose and face of a child with allergic rhinitis. Copyright © Logical Images, Inc.

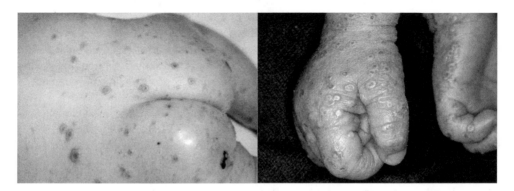

Figure 8. True generalized vaccinia. Note that each viremic lesion appears as a normal primary vaccination. Copyright © Logical Images, Inc.

eczema vaccinatum), progressive vaccinia, and, on occasion, mild erythematous rashes. As a result, the term has been misused in surveys attempting to define frequency. When defined by strict criteria, as above, this adverse event is rare and does not have the dire outcome associated with the diseases incorrectly identified as generalized vaccinia.

Moderate, Severe, and Life-Threatening Adverse Events

Eczema Vaccinatum (Contact Vaccinia in Atopic Individuals)

Contact vaccinia in atopic individuals, with or without current skin manifestations, can result in extensive vaccinal lesions and, prior to effective therapy, had 12 to 30% mortality (5, 9, 13) (Fig. 9). Atopic individuals are prone to this complication because they have both defective skin and an immunologic-modulation defect (9). In the past, this complication was called "eczema vaccinatum" because the term eczema was loosely applied to atopic dermatitis, as well as to seborrheic or other forms of extensive skin eruptions. We now know that the lethal complications most often occurred in atopic individuals because of the combined dermatologic and immunologic defects. Other types of skin eruptions may predispose to contact vaccinia, but it is often very limited in scope and severity. For

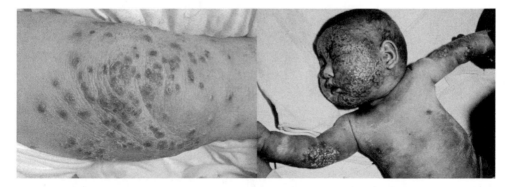

Figure 9. Eczema vaccinatum showing characteristic rash and distribution in patients with atopic dermatitis. Copyright © Logical Images, Inc.

example, diaper dermatitis, acne, traumatic wounds, and surgical wounds may become infected with vaccinia virus but do not have the same potentially lethal outcome seen in atopic persons. More extensive skin lesions, such as extensive burns or traumatized skin, can predispose to serious contact vaccinia. The exact extent of skin disruption that predisposes to serious disease is not known with certainty, and it is left to clinical judgment to determine the extent that constitutes a contraindication to vaccination.

Patients with Darier's disease, a keratitic genetic disorder of the skin, are uniquely susceptible to "eczema vaccinatum" if exposed to the virus (1, 22).

Another potentially dangerous complication is transmission of the virus to ocular structures (8, 13; http://www.cdc.gov/mmwr/preview/mmwrhtml/rr5010a1.htm) (Fig. 10). Rubbing of the eye (especially when irritated by allergic conjunctivitis) can infect surrounding skin and/or the conjunctiva and cornea. Periorbital vaccinia without corneal involvement should be recognized early, because prompt treatment with vaccinia immune globulin can avert corneal complications. Such treatment usually results in prompt healing with no residua. However, if the cornea is involved, treatment with VIG is controversial (2; http://www.cdc.gov/mmwr/preview/mmwrhtml/rr5010a1.htm). I believe, based on experience with patients and with experimental infection in rabbit corneas, that treatment with VIG can result in immune complex deposition, with attendant corneal clouding (13). Because of this possibility, I recommend treatment with antiviral medications alone. Some ophthalmologists believe that VIG can be safely given and that it is indicated in corneal infection if a life-threatening complication is present. This controversy has been summarized by the CDC as a result of a conference at which the varying viewpoints were presented and a consensus position was adopted (2; http://www.cdc.gov/mmwr/preview/mmwrhtml/rr5010a1.htm). The consensus currently is that isolated vaccinia keratitis should not be treated with vaccinia immune globulin, but if the keratitis is accompanied by potentially life-threatening or severe implantation, VIG should be used in conjunction with local ocular therapy.

Progressive Vaccinia

Vaccination of persons who are T cell deficient usually results in a progressive local vaccination and extensive viremic spread to other parts of the body with similar progressive

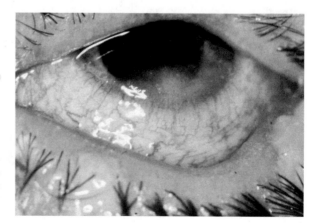

Figure 10. Vaccinia keratitis showing infection of the cornea and conjunctiva in a mother with allergic conjunctivitis whose infant was recently vaccinated. Copyright © Logical Images, Inc.

growth at all sites (10, 13, 14, 32). Essentially, there is no containment of the vaccinia virus infection, and contiguous cells become infected in a circumferential fashion and the blood stream is eventually invaded (Color Plates 5 and 6 [see color insert]).

It appears reasonable to assert that T-cell deficiency is the underlying pathogenic defect, but since most progressive vaccinia occurred prior to sophisticated immunologic testing, we cannot be certain that all patients were T cell deficient. In the cases we reported, we were able to determine T-cell deficiency with the diagnostic methods then available, but not all cases recorded in the literature were examined for T-cell deficiencies. Complicating the attempt to classify this disorder was the use of the term "generalized vaccinia" to define progressive diseases.

The infection proceeds inexorably. Each lesion grows circumferentially, with little or no evidence of surrounding inflammation (Color Plates 5, 6, and 7). Within the first week, viremic lesions appear, and each undergoes the same evolution as the primary lesion. In almost all instances, despite the therapy then available, the outcome was fatal, with multiple-organ failure or septic shock as the final event. Attempts to control the progression included VIG, the chemotherapy then available (thiosemicarbazones and interferon), and the usual high-level acute care. Unusual efforts included blood transfusions and infusion of lymphocytes or transfer of lymphatic tissue, which had an unexpected adverse outcome: the occurrence of graft-versus-host disease (14, 16). In these instances, all the signs of graft-versus-host disease appeared as terminal events, e.g., skin rash, hepatosplenomegaly, and anemia (Fig. 11).

A few reports listed B-cell deficiency as the underlying cause of progressive vaccinia. Most of these reports appeared before the dual nature of the immune system had been identified. Further, purely B-cell-deficient children (e.g., with Bruton-type hypogammaglobulinemia) had been vaccinated without incident in the past (19). We described several children with intact or near-intact antibody systems but deficient T-cell function who had

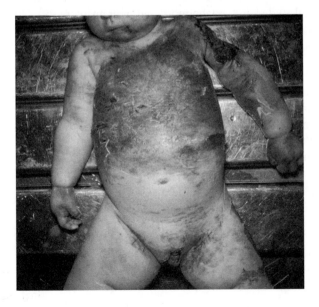

Figure 11. Graft-versus-host disease in a child with progressive vaccinia who received a blood transfusion with viable lymphocytes. Copyright © Logical Images, Inc.

progressive vaccinia (Color Plate 6) (14). Taken together, all the evidence supports T-cell deficiency as the underlying pathologic process. Hence, known T-cell-deficient individuals should not receive smallpox vaccination routinely. The CDC recommends that exposed individuals, irrespective of their T-cell-deficient status, should be vaccinated. I have great difficulty with this clinical dilemma. On one hand, smallpox will probably kill patients with T-cell deficiency, but vaccination is likely to produce progressive disease. My resolution depends on the availability of sufficient VIG, in which case vaccination can be immediately followed with treatment. The concept is that circulating antibody will neutralize viremia but will not have an effect on the local lesion (such as occurred in children with T-cell deficiency and intact antibody status). One can then treat the local lesion surgically, as was done successfully in one of our patients. Of course, there is still uncertainty of immunity following vaccination, whether or not this suggested method is employed.

A complicating feature of susceptibility in T-cell-deficient individuals is our lack of knowledge of the exact level of deficiency required for progressive vaccinia to occur. This is especially true for today's population of potentially T-cell-deficient individuals (organ transplant recipients, human immunodeficiency virus-infected and AIDS patients, cancer survivors with or without immunosuppressive therapy, and the multitude of patients with immunodeficiency diseases or undergoing treatment that renders them immunodeficient). There have been some instances of cure of progressive vaccinia in T-cell-deficient individuals (10, 14). Examination of these reports suggests that the deficiency was mild or that the disease was not progressive vaccinia. In our experience in Denver, we saw a few individuals with diseases that evoked T-cell deficiency, such as lymphoma, in whom we were able to "cure" the progressive lesions by diminishing or eliminating the immunosuppressive therapy, with concomitant treatment with VIG and antivirals (14). For some patients, however, the lesion was so extensive that this strategy failed (Color Plate 7). This experience and some of the reported cures in the literature suggest that there is a degree of reversible T-cell deficiency that does not necessarily lead to a fatal outcome.

Cidofovir, an antiviral effective for other virus infections, appears to offer some promise for vaccinia in early experimental studies in the laboratory and in animals (6, 29). No definitive statement can be made as to its efficacy, but the CDC has established a method for its experimental use in the event of a severe vaccinal reaction or in smallpox (2).

Postvaccinal Encephalitis

Although encephalitic disease has been reported in the interval after smallpox vaccination and has been labeled postvaccinal encephalitis (PVE), the exact extent of the disorder is uncertain (7, 15, 28). The problem is that many of the cases reported occurred at a time when we were unaware of the multitude of agents that produced inflammatory and infectious diseases of the nervous system and prior to our ability to diagnosis the exact cause, as can be done in many instances today. Further, there is no pathognomonic sign or set of laboratory findings that define PVE. Hence, the temporal association of encephalitis, or other neurologic diseases, after vaccination was sufficient to establish "causation" and a diagnosis of PVE.

The pathogenesis of PVE is unknown. Most believe that true PVE is either a parainfectious or postinfectious encephalitis. Autopsy results suggest that the midbrain, cerebrum, and medulla have lesions consistent with an autoimmune process. Myelitis has also been reported in a significant portion of cases. Nonspecific changes in the spinal fluid include increased pressure, lymphocytosis, and increased protein levels. There is no definitive diagnostic test or set of tests. The disease is reported to be fatal in one-third of instances, and the survivors often have significant neurologic defects. Recently, the military reported two patients with alleged PVE with mild illness, rapid recovery, and no residua.

Given the difficulty of diagnosis, the clinical descriptions vary somewhat. Symptoms usually appear 1 to 2 weeks after vaccination, with vomiting, drowsiness, severe headache, and fever as dominant manifestations. Some patients recover rapidly with no further difficulty. Others develop more severe and progressive symptoms, including paralysis, incontinence, urinary retention, coma, and convulsions. If death occurs, it often is sudden and within a week of onset.

There is no effective treatment for PVE, other than intensive care and supportive measures.

Cardiac Events after Vaccination

In the 1960s, a few reports from Europe suggested that military recruits experienced myopericarditis after smallpox vaccination. These data were not considered in the United States, as our experience did not indicate that heart problems were a risk. Of course, we were primarily immunizing infants, and it is conceivable that some experienced mild myopericarditis without recognition. Among the military population immunized recently, myopericarditis as a complication of vaccination became evident, verifying the earlier European experience (3). Experience among civilian vaccinees also affirmed myopericarditis as a complication. Among more than 650,000 vaccinated troops, 75 cases of myopericarditis occurred (1 in 8,367 vaccinations), a rate higher than that before the institution of smallpox vaccination. All the troops recovered, and among those tested after recovery, none had abnormal cardiac tests. The vaccinated civilian population appears to have paralleled the military, but the numbers were smaller.

Myocardial infarctions and other vascular cardiac events did occur in temporal relationship to vaccination, but the rates did not exceed those expected in nonvaccinees. As a result, it is not believed that this type of complication has any relationship to smallpox vaccination (3).

Congenital Vaccinia (Fetal Infection)

Fewer than 50 instances of congenital vaccinia have been reported, with only 3 in the United States, and many in the distant past (17, 23, 31). Recent experience suggests that vaccination of pregnant women is not associated with adverse events, although two instances of miscarriage have occurred among 6,374 vaccinated women of childbearing age, 6 of whom conceived close to the date of vaccination (2). These rates are the same as in unvaccinated individuals. Previous studies have also failed to show an association of vaccination with miscarriages, abortions, premature birth, low birth weight, and fetal anomalies. Despite these facts, a live-virus vaccine should not be administered to a woman who is pregnant or who intends to become pregnant within a month of vaccine administration.

Other Alleged Adverse Events

In the era of routine smallpox vaccination, there were reports of a variety of diseases and conditions that appeared within 1 to 4 weeks after vaccination. The list of disorders is long and includes diseases and conditions commonly seen in the general population (e.g., hemolytic anemia, thrombocytopenia, various cancers, and arthritis). No consistent pattern was determined for any of these entities, and most experts discounted them as true adverse events due to smallpox vaccination.

One such set of reports was ignored by most experts but appears to have been a true instance of an event caused by vaccination (myopericarditis, described above). No other event has surfaced in recent experience to justify inclusion as a complication of smallpox vaccination.

EPIDEMIOLOGY OF ADVERSE EVENTS

Lane, Neff, and colleagues attempted to define the frequency of complications in several surveys (20, 21, 25, 26) (Table 3). Complicating these surveys were the various reporting modes and definitions and their dependency on passive reporting from a variety of health professionals with differing degrees of knowledge and sophistication concerning adverse events after smallpox vaccination. Despite these limitations, they provide the only historical data with any reliability. The data were collected during a period when primary vaccination was largely confined to infancy and early childhood, and most adult data were from revaccination.

More recently, the military experience has provided some concept of the modern adverse-reaction rate among more than 650,000 adult vaccinees. One must recognize that many troops were excused from vaccination on the basis of a medical contraindication, so these results do not necessarily reflect what the rates might be among all adults, regardless of susceptibility status (2). This consideration is important if widespread vaccination becomes necessary in the future.

There were 5 deaths recorded among the 667,000 troops; 4 from vascular cardiac events not thought to be related to smallpox vaccination and 1 due to a lupus-like illness thought by a civilian review panel to probably be related to smallpox vaccination. In contrast, deaths occurred at a rate of 1 to 2 per million primary vaccinations in historical data.

Other adverse events in the military population included the following:

- No cases of eczema vaccinatum or progressive vaccinia
- 75 cases of myopericarditis
- Instances of "generalized vaccinia," none requiring treatment (see the discussion above of the misuse of this term for a variety of disorders, including benign rashes, which most of these appeared to be; vaccinia folliculitis and erythema multiforme appeared to have been labeled generalized vaccinia)
- 35 cases of contact vaccinia, all in family members or other close contacts
- Two instances of mild encephalitis
- Three instances in which individuals received VIG (two periocular and one burn)

It should be noted that 15 to 25% of those reporting for vaccination were excused due to medical contraindications or because there was a close contact with a medical contraindication. Therefore, the morbidity figures were skewed toward normal, healthy adult populations and might be considerably higher should vaccination be administered to everyone, irrespective of underlying susceptibility.

RECENT ADVANCES

Diagnostic Improvements

PCR and electron microscopy afford rapid early diagnosis of orthopoxvirus infections. Vaccinia virus, variola virus, and other orthopoxviruses can be specifically identified by these techniques and confirmed by culture of the virus. The CDC has established a network of public health laboratories across the country with appropriate materials and trained personnel. The CDC maintains extensive virologic capacity to verify preliminary results obtained by the network.

Immunologic techniques now enable investigators to specify the immune responses of susceptible individuals and those who suffer adverse events. These techniques should be employed to enable us to answer the multiple questions raised by our inability to measure immunologic capacity when both smallpox and vaccination were prevalent.

Imaging techniques provide an opportunity to identify pathologic states within each adverse event with precision, which was not possible in a previous era.

Dermatologic biopsies can be performed with greater ease than in the previous era and can provide vital pathologic, virologic, and immunologic information.

Therapy

Vaccinia immune globulin was initially prepared from vaccinated individuals whose sera were collected at the time of optimum immunologic response. It was purified as an intramuscular preparation, which could not be given intravenously. Currently, VIG stocks are available at the CDC in limited quantities. An intravenous preparation has been produced and should be available if needed in the immediate future. The CDC has developed protocols for the use of both the intramuscular and intravenous forms as investigational drugs.

The exact dosage should be determined in consultation with the CDC. In the past, initial doses for moderate disease started at 0.6 ml per kg of body weight, with a 15- to 20-ml maximum for adults. On occasion, much more VIG was administered to patients with severe complications, with such variable results that the adequate dose cannot be defined for such diseases as progressive vaccinia or eczema vaccinatum.

Currently, there is no antiviral therapy that is of proven value in clinical use. Various thiosemicarbazones have been used in an attempt to contain the virus in serious adverse events. Evidence for their efficacy cannot be determined from the uncontrolled trials in desperate clinical situations. In addition, vomiting occurred frequently, and often the dose given was not the dose absorbed. Also, multiple therapies were employed for seriously ill patients, limiting the determination of the exact roles of individual drugs or treatments.

Cidofovir is undergoing extensive testing in vitro and in animal models. It is possible that it may have a beneficial effect for vaccinal infections (2, 6, 29). The CDC has developed a protocol for cidofovir use as an investigational drug for severe forms of vaccinal infections.

CONCLUSIONS

Smallpox vaccine is very effective in preventing smallpox. It is a live-virus vaccine that is safe for almost all recipients. The vaccine is administered by insertion into the deep layers of the skin, usually in the posterior deltoid area, and results in a visible reaction, usually in 6 to 8 days.

Although it is safe for almost all persons, vaccination does result in local effects that are annoying but not life threatening. These consist of robust local reactions, some spread to local lymph channels and nodes, and occasional secondary pustules close to the original site of insertion. These reactions subside without incident.

Some individuals experience mild to moderate adverse reactions, including hypersensitivity rashes, local bacterial infections, contact spread to themselves or to other individuals, and a mild form of generalized vaccinia. Most require no treatment and are self-limited.

Rarely, more serious, even life-threatening, reactions can occur. Individuals with atopic dermatitis (or other severe skin diseases) may develop widespread lesions that can be life threatening. Persons with T-cell deficiencies are most likely to develop progressive vaccinia, a lethal complication, either from direct vaccination or from contact with a vaccinated person. A few individuals may experience postvaccinal encephalitis. Even rarer is the infection of a fetus by a pregnant women who has been vaccinated.

Therapy for serious complications employs vaccinia immune globulin and, possibly, cidofovir, although both are experimental at present. Investigative drug protocols, obtainable through the CDC, must be followed for the use of these agents.

Acknowledgments. I shall always be indebted to my mentor, the late C. Henry Kempe, then Chairman of the Department of Pediatrics, University of Colorado, and Director of the Smallpox Laboratory at the Hospital for Infectious Diseases, Madras, India. Kempe assembled a group of faculty in the Department, including William Hathaway, Jack Githens, Dave Pearlman, and others, who worked together to unravel the immunology and hematology underlying adverse events. Patients were referred to Denver from around the world with complications of smallpox vaccination, and a telephone consultation service for advice and dispensing of VIG was established. Eventually, the CDC took over these functions, with our unit and experts from around the country enlisted as consultants. All of us visited the laboratory and infectious-diseases wards in Madras, India, to gain knowledge and experience with smallpox, as well.

The photographs for this chapter are from my collection and from the estate of C. Henry Kempe. Art Papier of Logical Images, Inc., has processed the former images and contributed some illustrations from the University of Rochester. All images are copyright by Logical Images, Inc., and are reprinted with full permission of the author and the company.

REFERENCES

1. **Burge, S.** 1999. Management of Darier's disease. *Clin. Exp. Dermatol.* **24:**53–56.
2. **Centers for Disease Control and Prevention.** 2003. Smallpox vaccination and adverse reactions: guidance for clinicians. *Morb. Mortal. Wkly. Rep.* **52**(RR-4)**:**1–28.
3. **Centers for Disease Control and Prevention.** 2002. Smallpox vaccination and adverse events training module. [Online.] http://www.bt.cdc.gov/training/smallpoxvaccine/reactions/contraindications.html.
4. **Collier, A. D., P. D. Greenberg, and R. W. Coombs.** 1991. Safety and immunologic response to a recombinant vaccinia virus vaccine expressing HIV envelope glycoprotein. *Lancet* **337:**567–572.
5. **Copeman, P. W. W., and H. J. Wallace.** 1964. Eczema vaccinatum. *Br. Med. J.* **2:**906–908.
6. **DeClercq, E.** 2002. Cidofovir in treatment of poxvirus infections. *Antivir. Res.* **55:**1–13.
7. **Dixon, C. W.** 1962. *Smallpox.* J&A Churchill Ltd., London, England.

8. **Ellis, P. P., and L. A. Winograd.** 1962. Ocular vaccinia. *Arch. Ophthalmol.* **68:**56–65.

9. **Engler, R. J. M., J. Kenner, and D. Y. M. Leung.** 2002. Smallpox vaccination: risk considerations for patients with atopic dermatitis. *J. Allergy Clin. Immunol.* **110:**357–365.

10. **Fekety, F. R., S. E. Malawista, and D. L. Young.** 1962. Vaccinia gangrenosa in chronic lymphatic leukemia. *Arch. Intern. Med.* **109:**205–208.

11. **Fenner, F., D. Henderson, A. Z. Jezek, and I. D. Ladnyi.** 1988. *Smallpox and Its Eradication.* World Health Organization, Geneva, Switzerland.

12. **Fulginiti, V. A., A. Papier, M. Lane, J. Neff, and D. A. Henderson.** 2003. Smallpox vaccination: a review, part I. Background, vaccination technique, normal vaccination and revaccination, and expected normal reactions. *Clin. Infect. Dis.* **37:**241–250.

13. **Fulginiti, V. A., A. Papier, M. Lane, J. Neff, and D. A. Henderson.** 2003. Smallpox vaccination: a review, part II. Adverse events. *Clin. Infect. Dis.* **37:**251–271.

14. **Fulginiti, V. A., C. H. Kempe, W. E. Hathaway, et al.** 1968. Progressive vaccinia in immunologically deficient individuals, p. 129–151. *In* R. Good (ed.), *Birth Defects Original Article Series*, vol. IV. *Immunologic Diseases of Man.* The National Foundation March of Dimes, New York, N.Y.

15. **Gurvich, E. B., and I. S. Vilesova.** 1983. Vaccinia virus in postvaccinal encephalitis. *Acta Virol.* **27:**154–159.

16. **Hathaway, W., V. A. Fulginiti, C. W. Pierce, J. Githens, and C. H. Kempe.** 1967. Graft versus host reaction (human runt disease) following a single blood transfusion. *JAMA* **201:**139–144.

17. **Henderson, D. A., L. L. Borio, and J. M. Lane.** 2003. Smallpox and monkeypox. *In* S. A. Plotkin and W. A. Orenstein (ed.), *Vaccines.* W. B. Saunders Company, Philadelphia, Pa.

18. **Kempe, C. H., T. O. Berge, and B. England.** 1956. Hyperimmune vaccinal gamma globulin. *Pediatrics* **18:**177–181.

19. **Kempe, C. H.** 1960. Studies on smallpox and complications of smallpox vaccination: E. Mead Johnson Award address. *Pediatrics* **26:**176–189.

20. **Lane, J. M., R. H. Levine, J. M. Neff, F. L. Ruben, and J. D. Millar.** 1967. Complications of smallpox vaccination: national survey in the United States, 1963. *N. Engl. J. Med.* **276:**125–132.

21. **Lane, J. M., F. L. Ruben, J. M. Neff, and J. D. Millar.** 1970. Complications of smallpox vaccination, 1968: results of ten statewide surveys. *J. Infect. Dis.* **122:**303–309.

22. **Loeffel, E. D., and J. S. Meyer.** 1970. Eczema vaccinatum in Darier's disease. *Arch. Dermatol.* **102:**451–456.

23. **MacArthur, P.** 1952. Congenital vaccinia and vaccinia gravidarum. *Lancet* **ii:**1104–1116.

24. **Mack, T. M.** 1972. Smallpox in Europe, 1950–1971. *J. Infect. Dis.* **125:**161–169.

25. **Neff, J. M., J. M. Lane, J. P. Pert, R. Moore, and J. D. Millar.** 1967. Complications of smallpox vaccination. 1. National survey in the United States, 1963. *N. Engl. J. Med.* **276:**1–8.

26. **Neff, J. M., R. H. Levine, J. M. Lane, et al.** 1967. Complications of smallpox vaccination, United States, 1963, II: results obtained from four statewide surveys. *Pediatrics* **39:**916–923.

27. **Neff, J. M., J. M. Lane, V. A. Fulginiti, and D. A. Henderson.** 2002. Contact vaccinia—transmission of vaccinia from smallpox vaccination. *JAMA* **288:**1901–1905.

28. **Osuntokun, B. O.** 1968. The neurological complications of vaccination against smallpox and measles. *West Afr. Med. J. Niger. Pract.* **17:**115–121.

29. **Smee, D. F., K. E. Bailey, M. H. Wong, and R. W. Sidwell.** 2001. Effects of cidofovir on the pathogenesis of a lethal vaccinia virus respiratory infection in mice. *Antivir. Res.* **52:**55–62.

30. **Talbot, T. R., H. K. Bredenberg, M. Smith, B. J. LaFleur, A. Boyd, and K. Edwards.** 2003. Focal and generalized folliculitis following smallpox vaccination among vaccinia-naïve recipients. *JAMA* **289:**3290–3294.

31. **Tondury, G., M. Foukas, and A. Scouteris.** 1969. Prenatal vaccinia. *J. Obstet. Gynecol.* **76:**47–55.

32. **Virelizier, J. L., M. Hamet, J. J. Ballet, P. Reinert, and C. Griscelli.** 1978. Impaired defense against vaccinia in a child with T-lymphocyte deficiency associated with inosine phosphorylase defect. *Pediatrics* **92:**358–362.

INDEX